Veterinary Nursing

(Formerly Jones's Animal Nursing 5th edition)

TITLES OF RELATED INTEREST

Veterinary Handbook Series

Series Editor: A. T. B. EDNEY

BROWN
Aquaculture for Veterinarians: Fish Husbandry and Medicine

ANDERSON & EDNEY
Practical Animal Handling

EMILY & PENMAN
Handbook of Small Animal Dentistry, 2nd Edition

GELATT & GELATT
Handbook of Small Animal Ophthalmic Surgery, Vol. 1: Extraocular Procedures

GORREL, PENMAN & EMILY
Handbook of Small Animal Oral Emergencies

MORIELLO & MASON
Handbook of Small Animal Dermatology

PENMAN, EMILY & GORREL
Handbook of Advanced Small Animal Dentistry

SHERIDAN & McCAFFERTY
The Business of Veterinary Practice

WILLS & WOLF
Handbook of Feline Medicine

Other books

BURGER
The Waltham Book of Companion Animal Nutrition

GOLDSCHMIDT & SHOFER
Skin Tumours of the Dog and Cat

IHRKE, MASON & WHITE
Advances in Veterinary Dermatology, Volume 2

ROBINSON
Genetics for Cat Breeders, 3rd Edition
Genetics for Dog Breeders, 2nd Edition

THORNE
The Waltham Book of Dog and Cat Behaviour

WILLS AND SIMPSON
The Waltham Book of Clinical Nutrition of the Dog and Cat

WOLDEHIWET & RISTIC
Rickettsial and Chlamydial Diseases of Domestic Animals

Veterinary Nursing

(Formerly Jones's Animal Nursing, 5th edition)

Edited by

D. R. LANE

Leamington Spa, Warwickshire CV32 4EZ, UK

and

B. COOPER

College of Animal Welfare, Wood Green Animal Shelter
Huntingdon PE18 8LJ, UK

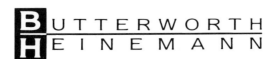

Butterworth-Heinemann
Linacre House, Jordan Hill, Oxford OX2 8DP
A division of Reed Educational and Professional Publishing Ltd

Ɑ̵ 'A member of the Reed Elsevier plc group

OXFORD   BOSTON   JOHANNESBURG
MELBOURNE   NEW DELHI   SINGAPORE

First published 1994
Reprinted with corrections 1995
Reprinted 1996, 1997 (twice)

British Library Cataloguing in Publication Data
Veterinary nursing: formerly Jones's animal nursing
    edited by D. Lane and B. Cooper
    p. cm.
    Includes bibliography and indexes
    1. Veterinary nursing   2. Pets - diseases   I. Jones, Bruce V.
    II. Lane, D. R.   III. Cooper, B.   IV. Jones's animal nursing
    SF774.5.V48   1994
    636.089'073-dc20   94-22434

ISBN 0 7506 3417 0

DISCLAIMER
Whilst every effort is made by the Publishers to see that no inaccurate or misleading
data, opinion or statement appear in this book, they wish to make it clear that the
data and opinions appearing in the articles herein are the sole responsibility of the
contributor concerned. Accordingly, the Publishers and their employees, officers and
agents accept no responsibility or liability whatsoever for the consequences of any
such inaccurate or misleading data, opinion or statement.

Drug and Dosage Selection: The Authors have made every effort to ensure the
accuracy of the information herein, particularly with regard to drug selection and
dose. However, appropriate information sources should be consulted, especially for
new or unfamiliar drugs or procedures. It is the responsibility of every veterinarian to
evaluate the appropriateness of a particular opinion in the context of actual clinical
situations, and with due consideration to new developments.

Printed and bound in Great Britain by Hartnolls Limited, Bodmin, Cornwall

Contents

15

Elementary Microbiology

J. JOWITT

The group of living things known as **micro-organisms** or **microbes** includes the bacteria, viruses, fungi, algae and protozoa. Micro-organisms are generally thought of as those organisms which are too small to be seen clearly with the naked eye. Microbiology is the study of these microscopic organisms, deriving its name from the Greek words: *mikros* (small), *bios* (life) and *logos* (science). Most micro-organisms are **unicellular**—that is, they consist of only one cell which carries out all the functions necessary for life—but a few (for example, some fungi) are **multicellular**. Viruses differ from other micro-organisms in that they have no cellular structure. Figure 15.1 shows the major similarities and differences between the different types of micro-organism.

Naming Micro-organisms

Most micro-organisms are named according to the **binomial system**, which gives them two names. The first part is the generic name, indicating the **genus** to which the organism belongs. Organisms within a given genus are closely related and possess many similarities. The generic name always begins with a capital letter. The second name is the specific name, indicating the **species**, and this is given a small initial letter. The generic name is often abbreviated; for example, *Escherichia coli* may be abbreviated to *E. coli*.

Viruses are not named in this way. Although most of the viruses affecting mammalian hosts have been assigned to virus families and genera, they are often referred to by the name of the disease they cause, e.g. feline leukaemia virus.

Measuring Micro-organisms

The unit most frequently used to measure the size of micro-organisms is the **micrometre** (or micron), written as μm. One micrometre is one thousandth of a millimetre or one millionth of a metre (10^{-6}m). Micro-organisms range in size from the relatively large Protozoa down to the very tiny viruses. Because viruses are so small they can only be seen with an electron microscope and are measured in **nanometres** (nm). One nanometre is one millionth of a millimetre or 10^{-9}m.

Saprophytes and Parasites

Micro-organisms can be described in terms of their nutritional requirements as either **autotrophs** (self feeders) which are able to synthesise their own food, or as **heterotrophs** (other feeders) which obtain organic molecules from their environment. Most micro-organisms are heterotrophs and are either **saprophytes**, a large, free-living group feeding on dead organic matter, or **parasites**, obtaining their nutrients from another living organism.

THE MAJOR SIMILARITIES AND DIFFERENCES BETWEEN THE DIFFERENT TYPES OF MICRO-ORGANISMS					
Characteristic	**Bacteria**	**Viruses**	**Fungi**	**Protozoa**	**Algae**
Size	0.5–5μm	20 – 300 nm	3.8μm (yeasts)	10–200μm	0.5–20μm
Cell arrangement	unicellular	non-cellular	unicellular or multicellular	unicellular	unicellular or multicellular
Cell wall	present; mainly peptidoglycan	absent	present; mainly chitin	absent	present; mainly cellulose
Nucleus	no true membrane-bound nucleus	absent	membrane-bound nucleus	membrane-bound nucleus	membrane-bound nucleus
Nucleic acids	DNA and RNA	DNA or RNA	DNA and RNA	DNA and RNA	DNA and RNA
Reproduction	asexual by binary fission	replicate only within another living cell	asexual and sexual by spores, budding in yeast	asexual and sexual	asexual and sexual
Nutrition	mainly heterotrophic – can be saprophytic or parasitic; A few are autotrophic	obligate parasites	heterotrophic – can be saprophytic or parasitic	heterotrophic – can be saprophytic or parasitic	autotrophic
Motility	some are motile	non-motile	non-motile except for certain spore forms	motile	some are motile
Toxin production	some form toxins	none	some form toxins	some form toxins	some form toxins

Fig. 15.1. Major similarities and differences between different types of micro-organism.

Parasitism

A parasite is an organism which lives on or in another living organism (the **host**) and derives nourishment from it. The parasite may feed on the host's tissues or body fluids or it may use the host's own food supply. Parasites can be divided into three main categories: pathogenic, commensal and mutualistic.

Pathogens harm the host, causing disease, but parasitism is not always harmful. In fact, the more successful parasites cause little or no damage to the host because if they are to survive then the host must survive too. Micro-organisms which lead a parasitic existence but neither harm nor benefit the host are called **commensals**. The surfaces of animal skin, gut and respiratory tracts carry large numbers of commensals which are harmless as long as they are confined to these places. The host's normal defence mechanisms keep these commensals in check. Many commensals, however, are **potential pathogens** or **opportunists** and will cause disease if the natural body defence mechanisms are breached or weakened. For example, *E. coli* is normally a harmless resident of the gut but will cause infection in a wound or in the urinary tract.

Some parasitic associations are of actual benefit to both the host and the parasite. These are **mutualistic** relationships. For example, ruminants such as cattle are unable to digest cellulose but their rumen contains micro-organisms which can break down cellulose into simple substances which the animal can then absorb. In return, the micro-organisms gain a warm environment with plenty of food.

The term **symbiosis**, meaning 'living together,' is sometimes used to describe any close, permanent association between different organisms, both beneficial and harmful. Therefore, commensalism, mutualism and parasitism are all examples of symbiotic relationships.

Bacteria

Size and shape

Bacteria (singular bacterium) are single-celled organisms. Most of them range from 0.5 to 5 μm in length, though there are some exceptions. Three basic shapes are generally recognised (though it should be noted that there are many variations) and these are sometimes used as a means of classification (Fig. 15.2):

- Cylindrical or rod-shaped cells called **bacilli** (singular bacillus). Some bacilli are curved and these are known as **vibrios**.
- Spherical cells called **cocci** (singular coccus). Some cocci exist singly while others remain together in pairs after cell division and are called **diplococci**. Those that remain attached to form chains are called **streptococci** and if they divide randomly

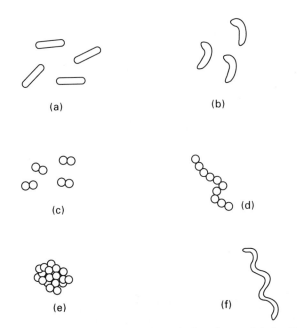

Fig. 15.2. Classification of bacteria by shape: (a) bacilli; (b) vibrios (curved bacilli); (c) diplococci; (d) streptococci; (e) staphylococci; (f) spirochaete.

and form irregular grape-like clusters that are called **staphylococci**.
- Spiral or helical cells are called **spirilla** (singular spirillum) if they have a rigid cell wall or **spirochaetes** if the cell wall is flexible.

Staining of Bacteria

Bacteria can also be classified on the basis of their reaction to certain stains. There are two basic types of microbial staining procedures: **simple** and **differential**. Simple stains such as methylene blue merely colour the cell and can be used to obtain a quick, general picture of the size and shape of the bacteria. Differential stains involve more than one dye solution and are used to show differences between bacterial cells or their internal structures. One of the most widely used differential stains is the **Gram's stain** developed by Christian Gram in 1884. Gram's method of staining enables us to divide bacteria into two groups:

- **Gram-positive**, which stain blue-purple
- **Gram-negative**, which stain red.

Structure

To find out how bacteria function in their environment, we need to look at the individual cell structures. Figure 15.3 shows the structure of a generalised bacterial cell; Fig. 15.4 gives a summary of bacterial cell structures. Some of the structures are common to all cells; others are only present in certain species or under certain environmental conditions.

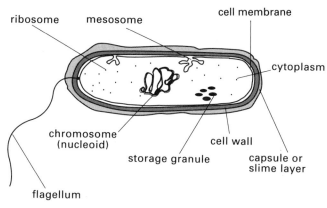

ribosome   mesosome   cell membrane

cytoplasm

chromosome
(nucleoid)   cell wall

storage granule   capsule or
slime layer

flagellum

Fig. 15.3. Cross-section of a generalised bacterial cell.

SUMMARY OF BACTERIAL CELL STRUCTURES

Structure	Functions
Cell wall	Maintains shape of cell Protects cell from bursting and from damage
Capsule/slime layer	Protects cell from environmental hazards Aids adherence to surfaces Aids in prevention of phagocytosis Contributes to virulence of some pathogens May act as food reserve
Cell membrane	Controls passage of substances into and out of cell Site of enzyme activity
Cytoplasm	Site of synthesis processes
Chromosome	Carries hereditary information of the cell
Flagella	Movement
Pili and fimbriae	Attachment to surfaces Involved in transfer of genetic material

Fig. 15.4. Summary of bacterial cell structures.

Cell wall

Most bacteria have a cell wall which is a rigid structure made mainly of a substance called **peptidoglycan** (sometimes called **murein**). It maintains cell shape and prevents the cell from bursting. Cell walls vary in thickness and in composition, and these differences help to explain the different response to Gram's stain.

The cell wall is chemically unlike any structure found in animal cells and is therefore the target for certain drugs that can attack and destroy bacteria without harming the host. For example, the antibiotic penicillin prevents the synthesis of the cell wall, especially in Gram-positive bacteria. Without a cell wall, the cell takes up water and bursts.

Capsules and slime layers

Some bacteria secrete a gelatinous **capsule** outside the cell wall. These capsules can vary considerably in thickness. Other species produce a more fluid secretion called a **slime layer** which adheres less firmly to the cell. Capsules and slime layers can serve a number of functions. They act as a barrier between the bacterium and its environment, protecting the cell from hazards such as drying out and chemicals. The presence of a capsule may protect pathogenic bacteria from being engulfed by the host's phagocytic white blood cells because the phagocyte is prevented from forming close enough contact with the bacterium to engulf it. The chances of infection are therefore increased. Capsules assist the adherence of bacteria to surfaces and may also serve as a food reserve.

Cell membrane (plasma membrane)

This lies just inside the cell wall. It is selectively permeable and controls the passage of substances into and out of the cell. In many bacteria, folds of the cell membrane called **mesosomes** project into the cytoplasm. This folding gives the membrane a larger surface area which is important since mesosomes are thought to be the site of cell respiration. Mesosomes may also be involved in cell division by serving as the site of attachment for the bacterial chromosome.

Cytoplasm

Inside the cell membrane is the cytoplasm, a thick fluid containing dissolved substances such as nutrients, waste products and enzymes. Within the cytoplasm are numerous small, rounded bodies called **ribosomes** which contain ribonucleic acid (**RNA**) and are the site of protein synthesis. It also contains various **inclusion granules**, some of which function as food reserves.

Bacterial chromosome

Suspended within the cytoplasm is the genetic material of the bacterium. A bacterial cell, unlike the cells of other organisms, lacks a distinct membrane-bound nucleus. Instead, the nuclear material or **nucleoid** consists of a single chromosome. The chromosome is a circular, extensively folded molecule of deoxyribonucleic acid (**DNA**) and contains the hereditary information of the cell.

Plasmids

Many bacteria also contain one or more **plasmids**. A plasmid is a small 'extra' piece of DNA which can replicate independently from the chromosome. The importance of plasmids will be discussed later.

Flagella, pili and fimbriae

Some bacteria also possess various appendages which are found outside the cell wall. Many species of bacteria move by means of one or more thread-like structures called **flagella** (singular flagellum). Flagella are long, hollow tubes of a contractile protein which extend from the plasma membrane and through the cell wall. They function by rotating in a corkscrew fashion, moving the bacterium through liquid. Flagella can propel bacteria through liquid sometimes as fast as 100 μm per second or about 3000 body lengths per minute.

Many bacteria, particularly those that are Gram-negative, have numerous straight hair-like appendages called **pili** (singular pilus) or **fimbriae** (singular fimbria) which have nothing to do with movement. Different types of pili have different functions. Some play an important part in enabling bacteria to stick to host cells. For example, in infection, pili help pathogenic bacteria to attach to the cells that line the respiratory, intestinal or urinary tracts, thus preventing them from being washed away by body fluids. Other pili, sometimes called sex pili, are involved in the transfer of genetic material from one bacterial cell to another during bacterial conjugation. Some microbiologists now use the term fimbriae to refer to the appendages involved in attachment and restrict the term pili to those involved in the transfer of DNA during conjugation.

Endospores

Some species of bacteria produce dormant forms called **endospores** (or simply **spores**) that can survive in unfavourable conditions. They are formed when the vegetative (growing) cells are deprived of some factor, for example when the supply of nutrients is inadequate. They are most common in the genera *Bacillus* and *Clostridium*. These genera contain the causative agents of tetanus, anthrax and botulism. The spore develops *within* the bacterial cell and appears under the microscope as a bright round or oval structure.

During spore formation the bacterial chromosome replicates, and the cell membrane grows inwards to form a **septum**. This divides the cell into two unequal parts, each containing one chromosome; the smaller of the two will become the endospore and is called the **forespore**. A series of coats are then synthesised around the forespore and, as it matures, the cell wall of the original vegetative cell disintegrates and the endospore is freed (Fig. 15.5). When favourable conditions return the endospore begins to grow or **germinate** and becomes an active vegetative cell. Many things, such as brief exposure to heat, can bring about germination.

Many endospore-forming bacteria are inhabitants of the soil but they can exist almost everywhere, including in dust. They are extremely resistant structures that can remain viable for many years. They can survive extremes of heat, pH, desiccation, ultraviolet radiation, and exposure to toxic chemicals such as some disinfectants. The reason why endospores are so resistant is not completely understood but heat resistance is thought to be due a dehydration process that occurs during spore formation and expels most of the water from the spore. The fact that they are so hard to destroy is the principal reason for the various sterilisation procedures which are carried out in veterinary practice. It is important to note that endospore formation (or **sporulation**) is *not* a method of reproduction; one vegetative cell produces a single spore which, after germination, is again just one vegetative cell.

Conditions Necessary for Bacterial Growth

Bacteria can grow and reproduce only when environmental conditions are suitable. The essential requirements for growth include:

- A supply of suitable nutrients.
- The correct temperature. The temperature at which a species of bacteria grows most rapidly is the **optimum growth temperature**. Most mammalian pathogens grow best at normal body temperature.
- The correct pH. The majority of mammalian pathogens grow best at pH 7–7.4.
- Water.
- The correct gaseous environment. Many species of bacteria can grow only when oxygen is present and are called **strict or obligate aerobes**. Some, the **obligate anaerobes**, can only grow in the absence of oxygen; others, the **facultative anaerobes**, grow aerobically when oxygen is present but can also function in the absence of oxygen. A few species, the **microaerophiles**, grow best when the concentration of oxygen is lower than in atmospheric air.

Reproduction of Bacteria

If their environment is suitable, bacteria can grow and reproduce rapidly. The sequence of events in which a cell grows and divides into two is called the **cell cycle** and the time interval between successive divisions is called the **generation time**. In some bacteria the generation time is very short; for others it is quite long. For example, under optimum conditions the generation time of *E. coli* is 20 minutes, whereas for the tuberculosis bacterium *Mycobacterium tuberculosis* it is approximately 18 hours.

Binary fission

Bacteria reproduce asexually by simply dividing into two identical daughter cells, a process called **binary**

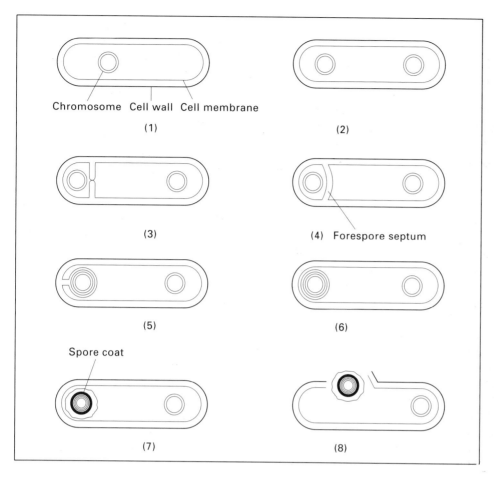

Fig. 15.5. Formation of a bacterial endospore. (1) A vegetative cell is about to sporulate. (2) The bacterial chromosome replicates. (3) The cell membrane grows inwards to form a septum, dividing the cell into two unequal parts. (4) The septum is complete; the smaller of the two parts will become the endospore and is called the forespore. (5) The cell membrane invaginates to engulf the forespore. (6–7) Further coats are synthesised around the forespore. (8) The cell wall of the original vegetative cell disintegrates, freeing the endospore.

fission. Prior to cell division, the cell grows; once it has reached a certain size, the circular chromosome or nucleoid replicates to form two identical chromosomes. As the parent cell enlarges, the chromosomes are separated and the cell membrane grows inwards at the centre of the cell. At the same time, new cell wall material grows inwards to form the septum and this divides the cell into two daughter cells (Fig. 15.6). These may separate completely but in some species (e.g. streptococci and staphylococci) they remain attached to form the characteristic chains or clusters. Replication of pathogenic bacteria usually takes place outside the host's cells, unlike in viruses where reproduction is intracellular.

Conjugation

The process of conjugation involves the passage of DNA from one bacterial cell, the **donor**, to another, the **recipient**, while the two cells are in physical contact. The cells are pulled together by an appendage called the **sex pilus** which is formed by the donor cell. Once contact has been made, the pilus retracts so that the surfaces of the donor and recipient are very close to each other. The cell membranes fuse forming a channel between the two cells, and DNA then passes from the donor to the recipient (Fig. 15.7).

Frequently, a **plasmid** is transferred from the donor to the recipient but sometimes part of the donor cell chromosome, or even the whole chromo-some, is transferred. Conjugation is important because the recipient acquires new characteristics. For example, one plasmid, the R plasmid, carries genes for resistance to antibiotics.

Conjugation is rare among Gram-positive bacteria but common among those which are Gram-negative. It is sometimes regarded as a primitive type of sexual reproduction but this is misleading because, unlike sexual reproduction in other organisms, it does not involve the fusion of two gametes to form a single cell.

Bacterial Cultivation in the Laboratory

The cultivation of bacteria in the laboratory requires an appropriate nutrient material or **culture medium**. This term is used to describe any solid or liquid on or within which bacteria can be grown. A culture medium must contain a balanced mixture of the essential growth requirements, namely carbon, nitrogen and water. Figure 15.8 summarises the uses of common media, and their role in diagnosis is described in Chapter 22 (Diagnostic tests).

Media are of two basic types:

- **Liquid media** or **broths** in which all the required nutrients are included in a fluid.
- **Solid media** which consist of a nutrient solution hardened to a jelly-like consistency by the addition of **agar**, a substance which is derived from seaweed.

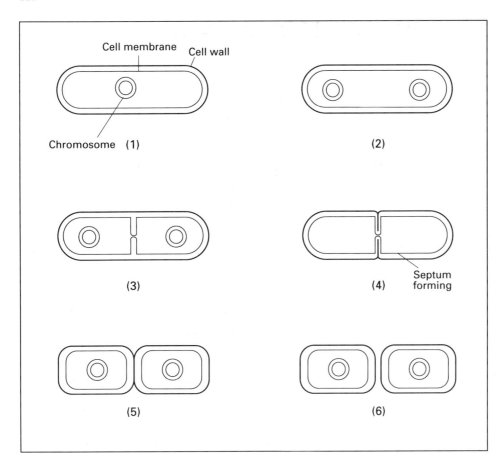

Fig. 15.6. Replication of bacteria by binary fission. (1–2) The cell grows and the chromosome replicates to form two identical chromosomes. (3) As the cell enlarges, the chromosomes are separated and the cell membrane grows inwards at the centre of the cell. (4) At the same time, new cell wall material grows inwards to form the septum. (5–6) The cell divides into two daughter cells.

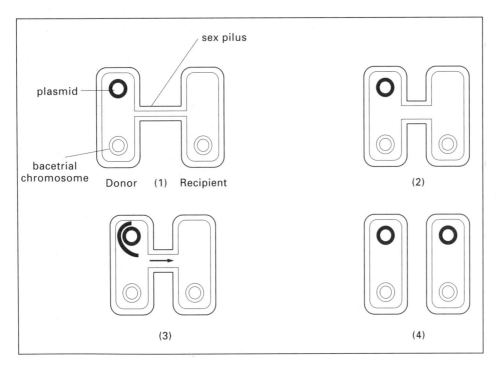

Fig. 15.7. Sequence of events in conjugation. (1) Donor and recipient cells are pulled together by the sex pilus, which is formed by the donor cell. (2) The pilus retracts, bringing the two cells very close to each other, and the cell membranes fuse to form a channel between the two cells. (3) The plasmid replicates and one strand passes through the channel to the recipient. (4) The two cells separate. The recipient becomes a donor because it now has the plasmid.

Solid media are usually used in flat dishes with lids called **petri dishes**; a petri dish containing the solid medium is called a **plate**. Solid media have the advantage that differences in size, shape and colour of bacterial **colonies** (a visible growth of bacteria) can be used for identification and individual colonies can be separated.

Types of media

Simple media (basal media). As the name suggests, this type of medium provides the basic growth requirements for bacteria. Examples of simple media include **nutrient broth**, **nutrient agar** and **peptone water**.

SUMMARY OF THE USES OF COMMON BACTERIOLOGICAL MEDIA		
Medium		**Use**
Plates	Nutrient agar	Growth of nutritionally undemanding species, e.g. *E. coli*
	Blood agar	Enriched medium to support the growth of most pathogens and to detect haemolysis
	Chocolate agar	Enriched medium which is more suitable for certain pathogens, e.g. *Neisseria* species
	Deoxycholate-citrate agar	Selective medium for growing *Salmonella*
	MacConkey's agar	Selective and differential medium used to distinguish those enteric species which ferment lactose (e.g. *E. coli*) from enteric species which do not (e.g. most strains of *Salmonella*)
	Sabouraud's agar	Selective medium for growing fungi
Broths	Nutrient broth	Standard broth for growth of bacteria in fluid
	MacConkey's broth	Selective medium used to isolate enteric from non-enteric bacteria
	Selenite broth	Enrichment medium for growing *Salmonella*

Fig. 15.8. Summary of the uses of common bacterial media.

Enriched media. Some more fastidious bacteria will not grow in simple media but will do so if it is supplemented with substances such as serum, blood or egg. For example, **blood agar**, produced by adding 5–10% blood to the nutrient medium, supports the growth of most mammalian pathogens and is also used to distinguish certain haemolytic bacteria. **Chocolate agar** is made by heating blood agar to 80°C until it becomes chocolate brown in colour. This ruptures the red blood cells, releasing the haemoglobin, therefore making the blood more nutritious.

Selective media. Selective media are designed to inhibit the growth of certain bacteria while not affecting the growth of others. An example is **MacConkey's broth**, which contains bile salts that inhibit non-enteric bacteria but do not affect the growth of enteric species. It is therefore used to isolate enteric from non-enteric bacteria when both are present in a sample. **Sabouraud's agar** is another example of a selective medium: it selects for fungi because it has a high glucose content and a low pH of 5.6. **Deoxycholate-citrate agar** (**DCA**), another selective medium, inhibits the growth of many non-enteric bacteria but most strains of *Salmonella* will form colonies on it.

Differential media. A differential medium is used to distinguish between different species of bacteria on the same agar plate. **MacConkey's agar** is a typical example of a differential medium. It contains a pH indicator (neutral red) as well as the carbohydrate, lactose. Any lactose-fermenting bacteria such as *E. coli* (a normal inhabitant of the gut) produce acidic products which affect the pH indicator and form red colonies. On the other hand, many enteric bacteria, such as most strains of *Salmonella*, do not ferment lactose and these give rise to colourless colonies.

MacConkey's agar also contains bile salts which inhibit the growth of non-enteric bacteria. It is therefore selective as well as differential.

Enrichment media. An enrichment medium (not to be confused with the enriched media discussed previously), is used when a required species of bacteria is only present in very small numbers in a mixed sample. It favours the growth of the wanted species, allowing it to become dominant. Unlike a selective medium, no inhibitory agent is used to prevent the growth of the unwanted species. For example, **selenite broth** is an enrichment medium which enhances the growth of *Salmonella* organisms.

Biochemical media. These are used to distinguish between different species of bacteria, by detecting differences in their biochemical reactions with the media. For example, in some genera the different species can be distinguished from each other by the types of sugar which they can ferment. To determine which sugars a particular organism can utilise they are grown in a series of media, usually peptone water or nutrient broth, each containing a different sugar and a pH indicator. If a particular sugar is fermented by the bacteria, acid will be produced and this is detected by the indicator.

Bacteria which produce the enzyme **urease** can be detected by growing them on solid media containing urea and a pH indicator. Urease-producing bacteria hydrolyse urea to carbon dioxide and ammonia. The ammonia raises the pH and causes the indicator to turn red.

Transport media. These are used for the transport or temporary storage of samples such as swabs. Their function is not to support growth but to ensure the survival of any organisms present until the material can be examined.

The Rickettsiae and Chlamydiae

The rickettsiae (singular rickettsia) and chlamydiae (singular chlamydia) are now classed as bacteria although they are not typical of the group.

The rickettsiae are smaller than most bacteria and are barely visible under the ordinary light microscope. Unlike bacteria, they are **obligate intracellular parasites** and can only be cultivated in tissue culture or in the yolk sac of embryonated eggs. Typically, they are rod shaped, about 0.8 to 2.0 μm long and appear to be structurally related to the Gram-negative bacteria. Most rickettsiae are transmitted from animal to animal by vectors such as the tick, louse, flea and mite which become infected when they ingest blood from an infected individual. *Haemobartonella felis* which causes feline infectious anaemia in cats, is a rickettsial disease.

The chlamydiae are also intracellular parasites. They are coccoid in shape and have a unique and complex developmental life cycle in which they exist in several forms. They are transmitted by inhalation of infectious dust and droplets and by ingestion. There is also evidence to suggest that vector borne infection may occur. Various strains of *Chlamydia psittaci* cause chlamydioses of animals. For example, *C. psittaci* causes psittacosis in psittacene birds (parrots, parakeets). It is a zoonotic infection which humans can acquire by inhaling chlamydia in the airborne dust or cage contents of infected birds. Feline pneumonitis is a frequent infection of cats caused by *C. psittaci*.

Viruses

Although viruses were first discovered in the 1890s, it was not until the development of the electron microscope in the 1940s that microbiologists first saw them. Viruses are much smaller and simpler than bacteria. They range in size from 20 to 300 nm in diameter, parvovirus (20 nm) being at the lower end of the range.

All viruses are **obligate parasites** and depend on host cells for reproduction (replication) and to carry out other vital processes. Viruses outside the host cell are inert particles called **virions** (but the terms, virus and virion, tend to be used interchangeably). Virions are the infectious forms which carry the genetic material from one cell to another.

Structure

All viruses consist of two basic components (Fig. 15.9):

- The **genome**—a central core of nucleic acid, either DNA or RNA (but never both in the same virus).
- The **capsid**—a protein coat which gives shape to the virus and provides a protective covering for the genome. The capsid is made up of individual protein sub-units called **capsomeres** which link together to give the capsid its characteristic symmetry. The number of capsomeres varies from virus to virus.

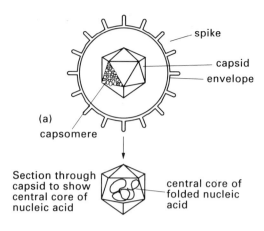

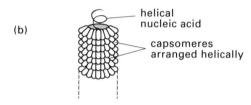

Fig. 15.9. General structure of viruses: (a) an enveloped virus with icosahedral symmetry; (b) part of a rod-shaped virus with helical symmetry.

In addition, many animal viruses are surrounded by a lipoprotein membrane known as an **envelope**, which they acquire as they bud through the host cell membrane. In some viruses the envelope may have projections called **spikes** which are involved in the attachment of the virion to the host cell.

Shapes of viruses

There are three basic viral shapes:

- **Icosahedral**, with 20-sided capsids (e.g. adenovirus, parvovirus).
- **Helical** (e.g. the rabies virus).
- **Complex**, where the symmetry is more complex than the above, or is uncertain.

Replication of Animal Viruses

Reproduction of viruses takes place by **replication**, a process in which the virion invades a susceptible host cell, takes over control of the metabolism of the cell and produces copies of itself (Fig. 15.10). The cycle starts with virus entry.

The virion attaches to receptor sites on the host cell membrane and then either the whole virus or the viral nucleic acid enters the cell. If the whole virus has entered the cell, uncoating of the virus must first take place to release the nucleic acid. The nucleic acid contains all the genetic information needed to take over control of the cell's metabolism, and redirect it to the production of large numbers of viral components. These are assembled into fully infective virus particles which are then released into the surroundings. Some are released by rupture or **lysis** of the host cell membrane while others bud through the cell membrane, picking up an envelope on the way.

Once a virus begins to replicate, the host cell does not usually continue to function normally. There may be obvious damage and cell death or a proliferation of infected cells, sometimes with changes of a malignant nature. Sometimes, though, infected cells show no visible change.

An important part of viral replication in animal cells is attachment of the virus to a specific receptor site on the surface of the cell. A cell lacking such receptor sites will obviously be resistant to infection by that particular virus. This explains why certain viruses only attack particular types of cells. Moreover, as the receptor sites are inherited characteristics, they will vary from animal to animal and this may account for the greater susceptibility of some individuals to a particular virus and the resistance of others.

Viral infections are usually difficult to control and treat because any drug that interferes with viral replication is almost certain to also have a harmful effect on the host cells. Prevention through the use of education and immunisation is still the main method for the control of human and animal viruses.

Fungi

Fungi (singular fungus) range in size from microscopic, unicellular forms to large multicellular organisms which can easily be seen with the naked eye. Most of the vast numbers of different fungi cause no harm to humans or animals but a few are recognised as pathogens (organisms that cause disease). Chapter 21 considers the diagnosis and treatment of fungal pathogens seen in veterinary practice.

Fungi that are classified as micro-organisms can be divided into two groups: yeasts and moulds.

Yeasts

Yeasts are unicellular fungi, usually round or ovoid but they may be other shapes. They are larger than the average bacterial cell and usually reproduce asexually by a process called **budding**, during which the cell becomes swollen at one end and the nucleus divides by constricting. Part of it enters the bud, which continues to enlarge until it is about the same size as the parent cell. The bud then breaks free. *Candida albicans* is a yeast-like fungus which is often present in the intestinal tract of healthy humans and animals, where it lives without causing disease. However, when the host's resistance is lowered or when changes occur in the normal body flora, it can flourish and spread to other parts of the body, becoming pathogenic.

Moulds

Moulds are multicellular organisms composed of long filaments called **hyphae** (singular hypha). Many moulds have septa (cross walls) in their hyphae which divide the hyphae into many cells, each with

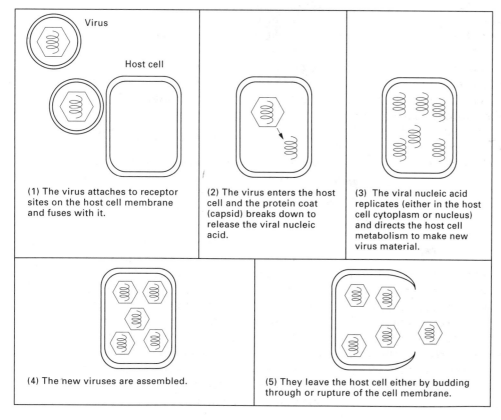

(1) The virus attaches to receptor sites on the host cell membrane and fuses with it.

(2) The virus enters the host cell and the protein coat (capsid) breaks down to release the viral nucleic acid.

(3) The viral nucleic acid replicates (either in the host cell cytoplasm or nucleus) and directs the host cell metabolism to make new virus material.

(4) The new viruses are assembled.

(5) They leave the host cell either by budding through or rupture of the cell membrane.

Fig. 15.10. Replication of animal viruses.

its own nucleus. Others are **aseptate** (they have no septa) and are essentially one long cell containing many nuclei (Fig. 15.11). As the hyphae grow, they intertwine and become a thick mass called the **mycelium**.

Moulds reproduce either asexually or sexually by the production of spores. Some moulds are parasitic and these include the ringworm fungi or **dermatophytes** which cause fungal diseases of the hair, skin and nails (e.g. *Microsporum canis*).

Micro-organisms as Pathogens

Micro-organisms that cause disease are called **pathogens**. With few exceptions, pathogens are parasites, living on or in the host and interfering in some way with the host's metabolism. When a pathogenic micro-organism invades a host (i.e. enters its body tissues) and starts to multiply, it establishes an **infection**. Disease results if the host is susceptible to the infection. Parasites vary greatly in their ability to cause disease. Some will almost always cause serious disease while others are less pathogenic and cause milder illnesses. Others are opportunistic pathogens and only become pathogenic when the body defence mechanisms are weakened. Whether disease develops or not depends on various factors such as the ability of the host to resist infection and the **virulence** of the pathogen, i.e. the *degree* of pathogenicity.

Virulence

Virulence is determined by factors such as:

- the parasite's **invasiveness**—its ability to invade particular cells and tissues and cause damage;
- the parasite's **toxigenicity**—its ability to secrete poisonous substances (**toxins**) which disrupt physiological processes in the body.

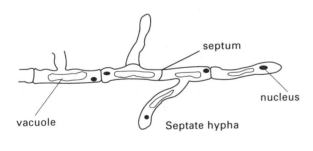

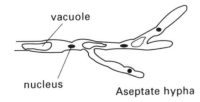

Fig. 15.11. Mould hyphae: (a) septate; (b) aseptate.

The presence of a capsule around the cell wall may contribute to the virulence of some bacteria by preventing **phagocytosis** (destruction by white blood corpuscles known as phagocytes). Pili may also enhance virulence by making the organism better able to adhere to the surface of host cells. In general, though, the factors determining virulence are poorly understood.

Toxins

Toxins are poisonous substances which have a damaging effect on the cells of the host. The effects of the toxin are felt not only in the affected cells and tissues but elsewhere in the body as the toxin is transported through the tissues.

Two types of toxin are recognised:

- **Exotoxins**, which are manufactured by living micro-organisms and released into the surrounding medium.
- **Endotoxins**, which are retained within the micro-organism and only liberated when it dies.

Exotoxins

Exotoxins are proteins produced mainly by Gram-positive bacteria during their metabolism. They are released into the surrounding environment as they are produced. This can be into the circulatory system and tissues of the host or, as in food poisoning, into food which is then ingested. Microbial toxins include many of the most potent poisons known to man and may prove lethal even in small quantities.

The effects of toxins are usually very specific. For example, when spores of the anaerobic tetanus bacilli *Clostridium tetani* get into a wound that provides favourable conditions, they may germinate and grow in the tissues. The bacteria do not spread through the tissues but secrete an exotoxin which travels along peripheral nerves to the central nervous system, where it interferes with the regulation of neuro-transmitters that control the relaxation of muscle. This leads to uncontrollable muscle spasms and paralysis. Tetanus toxin is called a **neurotoxin** because of its activity in the nervous system.

Unlike tetanus (which is caused by exotoxins produced while the organism is growing *within* the host), botulism (caused by the saprophytic bacterium, *Clostridium botulinum*), is the result of *ingestion* of food containing the toxins. In botulism, the exotoxin affects the nervous system leading to paralysis; it too is therefore a neurotoxin.

Other exotoxins formed outside the body include those produced by *Staphylococcus aureus*, the bacteria which cause staphylococcal food poisoning. This is an **enterotoxin** because it functions in the gastrointestinal tract, causing vomiting and diarrhoea.

The body responds to the presence of exotoxins by producing antibodies called **antitoxins** which neutralise the toxins, rendering them harmless.

Exotoxins, being proteins, are destroyed by heat and some chemicals. Chemicals such as formaldehyde are used to treat toxins so that they lose their toxicity but not their ability to elicit an immune response. These treated toxins are called **toxoids** and will stimulate the production of antitoxins if injected into the body. For example, tetanus toxoid is used to provide immunity to tetanus.

Endotoxins

Endotoxins are part of the cell wall of certain Gram-negative bacteria and are released only when the cells die and disintegrate. Compared with exotoxins, they are less toxic, do not form toxoids and are able to withstand heat. Blood-borne endotoxins are responsible for a range of non-specific reactions in the body, such as fever. They also make the walls of blood capillaries more permeable, causing blood to leak into the intercellular spaces; this sometimes results in a serious drop in blood pressure, a condition commonly called **endotoxic shock**.

Aflatoxin

Toxins are not made exclusively by bacteria. The saprophytic fungus, *Aspergillus flavus*, produces a toxin called **aflatoxin**. The fungus grows in warm, humid conditions and contaminates a variety of agricultural products such as peanuts, cereals, rice and beans. Aflatoxin has been implicated in the deaths of many farm animals that have been fed on mouldy hay, corn or peanut meal. When animals are fed on meal containing the toxin, it accumulates in their body and passes along the food chain.

How Micro-organisms Cause Disease

In order to cause infectious disease, a pathogen must:

- gain entry into the host;
- establish itself and multiply in the host tissue;
- overcome the normal host body defences for a time;
- damage the host in some way.

Some micro-organisms cause disease by releasing toxins that disrupt specific physiological processes in the host (as described above). Others invade tissue cells and destroy them. Viruses, for example, cause cell damage because they interfere with the normal cell metabolism and many leave the host cell by rupture of the cell membrane. Many micro-organisms produce toxic enzymes to assist in the process of invasion and tissue destruction. For example, the enzyme **hyaluronidase** helps the pathogen to penetrate the tissues of the host by breaking down the 'tissue cement' that holds the cells together. Hyaluronidase is an important virulence factor in certain species of streptococci and staphylococci. Another enzyme, **lecithinase**, lyses or disintegrates tissue cells, especially red blood cells.

Once they have invaded the host, some micro-organisms can grow and multiply in any tissue of the body, spreading through it (**systemic spread**) usually via the lymphatic system and blood circulation. However, many are more selective and localise in a particular tissue or organ, perhaps at the site of entry. For example, *Staphylococcus aureus*, which causes abscesses in the skin, generally attacks in this way. If these exacting organisms do not reach the specific cells in which they can live, they will not produce disease. Viruses in particular often have an affinity for a specific tissue or organ.

In some diseases, symptoms occur because of an overreaction of the host's own defence mechanisms, which can lead to cell damage or an allergic reaction.

The term **bacteraemia** is used to describe the presence of bacteria in the blood; **viraemia** denotes the presence of viruses; and **toxaemia** indicates the presence of toxins in the bloodstream. The word **septicaemia** is used when bacteria are actively multiplying in the blood, and **pyaemia** describes the presence of pus in the blood.

Epidemiology

Epidemiology is the study of the occurrence and distribution of disease. An infection is said to be **endemic** (or more correctly **enzootic**) if it is constantly present in a locality. For example, rabies was endemic in wild carnivores throughout Europe except in the British Isles. A disease is said to be **epidemic** (or more correctly **epizootic**) when its incidence increases sharply and involves large numbers of individuals in an area, e.g. parvovirus disease. **Pandemic** diseases are those that occur world-wide. A **zoonotic infection** or **zoonosis** is an animal disease that can be transmitted to humans.

16

Elementary Mycology and Parasitology

M. FISHER

DEFINITIONS

- **Parasite**: one eukaryotic organism living off another (the **host**) to the advantage of the parasite.
- **Ectoparasites** live on the outside of the host.
- **Endoparasites** live inside the host.
- **Eukaryote**: organism in which the chromosomes are enclosed in a nucleus (e.g. animals, plants, fungi).

Fungi

The division of fungi into unicellular yeasts and multicellular moulds is discussed in Chapter 15 (Elementary Microbiology). The fungal pathogens seen in small animal veterinary practice include both categories:

- Moulds: the 'ringworm' dermatophytes ('skin-eaters').
- Yeasts: *Candida albicans*, the 'thrush' yeast, is often present in the intestinal tract of animals without causing disease but it can become pathogenic in certain circumstances.

Dermatophytes

Fungal infection of **keratin** (the horny tissue that forms nail, hair and skin) can affect cats, dogs, rabbits and guinea pigs, for example. The condition broadly known as **ringworm** is caused by dermatophytes such as species of *Trichophyton mentagrophytes* (dog, cat, rabbit and guinea pig) and *Microsporum canis* (dog and cat), among others.

In its most obvious form, ringworm appears as circular areas of hair loss with active fungal infection around the edge of the lesion. The lesions may be small and discrete or large and coalescing, with an irregular outline. Some infections are not very inflamed and cause little irritation, whilst others may cause severe inflammation. A more marked reaction is common in dogs.

Transmission may be directly from affected animal to animal, or to humans (many dermatophytes are zoonotic). Long-haired cats, in particular, may appear normal but may be carriers of infection. There may also be indirect transmission via bedding, cages etc. Ringworm spores can remain viable in the environment for prolonged periods.

Diagnosis

- Place hair pluck or skin scrape on a slide and stain with lactophenol cotton blue or Quink. Affected material, including hair shafts, will stain blue (Fig. 16.1).
- Use Wood's lamp in a darkened room. Once the lamp has warmed up sufficiently, it produces ultraviolet light and some 50% of the *Microsporum canis* isolates will usually fluoresce and appear apple-green in colour. (Other matter, such as surface scale, may also fluoresce but will not be apple-green.)
- Culture a sample of the suspect hair and/or scale on specialist medium—for example, Sabouraud's or dermatophyte test medium (DTM). The latter contains a colour indicator that turns from yellow to red in the presence of dermatophytes. The culture should be incubated at room temperature and any dermatophytes should grow within 3 weeks.

Treatment

Topical

- Fungicidal wash such as enilconazole.
- Paint the affected area with tincture of iodine.
- Whitfield's ointment, containing salicyclic and benzoic acid.

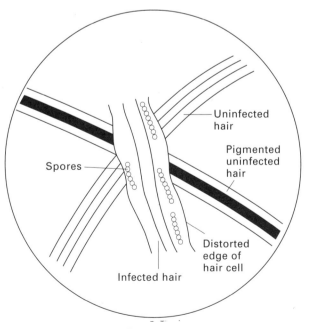

Fig. 16.1. Fungus infected hair.

Topical treatment is usually repeated after an interval to effect a full cure. It may be possible to treat the area of a discrete lesion only, or it may be necessary to wash the whole animal.

Systemic. Griseofulvin is administered orally in tablet form and has to be given for a prolonged period as the levels build up gradually in the skin. Care, including the wearing of gloves, should be taken when handling griseofulvin as it is **teratogenic** (i.e. it can cause malformation of a foetus).

Candida albicans

Candida infections are usually opportunistic, that is they take advantage of a young or debilitated animal and cause infection. The infection is known as 'thrush' and is occasionally seen on mucous membranes, particularly in the mouths of puppies or kittens.

Identification is by means of the appearance of a white growth on the affected area. Infection of the mouth in a puppy or kitten may be associated with unwillingness to suck and therefore a wimpering animal. Very rarely these yeasts may infect the skin, though *Candida* is not usually included in the dermatophytes.

Ectoparasites

Except for certain important fungi mentioned previously, most ectoparasites belong to the animal kingdom and have a hard outer shell or exoskeleton. They include:

- **Insects**, where the adult has three pairs of legs and the body is divided into head, thorax and abdomen (e.g. lice, fleas).
- **Arachnids**, where the adult has four pairs of legs and the body is divided into two parts only: cephalothorax and abdomen (e.g. mites, ticks).

Usually it is the adult stage that is parasitic, often together with the immature stages. There are two cases where only an immature form is parasitic: *Trombicula autumnalis* (a mite), and the larvae of the blowfly.

Insects

The diagnosis and control of insect ectoparasites are given in Fig. 16.2.

Lice

The lice are divided into biting and sucking lice (Figs 16.3 and 16.4), reflecting their manner of feeding.

INSECT PARASITES: DIAGNOSIS AND CONTROL		
	Diagnosis	**Control**
Lice	Demonstration of the eggs attached to hairs. Visualisation of the adult louse. The adult lice may be seen with the naked eye on close examination of an animal's haircoat or may be seen in a skin scrape/brush.	Thorough cleaning. Topical surface treatment with an insecticidal wash or spray.
Fleas	Demonstration of an adult flea or their faeces in the coat of a dog or cat by combing the coat thoroughly, preferably with a very fine tooth-comb (ideally a human louse comb). The animal may be brushed over a sheet of damp white paper. Flea faeces will be seen on the paper as small black dots. Since they contain a large amount of undigested blood, a ring of red is seen around the black spot when moistened. There is also a skin test for allergy to fleas.	Control of the environment stages: – hoovering, particularly around where the pet sleeps; – applying an environmental insecticide and/or an insect growth regulator such as methoprene to kill the immature stages. Chitin synthesis inhibitor (lufeneron) given orally to the dog or cat. It prevents egg hatching and/or larval development. Control of adult fleas on the animal: –thorough grooming, using a human louse comb; –applying an insecticide in the form of, for example, a spray, impregnated collar, powder, shampoo or spot-on. There is also an insecticide that comes in tablet form. The active ingredient in insecticides is often an organophosphate, carbamate or a synthetic pyrethroid.
Dipteran fly larvae	An affected animal will often stop eating and appear restless and depressed. The animal should be thoroughly examined to find the larvae and thus diagnose the problem.	In order to treat the infestation, the first step is to remove the larvae: Wash the affected area with a mild antiseptic solution, ensuring that the larvae are removed in the process. Lightly towel-dry the area. Apply wound powder, which will help both to dry the area and to prevent any infection developing. Any underlying problem (e.g. diarrhoea) that may have predisposed the animal to becoming 'fly blown' should be investigated and treated.

Fig. 16.2. Diagnosis and control of insect ectoparasites.

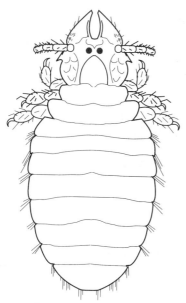

Fig. 16.3. Dorsal view of the biting louse (2 mm long, light to dark brown in colour). If viewed from the side, the louse would appear dorsoventrally flattened.

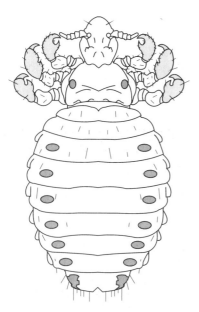

Fig. 16.4. Dorsal view of a sucking louse (approximately 2 mm long).

Infection is transmitted by close contact as the louse spends its entire life cycle on the host. Alternatively infection may be transferred by eggs collected on grooming equipment. However, lice are highly **host-specific** and will not survive if transferred to a host of a different species. (Other parasites, such as the cat flea, are more ubiquitous and will be found on a number of different hosts.)

Cats, dogs, rabbits, rodents and birds may be affected by lice, and often young or debilitated animals are the worst affected. Large numbers of lice cause intense irritation and concomittant self-inflicted injury. In addition, the sucking lice may cause anaemia if they are present in large enough numbers.

Life cycle

Adult female lice lay their eggs individually and cement them to hairs. The eggs ('nits') are just visible to the naked eye (Fig. 16.5). When these hatch, immature lice that are identical to the adult louse emerge; they become adults after several moults. The whole life cycle takes about 2–3 weeks.

Fleas

Adult fleas bite the host in order to take a blood meal. The area that has been bitten shows an inflammatory reaction and causes some irritation. A heavy flea infestation may cause anaemia.

Some animals become sensitised to **allergens** (particles that provoke an allergic reaction in sensitised individuals on repeat exposure) in the flea saliva and develop severe lesions after just a few bites. This is known as **miliary dermatitis** or **flea allergic dermatitis** in the cat and **flea allergic dermatitis** in the dog.

The species of flea may be identified by the appearance of the head (Fig. 16.6). Most fleas on cats and dogs are the 'cat flea' *Ctenocephalides felis*,

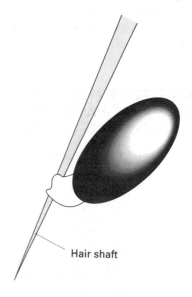

Hair shaft

Fig. 16.5. Louse egg ('nit') attached with 'cement' to the shaft of a hair.

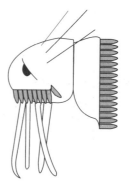

Fig. 16.6. Lateral view of the head of a cat flea, showing combs whose absence or presence and appearance are used in species identification.

but dogs in a dog-only situation (e.g. greyhound kennels) may be infected with the dog flea *Cteno-cephalides canis*. Infrequently other flea species (e.g. hedgehog fleas) are found on cats or dogs. Birds have their own species of flea, the immature stages of which live in the nest.

Life cycle of the cat flea

The life cycle of the flea is shown in Fig. 16.7. The adult is laterally compressed, which allows the flea to move readily between the host's hairs. The female flea mates on the host and then lays eggs. These are smooth and fall off into the environment, particularly around where the animal usually lies. After 2–14 days the eggs hatch out as larvae that look like small maggots. These feed off skin debris, the faeces of adult fleas and other organic matter in the environment. After about a week each matured larva spins a cocoon and pupates. The outside of the cocoon is sticky and so bits of debris from the environment stick to it. After a further 10 days (though this can be considerably longer in cold or dry conditions) the adult flea is fully developed inside the pupa. Before it emerges, it waits for signs of a host being available— e.g. vibration in the environment. (This is one explanation for the stories of new occupants going into an empty house and being bitten by fleas within hours.) Once emerged from its pupal case, the flea locates a host and jumps on to it.

Dipteran Flies

Myiasis is defined as parasitism by larvae of the dipteran flies (green, blue and black bottles). The life cycle is shown in Fig. 16.8. The flies lay their eggs on a suitable site, which might be (though not necessarily) on an animal, e.g. in the fleece of a sheep or around the anus of a rabbit. Flies are particularly attracted to smelly animals, such as those that are soiled with diarrhoea, etc.

The larvae (maggots) hatch after as little as 12 hours and begin to traumatise the skin suface and feed off the damaged tissue. After several moults the larvae drop to the ground. Here they may overwinter as larvae before pupating, or they may pupate immediately. Eventually the adult fly emerges from the pupal case.

Arachnids

The arachnids of veterinary importance are the ticks and the mites. The immature larvae that emerge from the eggs appear like a smaller version of the adult, except that they have only three pairs of legs, whereas the nymph and adult stages each have four pairs of legs.

Mites

The mites are all **permanent ectoparasites** (they spend their entire life cycle on the host), except for *Trombicula autumnalis*, where it is only the larva that is sometimes parasitic. Mites may be divided into the burrowing and the surface mites. Both types cause dermatitis, which may or may not be itchy, depending on the type of mite present. Diagnosis is usually by inspection of coat brushings or skin scrapes; specific guidance on diagnosis and treatment of each mite is given in Fig. 16.9.

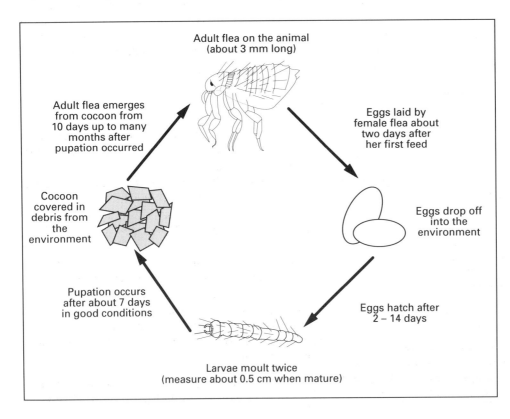

Adult flea on the animal
(about 3 mm long)

Adult flea emerges from cocoon from 10 days up to many months after pupation occurred

Eggs laid by female flea about two days after her first feed

Cocoon covered in debris from the environment

Eggs drop off into the environment

Pupation occurs after about 7 days in good conditions

Eggs hatch after 2 – 14 days

Larvae moult twice
(measure about 0.5 cm when mature)

Fig. 16.7. Life cycle of the flea.

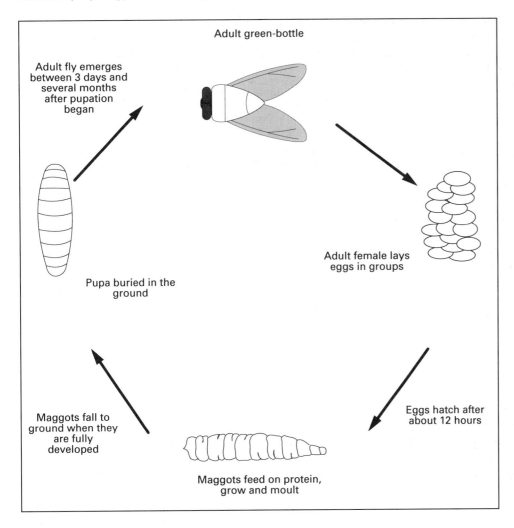

Adult green-bottle

Adult fly emerges between 3 days and several months after pupation began

Adult female lays eggs in groups

Pupa buried in the ground

Eggs hatch after about 12 hours

Maggots fall to ground when they are fully developed

Maggots feed on protein, grow and moult

Fig. 16.8. Life cycle of the blow fly.

SKIN SCRAPES

- Collection: Hold a scalpel blade at right angles to the skin surface and draw it repeatedly across a part of the edge of the affected area until the scraped area bleeds slightly. Debris will be collected in front of the scalpel blade: transfer it into a container such as a pill pot. Also place the scalpel blade into the container.
- Preparation: Place the material from the container, along with any debris attached to the blade, into a drop of 10% potassium hydroxide (KOH) on a microscope slide. Liquid paraffin is preferred by some but KOH helps to break down the skin and hair, thus allowing parasites to be spotted more readily. The KOH also helps to 'clear' the parasite, making its features more readily identifiable. The preparation may be heated to speed up the process. A coverslip is then placed over the preparation.
- Examination: The preparation is initially scanned under the low power (×4) objective to look for evidence of large parasites. It is then examined under the ×10 objective to search for smaller parasites such as *Demodex*.

Surface brushings are most readily examined in a petri dish under a low-power dissecting microscope. A portion of the sample may also be prepared and examined as detailed for skin scrapes.

Burrowing Mites

Burrowing mites live in small tunnels within the surface layers of the skin. They lay their eggs in small nests within these tunnels. There are three genera of burrowing mites typically seen in domestic pets:

- *Sarcoptes scabiei* var. *canis*
- *Notoedres*
- *Cnemidocoptes* sp.

Sarcoptes scabiei var. *canis*. This mite affects dogs and, very rarely, cats. (*Sarcoptes* species may also cause mange in rodents.)

Often the tips of the ears and then the face are the first areas affected but large areas of the body may be infected in severe cases. Affected areas become hairless, thickened and inflamed. This is due partly to the effect of the mites themselves and partly to the trauma that the animal causes by rubbing and scratching the affected area—the condition is very itchy. *Sarcoptes* infection in dogs will infect humans but normally the lesions are small and self-limiting. A separate type of *Sarcoptes* is responsible for causing scabies in humans, and another species may cause mange in rodents.

Notoedres. This burrowing mite of the cat (Fig. 16.11) is seen very rarely but it causes similar signs

MITES: DIAGNOSIS AND TREATMENT		
Diagnosis	**Presence of mite in:**	**Treatment**
Sarcoptes scabiei *Notoedres* *Cnemidocoptes* *Demodex* *Cheyletiella*	skin scrapes skin scrapes skin scrapes skin scrapes Coat brushings (adult mite and/or eggs)	Mite infections may be treated with a suitable acaricide. Where no licensed product is available, treat with e.g. selenium sulphide or an organophosphate preparation. Repeat treatments after 10–14 days to ensure all immature stages killed. Also treat the environment in *Cheyletiella* infection.
Otodectes cynotis	ear wax	Clean the ear canal; instil ointment containing suitable acaricide, often in combination with antibiotic. Also treat in-contact animals to clear reservoir of infection.

Fig. 16.9. Diagnosis and treatment of mites.

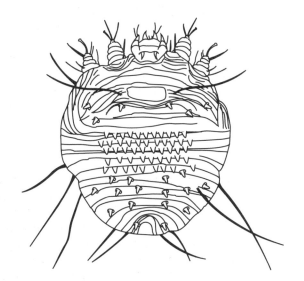

Fig. 16.10. Dorsal view of an adult *Sarcoptes* mite (0.4 mm long). Note the short, stubby legs that barely project beyond the body, spines and pegs, terminal anus, pedicles at end of legs with suckers on ends.

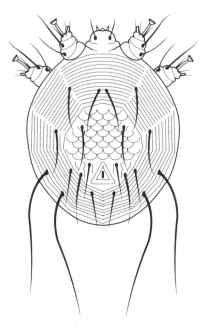

Fig. 16.11. Dorsal view of adult female *Notoedres* mite (0.36 mm long) showing concentric circles on body; containing an egg, dorsal anus.

to *Sarcoptes* in the dog. *Notoedres* sp. infection also occurs in rats.

Cnemidocoptes spp. These mites (Figs 16.12–16.14) are the cause of 'scaly leg' and 'scaly face' in birds, particularly budgerigars.

Demodex. This small, cigar-shaped mite may be found in normal hair follicles without necessarily causing any problem. In some individuals, particularly young dogs belonging to short-haired breeds, the numbers of *Demodex* increase dramatically and cause a dermatitis that is characteristically an area of non-itchy **alopecia** (loss of hair). Often the area around the eyes is first affected. It can be trickier to find than other burrowing mites as it is smaller and dwells deep within the hair follicle.

Demodex may also cause mange in hamsters and gerbils. The burrowing mite found in the guinea pig is *Trixacarus caviae*.

Surface Mites

Otodectes cynotis. These are the ear mites in dogs and cats. They live within the ear canal, often stimulating a dark brown waxy discharge. Mites may be seen on the surface as small white moving dots. Secondary bacterial infection may result in a pus-like discharge.

Most cats are infected, often without showing clinical signs. Some cats, and most dogs, show clinical signs of head-shaking and ear-rubbing when infection is present. This may result in trauma to the ears and haematoma formation in the ear flap.

Ear canker in rabbits is caused by *Psoroptes cuniculi*.

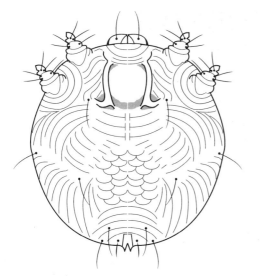

Fig. 16.12. Dorsal view of a *Cnemidocoptes* mite (0.2 mm long).

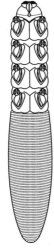

Fig. 16.13. Ventral view of *Demodex* mite showing cigar-shaped body (0.2 mm long).

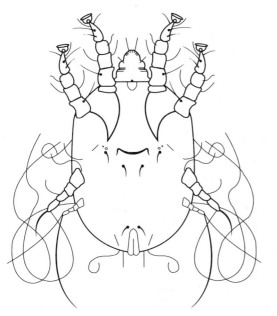

Fig. 16.14. Dorsal view of *Octodectes* mite (0.4 mm long). Note the longer legs protruding from the body and unjointed pedicles with suckers on the ends.

Cheyletiella. Animals infected with this fur mite are often said to be affected with 'walking dandruff' since infection often leads to the production of excess scale and since the mites are just visible with the naked eye (they are almost 0.5 mm long). Infection does not usually cause any marked loss of hair. Separate species affect rabbits, cats and dogs. Often the mites will move on to humans handling the animals and, though they will not survive for long periods, they will often bite. Small raised red spots appear in the affected areas of the human body.

Trombicula autumnalis. This mite (also known as *Neotrombicula autumnalis*) normally becomes a problem in late summer and autumn, particularly in chalky areas of southern England. The larval mites attach themselves to the legs of passing dogs and feed, causing intense irritation to the host.

Dermanyssus. This is the 'red mite' that sucks the blood of chickens and occasionally other animals. All stages live off the host—for example, in the eaves of poultry houses. The mites visit chickens to feed, particularly at night. Infection causes irritation and debility, with anaemia in heavy infections. Control is by cleaning the hen-house and treatment with an acaracide.

Ticks

Ticks on livestock are important in many parts of the world as carriers or vectors of disease. (A **vector** is a carrier of disease where no development of the disease occurs in the carrier—it simply transfers the infection from one host to the next.) A heavy burden may cause anaemia. In small animal practice it is more usual to encounter just one or two ticks on a cat or dog, with an owner who is concerned about how to get rid of them.

Several species of tick may affect dogs in the U.K. and one of them (*Ixodes canisuga*) is specific to the dog. However, by far the most common ticks seen on small animals are the sheep tick (*I. ricinus*) and the hedgehog tick (*I. hexagonus*). These ticks are remarkably cosmopolitan and will attach to many different hosts. Initially all that is visible is a small greyish swelling, firmly attached to the animal. Inspection reveals pairs of legs close to the attachment with the animal; the mouth parts are buried into the animal's flesh. Once the tick has fed fully it will drop off its host. The life cycle of the sheep tick is shown in Fig. 16.18. It should be noted that some other ticks, such as the dog tick, remain on the host from larva to adult and only drop off once they are fully fed adults.

Diagnosis is based on finding the ticks. The identification of the species of tick is a specialised skill.

Individual ticks may be removed by dabbing them with a cotton wool bud that has been treated with an acaricide. Once dead, they can be gently removed. A number of tick removal devices are available.

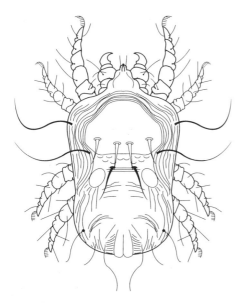

Fig. 16.15. Dorsal view of *Cheyletiella* (0.4 mm). Note the 'comb' on the end of each leg and the large palps either side of the head, each with a large claw.

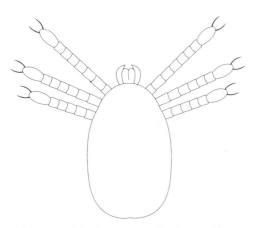

Fig. 16.16. *Trombicula autumnalis* larva (1 mm long, orange-brown in colour). Note that there are only three pairs of legs.

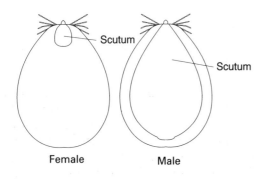

Fig. 16.17. Adult sheep ticks: (a) dorsal view of female, engorged (about 1 cm long); (b) dorsal view of male (about 3 mm long). Note four pairs of legs and backplate or scutum covering almost all of the abdomen.

> **WARNING**
> Never try to pull off a live tick, as its mouthparts may be left embedded in the animal and may become a focus for infection.

Endoparasites

Endoparasites may be divided into helminths and protozoa. The **helminths** are the worms and are subdivided into three types: the **flukes** (which are found in the livers of sheep and cattle but do not normally affect dogs or cats in the U.K.), the tapeworms or **cestodes**, and the round worms or **nematodes**. The **protozoal parasites** are small, unicellular organisms. Figure 16.19 lists the most common species in each category seen in small animal veterinary practice.

Helminths

Cestodes (tapeworms)

A cestode is tape-like and has no alimentary tract. It is composed of three parts (Fig. 16.20): the head or scolex; an area behind this where segments or proglottids form; and finally the maturing segments.

> **TAPEWORM DEFINITIONS**
> Adult tapeworm:
>
> - **Scolex**: head of a tapeworm—the part used for attachment to the host's intestine using suckers and the rostellum (where present) for attachment.
> - **Strobila**: the chain of individual segments.
> - **Rostellum**: the anterior part of the scolex, present in most tapeworms. It is a protrusible cone and is armed with hooks in some species.
> - **Proglottid**: name for each of the individual segments that make up the strobila.
>
> Immature tapeworm (**metacestode**)
>
> - **Cysticercus**: fluid-filled cyst containing a single invaginated scolex attached to the cyst wall.
> - **Cysticercoid**: single evaginated scolex (this is the form found in invertebrate intermediate hosts).
> - **Hydatid cyst**: large cyst containing many scolices, some loose in the fluid inside and some contained within 'brood capsules'.
> - **Coenurus**: a cyst with many invaginated scolices attached to the cyst wall.

Each tapeworm has an immature stage that develops in a separate or intermediate host, the exact structure varying according to the species of tapeworm.

The tapeworms in cats and dogs are *Echinococcus granulosus* (dogs), *Dipylidium caninum* (dogs and cats) and the *Taenia* species (one species in cats and

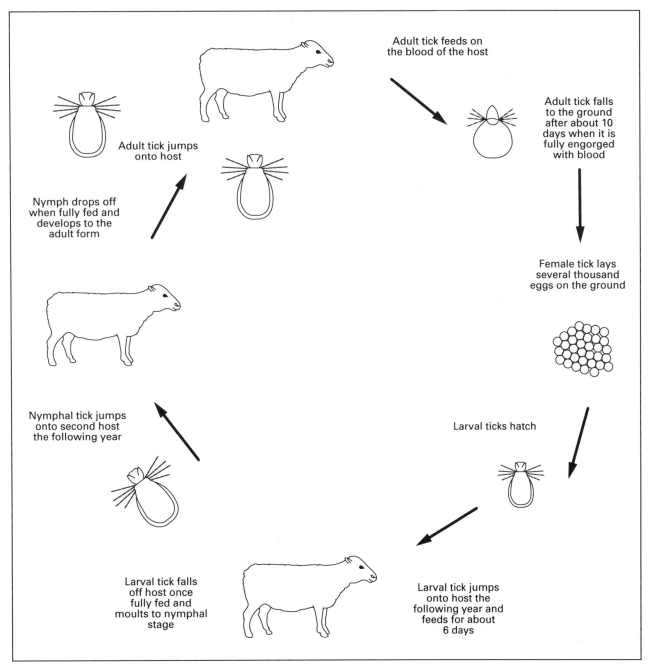

Adult tick feeds on
the blood of the host

Adult tick falls
to the ground
after about 10
days when it is
fully engorged
with blood

Adult tick jumps
onto host

Nymph drops off
when fully fed and
develops to the
adult form

Female tick lays
several thousand
eggs on the ground

Nymphal tick jumps
onto second host
the following year

Larval ticks hatch

Larval tick falls
off host once
fully fed and
moults to nymphal
stage

Larval tick jumps
onto host the
following year and
feeds for about
6 days

Fig. 16.18. Life cycle of the sheep tick.

several species in dogs). Their presence is not normally any problem to the final host, though the sight of tapeworm segments is repugnant to owners. There is more often a problem with infection of the intermediate host, either because the presence of the tapeworm cysts cause disease or because affected meat is condemned as unfit for human consumption.

Dipylidium caninum. This is probably the most common tapeworm of cats and dogs in the UK. The intemediate host is the flea, and the louse in the case of the dog. It is normally diagnosed by the presence of motile segments (shaped like rice grains) around the anus or in the faeces of a cat or dog.

Control depends on treating the existing infection and then eliminating any flea or louse problem to break the transmission cycle.

Taenia spp. Dogs and cats are affected with the taeniid tapeworms when they eat raw meat, either in the form of uncooked meat or offal or through catching and eating prey containing the intermediate stages of the parasite. The life cycle of *Taenia hydatigena* is shown in Fig. 16.22 and the names of the specific tapeworms with their final and intermediate hosts are shown in Fig. 16.23.

Diagnosis is based on seeing segments passed by the animal. More rarely eggs, liberated from the

ENDOPARASITES		
Helminths		
Flukes		
Cestodes (tapeworms)	*Echinococcus granulosus*	Dogs
	Dipylidium canium	Dogs/cats
	Taenia spp.	Cats/dogs
Nematodes (roundworms)		
Ascarids	*Toxocara canis*	Dogs
	Toxascaris leonina	Cats/dogs
	Toxocara cati	Cats
Hookworms	*Uncinaria stenocephala*	Dogs
	Ancylostoma caninum	Dogs
Whipworm	*Trichuris vulpis*	Dogs
Heart worm	*Dirofilaria immitis*	Dogs
Capillaria	*C. plica*	Dogs
	C. hepatica	
Lungworms	*Aelurostrongylus abstrusus*	Cats
	Angiostrongylus vasorum	Dogs
	Oslerus osleri	Dogs
Protozoa		
Coccidia	*Eimeria intestinalis*	Rabbits
	E. flavescens	Rabbits
	E. stiedae	Rabbits
		Dog/cats
Isospora		Dog/cats
Cryptosporidium parvum		Dog/cats
Sarcocystis spp.		Cats
Toxoplasma gondii		Cats
Hammondia		Dogs
Giardia		

Fig. 16.19. Common species of endoparasite.

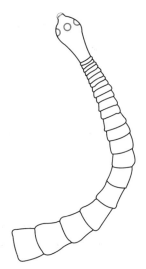

Fig. 16.20. Typical adult cestode, showing head or 'scolex' with ring of hooks on the rostellum and suckers for attachment to the wall of the intestine. Behind this is the neck, where new segments are formed. Further back is the strobila, consisting of maturing segments and, at the posterior end, the gravid segments full of fertilised eggs. These individually drop off the end of the worm and are passed in the faeces.

segments, are seen during microscopic examination of a faecal sample (Fig. 16.22). These eggs measure about 40 μm in diameter.

Control is based on treating the current infection and then preventing the animal having access to uncooked meat—which may be difficult if the infection is derived from wild prey.

Echinococcus granulosus granulosus. This organism has a dog-to-sheep life cycle (Fig. 16.24). It is an important zoonosis in the U.K. but is fortunately fairly rare—it is most common in rural areas, such as parts of Wales, where dogs have the opportunity to feed on sheep carcases on the hills.

The adult parasite is only about 6mm long, and several thousand may be present in the intestine of a single dog. Dogs in affected areas should be treated regularly with an effective anthelmintic and denied access to sheep carcases.

If a human ingests a proglottid or individual eggs, a hydatid cyst may develop in the liver or lungs in the same way as it will develop in the sheep. This forms a space-occupying lesion that may grow to a considerable size. Treatment of affected people is based on anthelmintic therapy followed by drainage of the cyst and then surgical removal the wall of the cyst. This is quite a hazardous procedure for the patient.

Echinococcus granulosus equinus is a separate tapeworm that has a dog-to-horse life cycle. It occurs particularly where hounds are fed on horse offal. It is not believed to pose a zoonotic risk.

Cestode infections in other animals. Birds and other animals such as rabbits, mice, rats and hamsters may all be infected with adult tapeworms specific to the host species. In most cases infection has no effect on the host. Occasionally a heavy tapeworm burden in hamsters may be associated with weight loss and perhaps intestinal blockage. In each case the intermediate host is an invertebrate such as a beetle or mite.

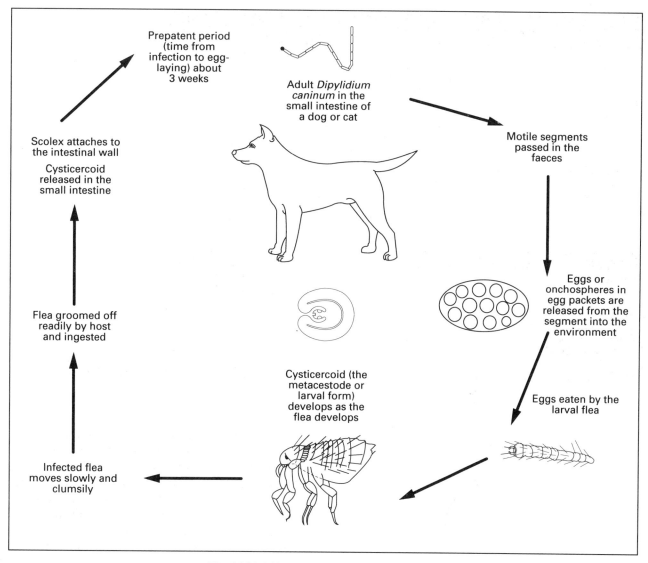

Fig. 16.21. Life cycle of *Dipylidium caninum*.

Treatment of cestode infections

It is difficult to kill the immature tapeworm infections in intermediate hosts and this is not usually attempted. However, the adult tapeworm can be killed by a number of anthelmintics. Products that only have activity against tapeworms are known as **cestocides**. Alternatively the preparation may have activity against other helminths, particularly nematodes, as well as tapeworms and these are known as **broad spectrum anthelmintics**. The active ingredients that have cestocidal activity are shown in Fig. 16.25.

Nematodes

Nematodes are round worms with a proper digestive tract. Most have a direct life cycle, though some (e.g. the lungworms) have a slug or snail as intermediate host. Others may be carried by a **paratenic host** (one that acts as a carrier only—no development of the parasite occurs in this host). Important nematode groups seen in small animal veterinary practice include:

- Ascarids (especially *Toxocara canis, Toxascaris leonina* and *Toxocara cati* in dogs and cats). Large, fleshy worms (Fig. 16.26), most numerous and frequent in young animals. Ascarids occur commonly in other animals including reptiles (e.g. tortoises) and birds (especially parakeets); in each case the ascarid species is host specific. Heavy burdens may be associated with poor growth or intestinal impactions.
- Hookworms (*Uncinaria stenocephala* and *Ancylostoma caninum*).
- Whipworm (*Trichuris vulpis*).
- Heart worm (*Dirofilaria immitis*).
- Bladder and liver worms (*Capillaria* spp.).
- Lungworms (*Aelurostrongylus abstrusus, Angiostrongylus vasorum* and *Oslerus osleri*—formerly known as *Filaroides osleri*).

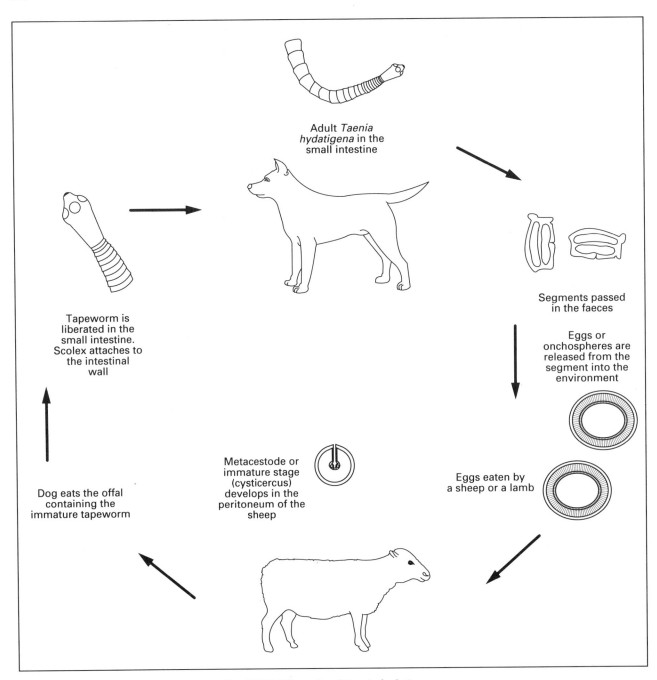

Fig. 16.22. Life cycle of *Taenia hydatigena*.

Toxocara canis. This is a very important worm since it is a zoonotic and can also cause disease in young pups. Its life cycle is shown in Fig. 16.27.

Pups are first infected before birth by **larvae** that pass from the bitchs' muscles to her uterus after about the 42nd day of pregnancy. The larvae migrate through the liver and lungs of the young pups and are then coughed up and swallowed. They remain in the small intestine, where they develop into **adult worms** by the time that the pups are 3 weeks of age. The pups can also receive further infection from embryonated eggs in the environment and by infective larvae that pass in the mother's milk. Usually the majority of the infection will have

occurred across the placenta. Pups that have a heavy *Toxocara* burden will typically be stunted with distended bellies; they may vomit and/or have diarrhoea, and severe infections may lead to a total blockage of the intestine.

The pups begin to expel their *Toxocara* infection spontaneously from about 7 weeks of age. Most have expelled all of their adult worms by 6–7 months of age. Further larvae that are ingested pass from the intestine to muscle, where they enter a resting state.

Adult worms pass large numbers of **eggs** (as many as several thousand eggs per gram of faeces in a 3-week-old pup). Each egg is surrounded by a thick wall (Fig. 16.28) which is very resistant to either physical or chemical damage. The eggs are not

Name of *Taenia* species	Final host	Intermediate host
THE TAENIID TAPEWORMS – INTERMEDIATE AND FINAL HOSTS		
T.taeniaeformis	Cat	Rat or mouse (*Cysticercus fasciolaris* in the liver)
T.serialis	Dog	Rabbit (*Coenurus serialis* in connective tissue)
T.pisiformis	Dog	Rabbit (*Cysticercus pisiformis* in the peritoneum)
T.ovis	Dog	Sheep (*Cysticercus ovis* in muscle)
T.hydatigena	Dog	Sheep/cattle/pig (*Cysticercus tenuicollis* in the peritonium)
T. multiceps	Dog	Sheep/cattle (*Coenurus cerebralis* in the central nervous system)

Fig. 16.23. Hosts of *Taenia* tapeworms.

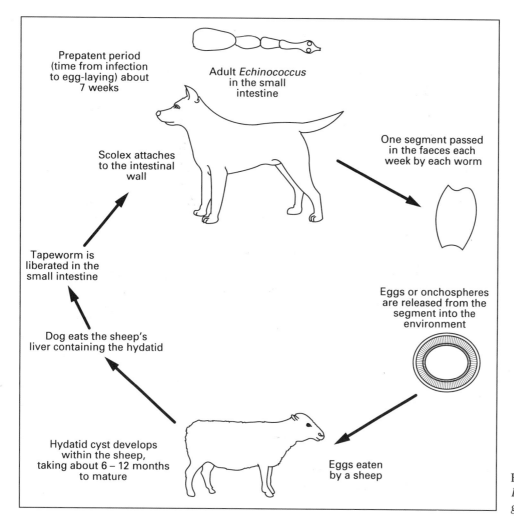

Prepatent period (time from infection to egg-laying) about 7 weeks

Adult *Echinococcus* in the small intestine

Scolex attaches to the intestinal wall

One segment passed in the faeces each week by each worm

Tapeworm is liberated in the small intestine

Eggs or onchospheres are released from the segment into the environment

Dog eats the sheep's liver containing the hydatid

Hydatid cyst develops within the sheep, taking about 6 – 12 months to mature

Eggs eaten by a sheep

Fig. 16.24. Life cycle of *Echinococcus granulosus granulosus*.

Name of active ingredient	Trade name	Animal	Activity
ANTHELMINTICS FOR USE IN THE DOG AND CAT			
Dichlorophen	Numerous	Dog, cat	C
Praziquantel	Droncit	Dog, cat	C
Fenbendazole	Panacur	Dog, cat	N C
Mebendazole	Telmin	Dog	N C
Oxfendazole	Bandit	Dog	N C
Nitroscanate	Lopatol	Dog	N C
Piperazine	Numerous	Dog, cat	N
Pyrantel	Strongid	Dog	N
Pyrantel/praziquantel /fenbantel	Drontal plus	Dog	N C

N, nematodes; C, cestodes. This indicates that these preparations have activity against some, though not necessarily all, nematodes or cestodes. The reader is directed to the NOAH Compendium for further details on individual products.

Fig. 16.25. Anthelmintics.

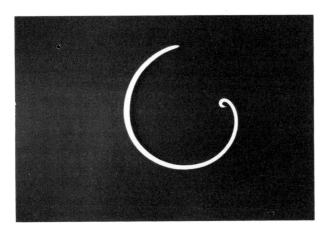

Fig. 16.26. Typical appearance of adult ascarid (approximately 6 cm long).

immediately infective but require time for a larva to develop inside. In ideal conditions this will take about 14 days but may take much longer in low temperatures. Since the larva remains in the shell until eaten by an animal, the eggs may remain infective in the environment for at least 2 years.

Larvae that are accidently eaten by **other animals** (including humans) migrate from the intestine and enter a resting state in other tissues. If a **human** ingests a large number of infective eggs and these all migrate together through the body, a condition known as 'visceral larval migrans' may develop, associated with signs of damage to the organs through which the larvae are migrating. If only a few larvae are ingested, they will usually migrate through the human body without any signs of illness except in the rare case where they come to rest in the eye, when blindness may result. Infection is usually seen in children, as they are the group that could have some unhygienic habits. If this animal happens to be a *bitch*, the larvae remain in this resting state until she becomes pregnant; some of the larvae will migrate to infect her pups, and others will remain to infect her subsequent litters.

To perpetuate their life cycle, dormant larvae in the tissues of birds or animals other than dogs depend upon their temporary host being eaten by a dog.

In about 10% of **adult dogs**, for one reason or another, adult worms will develop in the small intestine and create a patent infection there. Lactating bitches are particularly likely to have a patent infection, probably due to changes in their hormonal status. This infection may come from a number of sources, including young worms that are passed by the pups and are ingested by the bitch as she cleans up around the nest. Usually the bitch expels her remaining infection shortly after the pups are weaned.

CONTROL OF *TOXOCARA CANIS*

This is based on:

- control of infection in the dog to prevent disease in pups and reduce the number of eggs put into the environment;
- prevention of infection in children.

Prenatal infection in pups may be controlled by treating the bitch, prior to whelping, with a product that will kill the migrating larvae—for example, fenbendazole from the 42nd day of pregnancy to 2 days post-whelping.

Alternatively the pups may be treated at regular intervals with a suitable anthelmintic, starting from 2 weeks of age; the bitch should be treated at the same time.

Reducing the number of eggs in the environment is very difficult once the eggs are present. Scorching with a flame thrower has been found to be the most effective method, but education of the dog-owning public is the best way to reduce egg output in the future.

The most important methods in preventing children from becoming infected are to ensure that:

- dogs defecate in specified areas in parks;
- faeces are picked up ('pooper scooper') and disposed of;
- children wash their hands before eating;
- children are discouraged from handling young pups unless the animals have been thoroughly wormed.

Toxascaris leonina. This ascarid will infect both cats and dogs. Its life cycle is shown in Fig. 16.29. It has not been implicated as a zoonosis.

There is no prenatal infection, therefore infection is usually first seen in adolescent animals. The worm is not usually associated with clinical signs, since large burdens are reasonably well tolerated.

The egg (Fig. 16.30) can be distinguished by the smooth outer wall to the shell.

Toxocara cati. This organism is responsible for ascarid infection in cats, particularly kittens. It is transmitted to kittens by the mother's milk; infection also occurs through infective eggs in the environment and through ingestion of paratenic hosts (Fig. 16.31). A heavy infection may cause stunting of kittens and a pot-bellied appearance.

The adult worm can be distinguished by the appearance of the alae or 'wings' on either side of the head end (Fig. 16.32). The egg is grossly indistinguishable from that of *T. canis.*

Control is by regular treatment of kittens from 2–3 weeks of age until they are several months of age.

Hookworms. Hookworms are short, stout worms (Fig. 16.33) with hooked heads. *Uncinaria stenocephala* and *Ancylostoma caninum* occur in the small intestine of the dog. *Uncinaria* is the more common

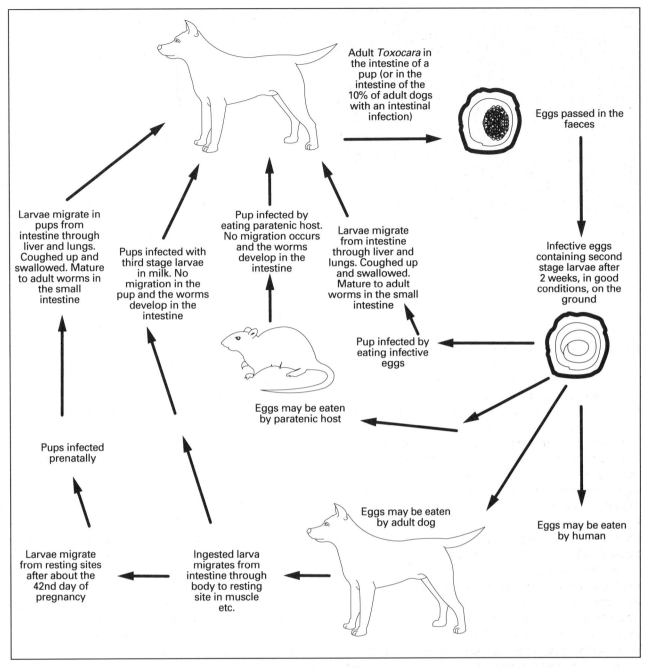

Fig. 16.27. Life cycle of *Toxocara canis.*

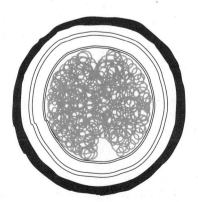

Fig. 16.28. *Toxocara canis* egg (approximately 80 μm diameter). Note the rough outer wall.

of the two in the UK and is known as the northern hookworm; it is particularly seen in greyhounds or hunt kennels.

The two species may be distinguished by the appearance of the head: *Ancylostoma* has large teeth (Fig. 16.34), while *Uncinaria* has plates in the mouth cavity. The life cycle is shown in Fig. 16.35.

The worms attach to the intestinal mucosa by their mouthparts. They use their teeth to damage the surface and then eat the damaged tissue. A heavy *Uncinaria* burden may cause a dog to be thin and *Ancylostoma* may cause anaemia. Eggs (Fig. 16.36) produced by the adult female worms are passed in the faeces.

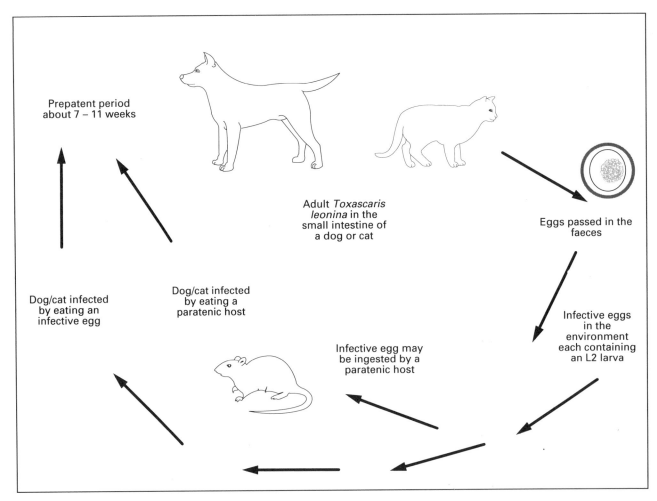

Prepatent period
about 7 – 11 weeks

Adult *Toxascaris
leonina* in the
small intestine of
a dog or cat

Eggs passed in the
faeces

Dog/cat infected
by eating an
infective egg

Dog/cat infected
by eating a
paratenic host

Infective egg may
be ingested by a
paratenic host

Infective eggs
in the
environment
each containing
an L2 larva

Fig. 16.29. Life cycle of *Toxascaris leonina.*

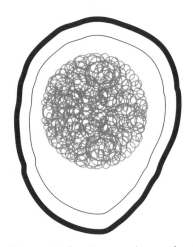

Fig. 16.30. *Toxascaris leonina* egg (approximately 85 μm long). Note the smooth outer wall. Contents are paler than those of Toxocara.

The infective larvae of both worms may penetrate the skin. *Uncinaria* larvae simply cause a dermatitis, as they are incapable of travelling further, but *Ancylostoma* larvae may travel to the intestine and develop into adults.

Whipworm. *Trichuris vulpis,* the whipworm of the dog, has a whiplike appearance (Fig. 16.37). The worms burrow into the mucosa of the large intestine, leaving the thicker caudal end in the intestinal lumen. A low burden is well tolerated but a heavy infection may be associated with a bloody, mucus-filled diarrhoea.

The eggs in which the larvae develop are characteristic (Fig. 16.38) and are covered in a thick shell which makes them resistant to damage in the environment. Eggs containing infective larvae may survive for several years in the ground. *Trichuris* therefore tends to cause problems when dogs have access to permanent grass runs but clinical signs are rarely seen in the UK.

The heartworm. *Dirofilaria immitis* does not occur in the UK but may be seen in dogs imported from warmer countries. The adult worms live in the heart and produce larvae known as microfilariae. These are dispersed in the host's blood and transmission occurs when a mosquito transfers the microfilariae from one host to another.

Bladder and liver worms (Capillaria spp.). Adult *C. plica* worms live in the bladder and so the eggs are passed in the urine of affected dogs. The eggs appear

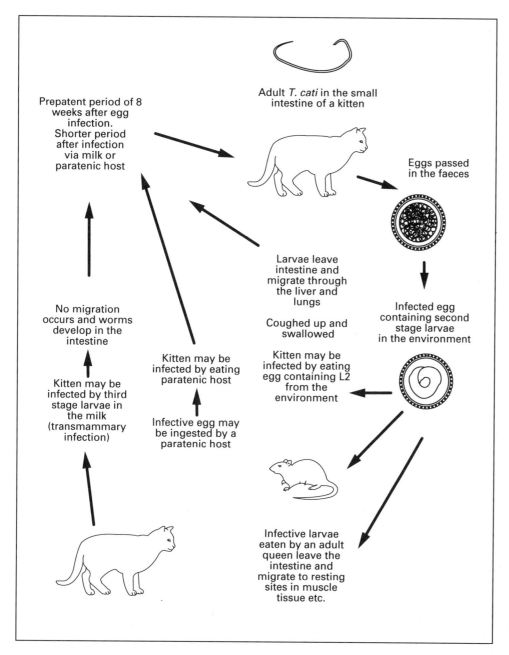

Fig. 16.31. Life cycle of *Toxocara cati*.

very like those of *Trichuris* but are smaller, with less distinct plugs. Infection is rarely seen in the U.K.

Capillaria hepatica is a parasite of rats, particularly wild rats. The adult worm lives in the liver of the host, where it lays its eggs. These are only released when the rat dies or is eaten by another animal. Cats, dogs and man may be infected, but this occurs very rarely.

Other *Capillaria* species specific to birds may cause diarrhoea in pigeons.

Lungworms. Aelurostrongylus abstrusus (cat lungworm). Cats become infected with this lungworm by eating slugs and snails containing the infective larvae. The adult worm lives within the cat's lung tissue. Infection with many worms may cause coughing, but a few worms often go unnoticed.

Adult females produce larvae (rather than eggs) and these are coughed up and swallowed. Diagnosis is confirmed by finding larvae in the faeces using the Baermann technique.

Angiostrongylus vasorum. Infection is acquired when a dog eats a snail containing the infective larvae. Transmission in England used to be confined to Cornwall and South Wales but it is now being seen in south-east England as well.

The slender adult worms live in the pulmonary artery of the dog and may cause signs of coughing and dyspnoea. The adult females produce eggs that travel to the alveoli, hatch and then penetrate through the alveolar walls. The larvae are coughed up, swallowed and passed in the faeces.

Faeces may be examined for presence of the larvae using the Baermann technique.

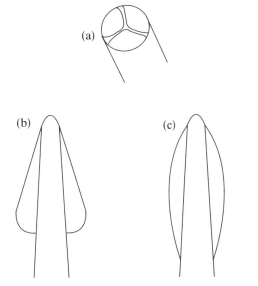

Fig. 16.32. (a) Head of an ascarid, anterior end showing three lips. (b) Head of *Toxocara cati*, showing arrow-shaped lateral 'wings' or alae. (c) Head of *Toxascaris leonina*, showing lateral alae.

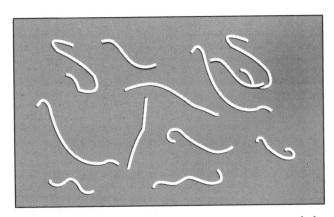

Fig. 16.33. Adult hookworms (*Uncinaria stenocephala*, approximately 1 cm long).

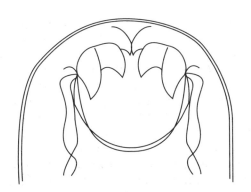

Fig. 16.34. Head of *Ancylostoma caninum*, showing two pairs of teeth at the entrance to the buccal capsule. *Uncinaria stenocephala* has a similar sized buccal capsule but with cutting plates instead of teeth.

Oslerus osleri (formerly *Filaroides osleri*). The adult worms live in small nodules at the bifurcation of the trachea in dogs, particularly greyhounds. The nodules can be seen on endoscopy and they may cause coughing in some dogs but others tolerate their presence without showing symptoms.

The adult female worms produce larvae that are coughed up and swallowed. The life cycle is direct (i.e. the parasite passes directly from one host to the next, without having to infect an alternative or intermediate host) and the bitch may infect her pups as she grooms them.

Diagnosis of nematode infections

It is important that faecal samples are fresh and are quickly picked up from the ground, otherwise they can become contaminated with free-living nematodes and their eggs from the environment. The main diagnostic tools are modified McMaster techniques to detect nematode eggs in faeces and the Baermann technique to detect larvae.

Treatment of nematode infections

Treatment of nematode infections is carried out in three main situations:

- Regular treatment to remove any infections that may have accumulated since the animal was last wormed. A broad spectrum anthelmintic with additional cestocidal activity is often used. Adult dogs and cats will usually be treated at intervals of 3–6 months.
- Control of *Toxocara* infections in puppies and kittens. Since these infections occur in the great majority of litters, it is normal to treat all puppies and their dams and kittens regularly.
- Treatment of an animal where the presence of a nematode infection has been diagnosed as the cause of a clinical problem. Here the product with the best activity against that infection will usually be chosen.

Protozoal Parasites

Coccidia

Eimeria spp. cause coccidiosis in livestock, horses and birds. Coccidia may cause marked diarrhoea in young animals, particularly lambs, birds and rabbits.

Coccidia in the rabbit. Rabbits may be infected with three *Eimeria* spp., all of which have the typical coccidian life cycle shown in Fig. 16.39.

- *E. intestinalis* and *E. flavescens* infect the caecum, causing diarrhoea and emaciation.
- *E. stiedae* infects the bile ducts in the liver, causing wasting, diarrhoea and excess urine production.

Diagnosis is based on finding oocysts present in the faeces. Small rod-like organisms may be found in the faeces of sick rabbits but these are not coccidia and are not believed to be significant.

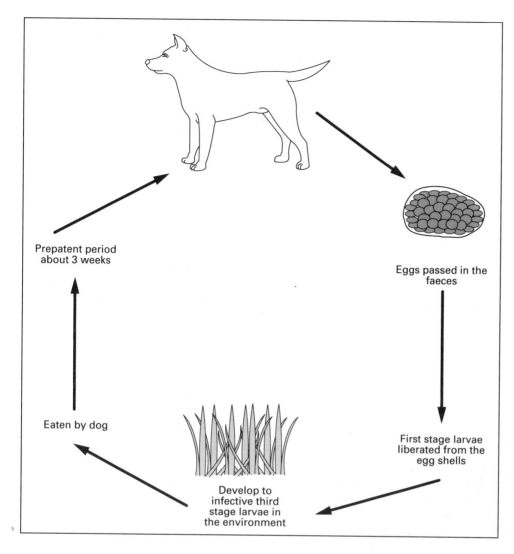

Prepatent period
about 3 weeks

Eggs passed in the
faeces

Eaten by dog

First stage larvae
liberated from the
egg shells

Develop to
infective third
stage larvae in
the environment

Fig. 16.35. Life cycle of
Uncinaria stenocephala.

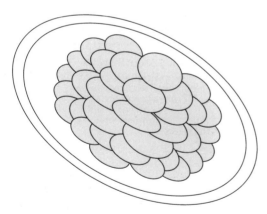

Fig. 16.36. Hookworm egg (approximately 70 μm long).

Treatment may be given in the rabbits' drinking water, for example using sulphamezathine. Control is based on making sure that the rabbits have clean bedding and that droppings and/or diarrhoea are not allowed to build up in the feeding area.

Isospora. This protozoan is also known as *Levineia.* Two species infect cats and another two infect dogs. The animals are infected when they ingest either sporulated oocysts (oocysts are not sporulated until a few days after they have been passed in the faeces) or infected intermediate hosts. Reproduction occurs in the cells lining the small intestine.

Infection is usually associated with few clinical signs—perhaps transient diarrhoea—but there may be severe diarrhoea in puppies and kittens.

Cryptosporidium parvum. This small protozoan parasitises epithelial cells in the small intestine. Both asexual and sexual reproduction occurs in the intestine and small oocysts, the result of sexual reproduction, are passed in the faeces. Infection occurs when animals ingest sporulated oocysts. This has been associated with diarrhoea in young puppies and kittens and the young of other domestic animals. Humans may be infected: usually there is only a transient diarrhoea, but severe diarrhoea may be associated with infection in immunocompromised individuals.

Diagnosis is based on finding the oocysts (4.5–5 μm in diameter) in the faeces. Identification may be assisted by staining with Ziehl–Nielsen, as the

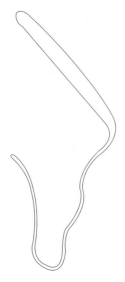

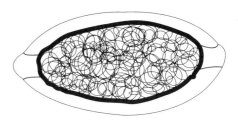

Fig. 16.38. *Trichuris* egg (approximately 70 μm long). Note plugs at both ends.

Fig. 16.37. Whipworm *Trichuris vulpis*. Note the wide posterior end and the narrow anterior end normally buried in the mucosa of the large intestine.

oocysts are acid-fast, or by immunofluorescence techniques.

There is currently no treatment for the infection.

Sarcocystis. This organism has a more complex life cycle than the coccidia and is therefore classified separately. The intermediate hosts are ruminants, pigs and horses. Large unsightly cysts are formed in muscle and so infected meat is condemned. The final host for each species is the dog or the cat and the species name reflects the two hosts in the cycle: in *Sarcocystis ovicanis*, for example, sheep are intermediate hosts and dogs are final hosts.

Reproduction occurs in the small intestine of the final host without clinical signs. The oocysts, measuring approximately 10 × 15 μm, are already sporulated when passed.

Toxoplasma gondii. The final host for *Toxoplasma* is the cat (Fig. 16.40). Sexual reproduction occurs in the epithelial cells of the small intestine. Oocysts are

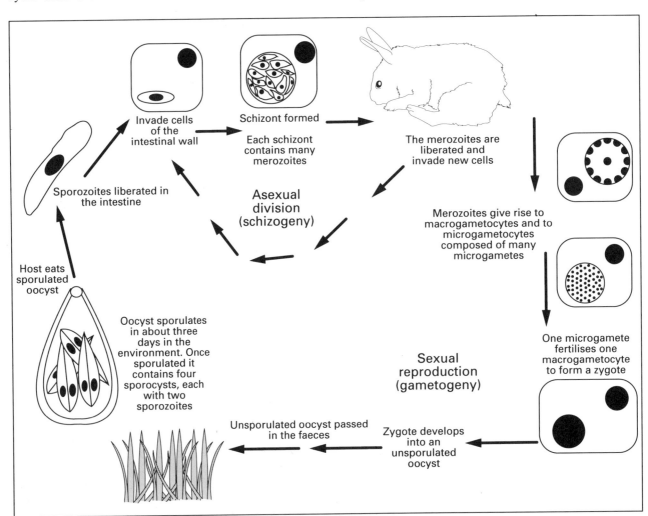

Fig. 16.39. Life cycle of *Eimeria* sp.

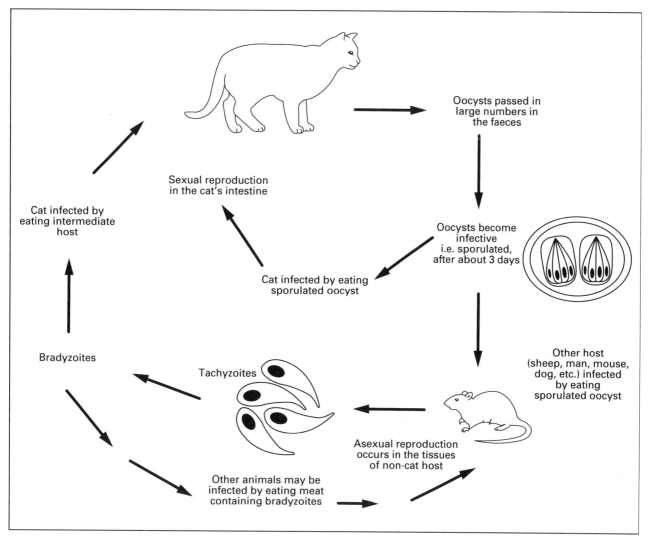

Cat infected by
eating intermediate
host

Sexual reproduction
in the cat's intestine

Oocysts passed in
large numbers in
the faeces

Cat infected by eating
sporulated oocyst

Oocysts become
infective
i.e. sporulated,
after about 3 days

Bradyzoites

Tachyzoites

Other host
(sheep, man, mouse,
dog, etc.) infected
by eating
sporulated oocyst

Asexual reproduction
occurs in the tissues
of non-cat host

Other animals may be
infected by eating meat
containing bradyzoites

Fig. 16.40. Life cycle of *Toxoplasma*.

produced and are passed in the faeces. The cat usually shows no sign of infection and normally, after excreting oocysts for about 10 days, becomes immune and stops production.

Asexual reproduction occurs in the extraintestinal (outside the intestine) tissue of almost any animal. Following ingestion of oocysts or asexual stages the sporozoites leave the intestine and travel to tissue, particularly muscle or brain. Here they divide to form **tachyzoites**. Once an immune response is started by the host these undergo slower division and are then known as **bradyzoites**. These remain in the tissue, waiting to be eaten by a cat.

The cysts in tissue are minute and cause little problem except in certain circumstances:

- A ewe is infected for the first time during pregnancy. Some cysts may occur in the placenta and may cause abortion.
- A woman is infected for the first time during pregnancy, for example by eating meat containing bradyzoites or accidently swallowing sporulated oocysts. The foetus may become infected and,

depending on the stage of pregnancy, this may result in abortion, severe fetal abnormalities or no clinical signs at all. Fortunately, infections during human pregnancy are not common.

- Infection in humans, dogs and other animals may be associated with malaise and 'flu-like symptoms that vary in severity from individual to individual.
- Cysts in immunosuppressed individuals may begin to undergo rapid division and cause severe tissue lesions.

In order to try to prevent these infections occurring:

- Farmers are advised to prevent cats, particularly young ones, from getting into food stores intended for sheep. There is now a vaccine against *Toxoplasma* for sheep.
- Pregnant women are advised to take precautionary measures. For example, they should not clean out cat litter trays; they should wear gloves when gardening; and they should ensure that all meat is thoroughly cooked before eating it.

There is no effective treatment to prevent oocyst shedding in the cat. Children that have been infected prenatally are treated with antibiotics.

Hammondia. This is another protozoan parasite where the cat is the final host. Infection is not normally associated with clinical signs. Sexual reproduction occurs in the intestine of the cat and oocysts are produced that appear similar to those of *Toxoplasma.* The intermediate hosts for *Hammondia* are rodents and so the presence of these oocysts does not provide a human health risk.

Giardia. This flagellate protozoan may parasitise the small intestine of humans and domestic animals. It is still unknown how important *Giardia* infection in pet animals is as a source of human infection, but it may cause death in cage birds such as cockatiels and budgerigars.

Infection may be asymptomatic or may be associated with transient or chronic diarrhoea. Diagnosis is based on demonstration of the cysts, which are small (approx 10 μm) and may be passed intermittently in the faeces. Even when a sample is positive, cysts may be present in only low numbers and so a sensitive detection technique is used, such as centrifugal flotation using saturated zinc sulphate solution. The cysts can then be stained with Lugol's iodine to increase visibility. It is suggested that collecting samples for 3 days and pooling them may help to overcome the problem of intermittent excretion.

17
Nutrition of Companion Animals

B. TENNANT

Nutrition is one of the more important considerations when maintaining optimal health. The need for adequate nutrition comes second only to the need for air. This chapter introduces those concepts of nutrition which are essential for the determinination of the correct diet for companion animals. It is divided into three main sections. The first is concerned with the individual nutrients, their requirements and sources. The second and third sections discuss the feeding of healthy and diseased animals respectively.

Nutrition refers to the science of the interaction of a substance with a part of an animal to promote optimal performance and/or function. These substances, assimilated from the gastrointestinal tract and utilised by cells of the body to support life, are the **nutrients**. Some nutrients are manufactured within the body and are therefore **non-essential**, whereas those that are **essential** must be provided in food because either they are not synthesised by the body at all or the rate of synthesis is too slow to meet demands. Certain components of food, such as fiber, are not strictly nutrients as defined above, but do have a role to play in optimising health. **Clinical nutrition** is the application of nutrition in the treatment of diseased patients.

Dietetics is the provision of foods in order to supply nutrients in the amounts and proportions that promote a specified performance, in both healthy and sick individuals. Alteration of a diet may be required to treat or manage diseases that are either diet induced or nutrient sensitive:

- **Diet-induced diseases** develop as a consequence of an animal's reaction to foods (e.g. dietary intolerances) or in association with malnutrition (e.g. an imbalance in the nutrient profile with respect to the animal's physiological status). Malnutrition leads to suboptimal function, but whether signs of illness develop depends on the nutrient(s) involved and the severity of the nutrient derangement. Its prevention and management requires an understanding of the normal nutrient requirements of an animal.

- **Nutrient-sensitive diseases** are physiological states where the animal's nutrient requirements have been altered by a disease process, e.g. renal failure, hepatic failure, cardiac failure and intestinal disease. Dietary alterations may help to maintain the animal's health. Management of such diseases relies on an understanding of the effect of the organ dysfunction on the animal.

Nutrients and their Requirements

The major classes of nutrients found in food are:

- Water
- Carbohydrate
- Fat
- Protein
- Minerals
- Vitamins.

They are essential for all body functions, including:

- Formation of the structural components of the body
- Enhancement/involvement in metabolism
- The transportation of substances around the body
- Temperature regulation
- Affecting food palatability
- The provision of energy.

Some nutrients (water and certain minerals) are involved in all the above functions, except for the production of energy. Carbohydrate, protein and fat are required for energy production and as structural components, whilst the use of vitamins is generally limited to metabolic reactions. Each of these classes comprises many different substances, some of which may be essential for one species but not for another. The requirements for each of the nutrients described below are derived from various published sources, including the recommendations of the National Research Council (NRC). Many of these recommendations, particularly for vitamins and minerals, are derived from the use of purified diets which have a higher nutrient availability than commercial pet foods. Therefore, where a range of requirements is provided, the lowest figure should be considered as the absolute minimum level for the normal healthy animal.

Relationship of Nutrient Intake to Function

The amount of a nutrient required is directly related to its importance for optimal bodily function. The order of precedence when evaluating a diet's nutritional adequacy is:

(1) *Water* is required in the largest amount—approximately two to three times the dry matter requirement.
(2) *Energy-yielding nutrients* (carbohydrates, fats and proteins)—approximately 50–80% of the dry matter is used for energy.
(3) *Protein* and the essential amino acids usually comprise 20–50% of the dry matter.

(4) *Minerals* comprise around 2–3% of the dry matter.

(5) *Vitamins* comprise approximately 0.2–0.3% of the dry matter.

Figure 17.1 shows the relationship of nutrient intake to function. Where nutrients are provided suboptimally, a deficiency occurs; if provided supraoptimally, then toxicity may develop.

Optimal nutrition is represented in Fig. 17.1 by the plateau zone (X–Y). Within this zone, increasing the amount of a nutrient in a diet has no effect on response (e.g. increasing the taurine content of a kitten's food beyond level X does not result in a better rate of growth). The length of the plateau zone varies with individual nutrients: some have a relatively narrow range between adequacy (at X) and toxicity (at Y), e.g. methionine; whereas others have a very wide safety margin, e.g. thiamine. Optimal nutrition is a dynamic, not static, condition which is dependent upon an individual's physiological state and function. The criteria which affect the nutrient needs for optimal nutrition include factors such as:

- Age.
- Reproductive status.
- Degree of physical activity.
- Aesthetic factors such as coat condition, apparent contentment of the animal and owner satisfaction.

Within the **toxicity zone** in Fig. 17.1, the provision of excess nutrients has a deleterious effect on the animal's response. The fact that a nutrient is essential and a 'little is good' does not mean that 'more is better'. Nutritional excesses may be linked to nutritional deficiencies.

The **deficiency zone** generally shows a linear relationship between the level of the nutrient and the animal's response. A complete nutrient deficiency (**starvation**) is rare, but may develop in anorectic animals. Partial deficiencies occur when:

- Diets are deficient in particular nutrients (e.g. meat only diets are deficient in calcium, riboflavin, vitamin A, iodine and copper; cereals are deficient in calcium, riboflavin, niacin and fat).
- Diets are complete but unbalanced. With such diets an excess of one nutrient may induce a deficiency of one or more other nutrients. Such interactions may involve several nutrients. For example:

—Nutrients may bind to indigestible materials in the intestinal tract, making them unavailable for absorption (e.g. mineral oil may carry away all the vitamin D; phytate binds iron, copper and zinc; and avidin (egg white) binds biotin).

—Nutrients, particularly divalent metals, may compete for carrier or transport systems (e.g. transferrin binds copper in preference to iron; metallothionein binds zinc in preference to copper or iron; copper deficiency may be caused by an excess of calcium, molybdenum, sulphur or zinc; and calcium deficiency may develop if high-phosphate diets are fed).

—In the gastrointestinal tract phytate binds zinc and calcium competes with zinc for absorption. Where the level of zinc in such diets is marginal, then zinc deficiency will occur.

—During the development of bone, cartilage in growth plates is calcified. Calcium, phosphorus, magnesium and fluorine interact with several hormonal systems at this time. A deficiency or excess of one or more of these minerals during growth will cause skeletal abnormalities.

Figure 17.2 summarises some of the possible interactions that occur between minerals.

Expression of Nutrient Requirements and Food Nutrient Content

Nutrient requirements may be expressed in terms of either the animal or the diet:

- *In animal terms*, the unit may be the individual or a function of its body weight or energy requirements (g/kg body weight, g/kcal or g/kJ **metabolisable energy (ME)** required).
- *In dietary terms*, requirements may be expressed per unit weight of food (g/100g dry matter (**% DM basis**) or g/100g as fed), per unit energy content (g/100kcal or g/100kJ ME content of the diet) or on the basis of the relative amount of energy supplied by the nutrient (protein, carbohydrate or fat) (%kcal ME or %kJ ME).

Energy is measured in units of calories or joules. In traditional units, 1 calorie is defined as the amount of heat required to raise the temperature of 1g of water from 14.5°C to 15.5°C.

One **kilocalorie** (kcal or Calorie) is equal to 1000 calories and is equivalent to 4184 **joules** (4.184kJ).

To convert % ME to g/per unit energy:
% ME = (energy/g of nutrient × g of nutrient/100kcal or 100kJ) × 100
EXAMPLE:
The fat content of a diet is 0.04g/kcal (0.0096g/kJ). Fat provides 8.5kcal (35.6kJ)/g.
%kcal ME of fat in the diet = 8.5 × 0.04 × 100 = 34% kcal ME.
%kJ ME of fat in the diet = 35.6 × 0.0096 × 100 = 34% kJ ME.

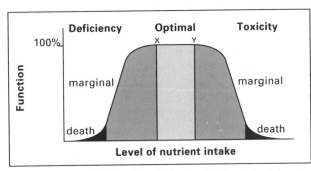

Fig. 17.1. Relationship of nutrient intake to health.

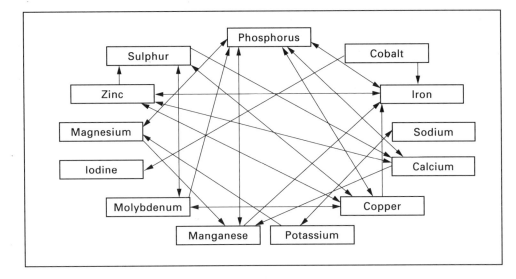

Fig. 17.2. Influence of mineral interactions on their absorption from the gastrointestinal tract. The arrows indicate an adverse effect of one mineral on another. Some interactions only act in one direction, e.g. cobalt influences iodine, but not vice versa. In contrast, iron and zinc may affect each other.

To convert nutrient content 'as fed' to % DM basis:
% DM = (% nutrient as fed ÷ % dry matter [100% −% water]) × 100
EXAMPLE:
A diet contains 5g protein and 80g water/100g of food as fed. What is the % protein on an as fed and dry matter basis?

If the water is removed the 5g protein is contained within 20g dry matter. Thus:
% protein as fed = (5g ÷ 100g) × 100 = 5%
% protein on a DM basis = (5g ÷ 20g) × 100 = 25%

Requirements expressed per kcal or kJ ME, or % ME, are the most accurate as they take account of the animal's physiological status. As accurate measures of a diet's energy density are often unavailable and there is little variation in dry matter energy densities between commercial pet foods, many recommendations on nutrient requirements are generally made on the basis of % DM, rather than % ME. However, care must be taken in interpreting the adequacy of a diet solely on the % DM of a nutrient, as the amount eaten will be determined by the energy density of the diet.

Water

Water is the most important nutrient required for life. It is found inside and outside cells, circulating and non-circulating. Since water is everywhere in the body, it is involved in practically every body process and biochemical reaction.

- Physiological activities occurring within body fluids occur because they are adapted to aqueous solutions. The high solvent activity and high dielectric constant permit reactions to occur rapidly.
- Water maintains normal electrolyte concentrations in body fluids.
- Water is essential in thermoregulation, lubrication of body tissues and as a fluid medium for blood and lymph.

- Water requirements vary but generally dogs and cats require approximately 33–66ml of water/kg body weight/day. It may be ingested or formed during the metabolism of carbohydrates, proteins and fats. Approximately 10–16g of water are produced for each 100kcal (418kJ) of energy metabolised, with fats producing about twice the water per unit weight as carbohydrates or protein.
- Water deficits of more than a few percent of body weight are incompatible with normal function and therefore need to be addressed promptly (see Chapter 21, Fluid Therapy).

Energy

Energy is the driving force in metabolic reactions, thereby allowing the utilization of nutrients. Dietary energy is the prime regulator of food consumption in most species and is therefore of prime importance when formulating a diet.

It is important to note that animals are unable to extract all the energy from food. Figure 17.3 shows the partition of energy in food.

- **Gross energy** (GE) is the total potential energy of a food. This is measured by direct calorimetry in a bomb calorimeter. During digestion and absorption, part of the gross energy is lost in faeces.
- **Faecal energy** (FE) can be measured by collecting all faecal material and burning it in a bomb calorimeter.
- The remaining energy is known as the **digestible energy** (DE), i.e. DE = GE − FE.
- **Gaseous products of digestion** (GPD) are gases which escape from the body during digestive and absorptive processes. These are only important in the nutrition of herbivorous animals.
- **Urinary energy** (UE) is the loss of energy in urine from food and endogenous sources.
- **Metabolisable energy** (ME), sometimes referred to as the usable portion of the ingested energy, is that energy remaining once account has been taken of UE, FE and GPD losses. ME = GE − (UE + FE + GPD).

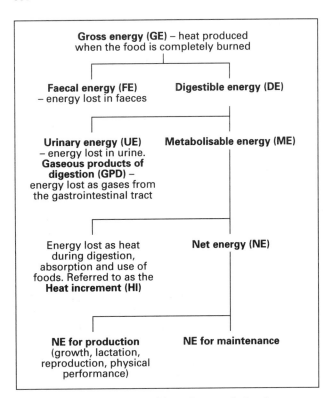

Fig. 17.3. The partition of energy in foods.

- **Heat increment** (HI) is the increase in heat production following consumption of food. It consists of **heat of fermentation** (HF) produced in the digestive tract by microbial fermentation and **heat of nutrient metabolism** (HNM) produced by intermediary metabolism of absorbed nutrients. The energy of HI is wasted, except when the environmental temperature is below the animal's critical temperature, when this heat may be used to keep the body warm and so becomes part of the net energy required for maintenance.
- **Net energy** (NE) is that energy available to the animal for maintenance (NE_m), production (NE_p) or maintenance and production (NE_{m+p}).
- **Net energy for maintenance** is that portion of total NE expended to keep the animal in energy equilibrium and includes:
  —basal metabolism (energy used to maintain cellular activity in the resting state);
  —energy of voluntary activity (energy to stand up, lie down, eating, drinking etc);
  —energy to keep the body warm;
  —energy to keep the body cool (panting, increased respiratory rate, increased heart rate etc).
- **Net energy of production** is that portion of the NE required for physical performance, growth, reproduction or lactation. Net energy is used first for maintenance. Only if additional energy is available will production occur.

As most animals consume only enough food to satisfy their energy needs, non-energy nutrients should be balanced to the energy density of the diet. This ensures that, if an animal consumes its energy needs, the requirements for non-energy components

are automatically met. When a diet of low energy density is fed, food intake is limited by the capacity of the gastrointestinal tract and the diet is said to be 'bulk limited'. Bulk-limited diets are most commonly encountered when low-energy foods of poor quality are fed during growth or lactation. Some diets for the management of obesity are intended to be bulk limited for energy, but not for non-energy nutrients. If the diet contains excess energy, food intake is limited by the animal's energy requirements and the diet is therefore 'energy limited'. This most commonly occurs when fat and/or carbohydrate supplements are added to a balanced diet leading to a reduction in the amount of food consumed.

Several terms are used to describe the energy requirements of an animal:

- **Basal energy requirement** (BER), also referred to as **basal metabolic rate** (BMR) or **basal energy expenditure** (BEE), is the amount of energy expended when an animal is completely inactive in a thermoneutral environment.
- **Resting energy requirement** (RER) is the energy expended by an animal at rest in a thermoneutral environment. It ranges from 1 to 1.25 times BER.
- **Maintenance energy requirement** (MER) is the amount of energy used by an active animal in a thermoneutral environment. It includes energy used to obtain food but would not support the energy required for increased work or production (growth, gestation or lactation). The MER for the dog is approximately twice the RER. Figure 17.4 lists factors that should be applied to the MER to obtain daily energy requirements for various production levels of the dog. Estimation of the feline MER are listed in Fig. 17.5. The lower MER for cats is possibly due to their quieter life cycle—it has been reported that cats spend approximately 15 hours a day sleeping.

ESTIMATED ENERGY REQUIREMENTS OF HEALTHY DOGS IN VARIOUS PHYSIOLOGICAL STATES	
Physiological state	**Energy requirement**
Work 1 hour light work	MER x 1.1
1 full day light work	MER x 1.5
1 full day heavy work (sledge dog)	MER x 2–4
Gestation (<42 days)	MER x 1
(>42 days)	MER x 1.1–1.3
Peak lactation (21–42 days)	MER x (1 + [0.25 x nos. in litter]
Growth birth to 3 months	MER x 2
3 months to 6 months	MER x 1.6
6 months to 12 months	MER x 1.2
Cold wind chill factor of 8.5°C	MER x 1.25
wind chill factor of <0°C	MER x 1.75
Heat – tropical climates	MER x 2.5
Inactivity	RER x 1.3

RER = resting energy requirement (kcal) = 70 x BW$^{0.75}$[kg]
RER (KJ) = 4.184 x (70 x BW$^{0.75}$[kg]
MER = maintenance energy requirement = RER x 2

Fig. 17.4. Estimated energy requirements of healthy dogs in various physiological states.

ESTIMATED ENERGY REQUIREMENTS OF HEALTHY CATS IN VARIOUS PHYSIOLOGICAL STATES		
Age	**Physiological state**	**MER* (kcal [KJ]/kg BW)**
10 weeks	Growth	250 [1046]
20 weeks	Growth	130 [544]
30 weeks	Growth	100 [418]
40 weeks	Growth	80 [355]
Adult	Inactive	70 [293]
Adult	Active	80 [335]
Adult	Gestation	80 [335] x 1.1–1.3
Adult	Lactation	80 [335] x (1+ (0.25 x nos. in litter)

* Maintenance energy requirement

Fig. 17.5. Estimated energy requirements for healthy cats in various physiological states.

Energy requirements vary considerably both between and within species but an estimate of an animal's energy requirement can be made on the basis of its body surface area. Most of the energy used by the body is lost by convection and radiation from the skin so that heat loss (and therefore energy expenditure) is directly related to body surface area. The RER is approximately 1000kcal (4184kJ) per square metre of body surface area. Smaller animals have greater body surface area per unit weight and therefore an increased heat loss and RER per unit weight, but the relationship is a logarithmic rather than a direct one—the smaller the animal, the greater its heat loss per unit of bodyweight. In dogs, it seems that body surface area is related to body weight (W) to the power of 0.75 ($W_{kg}^{0.75}$) and this modified weight is usually referred to as the **metabolic body size**.

The RER in the dog and cat may be derived as follows:

$$RER\ (kcal) = 70 \times (W_{kg}^{0.75})$$
$$RER\ (kJ) = 292 \times (W_{kg}^{0.75})$$

To estimate $W_{kg}^{0.75}$, take the square root of the weight twice and then cube the result (using a calculator). If fractional exponents are awkward to use, the RER may also be estimated in dogs and cats weighing between 2 kg and 50 kg as follows:

$$RER\ (kcal) = (30 \times W_{kg}) + 70$$
$$RER\ (kJ) = [(30 \times W_{kg}) + 70] \times 4.184$$

Carbohydrate

Plants are the main source of dietary carbohydrate. Carbohydrates are predominantly oxidised to form energy (1g yields 3.5–4 kcal, or 14.6–16.7 kJ) but they may also be converted to other compounds. There are four groups of carbohydrates:

- **Monosaccharides**, generically called sugars, are single molecules. The most common are fructose and glucose. They are absorbed directly from the intestinal tract and are the main carbohydrates used by animals.

- **Disaccharides** (sucrose, maltose and lactose) comprise two sugar molecules linked by an alpha bond which is hydrolysed by the intestinal brush border enzymes sucrase, maltase, lactase and isomaltase to yield monosaccharides. The digestibility of disaccharides varies with the activity of these enzymes. For example, the enzyme lactase has a lower activity in adults than the young, resulting in a lower digestibility for lactose.

- **Oligosaccharides** consist of chains of 3–10 monosaccharide units, either of the same type or a mixture.

- **Polysaccharides** are made from thousands of monosaccharide units and are present in plants (starch, cellulose, pectins, mucilage and hemicelluloses) and animals (glycogen).

Digestible carbohydrates (starch, glycogen) comprise monosaccharide units linked by alpha-1,4 glycosidic bonds, which are hydrolysed by amylase (starch granules require to be degraded by cooking first). **Undigestible carbohydrates** (dietary fibre or non-starch polysaccharides) found in most other plant polysaccharides are linked by beta-1,4 glycosidic bonds which are resistant to the action of mammalian gastrointestinal enzymes; therefore they are not sources of energy for animals.

Carbohydrates are physiologically essential for tissues which preferentially utilise glucose for energy production, such as the central nervous system, fibroblasts and red and white blood cells. However, it is not an essential dietary component as it may be manufactured from gluconeogenic amino acids. Carbohydrates compose a moderately high proportion of most pet foods, other than those composed entirely of meat, fish or viscera. They are used in pet foods because:

- They are a source of readily digestible inexpensive calories.
- They play an important part in sparing dietary protein.
- They provide fibre.

The digestibility of a mixture of carbohydrates and animal tissue in a cooked diet may be as high as 94%. However, the digestibility of carbohydrates in commercial dog and cat foods is around 85% and 75% respectively. Carbohydrates usually provide:

- 40–50% of the metabolisable energy in the diets of normal dogs.
- 30% of the metabolisable energy in the diet of cats.

Cats' requirements for carbohydrate are lower than other species because they are adapted to low carbohydrate levels in meat. Cats are unable to metabolise large amounts of carbohydrate rapidly because of low hepatic glucokinase enzyme activities. They obtain much of their energy from protein and fats.

Dietary fibre

Dietary fibre is referred to as soluble or insoluble (Fig. 17.6). Fibre is not strictly a nutrient and is therefore not an essential dietary component. However, it does perform several functions:

- Fibre binds water, thereby increasing the water content of the faeces. Soluble fibre has a greater water-holding capacity than insoluble fibre.
- Fibre influences nutrient absorption and adsorption.
- Fibre increases faecal bulk by increasing the undigested residue, increasing the mass of water in intestinal contents and increasing microbial dry matter.
- Fibre maintains the structural integrity of the intestinal mucosa.

The nutritional consequences of these effects are:

- Decreased protein, fat and carbohydrate digestibility.
- Decreased absorption of some minerals (calcium, zinc) with high fibre levels.
- Reduced rate of carbohydrate digestion and absorption.
- Decreased dry matter digestibility.
- Increased faecal volume and faecal frequency.
- Normalise gastrointestinal transit times—increased transit rates (diarrhoea) are reduced, decreased transit rates (constipation) are increased.

The adverse effects of high-fibre diets, particularly with rapid changes to such diets (< 1 week), include:

- Flatulence.
- Increased borborygmi.
- Increased faecal output.

It is recommended that normal healthy animals should receive a minimum of 0.28g of crude fibre/100kcal (418kJ) ME. There are several diseases for which high-fibre diets are indicated. e.g. diabetes mellitus.

Protein

Proteins are chains of amino acids linked by peptide bonds in varying quantities and sequences. Each protein has a precise combination and arrangement of amino acids. There are 23 amino acids in proteins, of which 11 are classed as essential for the dog and cat as they are not synthesised in the body in sufficient quantities (Fig. 17.7). Of these 11, however, two (cystine and tyrosine) may be manufactured in the body from methionine and phenylalanine respectively and are therefore only essential if the precursors are deficient.

Protein quality varies with the number and amount of essential amino acids present. It is best assessed using amino acid profiles. The most common measure in estimating quality is the **biological value** (BV) (Fig. 17.8), which is only relevant if there is sufficient intake of non-protein calories to meet the animal's energy requirements and the animal remains at a constant weight. The protein BVs of various foods are shown in Fig. 17.9. The higher the BV of a protein, the lower the amount required in the diet to meet all of an animal's essential amino acid requirements.

Some proteins contain insufficient levels of one or more essential amino acids. Since optimal protein usage requires a full complement of essential amino acids, a deficiency of just one will limit the utilisation of the others. The most deficient amino acid is known as the '**first limiting**' amino acid of that protein. In commercial pet food ingredients, the most common limiting amino acids are methionine, arginine, threonine and leucine.

To optimise protein intake, two or more complementary proteins should be provided to ensure that each of the essential amino acids is present at optimal levels. This is demonstrated in Fig. 17.10, where the addition of a single amino acid to a protein source (i.e. methionine to casein and lysine to gluten) decreases the amount of that protein required to maintain nitrogen equilibrium.

DIETARY FIBRE		
Classification	**Type**	**Foodstuffs**
Soluble fibre	Pectin	Fruits Vegetables Oats Beans Lentils
	Gums	
	Mucilages	
	Hemicelluloses	
Insoluble fibre	Celluloses	Vegetables
	Lignin	Cereal grains

Fig. 17.6. Dietary fiber classification, type and common sources.

ESSENTIAL AMINO ACIDS FOR DOGS AND CATS		
Amino acid	Dog	Cat
Arginine	✓	✓
Histidine	✓	✓
Isoleucine	✓	✓
Lysine	✓	✓
Methionine	✓	✓
Cystine	✓	✓
Phenylalanine	✓	✓
Tyrosine	✓	✓
Threonine	✓	✓
Tryptophan	✓	✓
Valine	✓	✓
Taurine	✗	✓

✓ = essential. ✗ = non-essential

Fig. 17.7. Essential amino acids for dogs and cats.

Protein is required for:

- Formation of tissues.
- Enhancement of metabolic reactions (enzymes).
- Transport of oxygen (haemoglobin).
- Protection of the body against infection (immuno-globins).
- Energy production.

Following the digestion of protein and absorption of amino acids in the small intestine, the amino acids are transported to the liver where they are either combined to form specific proteins or are deaminated. The carbon skeletons are used for energy (1g of protein yields 3.5–4 kcal, or 14.6–16.7 kJ), glucose or fat production, whilst the amino group is converted to urea. Protein digestibility in most commercial foods ranges from 70% to 85%.

THE PROTEIN BIOLOGICAL VALUES OF SELECTED FOODS	
Food	Biological value
Egg	100
Casein and methionine	100
Fish meal	92
Milk	90–92
Cottage cheese	90
Chicken	90
Liver	79
Beef	79–84
Casein	78
Fish	75
Rice	72
Soyabean meal	67–75
Oats	66
Yeast	63
Meat and bone meal	50 (approximately)
Whole wheat	48–60
Whole wheat + lysine	80
Whole corn	45–54
Gelatin	0 (contains no tryptophan)

Fig. 17.9. The protein biological values of selected foods.

Most animals receive excessive protein in their diet. This should be avoided for several reasons:

- The body is unable to store amino acids.
- Although the evidence is not clear-cut, it has been suggested that chronic excess protein intake may result in renal damage (glomerulosclerosis and premature renal aging).
- High protein intake in young dogs of large breeds has been suggested as a possible causal factor in the development of various orthopaedic problems such as osteochondrosis and cervical spondylo-myelopathy.

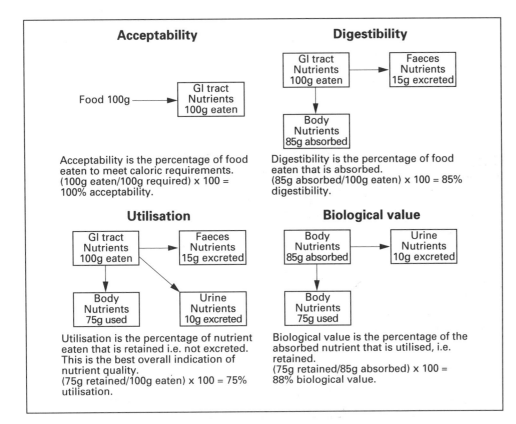

Fig. 17.8. Relationship between acceptability, digestibility, palatability and biological value.

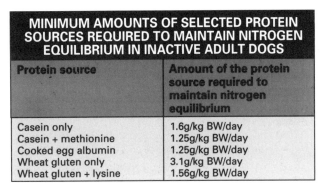

MINIMUM AMOUNTS OF SELECTED PROTEIN SOURCES REQUIRED TO MAINTAIN NITROGEN EQUILIBRIUM IN INACTIVE ADULT DOGS	
Protein source	Amount of the protein source required to maintain nitrogen equilibrium
Casein only	1.6g/kg BW/day
Casein + methionine	1.25g/kg BW/day
Cooked egg albumin	1.25g/kg BW/day
Wheat gluten only	3.1g/kg BW/day
Wheat gluten + lysine	1.56g/kg BW/day

Fig. 17.10. Minimum amounts of selected protein sources required to maintain nitrogen equilibrium in inactive adult dogs.

Inadequate protein intake may result in reduced production (decreased growth rates, weight gain, milk production), biochemical (low serum protein) and haematological (anaemia) abnormalities, and reduced food intake. Protein deficiencies are caused by:

- Inadequate food intake.
- Dietary protein of poor quality or low digestibility.
- Insufficient total protein in the diet.
- High-fibre, low-energy diets.
- Inability to digest or absorb protein.
- Excessive protein losses.
- Illness.

Some of these may be associated with the feeding of low-cost commercial pet foods of low quality, or high-carbohydrate foods such as corn, cereal-based biscuits, oatmeal and boiled potatoes. Inexpensive proteins of low biological value (e.g. gelatin, collagen or those in low-quality meat and bone meal and cereal wastes) are often present in poor-quality pet foods.

Cats have a high requirement for protein as they are unable to conserve nitrogen when fed low-protein diets. Their transaminase and urea cycle enzymes are permanently set at intermediate to high levels as an adaptation to a carnivorous diet. In contrast, transaminase activity in most other animals decreases when they are fed low-protein diets, to conserve nitrogen and increases when they are on high-protein diets, in order to excrete nitrogen.

Cats also have a dietary requirement for arginine and taurine. A taurine deficiency causes central retinal degeneration (taurine stabilises photoreceptor membranes), poor prenatal and neonatal development (cerebellar dystrophy, skeletal abnormalities and reduced growth rate) and dilated cardiomyopathy. Taurine is found only in animal products.

Fat

Fats, also referred to as oils, **lipids** or ether extract, are formed from **fatty acids** and glycerol. The majority of the fat in food is present as **triglyceride** (one glycerol and three fatty acids). Fatty acids comprise carbon chains which may be **saturated** (no double bonds) or **unsaturated** (one or more double bonds). Fats are required for several reasons:

- For the absorption of the fat-soluble vitamins A, D, E and K.
- To enhance palatability.
- As a source of essential (unsaturated) fatty acids (**EFAs**).
- To supply energy.
- For the formation of cell walls.
- For the manufacture of eicosanoids.
- For controlling water loss from the skin.

If a diet contains sufficient protein and carbohydrate, fats are not required for energy production. However, they are excellent sources of energy, with each gram providing approximately 8.5–9 kcal (36–37.5 kJ), and they have a high digestibility of around 90% in commercial foods. The type and quantity of fats and oils in a diet are important as they influence:

- Palatability.
- Appetite.
- Food intake.
- The dietary levels of minerals, vitamins and protein necessary to provide adequate nutrition.
- The ability to perform muscular work.
- Haircoat condition.
- Type of fat deposited in the body.

Dogs and cats can readily use most fats and oils of animal or plant origin, although a few hydrogenated fats (including hydrogenated coconut oil) are poorly digested. Fat is synthesised in the body from fatty acids, carbohydrate and protein. Certain fatty acids cannot be manufactured and are essential items in the diet; these include linoleic, alpha-linolenic and arachidonic acids. Linoleic and alpha-linolenic are the parent compounds for the manufacture of the more complex unsaturated fatty acids in the dog. The causes and clinical signs of EFA deficiency are shown in Fig. 17.13.

Minerals (Ash)

Ash is the non-combustible residue that remains after a food is burned at 600°C for 120 minutes. It contains all the essential minerals. All animals require a selection of inorganic materials in their diet.

The **macrominerals** are those which maintain:

- Acid–base balance.
- Osmotic pressures required for maintaining body fluid balance.
- Transmembrane potentials for various cellular functions.
- Nerve conduction.
- Muscle contraction.
- Structural integrity.

Dietary requirements are best expressed as a percentage or parts per hundred.

ESTABLISHED FUNCTIONS OF MINERALS IN THE DOG AND CAT	
Element	Function
Macrominerals	
Calcium	Bone and teeth development. Required for blood clotting, nerve and muscle function.
Chloride	Maintains osmotic pressure, acid-base and water balance.
Magnesium	Bone and teeth development. Energy metabolism.
Phosphorus	Bone and teeth development. Required for energy utilisation and various enzyme systems.
Potassium & Sodium	Maintain osmotic pressure, acid-base and water balance. Required for nerve and muscle function.
Microminerals	
Arsenic	Required for growth and red blood cell formation.
Chromium	Required for carbohydrate metabolism.
Cobalt	Component of Vitamin B12.
Copper	Required for haemoglobin synthesis, structure of bones and blood vessels, melanin production and various enzyme systems.
Fluoride	Bone and teeth development.
Iodine	Thyroid hormone production.
Iron	Component of haemoglobin and myoglobin. Needed for the utilisation of oxygen.
Manganese	Required for chondroitin sulphate and cholesterol synthesis. Various enzyme systems associated with carbohydrate and fat metabolism.
Molybdenum	Various enzyme systems.
Nickel	Function of membranes and nucleic acid metabolism.
Selenium	Component of glutathione peroxidase.
Silicon	Bone and connective tissue development.
Vanadium	Growth, reproduction and fat metabolism.
Zinc	Various enzyme systems including alkaline phosphatase, carbonic anhydrase and digestive enzymes. Maintenance of epidermal integrity and immunological homeostasis.

Fig. 17.11. Established functions of minerals in the dog and cat.

The **microminerals (trace minerals)** are those which are needed in smaller quantities for a variety of metabolic processes. Requirements are best expressed as parts per million, mg/kg of diet, or mg/100kcal. Figure 17.11 lists the major minerals required by animals, along with their functions. Dietary requirements for cats and dogs are given in Fig. 17.12.

Calcium and phosphorus

These two elements are often considered together as their functions are often closely related. Most of the body's calcium and phosphorus (99% and 85% respectively) is found in bones and teeth.

Several nutritional factors are critical to calcium homeostasis during growth, pregnancy and lactation. They include:

- Adequate intakes.
- The correct balance of calcium and phosphorus.
- The availability of the two minerals.
- A source of vitamin D.

If one or more of these factors are suboptimal, nutritional secondary hyperparathyroidism may develop. Calcium or phosphorus deficiency in growing dogs will result in weak bones and skeletal deformities, such as joint laxity and pathological fractures. Radiologically there is poor bone density and thin cortices. Calcium deficiency in the lactating bitch results in post puerperal hypocalcaemia. These diseases are most commonly seen when pure meat diets are fed, as they are deficient in calcium and have an adverse calcium:phosphorus ratio of 1:20. The recommended optimal calcium:phosphorus ratio for dogs and cats is 1.0–1.5:1.

Supplementation with calcium or calcium and phosphorus is only appropriate if the animal's diet is deficient in these minerals, i.e. fresh meat. Bone meal (30% calcium and 17% phosphorus w/w) and dicalcium phosphate (23% calcium, 17% phosphorus w/w) are suitable supplements in home-made diets. However, supplementation of balanced commercial diets is not only unnecessary but also dangerous. Excess dietary calcium and phosphorus may be a factor in the development of skeletal abnormalities.

Copper

Copper is present in many foods, although its availability may be reduced by phytates, elevated levels of vitamin C, cadmium, calcium, silver, lead, zinc, iron and sulphur. It is absorbed in the stomach and upper small intestine and stored primarily in hepatocytes.

Copper deficiency prevents maturation of collagen and elastic connective tissue and may result in rupture of major elastic blood vessels, osteoporasis, skeletal deformities and coat colour changes. Toxic copper doses are in the range of 500–800 mg/kg of diet.

Iodine

The only known metabolic role for iodine is in the synthesis of thyroid hormone (thyroxine (T4) and triiodothyronine (T3)), the primary function of which is the regulation of cellular oxidation. Iodine deficiency results in signs of hypothyroidism.

Iodine is found in high concentrations in meat and fish, and most commercial foods are supplemented with iodine, so that a nutritional deficiency is rare. However, it may occur in animals fed cereal diets, as cereals have a low iodine content, or diets containing large amounts of calcium, as hypercalcaemia interferes with the uptake of iodine by the thyroid gland.

MINERALS: DIETARY REQUIREMENTS

Mineral	Cat		Dog	
Calcium	Growth:	110–173 mg/kg BW/day or approximately 160–250 mg/100kcal (418KJ) ME.	Growth:	320 mg/kg BW/day or approximately 275 mg/100kcal (418KJ) ME.
	Maintenance:	87–156 mg/kg BW/day or approximately 125–200 mg/100kcal (418KJ) ME.	Maintenance:	119 mg/kg BW/day or approximately 130–160 mg/100kcal (418KJ) ME.
Phosphorus	Growth:	90–150 mg/kg BW/day or approximately 120–200 mg/100kcal (418KJ) ME.	Growth:	240 mg/kg BW/day or approximately 200–225 mg/100kcal (418KJ) ME.
	Maintenance:	90 mg/kg BW/day or approximately 120 mg/100kcal (418KJ) ME.	Maintenance:	89 mg/kg BW/day or approximately 120–160 mg/100kcal (418KJ) ME.
Copper	Growth:	100–160 µg/kg BW/day or approximately 300–460 µg/100kcal (418KJ) ME.	Growth:	160–500 µg/kg BW/day or approximately 150–440 µg/100kcal (418KJ) ME.
	Maintenance:	75 µg/kg BW/day or approximately 100 µg/100kcal (418KJ) ME.	Maintenance:	80 µg/kg BW/day or approximately 150 µg/100kcal (418KJ) ME.
Iodine	Growth:	20–30 µg/kg BW/day or approximately 27–33 µg/100kcal (418KJ) ME.	Growth:	30–50 µg/kg BW/day or approximately 16–25 µg/100kcal (418KJ) ME.
	Maintenance:	7–15 µg/kg BW/day or approximately 10–20 µg/100kcal (418KJ) ME.	Maintenance:	12 µg/kg BW/day or approximately 16–24 µg/100kcal (418KJ) ME.
Iron	Growth:	4–4.5 mg/kg BW/day or approximately 12–18 mg/100kcal (418KJ) ME.	Growth:	1.74–2.3 mg/kg BW/day or approximately 1–2 mg/100kcal (418KJ) ME.
	Maintenance:	1.2 mg/kg BW/day or approximately 1.6 mg/100kcal (418KJ) ME.	Maintenance:	0.65 mg/kg BW/day or approximately 100–130 mg/100kcal (418KJ) ME.
Magnesium	Growth:	7.5–9.4 mg/kg BW/day or approximately 10–12.5 mg/100kcal (418KJ) ME.	Growth:	22 mg/kg BW/day or approximately 25 mg/100kcal (418KJ) ME.
	Maintenance:	6 mg/kg BW/day or approximately 8 mg/100kcal (418KJ) ME.	Maintenance:	5.5–8.2 mg/kg BW/day or approximately 11 mg/100kcal (418KJ) ME.
Manganese	Growth and Maintenance:	80–250 µg/kg BW/day or approximately 100–250 µg/100kcal (418KJ) ME.	Growth:	280–1000 µg/kg BW/day or approximately 200–600 µg/100kcal (418KJ) ME.
			Maintenance:	100 µg/kg BW/day or approximately 140–200 µg/100kcal (418KJ) ME.
Selenium	Growth:	5–13 µg/kg BW/day or approximately 2–5 µg/100kcal (418KJ) ME.	Growth:	6–13 µg/kg BW/day or approximately 3–8 µg/100kcal (418KJ) ME.
	Maintenance:	5 µg/kg BW/day or approximately 6 µg/100kcal (418KJ) ME.	Maintenance:	6 µg/kg BW/day or approximately 7 µg/100kcal (418KJ) ME.
Sodium	Growth:	15–30 mg/kg BW/day or approximately 20–40 mg/100kcal (418KJ) ME.	Growth:	30 mg/kg BW/day or approximately 20–25 mg/100kcal (418KJ) ME.
	Maintenance:	14 mg/kg BW/day or approximately 18 mg/100kcal (418KJ) ME.	Maintenance:	14 mg/kg BW/day or approximately 18 mg/100kcal (418KJ) ME.
Chloride	Growth and Maintenance:	29 mg/kg BW/day or approximately 38 mg/100kcal (418KJ) ME.	Growth:	46 mg/kg BW/day or approximately 40 mg/100kcal (418KJ) ME.
			Maintenance:	17 mg/kg BW/day or approximately 21–30 mg/100kcal (418KJ) ME.
Potassium	Growth and Maintenance:	100–125 mg/100kcal (418KJ) ME.	Growth and Maintenance:	100–125 mg/100kcal (418KJ) ME.
Zinc	Growth and Maintenance:	2.5–3.9 mg/kg BW/day or approximately 1–2 mg/100kcal (418KJ) ME.	Growth:	1.9–3.3 mg/kg BW/day or approximately 0.97–2 mg/100kcal (418KJ) ME. 0.72 mg/kg BW/day or approximately 0.92–1.2 mg/100kcal (418KJ) ME.

Fig. 17.12. Dietary requirements: minerals.

Iron

Although animal bodies contain only about 0.004% iron, it is essential for optimal health. Iron deficiency causes anaemia. A nutritional deficiency in healthy animals is unlikely as iron is held tenaciously in the body. The exceptions are young suckling animals as they have little reserve and milk is low in iron. Secondary iron deficiency may develop in animals with chronic haemolysis or blood loss (e.g. chronic severe haemorrhagic colitis). In these cases iron reserves can be depleted after a few months. An excess of iron in the diet may interfere with phosphorus absorption by forming an insoluble phosphate.

Magnesium

Magnesium is required for both structural (bone) and metabolic (e.g. phosphokinases, acetyl CoA) functions. Approximately 55% of the body's magnesium is in bone and 27% in muscle. Magnesium is present in many foods, particularly vegetables and thus a dietary deficiency is unlikely. A deficiency causes depression and muscle weakness. The major interest in magnesium is its role in the formation of struvite calculi.

Manganese

Manganese is found in many foods and a nutritional deficiency is unlikely unless excess calcium and phosphorus interfere with its absorption. A deficiency results in poor growth, abnormal bone formation, impaired reproduction and infertility. The dietary requirements for dogs and cats are unknown; those suggested in Fig. 17.12 are based upon information from other animals.

Selenium

High-protein plants such as cereals contain the highest concentration of selenium. Meat is generally a good source of this mineral, unless the food animal consumed a low-selenium diet. Selenium deficiency appears to be rare in dogs and cats. Signs of deficiency include muscle weakness and a haemolytic anaemia. Large intakes of polyunsaturated fatty acids may predispose to a selenium deficiency.

Selenium is extremely toxic and intakes as low as two parts per million (2 mg/kg of diet) may result in listlessness, hair loss, hepatic necrosis and a hypochromic microcytic anaemia. Since dog and cat foods are based on meat and to a lesser extent cereals, and since fresh water contains very little selenium, toxicity is extremely unlikely.

Sodium, chloride and potassium

These three minerals are found in body fluids and serve largely as fluid-regulating minerals. Sodium and chloride are found in high concentrations extracellularly, whilst 98% of the body's potassium is found intracellularly. Sodium balance is controlled by aldosterone; potassium balance is regulated by the kidney.

Sodium chloride deficiency results from prolonged electrolyte losses associated with diarrhoea, vomiting or hypoadrenocorticism. Deficient dogs are depressed, are unable to maintain water balance, have a decreased water intake and are hypovolaemic. Salt toxicosis is extremely rare in small animals as long as good quality drinking water is available.

Potassium deficiency is rare in animals fed meat, but may develop if a large percentage of the diet is plant based. Potassium depletion may also occur with diarrhoea, vomiting, chronic renal failure or prolonged starvation. Deficiency signs in the dog include poor growth, restlessness, muscular paralysis and a tendency to dehydration. In the cat potassium deficiency causes anorexia, retarded growth, lethargy, muscle weakness and unkempt fur. A particular feature of hypokalaemia in the cat is ventroflexion of the head due to weakness of the neck muscles. This hypokalaemic myopathy has been reported in several breeds but Burmese cats appear to be more susceptible. Potassium toxicity is seen following excessive intake, as a result of acute renal failure or with hypoadrenocorticism. Hyperkalaemia causes cardiac arrhythmias and death.

Zinc

Zinc is present in many foods. Alaskan malamutes, Siberian huskies, Samoyeds, Bull Terriers and Great Danes may have an inherited defect in zinc absorption, resulting in zinc deficiency. Many other breeds may develop zinc deficiency signs when fed diets containing sufficient zinc. This develops as a result of a reduction in zinc availability due to the presence of fibre, iron, copper, calcium or phytates (particularly with dry dog foods).

Other trace minerals

There are a number of other minerals which are essential nutrients but for which requirements have not been determined.

| ESSENTIAL FATTY ACID DEFICIENCIES ||
Cause	Result
Animals fed on low-fat foods	– Skin changes – Skin scaliness – Coarse coat
Cheap or improperly stored food	– Pyoderma ulceration – Impaired reproductive performance
Food with inadequate levels of antioxidants	
Cats not fed enough dietary fat of animal origin (cats are unable to manufacture arachidonic acid from linoleic acid due to a lack of an effective delta-6 desaturase)	– Arachidonic acid deficiency in the cat is associated with fatty infiltration of kidney and liver, mineralisation of kidney and platelet aggregation

Fig. 17.13. Essential fatty acid deficiency: causes and clinical signs.

ESSENTIAL FEATURES OF THE MAJOR VITAMINS

Vitamin	Features
A	Fat soluble. Essential in diet. Found in liver, fats, oils, egg yolks and cereal grain germ. Exists as a pro-vitamin in vegetable sources. Stored in the body. Deficiencies affect vision, hearing, respiratory tract lining, skin and bones. Excesses are toxic.
B group	Comprises, Thiamine (B_1), Riboflavin (B_2), Niacin, Pyridoxine (B_6), Pantothenic acid, Folic acid, Biotin, Cobalamin (B_{12}). Water soluble. Many are produced by intestinal bacteria. Found in liver, egg yolks, yeast and whole cereal grains. Exists as the active form in vegetables. Not stored in the body, except vitamin B_{12}. Deficiencies affect appetite and metabolism. Excesses are not usually toxic.
C	Water soluble. No dietary requirement in healthy dogs and cats. Found in fresh fruit and vegetables. Found as the active form in vegetables. Not stored in the body. Deficiencies affect wound healing and capillary integrity. Excesses are not toxic.
D	Fat soluble. Essential in diet. Found in liver, fats, oils, egg yolks and cereal grain germ. Exists as a pro-vitamin in vegetable sources. Stored in the body. Deficiencies affect bone, teeth and calcium/phosphorous absorption/utilisation. Excesses are toxic.
E	Fat soluble. Essential in diet. Found in liver, fats, oils, egg yolks and cereal grain germ. Found as active form in vegetables. Stored in the body. Deficiencies affect, muscle, fat and reproductive ability.
K	Fat soluble. Minimal requirement in diet as it manufactured by intestinal bacteria. Found in liver, fats, oils, egg yolks and cereal grain germ. Exists as a pro-vitamin in vegetable sources. Not stored in the body. Deficiencies cause a coagulopathy.

Fig. 17.14. Essential features of the major vitamins.

Vitamins

Vitamins are essential organic micronutrients. Those of importance and their characteristics are listed in Fig. 17.14; dietary requirements are given in Fig. 17.15.

Vitamins may be classed as fat-soluble or water-soluble. The absorption, storage and metabolism of the **fat-soluble vitamins** A, D, E and K are well-regulated, although excessive intake may lead to toxicity. The **water-soluble vitamins**, B and C, must be supplied continuously as they are readily excreted and poorly stored.

Most vitamins or their derivatives are involved in specific biochemical reactions and, with the exception (in most species) of niacin and retinol, are not synthesised in the body. **Vitamin enhancers** (vitamin P) are bioflavonoids that are not essential when vitamin C is abundant, but may be useful if the supply of vitamin C is limited. Other vitamin-like substances are inositol, *para*-aminobenzoic acid, lipoic acid, ubiquinone and carnitine. **Antivitamins** include thiaminases (which degrade thiamine) in tea and certain fish, linatine (which binds pyridoxine) in flax seed and avidin (which binds biotin) in egg white.

Choline

Choline can be synthesised by all mammals from serine and therefore does not qualify as a vitamin. In addition, the body uses considerably more choline than conventional vitamins. However, a dietary choline deficiency can affect fat metabolism and lead to the development of a fatty liver. Choline supplementation may be necessary when high-fat diets are fed (required for extensive lipid transport), when low-protein diets are fed to growing animals or when its synthesis from methionine is limiting.

B-complex vitamins

The vitamins in this group are water-soluble, so that a daily intake is required to avoid depletion. The potential results of deficiences for the group are given in Fig. 17.16.

Biotin. Biotin is essential for metabolism in all animals. It participates in the prosthetic group of enzymes which perform carbon dioxide fixation and transfer reactions (e.g. pyruvate carboxylase, acetyl-CoA carboxylase, propionyl-CoA carboxylase and 3-methylcrotonyl-CoA carboxylase). However, a dietary requirement has not been demonstrated unless antimicrobial agents or antivitamins are present in the diet. Biotin deficiency leads to a reduced growth rate.

Primary biotin deficiency is a rarity in animals as the vitamin is found in many foods and is synthesised by gut flora. Secondary biotin deficiency has been described in mammals fed a diet containing raw egg white, as it contains high levels of avidin which binds biotin and makes it unavailable for absorption.

Cobalamin (vitamin B_{12}). Cobalamin, which contains cobalt, is involved in nucleotide synthesis in a similar manner to that of folate. In many species, cobalamin absorption requires **intrinsic factor**, a glycoprotein secreted by gastric parietal cells. Although dogs and cats secrete this factor, they are able to absorb the vitamin directly in the ileum and may also produce a pancreatic factor which enhances its absorption. This ability to absorb the vitamin without intrinsic factor may be an adaptation to the high concentration of the vitamin in meat. Intrinsic factor is not required by several herbivorous species in which large amounts of vitamin B_{12} are made by intestinal bacteria. The vitamin is not found in plants as it is only manufactured by micro-organisms. Good sources include fish, liver, kidney and heart.

A primary deficiency of this vitamin is unlikely. However, secondary deficiencies are quite common in animals with severe ileal disease or small intestinal bacterial overgrowth (SIBO), often resulting in markedly reduced serum cobalamin levels.

Folic acid. The derivatives of folic acid are coenzymes in several metabolic pathways involving the transfer of carbon units, e.g. the synthesis of nucleic acids. Fish products, kidney, liver and yeast are all rich in folic acid and it is also synthesised by

VITAMIN DIETARY REQUIREMENTS					
Vitamins	**Cat**			**Dog**	
Vitamin B		per kg BW/day	per 100kcal (418KJ)		per kg BW/day	per 100kcal (418KJ)
Choline	Growth:	120–130mg	48mg	Growth:	50mg	34mg
	Maintenance:	120–130mg	48mg	Maintenance:	25mg	34mg
Biotin	Growth:	1.5–3µg	1.4–3.2µg	Growth:	20µg	12.5µg
	Maintenance:	1.5µg	1.4µg	Maintenance:	20µg	12.5µg
Cobalamin	Growth:	1µg	0.4–1.25µg	Growth:	1µg	0.7µg
	Maintenance:	0.32µg	0.4–0.5µg	Maintenance:	0.5µg	0.7µg
Folate	Growth:	25–40µg	16–25µg	Growth:	8µg	5.4µg
	Maintenance:	16–20µg	27µg	Maintenance:	4µg	5.4µg
Niacin	Growth:	1.8mg	1.8–2.4mg	Growth:	0.45mg	0.3mg
	Maintenance:	0.9mg	1.8mg	Maintenance:	0.225mg	0.3–0.45mg
Pantothenic acid	Growth:	75–180µg	100–250µg	Growth:	400µg	270–330µg
	Maintenance:	75–180µg	100–250µg	Maintenance:	200µg	270–400µg
Pyridoxine	Growth:	0.128–0.2mg	0.08–0.16mg	Growth:	0.06mg	0.03mg
	Maintenance:	0.07mg	0.08–0.1mg	Maintenance:	0.022mg	0.03mg
Riboflavin	Growth:	150–320µg	130–280µg	Growth:	100µg	68-80µg
	Maintenance:	90µg	120µg	Maintenance:	50µg	68µg
Thiamine	Growth:	100–250µg	0.125–0.16mg	Growth:	54µg	27–40µg
	Maintenance:	80µg	0.1mg	Maintenance:	20µg	27µg
Vitamin A	Growth:	64–75U	80–100U/kg	Growth:	202U	100–170U
	Maintenance:	64–75U	80–100U/kg	Maintenance:	75U	100–150U
	Reproduction:	90–100U	120–140U/kg			
Vitamin D	Growth:	18–22U	15–25U	Growth:	22U	11–18U
	Maintenance:	8U	10U	Maintenance:	8U	11–15U
Vitamin E	Growth:	1–1.5U	0.9–1U	Growth:	1.4U	1.25U
	Maintenance:	0.45U	0.6U	Maintenance:	0.5U	0.6–1U
Vitamin K	Growth:	16–60µg	2–20µg	Growth:	16–60µg	2–20µg
	Maintenance:	16–60µg	2–20µg	Maintenance:	16–60µg	2–20µg

One international unit (1U) of Vitamin D is equivalent to 0.025mg.
One international unit (1U) of α-tocopherol is equivalent to 1mg.

Fig. 17.15. Dietary requirements: vitamins.

intestinal bacteria. Primary folic acid deficiency is unlikely. However, animals with proximal small intestinal disease often have low plasma folate levels due to folate malabsorption.

Niacin. Niacin is an essential component of the two coenzymes, nicotinamide adenine dinucleotide (NAD) and nicotinamide dinucleotide phosphate (NADP). These coenzymes function in oxidation–reduction systems, particularly those involved in the metabolism of protein, fat and carbohydrate. The main sources of the vitamin are meat, liver, fish, peanuts, beans and peas. The requirements of most species are met from preformed nicotinamides in the diet and from the endogenous conversion of trypto-phan to niacin. However, the activity of the enzyme picolinic carboxylase, which converts tryptophan to products other than niacin, is 30–50 times greater in the cat than other species. Thus cats are unable to manufacture sufficient niacin and are wholly depend-ent upon dietary nicotinamides. The high activity level of the enzyme picolinic carboxylase is thought to protect the cat from the toxic effects of high levels of tryptophan in meat.

As niacin may be manufactured from tryptophan in the dog, a deficiency does not occur unless the diet is also low in tryptophan. Niacin deficiency is uncommon as commercial foods are supplemented with this vitamin, but it may occur rarely when home-produced cereal diets are fed, particularly those based on maize, casein or boiled dried peas. There are no reports of niacin toxicity.

Pantothenic acid. Pantothenic acid is a component of coenzyme A which is essential for the utilization of fats, carbohydrates and proteins as energy sources. As pantothenic acid is present in most plant and animal foods and generous levels are added to most commercial foods a natural deficiency is extremely unlikely.

Pyridoxine (vitamin B_6). Pyridoxine has three components: pyridoxine, pyridoxal and pyridoxamine. Pyridoxine has the major nutritional value as the other two components are rapidly utilised by gastro-intestinal micro-organisms. The active metabolite of the vitamin is the coenzyme pyridoxal-5-phosphate. Enzymes containing this coenzyme are associated with the metabolism of amino acids (transaminases, amino acid decarboxylases and hydroxylases) and thus the requirement for pyridoxine is increased when high-protein diets are fed. The vitamin is widely distributed in yeast, muscle, cereals and vegetables. A deficiency is rare in dogs and cats.

Riboflavin (vitamin B_2). Riboflavin is a constituent of two co-enzymes, flavin mononucleotide and flavin-adenine-dinucleotide. Both of these play an important role in several oxidative enzyme systems. They are required by every cell for the metabolism of carbo-hydrates, fats and protein. Riboflavin is found in greatest quantities in liver, kidney and milk. Limited microbial synthesis in the intestinal tract occurs. There are no known toxic effects of riboflavin.

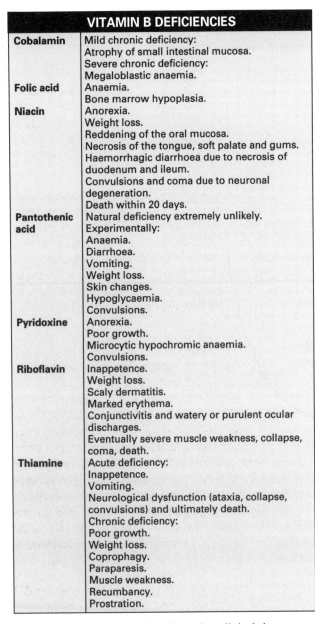

VITAMIN B DEFICIENCIES	
Cobalamin	Mild chronic deficiency: Atrophy of small intestinal mucosa. Severe chronic deficiency: Megaloblastic anaemia.
Folic acid	Anaemia. Bone marrow hypoplasia.
Niacin	Anorexia. Weight loss. Reddening of the oral mucosa. Necrosis of the tongue, soft palate and gums. Haemorrhagic diarrhoea due to necrosis of duodenum and ileum. Convulsions and coma due to neuronal degeneration. Death within 20 days.
Pantothenic acid	Natural deficiency extremely unlikely. Experimentally: Anaemia. Diarrhoea. Vomiting. Weight loss. Skin changes. Hypoglycaemia. Convulsions.
Pyridoxine	Anorexia. Poor growth. Microcytic hypochromic anaemia. Convulsions.
Riboflavin	Inappetence. Weight loss. Scaly dermatitis. Marked erythema. Conjunctivitis and watery or purulent ocular discharges. Eventually severe muscle weakness, collapse, coma, death.
Thiamine	Acute deficiency: Inappetence. Vomiting. Neurological dysfunction (ataxia, collapse, convulsions) and ultimately death. Chronic deficiency: Poor growth. Weight loss. Coprophagy. Paraparesis. Muscle weakness. Recumbancy. Prostration.

Fig. 17.16. Vitamin B deficiencies: clinical signs.

Thiamine (vitamin B₁). Thiamine is found in cereals, cereal brans, meat, legumes, green vegetables, fish, fruits and milk. Refined foods are poor sources of thiamine unless extra has been added.

Half of the body's thiamine is present in muscle (skeletal and cardiac), although brain, liver and kidney also contain large concentrations. Thiamine is predominantly found as thiamine pyrophosphate (TPP) which acts as a co-enzyme in several metabolic functions. These include:

- Oxidative decarboxylation of alpha-keto acids, pyruvate, alpha-ketoglutarate and branched chain amino acids. TPP converts pyruvic acid into acetyl CoA for entry into the citric acid cycle and alpha-ketoglutarate into succinyl CoA within the citric acid cycle.
- Production of ribose, required by cells for nucleic acid synthesis.

- Degradation of oxalate precursors.
- Conversion of carbohydrates to fat.
- Synthesis of acetylcholine.

Thiamine deficiency reduces the ability of cells, particularly those of the central nervous system and heart, to generate energy aerobically. Deficiencies may occur if thiamine is degraded by thiaminases or if thiamin antagonists (oxythiamin, pyrithiamin) are present.

Thiaminases are natural heat-labile enzymes found in high concentrations in some raw fish, such as smelt, bullhead, catfish, herring and carp. Prolonged storage of raw materials or inappropriate processing (undercooking) will promote the destruction of thiamine by thiaminases. There are no known toxic effects of thiamine.

The type of diet fed influences the amount of thiamine required. A high-fat, high-protein diet spares the need for thiamine, whereas a high-carbohydrate diet increases its requirement.

Vitamin A

Vitamin A is fat-soluble and therefore its absorption along with the other fat soluble vitamins is decreased where abnormalities in bile production, pancreatic function or fat absorption exist. It is found in several forms:

- Retinyl palmitate is found in the liver.
- Retinol is found in blood.
- Retinal or retinaldehyde is present in the eye.
- Retinoic acid is present in all tissues and is the active form.

In most species vitamin A may be synthesised from plant carotenoids, beta-carotene being the major one. However, cats lack a dioxygenase enzyme and as a consequence are unable to manufacture vitamin A. Therefore, they require preformed vitamin A, from meat and fish sources, in the diet.

Vitamin A is required for:

- Vision. In the retina, retinaldehyde combines with opsin to form rhodopsin, which is required for sight. Depletion of vitamin A intially causes a loss of visual acuity, particularly in the dark.
- Cell division. In many tissues vitamin A has a specific regulatory role affecting the rate of cell division and the specific pattern of differentiation.

Vitamin A deficiency is manifested mainly in tissues in which there is rapid or continuous cell division (i.e. testes, bone, skin, foetus). The consequences of vitamin A deficiency are many and varied:

- Failure of epithelial cell differentiation is responsible for xerophthalmia and keratomalacia in the eye, the loss of mucous-producing cells in the respiratory tract, reduced epithelial keratinization and a rough hair coat.
- Respiratory, digestive tract and urinary tract infections may develop as a consequence of decreased IgA secretion.

- Failure of bone cell differentiation results in altered patterns of bone remodelling. In young animals this is most evident in the skull bones and leads to deafness and facial nerve paralysis due to excessive periosteal bone growth and constriction of foraminae. Poor growth, lethargy, poor appetite and cachexia may also occur. Cleft palate, ataxia, stiff gait and hydrocephalus due to an increase in cerebrospinal fluid pressure may be seen in the neonate.
- Male animals may become sterile due to testicular hypoplasia and aspermatogenesis.
- Females are infertile due to a failure to ovulate or through resorption or abortion of foetuses.

Clinical signs of vitamin A deficiency are rare, as most dogs and cats eat sufficient meat and most adults have adequate reserves. However, a deficiency may occur in cats fed non-meat diets and in young animals (particularly orphans) born with low reserves who fail to ingest adequate amounts of the vitamin. Vitamin A supplementation should be limited to these indications. Liver and cod-liver oil are rich sources of vitamin A, although unlimited liver consumption should be avoided.

Natural hypervitaminosis A has been reported in cats fed large quantities of raw beef liver or fish for long periods, when 20,000–40,000 mg/kg body weight/day of vitamin A was ingested. The clinical features include cutaneous hyperaesthesia, forelimb lameness, pain, skeletal immobility due to bony exostoses of the cervical vertebrae and joints and fatty infiltration of the liver.

Vitamin C (ascorbic acid)

Vitamin C is very labile in solutions but is stable when dry. Normal dogs and cats are able to synthesise sufficient vitamin C from glucose and therefore do not have a dietary requirement. However, the average rate of ascorbic acid synthesis in dogs and cats is only half that of most mammals. A decrease in plasma ascorbic acid levels has been reported in working sledge dogs and in dogs with pain and hepatic disease. It has been suggested that supplementary dietary ascorbic acid may be beneficial to dogs under these circumstances (100 mg/100 kcal (418 kJ) ME). Guinea pigs, fish and primates are unable to synthesise vitamin C and thus require a dietary source.

Vitamin C is required for the synthesis of collagen and the function of osteoblasts. A deficiency results in a syndrome called 'scurvy' characterised by gingival haemeorrhage, anaemia, epiphyseal fractures and exophthalmos.

Vitamin D (cholecalciferol)

Vitamin D is fat-soluble and is one of the three major hormones involved in the regulation of calcium metabolism. Vitamin D_3 from dietary sources or from endogenous synthesis in the skin is activated by conversion to 25-hydroxycholecalciferol in the liver and then to the functional metabolite 1,25-dihydroxycholecalciferol in the kidney. The active metabolites are required for:

- Absorption of calcium from the proximal small intestine and phosphorus from the distal small intestine.
- Orderly growth and mineralization of cartilage in the growth plate of bones of young animals.
- Osteoclastic resorption and calcium mobilization from bone in adults.

A deficiency of vitamin D causes rickets in growing animals and osteomalacia in adults. Chronic over-supplementation with vitamin D may cause poor growth, depression and soft tissue mineralization. Acute vitamin D poisoning, following consumption of cholecalciferol containing rodenticides, causes anorexia, polyuria, polydipsia, bloody diarrhoea, excessive thirst and depression.

Vitamin E (tocopherol)

Vitamin E comprises a number of related compounds of which the most active is α-tocopherol. It is fat-soluble and is found in plant oils, particularly in association with polyunsaturated fatty acids (PUFA). Sunflower seeds and wheat germ are particularly rich in this vitamin. Liver and adipose tissue are sources for carnivores. Vitamin E acts as an antioxidant to protect unsaturated fatty acids in phospholipid membranes. Peroxides and superoxides produced in in the course of normal cellular metabolism are destroyed by antioxidants, such as vitamin E and the selenium-containing enzyme glutathione peroxidase. In the absence of such antioxidants, unsaturated fatty acids are degraded resulting in membrane breakdown and death of the cell. Tissues with a high PUFA content, such as testes, red blood cells, retina and adipose tissue, are most susceptible to vitamin E deficiency.

The most common manifestation of acute vitamin E deficiency is pansteatitis or 'yellow fat disease', characterised by extreme hyperaesthesia, pyrexia, anorexia, depression, palpable lumps in the fat, weight loss and a leucocytosis. It occurs in cats fed a diet high in PUFA (e.g. large quantities of oily fish such as tuna or pilchards). Chronic deficiency (rare in dogs and cats) causes intestinal lipofuscinosis (brown gut disease), progressive retinal atrophy, sterility and reproductive failure, nutritional muscular dystrophy and seborrheic skin disease.

There are no known adverse effects of excessive vitamin E intakes, due to its limited absorption. Supplementation with the vitamin is only indicated where diets high in PUFA are being fed. For example, some show dogs fed large quantities of wheat-germ oil or similar sources of PUFA (on the understanding that it improves the coat) are susceptible to vitamin E deficiency. Vitamin E requirements may need to be increased five-fold if high levels of PUFA are present.

Vitamin K

Three forms of this fat-soluble vitamin are recognised:

- Vitamin K_1 (phylloquinone), found in plants.
- Vitamin K_2 (menaquinone), synthesised by bacteria.
- Vitamin K_3 (menadione), the parent synthetic compound.

The gut flora can synthesise this vitamin, thereby reducing its dietary essentiality. Vitamin K is required for the formation of prothrombin and the clotting factors VII, IX and X. A deficiency results in a coagulopathy. A primary deficiency has not been recorded in dogs or cats, although it is possible that animals with severe fat malabsorption may become deficient in the fat-soluble vitamins. Secondary vitamin K deficiency does occur as a result of coumarin (e.g. warfarin) ingestion. These chemicals block the action of Vitamin K.

Vitamin K toxicity in animals has not been reported but the injection of pregnant women and new born infants with water soluble Vitamin K analogs has caused red cell haemolysis.

The actual requirements for Vitamin K have been difficult to determine as the gut flora are a source of this vitamin. Recommended dietary vitamin K requirements for growth and maintenance in cats and dogs are 16–160 µg/kg BW/day or approximately 2–20 µg/100 kcal (418 kJ) ME.

Pet Foods

There are many pet foods available. The suitability of a diet for a given physiological situation depends upon various factors. A satisfactory diet must be:

- Complete—contains all the necessary nutrients.
- Balanced—all nutrients included in the correct proportions.
- Digestible and utilisable—nutrients available for absorption and utilisation.
- Palatable—it is not food if it is not eaten.
- Acceptable.

Complete and Balanced Diets

A complete and balanced diet is one that contains all known essential nutrients and that, when fed to an animal, supports the particular physiological state for which it was designed. There is a need for different diets which satisfy the nutrient requirements of healthy animals at different stages of their life as well as for diseased animals.

The terms 'complete' and 'complementary' are often used on commercial products:

- A diet **complete** for all life stages contains all the essential nutrients for growth, pregnancy, lactation and maintenance, in contrast to some diets that may be complete for only growth or maintenance.

- A **complementary** diet is one that lacks one or more nutrients and is not balanced when fed as the sole source of food. Such diets are designed to be fed with another food. Thus, a company may produce complementary tinned and dry foods, which form a complete balanced diet when fed together.

Three methods are available to determine the nutrient content of a food:

- **Proximate or laboratory analysis** (Fig. 17.17) is the most accurate measure of nutrient content. The soluble carbohydrate fraction or nitrogen free extract (NFE) is determined by subtracting all other assayed components from 100%, i.e. NFE = 100% − (% moisture + % crude protein + % crude fat + % crude fiber + % ash). Any errors in these analyses will appear in the NFE value.
- **Guaranteed analysis**, as provided on the labels of all foods, is a less accurate measure of nutrient content. Such an analysis does not guarantee that the product contains the amounts listed; it only guarantees the minimum or maximum levels of a nutrient. For example if the pet food label states that the product contains a minimum of 10% protein as fed, it could have 15% protein as fed. Two foods with the same guaranteed analysis may contain markedly different levels of a nutrient (Fig. 17.18).
- **Calculation of the nutrient content** of the food from the average nutrient content of its ingredients is reasonably accurate but it is time-consuming and relies on knowing the nutrient make-up of the ingredients.

Digestibility

Although a diet may be chemically complete, the nutrients must be in a form which the animal can digest and utilise.

Digestibility is a measure of the proportion of consumed food that is absorbed and not lost in faeces. Digestibility data are obtained by feeding a diet to an animal and collecting all its faeces over a fixed period, often 2 weeks. The nutrient levels are measured in the faeces and are compared with those in the food. The difference between the quantity taken in and that excreted gives an indication of the digestibility (Fig. 17.8). If a food is indigestible, the animal will derive no benefit from it no matter how much it eats.

Two methods of calculating digestibility are used: apparent and true. True digestibility takes into account the amount of a nutrient in faeces that is derived from the host (e.g. shed epithelial cells) as well as the food. If this endogenous faecal loss = EFL, the amount ingested = AI and the amount in faeces = AF, then:

Apparent digestibility = (AI − AF) ÷ AI
True digestibility = [AI − (AF − EFL)] ÷ AI

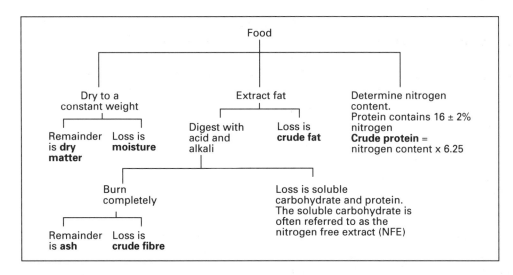

Fig. 17.17. Proximate analysis of food.

Utilisation is another term used to describe the quality of a food. It is the percentage of a nutrient that is eaten and retained in the body (Fig. 17.8). This is the better overall indicator of the quality of a food.

Biological value (BV) is the percentage of absorbed nutrient that is not excreted in urine or faeces and therefore is presumably utilised by the body (Fig. 17.8). It is commonly used when determining protein quality. Biological values of proteins are assessed by using total nitrogen as a measure of protein content and are calculated by measuring nitrogen intake and output in urine and faeces.

Palatability

Palatability is a measure of how well an animal likes a food. It is dependent upon several factors:

- Smell.
- Temperature.
- Taste.
- Consistency.
- Nutrient content of the food.
- The individual's appetite and feeding behaviour.

These palatability factors are interrelated. For example:

- Fat and water content affect both the odour and texture of the diet.
- Smell is important, and some animals, notably cats, exhibit preferences for particular odours. If the nasal passages are obstructed (e.g. in feline viral rhinotracheitis), warming the food may vaporise odours and so make a food more appealing.

- Temperature of the food. Warming tinned food from 0°C to 40°C increases palatability from 4% to 80%, but further increases in temperature to 50°C decrease palatability to 25%. As a general rule, food intake is optimal at body temperature.
- Texture. Cats tend to like canned or dried food, whereas dogs uniformly prefer canned to dry because of the higher water content. Adding water to a dry foods increases its palatability for dogs, but not usually for cats. Cats do not like sticky foods.
- The presence of certain nutrients increases palatability (e.g. sodium, fat and protein), whereas others will decrease the palatability (e.g. fibre). Cats also prefer acidic foods (pH 3.5–5). The palatability of dry foods is increased by spraying the product with 'digest'. 'Digest' is derived from proteolytic digestion of animal tissues and different formulations of digest are often used to justify different flavour descriptions for foods.

Acceptability of a diet is an indication of whether the amount of food eaten will be enough to meet the animal's caloric requirements (Fig. 17.8). A balanced diet need only be palatable enough to assure acceptability and therefore adequate nutrient intake. Highly palatable diets should not be used for free choice feeding as this may result in excess energy intake.

Commercial pet foods

Pet foods may be commercial or home-made. Commercial foods are generally balanced and complete and are preferred for most animals. When assessing commercial products, read the label, which should state:

COMPARISON OF THE GUARANTEED WITH THE ACTUAL ANALYSIS OF THE NUTRIENT CONTENT OF FOODS						
Diet	Guaranteed analysis (%)		Actual analysis (%)		DM Fraction	% DM sodium in diets
	Water	Sodium	Water	Sodium		
A	75 max	0.1 min	70	0.1	0.3	0.1/0.3 = 0.33
B	75 max	0.1 min	75	0.15	0.25	0.15/0.25 = 0.6

DM – dry matter

Fig. 17.18. Comparison between guaranteed and actual analysis of nutrient content of foods.

CALCULATION OF THE CALORIE CONTENT OF A COMMERCIAL CANNED FOOD

From the guaranteed analysis a food is known to contain:

Crude protein (CP)	8.8% = 8.8g/100g
Crude fat (CF)	4.0% = 4g/100g
Ash	1.8%
Fibre	0.4%
Moisture	80%
Total	95%

The nitrogen free extract (NFE) or carbohydrate = 5% = 5g/100g
Dry matter (DM) weight = 100 – % moisture = 20g/100g
Oxidation of protein or carbohydrate yields 3.5 kcal (14.5KJ)/g and fat 8.5kcal (35.6KJ)/g

Approximate kcal/100g as fed	= (8.8 x 3.5) + (4 x 8.5) + (5 x 3.5) = 82.3kcal
Approximate KJ/100g as fed	= (8.8 x 14.5) + (4 x 35.6) + (5 x 14.5) = 343KJ
Approximate energy content/g DM	= Energy content/100g ÷ DM weight
	= 82.3kcal (344kJ)/100g ÷ 20g DM
	= 4.1kcal (17.2kJ)/g DM

Fig. 17.19. Calculation of the calorific content of a commercial canned food.

- Whether the product is complete and balanced.
- The list of ingredients.
- The levels of protein, fat, ash, fibre and moisture.

Information that is often not available from the label includes:

- Overall digestibility.
- Protein BV.
- Quality.
- Contamination.
- Approximate caloric content. (This may be calculated as shown in Fig. 17.19.)

Three forms of commercial pet foods are available:

- Dry, containing 6–10% water.
- Semi-moist, containing 24–40% water.
- Canned, containing 68–80% water.

The advantages and disadvantages of each type are suggested in Fig. 17.20.

Pet foods may have open or closed formulations. An open formulation is one where the ingredients vary from batch to batch but the nutrient content remains the same. The choice of ingredients is determined by their cost and availability. Closed formulations utilise the same ingredients from batch to batch. The energy densities of commercial foods range from 3.5 to 5.5 kcal (14.6–23 kJ)/g of dry matter.

Dry foods

Several forms of dry foods are available including kibbles, meals and expanded particles. **Kibbled** foods are baked as a sheet, then broken into small pieces. A **meal-type** food is one in which prepared dry ingredients are simply mixed together. **Expanded** dry foods (the commonest form) are cooked in an extruder and forced through a die which results in expansion. During extrusion the products reach temperatures of around 150°C which cooks the carbohydrates, thereby increasing their digestibility, and flash-sterilises the product. Fat and digests are sprayed on to the foods after drying (Fig. 17.21).

Canned foods

Canned foods are cooked in the can at temperatures of around 120°C to achieve sterility.

COMMERCIAL FOOD CHOICES

Type of food	Advantages	Disadvantages
Dry	They are the least expensive to buy (approximately 1/2 to 1/3 the cost of canned foods). They may be fed free choice. Their abrasive effect reduces (but does not prevent) accumulation of dental tartar.	They may be less palatable. Palatability of dry dog foods (but not cat foods) can be increased by moistening them before feeding (1 cup of water/4–5 cups of dry food). They may have a lower digestibility. Thus, although cheaper to buy, they may not necessarily be the most economical as more food has to be fed. Harsh drying may reduce the nutrient content and digestibility of some ingredients. As most dry pet foods tend to be lower in digestibility and fat content, but higher in fibre, excretion of water in faeces is increased whilst its excretion through the kidney is decreased. Urine mineral concentrations will therefore rise, increasing the risk of urolithiasis. Short storage life.
Canned	Convenience. Increased palatability and digestibility.	They are more expensive per unit weight than dry foods. They may not keep teeth clean.
Semi-moist	A high energy digestibility in many cases because the carbohydrate portion contains corn syrup and porpylene glycol, included as antibacterial and antifungal agents. A large variety of ingredients can be used. However, in order to keep costs down, they often contain ingredients similar to those used in dry foods. Refrigeration is not required and they have a fairly long shelf life. High palatability.	Low energy densities. Expensive (approximately the same as canned foods). Propylene glycol preservative may be toxic to cats.

Fig. 17.20. Types of commercial petfood: advantages and disadvantages.

EXAMPLES OF THE INGREDIENTS USED IN COMMERCIAL PET FOODS		
Dry foods	**Canned foods**	**Semi-moist**
Ground cereals (corn, oats, wheat, sorghum)	Ground cereals (corn, oats, wheat, sorghum)	Ground cereals (corn, oats, wheat, sorghum)
Meat and bone meal	Meat and bone meal	Sucrose
Whey	Meat	Meat and bone meal
Soyabean meal	Meat by-products	Wheat bran
Animal fat	Liver	Meat
Iodised salt	Lung	Meat by-products
Vitamin/mineral mix	Corn flour	Tallow
	Heart	Milk
	Lard	Soy flour
	Blood	Proplyene glycol
	Vitamin/mineral mix	Iodised salt
		Vitamin/mineral mix

Fig. 17.21. Some ingredients used in commercial petfoods.

Both wet and dry ingredients are used in canned foods and most canned foods combine cereals with animal tissues (Fig. 17.21). The fat content is usually higher, thereby increasing the caloric density of the food.

Canned pet foods for both dogs and cats may be classed by type:

- **Ration type**. These are composed of a variety of animal tissues, soy products and cereals and are nutritionally balanced.
- **Gourmet or meat-type**. These are composed of animal by-products and textured vegetable protein (TVP) made to look like chunks of meat. They are relatively expensive when compared with the ration type. They tend to be very palatable and digestible.

Soft-moist foods

In soft-moist foods, preservation is achieved by reducing water activity by including humectants. Humectants tie up water, making it unavailable for micro-organisms. Some products may also be extruded.

Non-nutrient additives in pet foods

Non-nutrient additives are included in pet foods to enhance the quality and prevent deterioration after processing. The commonly used additives include:

- Anti-caking agents.
- Antimicrobial agents (including humectants).
- Antioxidants.
- Colours (organic food dyes and iron oxide).
- Emulsifiers.
- Flavours.
- Stabilisers.

Emulsifiers prevent fats and water from separating; **colour** contributes to the foods appearance. Whether such additives are beneficial to the animal is debatable. **Flavours** are required to assure acceptability of the diet.

Antioxidants prevent fat from becoming rancid in dry foods and include:

- Butylated hydroxyanisole (BHA).
- Butylated hydroxytoluene (BHT).
- Organic acids.
- Propyl gallate.

- Ethoxyquin.
- Tocopherols.

Antimicrobial agents and mould inhibitors (sorbates, organic acids) prevent spoilage. Some humectants, sucrose, salt and propylene glycol have a nutritive value as well as a preservative function.

Home-made Diets

Home-made diets are often unbalanced and incomplete because owners use cheap foods, or use inappropriate foods that they perceive the animal to like best. The use of home-made diets and indiscriminate supplementation are two of the most common causes of nutritional imbalances in dogs and cats.

However, home-made diets are required in circumstances in which an animal's nutrient requirements cannot be met from commercial foods. To formulate a diet, the nutrient content of the foods in the diet (proximate analysis) and the required amount of the nutrient of concern must be known. Figures 17.22 and 17.23 list some common ingredients used in home-made foods and their comparative protein or energy contents. Home-made diets should:

- Provide the correct balance of protein and energy.
- Include in the energy component 15ml (15g) of vegetable oil for dogs and cats weighing < 40kg and 30ml for dogs weighing > 40kg.
- Not contain more than 75g of cottage cheese or cheddar cheese per day.
- Not contain the following high sodium foods: anchovies, bacon, baked beans, breaded meat or fish, canned entrees, cheese foods (other than cottage cheese or cheddar cheese), canned or smoked fish, frankfurters, ham, kidney, luncheon meats, canned or smoked meats, meat extracts, meat pies, nuts, peanuts, processed cheese, salt pork, bran cereals, instant hot cereals, chocolate desserts, salted crackers, crisps, biscuits, pancakes, self-raising flour.
- Be complete and balanced for the particular physiological state of the animal.
- Provide 0.13–0.27g calcium and 0.11–0.23g phosphate/100kcal (418kJ) ME, i.e. approximately 0.75g bone meal or 0.6–1.2g dicalcium phosphate/100kcal (418kJ) ME.
- Include a multivitamin/mineral supplement each day.

SELECTED COMMON PROTEIN SOURCES AND QUANTITIES REQUIRED TO SUPPLY 10g OF PROTEIN

Type of food	Approximate amount (g) required to supply 10g protein*	Ca	P	Na	Cu	Fi	Fa	BV
Chicken – meat	50	L	M	L	L	L	L	H
Chicken – skin	62	L	M	L	M	L	H	M
Giblets	47	L	M	L	M	L	L	H
Cod	57	L	M	L	M	L	L	H
Haddock	53	L	M	L	L	L	L	H
Halibut	48	L	M	L	M	L	L	H
Shrimp	55	L	M	H	M	L	L	H
Tuna canned in oil	41	L	M	H	M	L	H	H
Tuna canned in water	36	L	M	L	M	L	L	H
Beef lean meat	48	L	M	L	H	L	M	M
Beef normal meat	56	L	M	L	H	L	H	M
Beef heart	59	L	M	M	–	L	L	M
Beef kidney	65	L	M	H	–	L	M	M
Beef liver	50	L	M	H	–	L	L	M
Lamb meat	65	L	M	M	–	L	H	M
Cottage cheese creamed	74	L	M	H	L	L	L	M
Cottage cheese non-creamed	59	L	M	H	L	L	L	M
Cheddar cheese	40	M	M	H	L	L	H	M
Egg whole	78	L	L	M	L	L	L	H
Egg white	92	L	L	M	L	L	L	H
Egg yolk	63	L	L	L	L	L	L	H

*The amounts required will vary between products. The amount required to supply 10g protein can be calculated in the following way:
Amount required in g = (100 ÷ protein content per 100g of the food) x 10
Ca – calcium. P – phosphorous. Na – sodium. Cu – copper. Fi – fibre. Fa – fat. BV – protein biological value.
L = low levels (provides <50% of daily requirements on an ME basis).
M = medium levels (provides >50–150% of daily requirements on an ME basis).
H = high levels (provides >150% of daily requirements on an ME basis).
– = unknown or variable levels.
The sodium levels are assuming food is cooked in unsalted water.

Fig. 17.22. Selected common protein sources and quantities required to supply 10g of protein in home-made diets.

SELECTED COMMON ENERGY SOURCES AND THE QUANTITIES REQUIRED TO SUPPLY 100kcal (418KJ)

Food	Approximate amount (g) required to supply 100kcal (418KJ) energy*	Ca	P	Na	Cu	Fi	Fa	BV
Bread white	37	L	L	H	M	H	L	L
Bread whole wheat	41	L	L	H	M	H	L	L
Corn flour	27	L	L	L	–	M	L	L
Corn meal	27	L	L	L	–	M	L	L
Corn flakes (breakfast cereal)	26	L	L	H	M	M	L	L
Macaroni, cooked	75	L	L	L	L	M	L	L
Oatmeal, cooked	181	L	L	L	–	M	L	L
Potato, cooked	133	L	L	L	–	M	L	H
Rice long grain, cooked	80	L	L	L	L	M	L	L
Soybean flour high fat	26	L	M	L	–	–	L	L
Soybean flour low fat	28	L	M	L	–	–	L	L
Spaghetti (quick cook), cooked	77	L	L	L	L	M	L	L
Spaghetti (ordinary), cooked	91	L	L	L	L	M	L	L
Wheat dry	27	L	L	L	–	M	L	L
Wheat cooked	240	L	L	L	–	M	L	L
Wheat flour	30	L	L	L	–	M	L	L
Fat, trimmed from beef	14	L	L	L	L	L	H	0
Lard	11	L	L	L	L	L	H	0
Margarine	14	L	L	H	L	L	H	L
Oils – salad/cooking	12	L	L	L	L	L	H	0

*The amounts required will vary between products. The amount required to supply 100kcal can be calculated in the following way:
Amount required in g to supply 100kcal = 100 ÷ energy density kcal/g
Amount required to supply 418KJ = 418 ÷ energy density KJ/g
Key:
Ca – calcium. P – phosphorous. Na – sodium. Cu – copper. Fi – fibre. Fa – fat. BV – protein biological value.
L = low levels (provides <50% of daily requirements on an ME basis).
M = medium levels (provides >50–150% of daily requirements on an ME basis).
H = high levels (provides >150% of daily requirements on an ME basis).
– = unknown or variable levels.
0 = does not apply to these ingredients.
The sodium levels are assuming food is cooked in unsalted water.

Fig. 17.23. Selected common protein sources and quantities required to supply 100kcal (418kJ) in home-made diets.

Supplementation

Supplements are foods which are fed in addition to a normal diet. They are often given to pets by owners who believe them to be beneficial, even though the animal is fed a complete and balanced ration. Reasons given for the use of supplements include a lack of confidence in the basic diet, a wish to increase palatability, or to provide extra nutrients during periods of stress. However, nutritional supplements are only of benefit under two circumstances:

- Correction of a specific deficiency due to the animal's inability to use the normal level of a particular nutrient.
- Stimulation of food intake during periods of increased productivity.

Supplements will not improve a poor quality diet. If an owner insists on supplementing a pet's diet, advice should be given in order that they may select an appropriate supplement that is least likely to unbalance the diet. Figure 17.24 lists some commonly used supplements and their nutritional inadequacies. Some points to consider when using supplements are:

- The total proportion of supplements in the diet should not exceed 10% by weight of the food intake if a commercial pet food is also being fed.
- If whole fish is provided, the bones must be finely ground.
- Fats and oils increase the caloric density of the food. This may result in the energy needs being met with less food thereby causing multiple deficiencies. Vegetable oils may be used to improve the coat. The maximum that can be recommended is 3ml of vegetable oil, or 3g of lard/100kcal (418kJ) ME. If any effect is to be seen, 15ml of vegetable oil will supply sufficient linoleic acid to improve the coat.
- Eggs, cheese and cottage cheese are excellent sources of protein.
- Supplemental liver is particularly useful for sick, weak or anaemic animals as it contains high biological value protein, fat, carbohydrate, trace minerals and vitamins.
- Vegetables, when properly balanced in the diet with protein and mineral-supplying ingredients, are good foods for dogs but not cats.

- Medical problems resulting from oversupplementation with vitamins and minerals are more common than deficiencies. Vitamin/mineral supplements should only be used to balance home-made diets or for specific medical conditions.
- Bones should not be given to dogs because of the risks of obstruction of the mouth or gastrointestinal tract, and the potential of breaking teeth.
- Table scraps should not be used as a dog's primary diet. Fat trimmings may be fed as long as they do not comprise more than 10% of the diet by weight.
- Most dogs eat chocolate readily. However, excessive chocolate may diminish an animal's appetite quite significantly. In addition, the high energy intake may cause obesity and the high sugar content may cause dental caries. Chocolate also contains theobromine, which is toxic to dogs and cats. Milk chocolate contains about 1.5mg theobromine/g and unsweetened cooking chocolate contains 16mg/g. The lethal dose for theobromine in dogs is reported to be 240–500mg/kg body weight. However, death may occur following the ingestion of only 114mg/kg body weight. To reach a potentially fatal dose of 100mg/kg, a dog weighing 10kg would have to ingest 63g of cooking chocolate or 670g of milk chocolate.
- Feeding onion and garlic will not control worms or fleas but will cause halitosis. Consumption of 0.5% of the body weight in onions (i.e. 50g for a 10kg dog) results in toxic levels of the alkaloid n-propyldisulphide causing a haemolytic anaemia, pyrexia, dark urine and death.
- Health foods consumed by humans are not suitable for pets, due to the different nutritional requirements of dogs and cats.
- Chews are useful for reducing tartar on teeth and improving the health of gums.

Toxins

The consumption of toxins or poisons in food is rare. It may occur if toxins are present in the raw ingredients, or following improper storage. Commercial products are quality controlled before release of the product on to the market. With respect to home-

NUTRIENT IMBALANCES OF SELECTED FOODS		
Food	Deficiencies	Excesses
Meat	Calcium, Phosphorus Sodium, Iron, Copper, Iodine, vitamins A, D, E	Protein
Fish (bones removed)	Calcium, Phosphorus, Iodine, vitamins A, D, E	
Fish (including bones)*	Iron, vitamins A, D, E	
Fats and oils		Calcium, Phosphorus Energy, vitamin D (fish oils)
Eggs	Calcium, Phosphorus	Fat, Avidin
Milk		Lactose
Cheese, cottage cheese	Calcium, Phosphorus	
Liver	Calcium	Vitamin A
Vegetables	Calcium, Phosphorus Protein, Fat	
Cereals	Calcium, Phosphorus	

*Cooked and finely ground fish.

Fig. 17.24. Nutrient imbalances of selected foods.

produced foods, toxicity should not be a problem as long as the raw materials are stored in an appropriate manner and the food has been thoroughly cooked.

Feeding

Many different species of animals are kept as pets, including dogs, cats, small mammals, birds, reptiles, fish and invertebrates. A number of biological differences between species alter their nutritional needs, including:

- Morphology of the gastrointestinal tract.
- Dietary habits.
- Feeding behaviour.
- Life-cycle stages.

There are also nutritional similarities. These include:

- Universal nutrient requirements for water, energy, protein, vitamins and minerals in roughly similar proportions.
- Energy requirements that can be calculated from metabolic body size (Fig. 17.25).
- Similar increases in energy requirement for increased physiological activity (i.e. gestation, egg-laying, growth, activity).

Feeding Dogs and Cats

Feeding is an integral part of the human–animal relationship. Ideally it should be:

- At a time convenient to the owners when they are least likely to be hurried or have to change or delay the process.
- Not too late, as ingestion of the meal causes increased intestinal peristalsis and is associated with increased fluid intake. The need to defecate and urinate 3–4 hours after eating should be recognised and sufficient opportunity given.

There are three commonly used methods of feeding:

- **Free-choice** or ad lib feeding—fresh food and water are always available and the animal can eat as much as it wishes, whenever it wishes.
- **Time-restricted** meal feeding—providing more food than the animal requires for a specified time, generally 5–30 minutes, after which time the food is removed.

RESTING ENERGY REQUIREMENTS OF DIFFERENT CLASSES OF ANIMALS	
Class of animal	**Resting energy requirement (kcal)**
Passerine birds	$210 \times$ body weight$^{0.75}$ [kg]
Non-passerine birds	$140 \times$ body weight$^{0.75}$ [kg]
Placental mammals	$70 \times$ body weight$^{0.75}$ [kg]
Marsupial mammals	$50 \times$ body weight$^{0.75}$ [kg]
Reptiles (@ 37°C)	$30 \times$ body weight$^{0.75}$ [kg]

Multiply by 4.184 to convert kcal to KJ

Fig. 17.25. Resting energy requirements of different animals.

- **Food-restricted** meal feeding involves feeding the animal less food than it would eat if the amount were not restricted.

Food-restricted or time-restricted meal feedings may be repeated at regular intervals during the day.

Most adult cats and dogs will consume adequate food for optimal health if meal-fed once a day. However, for both social and health reasons, it is recommended that growing and adult dogs should be fed at least twice a day; that toy breeds (especially those less than 6 months old) should be fed three or more meals a day; and that cats of all ages should be fed free-choice.

The advantages of free-choice feeding are:

- It takes the least amount of work, thought and knowledge on the part of the owner.
- It ensures that the animal receives an adequate quantity of food.
- It has a quietening effect in kennels.
- It discourages coprophagy.
- In a group, the animal lowest in the social hierarchy has a better chance of obtaining its share of the food.

Disadvantages to free-choice feeding are:

- Anorexic animals may not be noticed, particularly if two or more animals are fed together.
- Overeating.

Dogs are pack hunters and therefore tend to eat voraciously, particularly if there is competition for the food. If fed free-choice, they are more likely to overeat and develop obesity. This is particularly so with puppies and it is recommended that puppies are not fed free-choice until they have attained 90% of their adult weight. Cats, on the other hand, are solitary hunters, eating every few hours during a 24-hour period and are therefore unlikely to overeat when offered food free-choice.

The amount to feed is determined by the animal's energy requirements and the caloric density of the food. However, it must be appreciated that the figures recommended are only averages and that there is considerable variability in needs, particularly of dogs. Physical assessment of the animal—i.e. body weight and the extent of subcutaneous fat—are the best guides as to whether sufficient food is being provided. Feed to a body condition that allows the ribs to be felt but not seen, without noticing appreciable subcutaneous fat. Generally, dogs should have an hour-glass shape when viewed from above. The amount of food required for optimal health is influenced by:

- Individual variation.
- Environmental temperature, humidity and air movement.
- Stress.
- Physical activity.
- Stage of life.
- Health status.

The variation in energy needs for dogs in different physiological states are listed in Fig. 17.4. The requirements for other nutrients are given in the sections on the individual nutrients. Figures 17.26 and 17.27 summarise the nutrient profiles recommended for the various life stages of dogs and cats.

Feeding for reproduction in the dog

Malnourishment of the bitch before and during gestation is thought to contribute to a 20–30% neonatal mortality. Nutritionally related gestational or lactational problems may be associated with one of the following feeding practices:

- **Feeding insufficient digestible nutrients** to the bitch, either because the quantity of food has not been increased during late gestation and lactation or because only a maintenance diet has been fed. The latter will induce nutrient depletion during pregnancy and overt nutritional deficiency during lactation.
- **Feeding an imbalanced diet**. This may not cause problems when fed for maintenance but does during lactation because of the greater nutrient demand.

A growth or lactation diet should be fed throughout pregnancy (Fig. 17.26) without supplementation (meat, milk, calcium, phosphorus or vitamins). Calcium or vitamin D supplementation may cause soft tissue calcification and physical anomalies in pups and does not prevent post puerperal hypocalcemia. During the last 3–4 weeks of pregnancy, foetal size increases rapidly and the bitch's food intake should be 15–25% greater than her normal maintenance requirements to compensate for this increased demand. Meal-feed at frequent intervals or feed free-choice during the last 10 days of gestation, as the capacity of the stomach may be limited by the enlarged uterus. Lactation puts a considerable demand on the bitch's nutrient status. During peak lactation (weeks 3–6) there is an extra energy requirement of 200kcal (840kJ)/kg of litter/day. This may be provided by increasing the amount fed by 25% for each puppy (Fig. 17.4). A bitch with an average litter will generally require 1.5 times the amount needed for maintenance for the first week, increasing to 2 and 3 times maintenance requirements during the second and third week respectively. At this stage she should be fed free-choice and clean drinking-water must be available at all times.

Post puerperal hypocalcemia, characterised by muscle tremors, ataxia and convulsions, is a particular problem in bitches with large litters. To prevent it puppies should be encouraged to eat growth diets from 3 weeks of age to reduce the demand for milk and the bitch should be fed a diet containing at least 1.4% calcium on a dry matter basis and a calcium:phosphorus ratio of 1:1. During gestation both low calcium diets (e.g. unsupplemented meat), and calcium supplementation are contraindicated.

Feeding for reproduction in the queen

A growth/lactation diet (Fig. 17.27) may be fed throughout pregnancy but is particularly important during the 4 weeks prior to parturition. At parturition the queen needs approximately 25% more food than that required for maintenance. During lactation the energy requirements are 2–3 times those required for maintenance. The queen should be fed free-choice at all times.

Feeding the growing dog

In the first few weeks of life puppies derive all their nutrition from the dam's milk. Feeding in preparation for weaning at 6 weeks can start at 3–4 weeks of age. Pups may be fed the bitch's food with sufficient water added to make it mushy but not sloppy. The nutrient requirements for growth are summarised in Figs 17.4 and 17.26, and in the appropriate sections for each nutrient.

The aim when feeding weaned puppies is to attain a growth rate of 2–4g/day/kg of their anticipated adult weight, for the first 5 months of life. Overfeeding to increase growth rates is detrimental to health. Slight underfeeding is preferable to overfeeding. To reduce the risk of excessive growth, diets adequate for maximum growth should not be fed free-choice until the dog has attained 80–90% of its anticipated adult weight. Twice daily time-restricted meal-feeding is

RECOMMENDED NUTRIENT REQUIREMENTS FOR THE DOG ACCORDING TO PHYSIOLOGICAL STATUS

Status	Min. ME density (kcal (KJ)/g)	Dig (%)	Prot (%ME)	Fat (%ME)	Fibre (%DM)	Ca (mg/100kcal (418KJ)	PO₄	Na
Maintenance	3.5 (14.6)	>75	16–20	30–50	5	130–160	110–160	15
Growth Gestation Lactation	3.9 (16.3)	>80	22–28	30–50	5	280	200–250	23
Geriatric	3.75 (15.7)	>80	14–18	30–50	4	130–150	110–140	15
Stress: Environmental Psychological Physical	4.2 (17.6)	>82	20–25	30–50	4 max	150–250	130–230	23

%ME – The proportion of energy supplied by that nutrient.
%DM – g/100g dry matter. ME – metabolisable energy.
Dig – Digestibility. Prot – Protein. PO₄ – Phosphate. Na – Sodium. Ca – Calcium. max – maximum

Fig. 17.26. Recommended nutrient requirements for the dog, according to physiological status.

RECOMMENDED NUTRIENT REQUIREMENTS FOR THE CAT ACCORDING TO PHYSIOLOGICAL STATUS									
Status	Min. ME density (kcal (KJ)/g)	Dig (%)	Prot (%ME)	Fat (%ME)	Fibre (%DM)	Ca (mg/100kcal	PO$_4$ (418KJ)	Mg	Na
Maintenance	>3.7 (15.7)	>75	24–26	>25	5	130–200	120	80	15
Growth Gestation Lactation	3.9 (16.3)	>80	30–35	>40	5	160–250	120–200	150	30
Geriatric	3.75 (15.7)	>80	24–26	>34	5	130–150	120	80	15

%ME – The proportion of energy supplied by that nutrient.
%DM – g/100g dry matter. ME – metabolisable energy.
Dig – Digestibility. Prot – Protein. PO$_4$ – Phosphate. Na – Sodium. Ca – Calcium. Mg – Magnesium
max – maximum

Fig. 17.27. Recommended nutrient requirements for the cat, according to physiological status.

recommended for most breeds. Toy breeds should be fed 3–4 times per day until 6 months of age as they are susceptible to hypoglycaemia. At each feed the puppy should be allowed 20–30 minutes to eat. Vitamin, mineral or protein supplementation is unnecessary if commercial diets designed to support growth are fed and in many instances may be harmful.

Orphan puppies may be fed commercial milk replacers or home-made diets (Fig. 17.28). Cow's milk alone is unsuitable; when compared with bitch's milk it contains 3 times as much lactose and is deficient in protein (Fig. 17.29). Lactose may cause diarrhoea in some pups. Figure 17.30 indicates the recommended amounts to feed pups. It is important that orphans are not overfed. Administer food with a bottle or through a stomach tube. When bottle fed the animal will refuse food when full. With tube feeding, administer a maximum of 50ml/kg body weight at each feed. Healthy orphans should be fed 4 times a day at 6-hourly intervals and can be weaned onto an appropriate growth diet from 3 weeks of age.

SUITABLE FOODS FOR ORPHAN PUPPIES AND KITTENS
Puppies
Commercial milk replacer
3 parts evaporated milk (not skimmed): 1 part water
2 parts tinned puppy food blended with 1 part water
1 litre whole cows milk, 4 egg yolks, 1 tablespoon corn oil
800ml cows milk, 1 egg yolk, 200ml cream, 6g steamed bone flour, 2.000iu vitamin A, 500iu vitamin D, 4ml citric acid
1 cup whole cows milk, 1 tsp. vegetable oil, 1 drop multivitamins and 2 egg yolks blended together
Milk mixed with a diet suitable for growth
Kittens
Commercial milk replacer
0.5 cup whole cows milk, 1 egg yolk, 1 drop multivitamins, 1500mg calcium carbonate tablet blended together
Milk mixed with a diet suitable for growth

Fig. 17.28. Suitable foods for orphan puppies and kittens.

Feeding the growing cat

Kittens may be fed free-choice, on a diet suitable for growth, from 3 weeks of age. Supplementation should be avoided. Suitable diets for orphan kittens are listed in Fig. 17.28—note that cow's milk is unsuitable (Fig. 17.29). Figure 17.30 indicates the recommended amounts to feed kittens, either by bottle or by stomach tube. The food should be mushy but not sloppy.

Feeding the geriatric dog or cat

The objectives of feeding the older dog or cat may include:

- Reducing the symptoms of disease.
- Reducing or preventing the progression of disease.
- Maintainance of optimal nutritional status.

Figure 17.31 lists some of the changes that occur with ageing and their possible effect on the animal's nutritional status. Other diseases that may alter an animals nutritional requirements are discussed in the clinical nutrition section below. The general characteristics of diets suitable for geriatric dogs and cats are listed in Figs 17.26 and 17.27.

The geriatric patient has special requirements:

- Dietary energy intake may need to be reduced, as with ageing there is a decrease in lean body mass, an increase in body fat, a reduction in metabolic activity, a reduction in exercise and an increased likelihood of obesity.
- Reduction of protein intake in healthy geriatrics is controversial. Some authors suggest that the feeding of reduced protein diets may possibly prevent degenerative renal changes. Protein intake should certainly be no greater than that required for maintenance and ideally should be of high quality to reduce nitrogenous waste.
- Reduction in fat intake may be necessary to prevent obesity.
- Increasing the fibre intake may reduce the incidence of constipation in older animals.
- A reduced intake of phosphorus and sodium may be required.
- The diet should be highly palatable and digestible.

NUTRIENT CONTENT OF MILK FROM DIFFERENT SOURCES					
	% Nutrient as fed (g/100kcal (418KJ) ME)				
Nutrient	Bitch's milk	Cow's milk	Queen's milk	Goat's milk	Evaporated* milk + water
Water	77 (0)	88 (0)	81.5 (0)	87 (0)	80 (0)
Protein	8.2 (6.6)	3.2 (5.4)	7.4 (8.4)	3.5 (5.5)	5.3 (5.5)
Fat	9.8 (7.8)	3.7 (6.3)	5.2 (5.9)	4.2 (6.6)	6.1 (6.3)
Lactose	3.6 (2.9)	4.6 (7.8)	5.0 (5.7)	4.5 (7)	7.6 (7.8)
Calcium	0.28 (0.22)	0.12 (0.2)	0.035 (0.04)	0.13 (0.2)	0.19 (0.2)
Phosphorus	0.22 (0.18)	0.1 (0.17)	0.07 (0.08)	0.11 (0.17)	0.15 (0.16)
ME					
kcal/100g**	125	59	88	64	97
kJ/100g**	522	246	360	267	406

* 3 parts whole evaporated milk diluted with 1 part water
** ME content as fed was estimated using nutrient energy densities of 3.5kcal (14.6KJ)/g for protein and lactose, and 8.5kcal (35.6)/g for fat.

Fig. 17.29. Nutrient content of milk from different sources.

- Alterations to the gastrointestinal tract and general metabolism may result in an increased requirement for vitamins A, B_1, B_6, B_{12} and E.

Feeding dogs for work

Working dogs (e.g. racing, hunting, police and guarding duty, herding, guiding the blind and other assistance-dog work) are exposed to a variety of stressful situations which increase their nutritional requirements and impart physical and psychological stresses on the dogs in different proportions. The greatest need for nutrients is seen in physically stressed dogs. However, malnutrition is uncommon in such dogs because they usually have increased appetites and are able to satisfy their nutrient requirements. In contrast, psychologically stressed dogs may have a lower nutrient requirement than physically stressed dogs, but are at greater risk from developing malnutrition because their appetite is often reduced.

Provision of adequate water is the most important dietary consideration, particularly for dogs working in higher ambient temperatures. Dogs lose heat primarily by evaporation of water from the tongue and upper respiratory tract. The provision of fresh, cool water early in the working period is recommended to prevent dehydration. Cool water (4–10°C) is preferable to warm water as it is more palatable, empties from the stomach quicker and cools the body. Water is also produced endogenously through the metabolism of carbohydrate, protein and fats. Approximately 10–16ml of water is produced for each 100kcal (418kJ) expended. In addition, around

3–4g of water are released for each gram of glycogen used. It is therefore important that glycogen stores are adequate prior to endurance exercise.

The nutrient profile for a diet suitable for stressed or working dogs is given in Fig. 17.26. These diets are highly digestible more energy dense and they have greater concentrations of non-energy nutrients.

Increasing carbohydrate intake decreases the performance of working dogs as it displaces fat from the diet, thereby reducing the caloric content of the food. There is no evidence at the present time to support the suggestion that protein or vitamin requirements are increased for stress or work, providing a complete and balanced diet is fed.

MILK SUBSTITUTE REQUIREMENTS OF ORPHANED PUPPIES AND KITTENS	
Age (weeks)	Approximate daily amount of milk substitute by neonatal animals (ml/100g BW)*
1	13
2	17
3	20
4	22

*divide the daily amount into four or five feeds

Fig. 17.30. Milk substitute requirements of orphaned puppies and kittens.

AGEING CHANGES AND THEIR EFFECTS ON THE ANIMAL'S NUTRITIONAL STATUS	
Ageing change	Effect on nutritional status
Metabolism	
Reduced sensitivity to thirst	Dehydration
Reduced thermoregulation	Increased energy expenditure with extremes of heat
Reduced immunological competence	Increased susceptibility to infection
Decreased activity and metabolic rate (possibly due to decreased thyroid function)	Decreased energy needs predisposes towards obesity
Increased body fat	Predisposes towards obesity
Special senses	
Decreased olfaction	Reduced food intake which
Decreased ability to taste	may lead to a loss of weight
Decreased visual acuity	and condition
Oral cavity	
Dental calculus	
Periodontal disease	Reduced food intake which
Loss of teeth	may lead to a loss of weight
Decreased saliva production	and condition
Gingival hyperplasia	
Urinary system	
Decreased renal function	
Decreased renal blood flow	Decreased protein
Decreased glomerular filtration rate	requirement
Skeletal system	
Osteoarthritis	Decreased mobility reduces energy requirements.
Reduced muscle mass	Decreased protein reserves
Cardiovascular system	
Congestive cardiac failure	Decreased salt intake

Fig. 17.31. Ageing changes and their effect on the animal's nutritional kittens.

Feline nutritional peculiarities

Cats are not small dogs! The cat has several unique dietary needs because it evolved as a strict metabolic carnivore, whereas dogs are naturally omnivorous. These nutritional peculiarities are listed in Fig. 17.32 and are discussed in detail under the appropriate nutrients.

Feeding Small Animals and Exotics

The needs of exotic pets, including their nutrition, are discussed in Chapter 4. Figure 17.33 gives a summary of the types of food that are acceptable for various groups of mammals, reptiles, amphibians, fish and invertebrates. The literature on cage-bird nutrition is varied and contradictory; it depends largely on personal opinion and superstition, or is extrapolated from research into poultry nutrition—which is not necessarily appropriate. Some suggested food items and energy requirements for birds are given in Fig. 17.33.

Clinical Nutrition

The importance of nutrition as an adjunctive therapy for the successful management of disease has been recognised for over a century. When reviewing a patient's nutritional requirements in the light of any disease process, it is essential that a nutritionally relevant history is taken. Information that should be determined includes:

- The type and quantity of food and fluid consumed.
- The frequency of feeding.
- Who feeds the animal.
- The presence of any food aversions or food intolerances.
- Changes in intake of food or fluid.
- Type and amount of exercise.
- Appropriateness of the present diet.
- Recent dietary changes.
- The use of drugs and/or supplements.
- Current body weight versus usual body weight.
- Age.
- Changes in urine output.

NUTRITIONAL ADAPTATIONS OF THE CAT TO A CARNIVOROUS DIET

Inability to convert carotene to vitamin A.
Inability to synthesise adequate niacin from tryptophan.
Inability to synthesise adequate taurine.
Inability to synthesise arachidonic acid from linoleic acid.
Inability to synthesise ornithine or arginine.
Inability to conserve nitrogen which results in an increased protein requirement.
Limited ability to metabolise carbohydrate.
Pyridoxine (vitamin B_6) requirements are four times that of the dog.

Fig. 17.32. Nutritional adaptations of the cat to a carnivorous diet.

- Changes in gastrointestinal function, e.g. the presence of signs related to nausea, vomiting, diarrhoea or abdominal pain.
- Previous gastrointestinal problems or surgery.
- Abnormalities of the special senses (taste, sight, smell).
- The animal's social status and the presence of other animals.
- The animal's productivity level; growth, pregnancy, lactation and exercise.

In general, diets are used to support or to spare the workload of failing organs. The nutrient requirements of ill animals often differ from those of their healthy counterparts in many ways. Various commercial veterinary clinical diets are available to aid in the management of disease. The choice of diet depends upon an understanding of how a particular illness affects the normal physiology (see Chapters 14 and 23) but it is beyond the scope of this chapter to describe these physiological alterations in detail. The information given below is primarily intended as an overview of the nutritional recommendations.

Anorexia and Critical Care Nutrition

Anorexia is a complete lack of appetite with no desire to eat whereas **inappetence** is a reduced appetite. Such a reduction in appetite may be associated with many metabolic conditions, pyrexia, sepsis, pain, surgery or trauma and may be complicated by increased nutrient requirements, e.g. for healing.

Starvation

In healthy animals, **starvation** is characterised by the mobilization of glycogen, fatty acids and metabolically labile proteins. After 48–72 hours, glycogen stores are depleted; thereafter glycerol and amino acids are used for gluconeogenesis to maintain blood glucose levels. Glucose is essential for normal metabolism of the cells of the nervous system, renal medulla, bone marrow and circulating blood as they have an obligate need for glucose. The amount of glycerol available from lipolysis is insufficient to meet the body's entire needs for glucose and the use of amino acids places the animal in a negative nitrogen balance. To safeguard energy and protein stores, the metabolic rate and therefore energy expenditure is markedly reduced. This is mediated by decreased serum levels of thyroid hormone, catecholamines and somato-medins and a reduction in physical activity. Fatty acids are exclusively used for energy production in most tissues; those tissues normally relying on glucose gradually adapt to the use of ketone bodies. Protein catabolism is minimised through inactivity and the sparing effect of triglyceride oxidation. However, once fat stores are depleted, protein utilisation is no longer spared and protein depletion occurs rapidly, resulting in a marked loss of lean body mass. Fasting dogs lose 1–3% of their body weight daily, although

FEEDING OF SMALL PETS	
Species	**Food requirements**
Small mammals: Chinchilla	20g/day. Avoid low-fibre diets. Wide range of vegetables (fresh carrot, cut grass, green vegetables), dried fruit and nuts. Standard rabbit or guinea pig pellets.
Chipmunk	Vegetables/fruit (25%), seeds nuts (75%). Wide variety of fruit – oranges, apples, grapes, blackberries, gooseberries, plums, raisins, sultanas, tomatoes. (Plum stones are toxic). Wide variety of vegetables – lettuce, dandelions, peas, sweetcorn, clover, chickweed. Seeds – sunflower, maize, rolled oats (not whole oats). Nuts – acorns, beech, hazel, pine, sweet chestnut (not peanuts). Twigs and branches to chew. Supplementary protein for sick, pregnant or lactating – milk and honey mixed with canine growth diet or chicken.
Ferret: true carnivore	20–40g/day food; 75–100ml/day water. Tinned or dried cat food (low carbohydrate, low fibre). Occasional whole carcase (mice, day old chicks, rabbit etc.)
Gerbil: herbivorous (seed and vegetables in the wild)	5–8g/day food; 2–10ml/day water. Complete and balanced proprietary mouse or rat diet. Sunflower seeds only as treats – will eat to excess (low calcium, high fat, may cause metabolic bone disturbances). Vegetables in small quantities.
Guinea pig: herbivorous	80g/kg BW/day food; 50–100ml day water (with succulent diets); 250–1000ml/day (including spillage and wastage). Complete and balanced commercial guinea pig diet. Supplement with hay and green vegetables. Vitamin C in diet essential.
Hamster: omnivorous	5–15g/day food; 7–10ml/day water. Complete and balanced proprietary hamster pellets or rodent foods – must be fresh. Seeds, grains, fruit and green vegetables but not to excess.
Rabbits	30–60g/kg/day food; 60–150ml/kg/day water. Complete and balanced commercial pellets. Supplement with hay and small quantities of fresh green vegetables, carrots, cabbage, salad crops. May browse on grass but do not feed grass cuttings.
Rats and mice	Adult rats require 10–20g/day dry food; 25–45ml/ day water, Adult mice require 5–10g/day dry food; 5–7ml/day water. Commercial pellets. Supplement with small amounts of biscuit, apple, tomato. Chocolate as treat but do not overfeed.
Amphibians	Almost all adults carnivorous. Aquatic: earthworms and mealworms. Terrestrial: crickets, maggots, baby mice. Arboreal: flies on the wing (*Drosophila, Stomoxys*). Some may adapt to fish pellets or dog food. Larval stages: aquatic vegetation, later small prey such as *Daphnia*.
Chelonians	May require vitamin/mineral supplements. (Vitamin A deficiency characterised by white cellular debris in conjunctival sacs). Mediterranean tortoises: omnivorous Wide variety of plants – cabbage, beans, cucumber, lettuce, peas, courgette, broccoli, clover, grass, dandelion, buttercup, bindweed, brassica leaves, parsnip, carrot, watercress, fruit (apple, pear, melon, strawberry, peach, tomato, blackberry, raspberry) etc. Avoid excess quantities of brassica and buttercup. Hard-boiled eggs and teaspoon of tinned dog food once a week. American box tortoises: diet varies with age Very young: carnivorous – meat or fish containing bone. Older: omnivorous – insects, mealworms, crickets, slugs, snails, earthworms, woodlice, fruit, vegetables; dogfood may be given. Terrapins: should always feed away from main tank in separate feeding container Fish (sprats, herring, mackerel, sardines, pilchards, whitebait). Tadpoles, water beetles, insect larvae, water snails, earthworms, prawns, shrimps. Some water plants, e.g. watercress. Trout pellets and dried catfood soaked in water

Fig. 17.33.—Continued ▶

FEEDING OF EXOTIC PETS	
Species	**Food requirements**
Lizards and Snakes	Entirely carnivorous – Rodents (gerbils, mice).
Fish	Commercial proprietary foods to avoid dietary imbalance (pellets, flakes, crumbs). Some species require fresh or live food. Live invertebrates should be non-aquatic source to reduce risk of disease, e.g. earthworms. Home-made diets: prawn, tuna, beef, vegetables, set with gelatin, plus vitamin supplement.
Invertebrates	Fresh, clean drinking-water essential: some will drink from bowl (but beware of drowning); some only drink from droplets sprayed on foliage. Carnivorous species (e.g. spiders) require living prey. Do not give good too large or unmanageable. Remove uneaten prey; do not allow to die in the cage. Do not present live food when spider is shedding its skin (it is very vulnerable to attack). Offer a variety of food to prevent deficiencies. Herbivorous species. Some feed only on certain plants (e.g. stick insects). Most require fresh food regularly – prevent wilting by placing foliage in sealed container of water. Avoid foods treated with herbicides or pesticides.
Cage-birds	Hardbills – seed/nut kernels and soft fruit. Softbills – insects, soft fruit, pollen, nectar. Variety for the sake of nutritional balance is vital – if not on balanced commercial pellets, diet should comprise at least six different foods. Commercial pelleted diets, if accepted. Fresh fruit, vegetables, seeds (of appropriate size). Supplementary foods to provide range of nutrients – green vegetables (lettuce, watercress, chickweed, parsley, etc.), sprouted seeds, solid vegetables (carrots, turnips, beetroot), fruit (oranges, apples, plums, grapes, tomatoes) – can be mashed with cooked egg, chicken, hard cheese or milk. Introduce gradually. Insectivores usually require live food (mealworms, crickets, fruit flies). Fruit/nectar eaters – fresh ripe fruit and/or substitute nectar (maltose/dextrose mixture with evaporated milk, honey, vitamin/mineral supplements and a little animal protein).

Fig. 17.33. Feeding of exotic pets.

the rate of loss diminishes with time. Up to 56% of the loss in body weight is from lean body mass. A similar response occurs in starvation associated with metabolic stress but at a more accelerated rate. There are three phases:

(1) The **ebb (shock) phase** lasts for around 48 hours. During this time, the metabolic rate is diminished, there is fluid sequestration, but nutritional support is a low priority.
(2) In the subsequent **flow (catabolic) phase**, nutrients are mobilised from body stores for healing. There is a marked increase in the metabolic rate, oxygen consumption, proteolysis and urinary nitrogen excretion. This phase peaks around 4 days and may last for as long as 4 weeks. It is during this time that nutritional support is important. A '**diabetes of injury**' often develops due to peripheral insulin resistance and low serum insulin levels, ultimately resulting in rapid and uncontrolled utilisation of fat and protein stores for energy production. Within 3–5 days, affected patients lose weight, may be immunocompromised and can eventually develop sepsis and organ failure. This type of malnutrition is referred to as **protein-energy malnutrition** (PEM).
(3) The final, **reparative phase** is one of anabolism and recovery.

The incidence of PEM in veterinary medicine is unknown but ranges from 25 to 65% in humans. It is one of the major causes of morbidity and mortality in metabolically stressed patients and it arises when there is inadequate food intake (inappetence or iatrogenic) or nutrient imbalance during the flow phase.

Malnutrition in the hospitalised animal. Malnutrition, if not present on admission, may develop during hospitalisation for a variety of reasons (Fig. 17.34). Every animal must be assessed to determine the likelihood of developing PEM. Assessment of nutritional status is difficult: clinical judgement is the main guide, although various biochemical parameters may be used for guidance. Some of the criteria used to judge a patient's need for nutritional support are listed in Fig. 17.35. If the risk of developing PEM is high, nutritional support must be instituted at an early stage of the disease process.

A common complication of malnutrition is **bacterial translocation and overgrowth** (BTOG) in which the enteric barrier is breached by bacteria. They then replicate in blood and tissues, causing a potentially fatal toxaemia. Degradation of the intestinal mucosa barrier results from atrophy of the mucosa and a loss of the enteric immune system, and so it is important that patients receive some food enterally to preserve the intestinal mucosa.

Previously well-nourished patients, with acute medical or surgical problems of anticipated short duration, will generally resume eating upon resolution of their disease and are not usually candidates for nutritional support. On the other hand, chronically debilitated patients, in whom food intake is likely to be reduced for an extended period, or that are anorectic and have an increased metabolic rate, will require nutritional support.

Objectives of nutritional support

The objectives of nutritional support are:

- To meet the animal's requirement for water.
- To reduce gluconeogenic drafting on endogenous amino acids.
- To meet the animal's energy requirements.
- To provide a large proportion of calories from fats, as they are more efficiently used by those organs essential for survival (heart, muscle, liver). High-fat diets are desirable for patients with respiratory failure, because fat metabolism results in a lower respiratory quotient (less carbon dioxide produced per unit of oxygen used) than does glucose, thereby decreasing the work load of the lungs.
- To satisfy protein requirements.
- To provide nutrients for the normal maintenance of the gastrointestinal mucosa, i.e. glutamine and glucose.

INDICATIONS FOR NUTRITIONAL SUPPORT

Decreased food intake, or anorexia for >3 days.
Current body weight <80% of normal.
Recent weight loss of >5%.
Poor body condition e.g. easily depilated hair, cracked/split nails, non-healing wounds, oedema, ascites and muscle atrophy.
Increased nutrient losses from diarrhoea, wounds, renal disease or burns.
Increased needs due to trauma, surgery, infection, hypoalbuminaemia (albumin <15g/l), anaemia, lymphopaenia, pyrexia or neoplasia.
Use of drugs that promote catabolism (eg. corticosteroids) or anorexia (eg. digoxin, chemotherapeutic drugs).

Fig. 17.35. Indications for nutritional support.

The nutrient requirements of sick animals are not known. To estimate their illness energy requirement (IER), the approximate resting energy requirements (RER) of healthy dogs and cats must be multiplied by an illness factor (Fig. 17.36). Protein requirements are based on the energy requirement as sufficient energy must be available for optimal protein usage. Insufficient protein results in poor healing, loss of lean body mass and immunoincompetence. Excess protein increases energy expenditure. Optimal protein requirements for ill animals are unknown. It is suggested that for the dogs protein should supply 20–22% of ME (5–6g protein/100kcal (418kJ)ME) and for dogs with increased requirements and cats, protein should supply 24–30% of ME (6–8g protein/100kcal (418kJ)ME). At these levels, the non-protein calorie: nitrogen ratio is 78–125:1. Where renal or hepatic disease exists protein intake should be reduced to 3g/100kcal (418kJ)ME for dogs and 5g protein/100kcal (418kJ) ME for cats.

Various foods are available for enteral feeding (Fig. 17.37). Many of these diets have non-protein calorie:nitrogen ratios that are below what is recommended, and may cause depression and vomiting.

FACTORS THAT MAY ADVERSELY AFFECT THE NUTRITIONAL STATUS OF SICK ANIMALS

Failure to record daily weight.
Failure to observe, measure and record the amount of food consumed.
Delay of nutritional support until the patient is in an irreversible state of depletion.
Withholding food for diagnosis procedures.
Failure to recognise and treat increased nutritional needs brought about by injury or illness.
Failure to appreciate the role of nutrition in the prevention of and recovery from infection: unwarranted reliance on drugs.
Prolonged administration of glucose and electrolyte solutions.
Rotation of staff at frequent intervals and confusion of responsibility for patient care.
Inadequate post-operative nutritional support.
Limited availability of laboratory tests to assess nutritional status.

Fig. 17.34 Practices that may adversely affect the nutritional status of sick animals.

APPROXIMATE ENERGY REQUIREMENTS OF SICK DOGS AND CATS

Reason	Illness energy requirements (IER)
Dog:	
Hospitalisation	RER x 1.3
Minor surgery/trauma	RER x 1.3–1.5
Major surgery/trauma	RER x 1.5–1.7
Neoplasia	RER x 1.5–1.8
Severe infections/sepsis	RER x 1.7–1.8
Major burns	RER x 2
Cat:	
(for any reason)	RER x 1.4–1.5

RER = 70 x body weight$^{0.75}$[kg]

Fig. 17.36. Approximate energy requirements of sick dogs and cats.

Methods of nutritional support

Prior to the provision of nutritional support, pre-existing fluid or acid-base deficits should be corrected (Chapter 21, Fluid Therapy). Only subsequently should the animal's nutrient requirements be addressed.

There are several methods available to improve an animal's nutritional status:

- Some animals may refuse to eat different food in strange surroundings. Returning an animal to its own environment may increase its appetite.
- Time spent hand-feeding patients may help.
- Ensure that food is at room temperature and in suitably shaped bowls (wide and shallow for cats, for example).
- The use of strong-smelling food is recommended for some animals (e.g. cats with upper respiratory tract disease), although such foods may not be suitable for nauseous animals.
- Dogs often prefer sweet foods.
- Intravenous diazepam or, in cats, oral oxazepam may stimulate the appetite.

If a patient is unable to eat (e.g. fractured jaw) or remains unwilling to eat, food must be provided by enteral or parenteral means.

Enteral nutrition

Enteral nutrition is the provision of a patient's nutritional requirements via a functional gastrointestinal tract. As a general rule, **if the gut works, use it**. Enteral feeding is contraindicated in patients with gastrointestinal failure, e.g. severe malabsorption, pancreatitis, gastric or intestinal obstruction, uncontrolled vomiting or severe upper gastrointestinal bleeding. Several routes are available for enteral nutrition.

Force-feeding. This is only suitable for short-term feeding. Soft tinned or liquid foods may be squirted into the mouth through a syringe or by placing preformed boluses on the back of the tongue.

Alternatively, food may be administered into the stomach through an orogastric tube. Liquids in particular should be administered carefully to reduce the risk of laryngotracheal aspiration. For both methods, a co-operative patient is required. If a patient is un-cooperative, or if nutritional support is intended to be prolonged, other techniques should be considered.

Nasal feeding tubes. These are probably the route of choice for most critically ill animals. Polyvinyl tubes may be passed through the external nares and oropharynx into the stomach.

Prior to tube placement, the nostril is anaesthetised with lignocaine or proxymetacaine drops. The tube is lubricated with a water soluble lubricant and is passed in a caudoventral, medial direction into the ventrolateral aspect of the external nares. A wire stylet may occasionally be needed to facilitate passage of the tube. The patient's head should be in a normal position. In cats, the tube is then advanced into the ventral meatus and subsequently into the pharynx. In dogs, digital pressure on the rhinarium, such that the external nares are deviated dorsally, facilitates passage of the tube into the ventral, rather than medial, meatus (Fig. 17.38). Advancement of the tube into the pharynx should elicit a swallowing reflex, allowing its passage into the oesophagus and subsequent placement in the stomach. If the tube enters the trachea, air will be aspirated and the infusion of a sterile saline solution will induce coughing.

Once in place, zinc oxide tape is wrapped around the tube and is glued to the hair using 'superglue', ensuring that the tube is tightly tucked into the alar fold (Fig. 17.39). The tube can then be taken over the top of the head or round the side of the face.

As a general rule the widest tube that the patient can accommodate should be used. 4 to 8 French tubes are suitable in most cases, although in large dogs size 10 tubes may be placed. An Elizabethan collar is required to prevent tube dislodgment. Nasal feeding tubes can be left in position for several weeks and are usually well tolerated. Commercial liquid diets are used with these tubes.

COMMERCIAL VETERINARY DIETS SUITABLE FOR ENTERAL NUTRITIONAL SUPPORT IN THE DOG AND CAT				
Product	Energy density kcal [KJ]/100g DM	Protein content g/100g DM	kcal:N ratio	KJ:N ratio
Hills a/d	493 [2062]	45.7	67:1	280:1
Hills p/d (dog)	490 [2050]	31.4	98:1	410:1
Hills p/d (cat)	510 [2133]	50	64:1	268:1
Pedigree canine concentration instant diet	437 [182]	41	67:1	280:1
Whiskas feline concentration instant diet	478 [2000]	42	71:1	297:1
Reanimyl (Virbac)	500 [2092]	29.5	100:1	418:1
Clinicare canine (PetAg)	550 [2301]	28	125:1	523:1
Clinicare feline (PetAg)	511 [2138]	39	83:1	347:1
Renal care canine (PetAg)	470 [1966]	12	245:1	1025:1
Renal care feline (PetAg)	441 [1845]	24	116:1	485:1

Fig. 17.37. Commercial veterinary diets suitable for enteral nutritional support in the dog and cat.

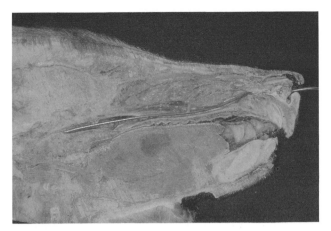

Fig. 17.38. A nasal feeding tube passing through the ventral meatus.

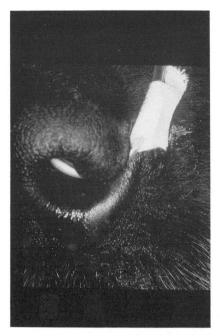

Fig. 17.39. Nasal feeding tube tucked into the alar fold so as to reduce the chance of dislodgement.

Pharyngostomy tubes. These are placed under general anaesthesia, through the lateral aspect of the oropharynx into the oesophagus. An 8–14 French tube is used in cats and small dogs; a 12–28 French tube is used in larger dogs. Such tubes can be left in place for several weeks. Liquidised tinned food or commercial liquid diets may be fed. The popularity of the pharyngostomy tube has declined in favour of other forms of feeding.

Gastrostomy tubes. These are becoming increasingly popular with the advent of techniques which allow their placement without the need for a laparotomy. Human purpose-made gastrostomy tubes are available but they are expensive. The materials required for the placement of **percutaneous endoscopically placed gastrostomy** (PEG) tubes are:

(1) Flexible endoscope with biopsy or foreign body retrieval forceps.
(2) Scalpel blade.
(3) Two strands of monofilament nylon (1 metric) and a cutting needle.
(4) An 18 gauge intravenous catheter.
(5) A 0.1 ml disposable pipette tip.
(6) A depezzer (mushroom tipped) urological catheter.

Fast the patient for 12 hours prior to PEG tube placement. Modify the depezzer catheter by discarding its wide end and making two 2 cm flanges from the end of the tube. One flange is slipped over the tube until it rests adjacent to the mushroom tip. The nipple tip of the mushroom is then removed. Place the anaesthetised patient in right lateral recumbency and surgically prepare the area of the left flank extending 15cm behind the last rib (depending on the breed). The stomach is inflated gently until the endoscope light is visible through the left flank. A stab incision is made in the skin caudal to the last rib in the dorsal two thirds of the flank and an intravenous catheter is passed through the skin into the stomach. It may be necessary to push the transilluminated spleen out of

the path of the intravenous catheter. Remove the stylet and pass nylon suture through the catheter into the stomach where it is grasped by the biopsy forceps. It is necessary to place a finger over the catheter to prevent deflation of the stomach.

After removing the endoscope and biopsy forceps, pass the nylon through the narrow end of the pipette tip and suture it securely to the gastrostomy tube. The second piece of nylon is sutured as a loop through the mushroom tip, but not tied. If any difficulty is encountered during placement, the tube can be removed by traction on this suture material. As the nylon exiting through the abdominal wall is pulled steadily, the tube passes down the oesophagus into the stomach. Resistance will be encountered as the pipette tip abuts the stomach wall. Firm application of digital counterpressure to the abdominal wall and the exertion of steady traction on the suture are required to pull the pipette tip out through the stomach and body wall.

Position the tube so that the internal flange gently abuts the mucosa. The second flange is slid over the tube until it lies on the skin. The endoscope can be re-introduced to ensure correct placement but do not insufflate the stomach further. Aspirate the air from the stomach and cap the tube.

To prevent flange removal or tube migration, a piece of zinc oxide tape is wrapped around the tube distal to the external flange; there is no need to suture the tube in place (Fig. 17.40). Antimicrobial ointment on a gauze swab may be applied to the exit site and a conforming stretch bandage can be used to protect the tube. This may need to be changed within the first 3 days but subsequently it should be checked regularly for leakage, displacement etc., and changed only if soiled or dislodged.

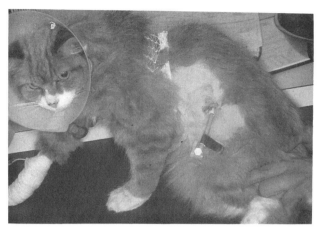

Fig. 17.40. Gastrostomy tube placed to provide nutrition to
a cat with empyema.

Gastrostomy tubes may be placed percutaneously without using an endoscope. The animal is prepared as above but, instead of passing an endoscope, a stomach tube is passed until its end visibly pushes the stomach and body wall out. A wide-bore intravenous catheter is advanced through the body wall into the lumen of the tube. A rigid piece of wire, to the end of which is attached the suture material, is passed through the catheter and up the stomach tube until it appears at the oral opening. Removal of the tube and wire will therefore bring the suture material to the mouth and the gastrostomy tube may be attached as described above.

Foley catheters placed during a laparotomy may also be used as gastrostomy tubes. The foley bulb should be inflated with water, not air, to reduce the risk of deflation and subsequent slippage. This tube should be sutured to the abdominal wall.

Gastrostomy tubes should be left in place for at least 5 days before removal. Percutaneously placed tubes and foley catheters can be removed in the conscious patient without the need for any sedation. To remove a percutaneously placed tube, exert firm traction on it whilst counterpressure is applied to skin around the ostomy site. The mushroom tip will collapse as it is pulled through the skin, whilst only the flange remains in the stomach. This flange will be passed in faeces at a later stage. Foley catheters are removed by deflating the balloon and pulling out the catheter. Food should be withheld for 12 hours prior to and following tube removal. The gastrocutaneous fistula which is present heals rapidly. These tubes may be left in place for several months with few complications. Liquidised canned food or commercial liquid diets can be administered with relative ease.

Methods of feeding. When using feeding tubes, check that the tube is in the correct position at each feed. For feeding, the animal should be standing in an upright position or placed in sternal or right lateral recumbency. Tube feeding may be administered continuously, by gravity or with an enteral pump, or more commonly by intermittent boluses.

In critically ill patients, continuous infusion is recommended at an initial flow rate of 1ml/kg/hr, increasing gradually over 48 hours until the total daily volume can be given over a 12–18 hour period. If there is overfilling of the stomach, the rate should be reduced.

With bolus feeding the required volume of food should be divided into three or four feeds initially. The volume given at each feed should not exceed 50ml/kg body weight nor should more than one-third of the total daily volume be given at any one time. The food should be at room temperature and the animal should be fed over a 5–10-minute period to reduce the incidence of vomiting or regurgitation. If either of these occur, stop feeding and clear the mouth of food. After, feeding flush the tube with 5ml of water and cap it.

The volume of food required is calculated as follows:

Volume of food (ml/day) = IER (kcal or kJ) ÷ energy density of the food (kcal or kJ/ml).

Observe the patient for a few minutes after feeding for signs of discomfort or vomiting. It is essential that all feedings are recorded on the patient's case record along with its daily weight and any problems encountered.

Animals with feeding tubes are usually able to eat voluntarily and should be offered food as they respond to treatment. The feeding tube can be removed once the patient voluntarily consumes 75% of its daily caloric intake. Hospitalisation is necessary during the initial stages of nutritional support but many patients can be discharged with the feeding tube in place as most owners are able to accept the presence of the tube and to manage it successfully.

Complications of enteral feeding. Mechanical problems include:

- Tube occlusion. Fragments of tablets are the most common cause. Tablets to be administered through tubes must be dissolved first. Other causes of occlusion should be infrequent as long as only liquid diets are used with fine-bore tubes and as long as liquidised tinned diets are sieved prior to use with wide-bore tubes. If occlusion does occur, the tube should be flushed with water or coca cola, or replaced.
- Pharyngostomy and occasionally nasal feeding tubes may compromise oropharyngeal function, causing gagging, regurgitation, airway occlusion or aspiration pneumonia. Susceptible patients, particularly brachycephalic dogs and cats, should be monitored regularly for any signs of oropharyngeal discomfort.
- Regurgitation of naso-oesophageal tubes is occasionally seen in dogs and more frequently in cats. The use of tubes with weighted ends may help to prevent this.

Gastrointestinal complications include:

- Vomiting and bloat due to rapid administration of food or obstruction of the pylorus by the mushroom tip if the tube should migrate into the stomach.
- Diarrhoea, which may be associated with a low fiber intake, lactose intolerance, too rapid delivery or, most likely, the administration of drugs.
- Constipation may occur if the fibre intake is too low.

Metabolic, fluid and electrolyte abnormalities are uncommon in uncomplicated cases where a food formulated specifically for dogs or cats is used. Human liquid diets should not be used. Careful attention to the dietary make-up is necessary where organ dysfunction, such as renal or hepatic failure, is present.

Infectious complications include:

- Necrosis and cellulitis at an ostomy site may occur if there is excessive pressure on, or too large an incision in, the skin. With percutaneously placed gastrostomy tubes, discharge from the ostomy site is commonly encountered for up to 7 days after tube placement. This is usually self-limiting but may occasionally develop into a more serious diffuse cellulitis. Cellulitis may also develop as a result of the leakage of gastric contents, if the exit site for gastrostomy tubes are too far ventral in the body wall.
- Aspiration pneumonia may develop if pharyngostomy, or occasionally a nasal feeding tube, compromises oropharyngeal function.

Parenteral nutrition (PN)

Parenteral nutrition is a specialised method of nutritional support where nutrients are administered intravenously. It requires specialised equipment and on-site laboratory facilities. The indications for PN are limited to those patients with conditions that severely limit the effectiveness or use of the gastrointestinal tract for feeding (protracted vomiting, inflammatory bowel disease, pancreatitis, peritonitis and gastrointestinal obstruction). It is contraindicated in patients with a functional gastrointestinal tract or when nutritional support will have no impact on the disease process (e.g. terminal neoplasia).

Nutrient requirements are calculated as for enteral feeding. The components of PN solutions are 50% glucose solution, 10% or 20% lipid emulsions, crystalline amino acid solution (usually 8% or $8\frac{1}{2}$%), trace element mix and a multivitamin solution. Figure 17.41 demonstrates a method of determining the required volumes of each constituent.

Method of feeding. For parenteral feeding, a silicone catheter is placed aseptically into the jugular vein with the catheter tip in the cranial vena cava or right atrium. This catheter should be dedicated to

---

CALCULATION OF THE PARENTERAL REQUIREMENTS FOR PROTEIN, CARBOHYDRATE AND LIPIDS IN DOGS AND CATS

RER (kcal) - 70 x (BW$^{0.75}$) = **a** kcal/day
RER (KJ) - (70 (BW$^{0.75}$)) x 4.184 = **a** KJ/day
Illness factor (Fig.17.36)

Energy requirement = IER = RER x illness factor = **b** kcal [KJ]/day.
Protein requirement = **c** g/day (see text).
Vol. of 8.5% **amino acid** (8.5g/100mls) required = (**c**/8.5) x 100 mls. = **d** ml amino acid.
Lipid and **glucose** provide 50% of the energy requirements each.
Vol. of 20% **lipid** (2kcal/ml) required = (0.5 x **b**)/2 = **e** ml lipid.
Vol. of 50% **glucose** (1.7kcal/ml) required = (0.5 x **b**)/1.7 = **f** ml glucose.

Example: 10kg dog is presented with a 7-day history of anorexia, vomiting and weight loss. Major abdominal surgery is performed.

RER = 70(BW$^{0.75}$) = 393 kcal.[1644KJ](a)
IER = 1.5 x RER 1.5 x 393 = **590** kcal [2467KJ](b)
Protein requirement = **23.6** g/day (c)
Vol. of 8.5% amino acid solution = (**23.6**/8.5g/ml) x 100 ml = **278** ml (d)
Vol. of 20% lipid solution = 0.5 x **590kcal** [2467KJ]/2kcal/ml [8.4KJ/ml] = **148** ml (e)
Vol. of 50% glucose solution = 0.5 x **590kcal** [2467KJ]/1.7kcal/ml [7.1KJ/ml] = **174** ml (f)

Thus this dog requires
278ml of an 8.5% amino acid solution +
148ml of a 20% lipid solution +
174ml of a 50% glucose solution =
600ml in total to be administered over 24 hours at a rate of 25ml/hour

Fig. 17.41. Calculation of parenteral nutritional requirements for protein, carbohydrate and lipid in dogs and cats.

---

parenteral nutrition solutions to minimise the risk of catheter sepsis developing. The parenteral nutrition solutions should be mixed aseptically. The solution, given at body temperature, should be administered by an infusion pump or other form of flow-limiting device, over a minimum of 18 hours and preferably 24 hours. For the first 24 hours a half-strength solution is given. Whilst feeding parenterally, serum biochemical parameters including blood glucose, triglycerides, electrolytes and urea should be monitored daily or every other day along with regular checks of the temperature, pulse and respiration. Haematology should be checked weekly.

Complications. Parenteral nutrition may be associated with several complications, of which catheter sepsis is potentially the most serious. The nutrition solution is an ideal culture medium for bacteria and infection of the catheter is a common cause of morbidity in parenterally fed patients. Mechanical or technical problems such as catheter occlusion, line disconnection and thrombophlebitis may occur. There may be metabolic derangements including hyperglycaemia, hypokalaemia, hypophosphataemia, elevated liver enzymes, hypomagnesaemia, acidosis or alkalosis, and dehydration may develop. Insulin may be required (0.25u/kg IV) to control hyperglycaemia.

Dietary Sensitivity

Food intolerance or dietary sensitivity are terms used to describe any abnormal reaction to food; usually diarrhoea and/or vomiting or dermatological signs (pruritus, urticaria and otitis externa). Food allergy specifically refers to an immunological reaction to a component of food, including preservatives and dyes. The term dietary sensitivity or intolerance is preferred unless a specific allergic response can be demonstrated. The intolerance appears to be predominantly related to the presence of glyco-proteins. Various protein sources have been documented as being responsible for dietary intoler-ances, including milk, soya bean, wheat, beef, egg, horse meat, chicken, pork and yeast in both dogs and cats and also fish in cats.

Demonstration of a food intolerance requires that an animal be fed a "hypoallergenic diet" for 3 weeks. This diet must be the animal's sole source of nutrients and must contain 'novel' ingredients to which the animal has not been previously exposed. Commercial or home-made foods may be used; commercial diets are preferred as they are complete and balanced.

Home-made foods should contain two compo-nents—carbohydrate and protein—mixed in the ratio of 2:1 to 3:1 carbohydrate to protein. Suitable carbohydrate sources include long-grain rice and boiled potato; the protein may be egg, poultry, lamb, cheese, fish, venison or rabbit. As home-made diets are unbalanced and incomplete, they require the addition of a hypoallergenic vitamin and mineral supplement. Note that most veterinary preparations are not hypoallergenic and therefore trial and error is required to select a suitable supplement.

Intestinal or dermatological changes resulting from dietary sensitivity are generally reversible, and clinical signs often resolve within 6 weeks. Once the patient is stabilised on a single protein source, other individual foods can be added in order to attempt to determine the particular food to which the animal is intolerant. In many cases the offending substance is not identified and animals will require "hypoallergenic" diets for the remainder of their lives.

Cardiac Disease

The nutritional consequences of congestive cardiac failure include:

- Retention of sodium and water, as a consequence of several neuroendocrine alterations, resulting in volume overload and hypertension.
- Development of cachexia due to anorexia (associa-ted with renal failure, hepatic dysfunction, drug therapy), malabsorption (due to reduced intestinal blood flow) and increased energy expenditure.

Treatment of congestive failure is aimed at decreas-ing cardiac workload and improving myocardial function. Drug therapy is the mainstay of most treatment protocols, but dietary manipulation is an important adjunctive therapy. It is important to main-tain lean body mass, reduce the volume overload and decrease the work of the gastrointestinal tract, kidney, liver and lung. The dietary aims include the following:

- Low salt diets are indicated to reduce sodium accumulation, thereby decreasing water reabsorp-tion. Sodium restriction should be implemented once cardiac disease is diagnosed even if clinical symptoms are not apparent.
- Total body potassium levels must be maintained when diuretics are used.
- Increased protein intakes (> 30% ME for cats and 18–25% ME for dogs) are often required to main-tain lean body mass. However, if renal failure is present the protein intake should be reduced to a level which prevents deterioration of the renal dysfunction but does not severely compromise the protein status. Protein should be of a high biological value.
- Highly digestible, low fibre diets should be fed little and often in order to decrease intestinal workload.
- Reduce metabolic stress on the congested liver by providing energy from carbohydrates and fats.
- Increase energy intake in order to compensate for the increased energy expenditure.
- Provide additional B-vitamins, particularly when diuretics are used.
- Provide an acid ash diet to aid in sodium excretion.
- Monitoring of the patients electrolyte is crucial.

Palatability may be a problem with low-salt diets. Any change to such a diet should be carried out slowly by mixing it with the animal's normal diet, warming it or adding flavour enhancers (e.g. garlic). Figure 17.42 lists foods which are permitted in salt-restricted diets and those which should be omitted. Most commercial pet foods have salt contents in the region of 0.26–0.8% DM, which are in excess of that recommended for an animal with congestive failure. Commercial low-salt diets are available or a suitable home-made diet may be formulated.

SALT-RESTRICTED DIETS	
Permitted foods* for salt-restricted diets	**Foods to be excluded from salt-restricted diets**
Beef meat	All processed meats, cheeses
Rabbit	breads and cereals
Chicken meat	Carrots
Lamb meat	Heart
Fresh water/white fish	Kidney
Egg yolks	Whole egg
Oatmeal	Salted fats (butter/margarine)
Corn	Salted snacks and nuts
Potato	Liver
Spaghetti/macaroni	

*Assuming foods are not cooked with any added salt

Fig. 17.42. Food which may be included in or should be excluded from salt-restricted diets.

Dermatological Diseases

The skin is a large metabolically active organ which is susceptible to nutritional imbalances. Where animals eat commercial foods, deficiencies are rarely causes of skin disease. Vitamins A and E, zinc and essential fatty acids appear to be the nutrients of most concern. These nutrients are discussed in more detail in the relevant sections.

Dietary hypersensitivity may result in dermatological changes, as already described.

Fibre-responsive Diseases

There are several fibre-responsive diseases:

- Diabetes mellitus.
- Obesity.
- Constipation.
- Colitis.
- Hyperlipidaemia.

The causes, symptoms and general treatment of the diseases are discussed in more detail in Chapter 23 (Medical Disorders). Nutritional management of the obese patient and those with colitis or constipation are discussed later in the sections on obesity and gastrointestinal disease, while this section looks at diabetes mellitus and hyperlipidaemia.

Diabetes mellitus

Dietary manipulation is a useful adjunctive therapy for diabetes mellitus. Diabetic patients should be fed a diet that is uniform with respect to both quality and quantity. The ideal nutrient profiles for diabetic animals have not been determined but humans are often recommended a diet that is high in complex carbohydrates and fibre and moderately restricted in fat.

Fibre delays the digestion and absorption of carbohydrates, by increasing gastric emptying time, modifying gut transit time and enhancing tissue sensitivity to insulin. Thus, post-prandial surges in blood glucose are smoothed out. Soluble fibre is considered to be of greater benefit than insoluble fibre.

Hyperlipidaemia

Dietary manipulation may be an effective adjunct to medical management. A low-fat diet is recommended to decrease the serum triglyceride levels. High-fibre diets have also been advocated by some to be beneficial but there is, as yet, no evidence that fibre plays a role in the reduction of serum lipids, although such an effect is possible.

Gastrointestinal Disease

Gastrointestinal disorders are common causes of malnutrition. Each disorder results from some alteration in the normal physiological function (Chapter 23). Dietary management of these disorders is directed at compensating for these altered functions. Figure 17.43 summarises the optimal nutrient profiles of patients with a variety of gastrointestinal disorders.

Regurgitation and vomiting

Regurgitation is the reflux of undigested food from the mouth or oesophagus before it has reached the stomach. Regurgitation should be differentiated from **vomiting**, which is defined as the forceful ejection of food from the stomach and often the proximal small intestine.

In patients with oesophagitis, or following surgery for oesophageal obstruction, food and water should be administered through a gastrostomy tube, and not orally, for 1 week to allow the oesophagus to heal. Patients with primary or secondary megoesophagus should be fed a canned or dry food (often preferable) from a raised position, with the patient standing at a minimum of 60° from horizontal. The animal should be maintained in this position for approximately 10 minutes. If regurgitation persists, soft sloppy foods can be fed.

DIETARY RECOMMENDATIONS FOR GASTROINTESTINAL DISORDERS	
Disorder	**Recommendations**
Vomiting	NPO for 24–48 hours. Then feed a highly digestible (>90%), low fat (<30% ME), low fibre (<2% DM) q4–8 hours. Return to a normal diet over 3 days.
GDV	Feed a highly digestible, low fibre (<2% DM), high-energy dense diet at least q12h. Avoid excitement during and for one after feeding. Do not give calcium supplements.
Diarrhoea	In acute cases NPO for 24–48 hours. Feed a highly digestible (>90%), low fat (<30% ME), low fibre (<2% DM) diet to acute and chronic cases. Supplement vitamins in chronic cases. Feed q6–8 hours. Return to a normal diet over 3 days (acute cases).
Dietary sensitivity	Limit protein sources. Gluten free, "hypoallergenic", highly digestible or elimination diets.
Malabsorption/ malassimilation	As for diarrhoea (+ MCTs?)
Coprophagy	High energy dense diets. High fibre (>10% DM).
Constipation	High fibre (>10% DM) or add bulking agent eg bran, isphaghula or sterculia.
Colitis	Acute: as for diarrhoea. Chronic: Highly digestible low fibre (<2% DM) diet, high fibre (>10% DM) diet or hypoallergenic diet.
Flatulence	Highly-digestible low fat (<6% DM), low fibre (<2% DM) diet. Avoid milk, soya and vegetables.

NPO – nil by mouth (nil per os). DM – dry matter.
GDV – gastric dilatation and volvulus. MCT – medium chain triglycerides.

Fig. 17.43. Dietary recommendations for gastrointestinal disorders.

Following severe protracted vomiting, significant quantities of water, potassium, sodium, chloride and bicarbonate are lost. The priority is to address this fluid and electrolyte imbalance (Chapter 21). The aims of nutritional management of vomiting are:

- To decrease gastric irritation, thereby decreasing the stimulus for vomiting.
- To increase the rate of gastric emptying.
- To feed a highly digestible diet to decrease feedback stimulation to the stomach.
- To provide proper nutrition to maintain optimum body weight and condition.

Food should be withheld from acutely vomiting patients for up to 72 hours. Water and electrolytes must be provided either orally or parenterally. Subsequently introduce a highly digestible, low-fat, low-fibre diet as shown in Fig. 17.44. Foods that contain highly digestible carbohydrates and proteins (Fig. 17.45) are suitable. Reducing the fat and fibre content results in rapid gastric emptying.

Chronically vomiting animals should be fed a similar diet to that used for acute vomiting. Nutrient requirements may have to be met parenterally in intractable cases.

Gastric dilatation and volvulus (GDV)

Predisposing dietary factors for GDV include:

- Long-term consumption of large amounts of food at a single meal. This results in laxity of the gastrohepatic ligaments and contributes to the development of hyperplasia and hypertrophy of the gastric musculature.
- Long-term excessive dietary calcium intake. This may predispose to the development of hyperplasia and hypertrophy of the gastric musculature.
- A build-up of gas in the stomach. Aerophagia is the primary source of the gas, not bacterial fermentation of food. It is associated with rapid food consumption, particularly when there is competition for food and/or excitement at feeding.

GDV does not appear to be associated with any particular diet. It has been reported in dogs fed meat or cereal-based diets and diets with or without soyabeans. Prevention of GDV may be achieved by feeding a low-fibre, highly digestible diet at least twice

FOODS SUITABLE FOR ANIMALS WITH VOMITING, DIARRHOEA, PANCREATITIS OR HEPATIC DISEASE	
Highly digestible carbohydrate foods*	**Highly digestible protein foods****
Rice	Egg
Glucose	Chicken
Cornstarch	White fish
Pasta	Cottage cheese
Potato	

* Digestibility of at least 85%
** Digestibility of at least 90%

Fig. 17.45. Foods suitable for animals with vomiting, diarrhoea, pancreatitis or hepatic disease.

daily or free choice. Avoid diets high in calcium. Minimise excitement and physical activity immediately before, during and for at least one hour after feeding. Dogs with a previous history of GDV should be fed alone.

Small bowel diarrhoea

Diarrhoea is the passage of unformed, loose or liquid faeces. It is the primary sign associated with loss of intestinal function and occurs secondarily to many disorders. Acute diarrhoea may be due to viral infections or dietary indiscretions whilst chronic diarrhoea is associated with many inflammatory or structural disorders. Diarrhoea may develop for several reasons:

- **Osmotic diarrhoea** occurs when osmotically active chemicals are present in the luminal contents, as is seen with various malabsorptive or maldigestive disorders (e.g. exocrine pancreatic insufficiency and villus atrophy).
- **Secretory diarrhoea** results from the excess secretion or decreased absorption of electrolytes. This may occur if bacterial enterotoxins are present (e.g. from certain types of *E.coli*).
- **Permeability diarrhoea** results from leakage of fluid, electrolytes or protein into the intestinal lumen (e.g. mucosal damage or lymphangiectasia).
- **Disordered motility** with a resultant decreased transit time for intestinal contents may cause diarrhoea. This may be secondary to other gastrointestinal diseases.

The aims of nutritional management are:

- To allow intestinal rest and healing.
- To provide a highly digestible diet to decrease the residue in the intestine, thereby decreasing intestinal work.
- To provide adequate nutrition to maintain optimal body weight and condition.

Acute enteritis is often associated with significant water and electrolyte losses, sufficient to cause dehydration. This should be treated first using lactated Ringer's or normal saline (Chapter 21). The patient should be starved for 24–72 hours, but

FOOD RE-INTRODUCTION SCHEDULE FOR ANIMALS RECOVERING FROM VOMITING, DIARRHOEA OR PANCREATITIS	
Day	**% of normal daily food quantity**
1	33%
2	66%
3	100%

Feed small, frequent meals (4–6/d) of a highly digestible, low fat (<15%DM; <30%ME), low fibre (<2%DDM; 0.5g/100kcal (418kJ)ME) diet.

Fig. 17.44. Food reintroduction schedule for animals recovering from vomiting, diarrhoea or pancreatitis.

given free access to water if vomiting is not a problem. For cases of simple diarrhoea, a highly digestible food may be re-introduced. The diet should be:

- Highly digestible.
- Low in fat for dogs, as fat malabsorption, due to bacterial deconjugation of bile salts, bacterial degradation of fats to fatty acids and hydroxylation of fatty acids to short chain fatty acids, exacerbate the diarrhoea. Clinically cats appear to do better with higher fat diets
- Lactose-free, as many animals are unable to digest lactose and it therefore causes an osmotic diarrhoea.

Where severe acute diarrhoea proves intractable (more than 3 days in duration), parenteral feeding should be considered. This will allow complete rest for healing. However, the presence of food in the small intestinal lumen is important:

- It provides nutrients to enterocytes as they obtain much of their nutrition directly from the gut lumen.
- It maintains the local gut immunity.
- It stimulates brush border enzyme activity.
- It stimulates villus development.

Prolonged gastrointestinal starvation, as occurs with parenteral feeding, results in mucosal atrophy and predisposes to bacterial translocation and overgrowth.

Chronic diarrhoea. Chronic diarrhoea results from **malassimilation**. The syndrome has two components, malabsorption and maldigestion, which may result from failure of several organ systems (Fig. 17.46):

- **Malabsorption** occurs when defects in the structure or function of the SI mucosa or lymphatics reduce the absorption of nutrients. Causes include lymphosarcoma, food intolerance, inflammatory bowel disease (IBD) and lymphangiectasia. Malabsorptive conditions may be associated with a protein-losing enteropathy.

THE EFFECTS OF ORGAN DYSFUNCTION ON THE ASSIMILATION (DIGESTION AND ABSORPTION) OF NUTRIENTS FROM THE GASTROINTESTINAL TRACT

Organ	Normal function	Nutrients affected by loss of function
Small intestine	Digestion and absorption	Fat, CHO Protein
Lymphatics	Transport (fat)	LCT
Pancreas	Digestion	Fat, CHO Protein
Liver	Micelle formation Absorption (fat)	LCT

LCT – long chain triglycerides. CHO – carbohydrate

Fig. 17.46. Effects of organ dysfunction on the assimilation (digestion and absorption) of nutrients from the gastro-intestinal tract.

- **Maldigestion** is due to defective intraluminal digestion. The defect may be due to impaired gastric, pancreatic and/or biliary function. Causes include exocrine pancreatic insufficiency (EPI) and IBD.

The aim in nutritional management of malabsorptive disorders is to provide nutrients in a form in which passive diffusion or absorption is sufficient to meet the nutrient requirements of the patient. With maldigestive diseases, the aim is to provide adequate nutrients in a readily digestible or previously digested form.

Various protocols have been advocated for the management of chronic diarrhoea:

- The nutrient profiles described above for acute diarrhoea would be suitable, i.e. a highly digestible, low-fat, low-fibre diet for dogs, and a highly digestible, low-fibre, high available fat diet for cats.
- It may be necessary to add medium chain triglycerides (MCT) in order to provide additional energy. However, MCTs are unpalatable and may result in a decrease in the volume of food eaten.
- High-fibre diets diets may sometimes be useful. Fibre may alleviate diarrhoea by binding water and so decreasing the amount of free faecal water. The viscous gel formed by water and soluble fibres prolongs intestinal transit time, allowing greater water absorption. The binding properties of dietary fibres may reduce the effect of toxins within the intestinal lumen. Carbohydrate tolerance improves, and small intestinal villus height and mucosal weight increase. Finally, alterations in the intestinal microflora may reduce the number of pathogenic bacteria in cases of primary or secondary bacterial overgrowth.
- Elemental diets are indicated for severe malassimilation. These diets consist of amino acids, simple sugars and fats in forms which require little further digestion and are easily absorbed. Such diets are expensive and are not formulated for dogs or cats.
- Animals losing large quantities of protein through the intestinal mucosa will require increased protein in the diet.
- Multiple vitamin deficiencies may also develop in animals with severe malassimilation (in particular deficiencies in vitamins B, K and folate have been reported). Supplementation with parenteral vitamins is indicated.
- Parenteral feeding may be required for short-term feeding, but is not practical for long-term management.

Colitis

Colitis is common problem in animals. Large bowel diarrhoea may be distinguished from small bowel diarrhoea on the following criteria:

- Increased frequency with blood or mucus.
- Possibly increased volume.

- Usually signs of urgency, tenesmus or painful defecation.
- Undigested food is rarely present.
- Weight loss, flatulence or borborygmus are rare.

The aims in treating colitis are:

- To reduce irritation to the LI mucosa.
- To normalise intestinal transit time.
- To allow healing of LI mucosa.

There are three possible approaches to the dietary management of colitis:

- **Low-residue diets**. A highly digestible, low-fibre diet decreases the residue presented to the large intestine and is most effective where there is significant damage to the large intestinal mucosa.
- **High-fibre diets**. High-fibre (10–25% DM; 3.8–6.2g/100kcal ME), low-fat diets (< 15%DM, < 30% ME) are useful when diarrhoea is due to increased colonic motility. Fibre increases faecal bulk, decreases colonic transit time and improves faecal consistency.
- **"Hypoallergenic" diets**. Dietary insensitivities may cause colitis. Single protein sources (lamb, chicken, cottage cheese, fish, commercial preparations) may be fed as described for dietary sensitivity.

Pancreatic disease

Exocrine pancreatic insufficiency and pancreatitis, an uncommon yet potentially life-threatening disorders, are the two main pancreatic diseases which require dietary management.

Exocrine pancreatic insufficiency is a common cause of chronic diarrhoea in the dog. In most cases, enzyme replacement results in weight gain and a reduction in appetite. Dietary management is an adjunct to drug therapy:

- A highly digestible, low-fibre but moderate fat diet is required, as the digestibility of food may be reduced by 10–15%, even with enzyme supplementation. The availability of nutrients may be too low in normal maintenance foods.
- A reduction in fibre is required as fibre binds bile acids and pancreatic enzymes, thereby reducing their effectiveness.

Pancreatitis usually occurs following a large meal but may be associated with surgery, glucocorticoid administration or excess stimulation of endogenous secretion by fat. Long-term feeding of high-fat diets may predispose to its development. The aims of treatment are to reduce pancreatic stimulation:

- The animal should be starved completely for 2–5 days. Water and electrolytes should be provided parenterally.
- Subsequently water and small amounts of food (if tolerated) should be provided orally for a further 3 days. Feed a highly digestible, low-residue, moderately fat-restricted diet.
- If food is withheld for more than five days nutrients must be provided parenterally.
- To prevent recurrences, feed a highly digestible, low-to-moderate fat-restricted but high-carbohydrate diet.

Lymphangiectasia

Dogs and cats with lymphangiectasia should be fed a high-fibre diet severely restricted in fat, as the absorption of long-chain fatty acids increases lymph flow and therefore lymph loss. If such a diet does not provide a clinical improvement in 2 weeks, the diets described above for acute diarrhoea should be tried. Medium-chain triglycerides may be included as a supplement to increase the energy density of the diet, if they are tolerated. These fats are not absorbed into the lacteals but directly into the portal system. They may be used to supply up to 25% of the dog's energy requirements.

Coprophagy

Coprophagy is fairly common in dogs. It is a normal phenomenon in wild dogs, which routinely consume faeces from herbivorous animals. This may be an important source of some nutrients but the cause of coprophagy in domestic dogs is often not determined. It may be a vice associated with boredom or possibly an indication of gastrointestinal disease. Dogs with a malassimilation syndrome, in particular EPI, are often coprophagic. Management of coprophagy includes removal of faecal material promptly to reduce the opportunity for coprophagia. Increasing activity will achieve a similar effect. Both highly digestible and high-fibre diets have been advocated to prevent coprophagy.

Flatulence

Flatulence is an objectionable chronic problem. Most of the gas in the intestines is derived from air swallowed during eating or panting. Some gases, particularly the odoriferous components, are formed from bacterial fermentation of poorly digested carbohydrate or fibre in the colon. Soyabeans, beans and peas (which contain large quantities of the non-absorbable oligosaccharides raffinose, stachyose and verbascose) are likely to produce large amounts of intestinal gas. Flatulence may be a sign of malassimilation. The goals in managing flatulence are to reduce the amount of air ingested and the amount of gas produced:

- Feed free-choice, or meal-feed at least 3 times a day.
- Encourage the consumption of small amounts of food.
- Reduce competition at feeding.
- Avoid diets high in fibre and those that contain soyabeans, wheat or lactose. Do not feed strongly-flavoured sulphur-containing vegetables (root vegetables), milk, high-protein diets or vitamin/mineral supplements.
- Feed a highly digestible, low-residue diet.

Constipation

Constipation is the inability to pass or difficulty in passing faeces. Retention of faeces in the colon results in excess water reabsorption from the colonic contents, resulting in faecal impaction and discomfort. Constipation is a common sequel to the ingestion of bones or hair, or to inadequate water intake. It may also result from obstruction to faecal passage (e.g. prostatic disease), pelvic damage, neurological problems or lack of exercise. Dietary management entails feeding a high fibre-diet so as to increase the water content and bulk of the faeces. Increasing faecal bulk decreases the tension and pressure needed by the colonic musculature to empty the colon. It should be noted that provision of fibre to a dehydrated, constipated patient could cause faecal impaction. Allow free access to the garden within 30 minutes of feeding to further stimulate defecation.

Liver Disease

Inflammatory/degenerative liver disease

The liver plays an important role in the metabolism of fats, protein, carbohydrates, vitamins and minerals and is also required for detoxification of many substances. Although there are various liver diseases (Chapter 23), the aims of nutritional therapy have a commonality of purpose, independent of the disease process. Failure of hepatic function results in a rapid deterioration in the animal's nutritional status:

- **Fluid and electrolyte disturbances** may develop in acute liver disease because of vomiting.
- **Hypoglycaemia** may result from a reduction in liver glycogen stores and a decreased ability to manufacture glucose by gluconeogenesis.
- **Nitrogenous wastes**, such as ammonia, accumulate due to failure of the urea cycle. Ammonia is absorbed from the gastrointestinal tract and is also produced endogenously when protein is used for energy production.
- **Plasma amino acid profiles** are altered. There is a relative increase in aromatic amino acids and a decrease in branched chain amino acids. Many aromatic amino acids are neurotoxic or act as false neurotransmitters and, along with mercaptans (derived from bacterial degradation of methionine) and octopamine, contribute to the depression of the central nervous system (hepatic encephalopathy).
- **Fat accumulation** in the liver may interfere with the urea cycle.
- **Reduced hepatic protein synthesis** results in hypoalbuminaemia.
- Clinical signs of **hypovitaminosis** (particularly vitamins B, K and E) may develop. This is due to increased urinary loss (B vitamins) and to decreased fat and therefore fat-soluble vitamin absorption as a consequence of reduced bile production.

- **Water retention** (ascites, peripheral oedema) may develop in association with hypoproteinaemia and sodium retention.

Dietary requirements of patients with liver disease are:

- Low-protein diets (3–4g/100kcal/day for dogs and 5–6/100kcal/day for cats) are required for animals with hepatic encephalopathy as an adjunct to drug therapy. In some cases a further reduction in protein intake is necessary. Extra protein may be supplied if there is hepatic regeneration or hypoproteinaemia, as long as blood ammonia levels are normal. Note that the animals with liver disease may not be able to tolerate protein levels above these because of a decreased ability to metabolise and excrete waste products.
- **Protein** must be of a high biological value and should contain high proportions of branched chain amino acids in order to attempt to normalise the serum amino acid profile. Foods rich in methionine should be avoided so as to reduce mercaptan production. Cottage cheese, egg and milk casein are good protein sources.
- **Sufficient energy** is required to reduce the catabolism of body protein for energy, for healing and to decrease the rate of release of fat from adipose tissue. An intake of 10–13g/100kcal ME of a highly digestible carbohydrate (boiled rice) protects liver function and spares protein. Moderate-fat diets may be fed as long as carbohydrate and protein intakes are adequate. High-fat diets should be avoided in cholestatic disease, where fat malabsorption due to reduced bile salt secretion develops and in degenerative or inflammatory conditions when they may worsen encephalopathic states.
- **Moderate sodium restriction** in conjunction with diuretics helps control portal hypertension and alleviate oedema and ascites associated with fibrotic or atrophic liver disease.
- **Vitamins** should be administered parenterally.

Copper storage disease

This particular cause of liver disease deserves special mention. The aim of dietary management is to prevent significant copper accumulation by providing a low-copper diet early in life in susceptible breeds (Bedlington terrier, Dobermann, Cocker spaniel, West Highland White, Kerry Blue and Sky terriers) and supplementing with zinc (2mg/kg/day) to reduce copper absorption. Table scraps, particularly viscera such as liver, and mineral supplements that result in copper intakes above 1.2mg/100g DM (<0.3mg/100kcal ME) should not be given.

Renal Disease

The role of diet in the pathogenesis of renal failure is controversial but, although the effects of excess dietary protein, phosphorus and sodium on renal function are unproven, it is prudent to recommend that their intakes should not exceed maintenance levels.

Chronic renal failure develops once 70% of the nephrons have been destroyed, irrespective of the aetiology. Surviving nephrons may hypertrophy, thereby compensating for the loss of some nephrons and delaying the progression of the disease. There is a limit to such compensation and eventually glomerular filtration and tubular function in the remaining nephrons are insufficient to cope with the workload.

The management of chronic renal failure depends upon decreasing the workload on the kidneys while meeting the animal's nutritional needs. The major considerations include:

- **Water**. Fresh clean water should be provided at all times.
- **Energy**. The energy density of the diet should be increased to reduce protein catabolism and maintain body weight. Where low-energy diets are fed, protein catabolism is required to provide energy. This results in an increase in the amount of nitrogenous waste to be excreted.
- **Protein**. In animals with chronic renal failure, but without significant proteinuria, a reduction in protein intake decreases nitrogenous waste and therefore contributes to the amelioration of some of their toxic effects. However, there is controversy as to when dietary protein should be reduced. Until further information is forthcoming, it is recommended that protein intake be individualised for each patient. As a general rule protein intake should be reduced to that level which prevents clinical and biochemical signs of uraemia, i.e. the animal's response to the diet governs the amount fed. In the majority of cases, protein intakes will be in the order of 3–4g/100kcal (418kJ) ME for dogs and 5–6g/100kcal (418kJ) ME in cats. If these protein levels do not result in a clinical or biochemical improvement they can be reduced further—but cautiously, as protein malnutrition is likely to develop.
- The level of protein intake required by patients with **nephrotic syndrome** is also controversial. Although such patients are losing protein in urine, an increase in protein intake only results in increasing the amount of protein lost in urine and may hasten the progression of glomerular disease by promoting renal blood flow. However, decreasing protein intake may contribute to a worsening of the hypoproteinaemia. Thus, nephrotic patients without uraemia should be fed a level of protein that stabilises serum protein without increasing the amount lost in urine. Nephrotic patients with uraemia should be fed the lowest level of protein that maintains serum protein and blood urea at levels consistent with a reasonable quality of life. The protein source should be of a high biological value (> 80%).
- **Phosphorus** levels should be reduced. Meat contains high levels of phosphorus and protein and so a low-meat diet should be fed. A reduction in phosphorus absorption is required to normalise the serum calcium:phosphorus ratio and to limit the development of renal secondary hyperparathyroidism. This may be achieved by feeding a phosphate binder (aluminium hydroxide) but its prolonged use may induce a zinc deficiency.
- **Sodium** intake should be reduced to restrict the development of hypertension.
- **B vitamin** supplementation is recommended to offset increased losses.
- **Potassium** supplementation may be required in some cases due to renal potassium wasting. Potassium depletion results in muscle weakness, ventroflexion of the neck, depression and anorexia.
- Dietary potassium restriction is necessary in other cases if hyperkalaemia develops.
- **Calcium** supplementation may be required in some cases (once the calcium:phosphorus ratio has been corrected).

Urolithiasis

Urolithiasis is a disease characterised by the presence of calculi or crystals in the urinary tract (Chapters 22 and 23).

Uroliths or crystals may be composed of six different substances. The most common is struvite (ammonium magnesium phosphate), followed in decreasing order of incidence by calcium oxalate, ammonium urate, silicate, cystine and calcium phosphate. Mixed calculi may be found in some cases.

- **Struvite calculi** form in an alkaline urine and are composed primarily or exclusively of magnesium--ammonium–phosphate hexahydrate. The levels of magnesium and phosphate in urine relates directly to the amount consumed, whereas urine ammonium and urea relate directly to the amount of protein consumed. Thus, the higher the intake of these minerals and protein, the greater the risk of struvite uroliths forming.
- **Ammonium urate uroliths** form in an acid urine and most commonly occur secondarily to hepatic disease in any breed, as a consequence of the decreased metabolism of ammonia and urate. They may also occur in the absence of hepatic disease in Dalmatians and English bulldogs. Dalmatians normally excrete high levels of urate in their urine so favouring the formation of crystals. Urine ammonia and urate levels are directly related to protein intake.

- **Calcium oxalate uroliths** form when there is increased urinary excretion of the components in urine or a reduction in urinary calcium oxalate inhibitors. Many factors may predispose to their formation.

- **Silicate uroliths** form when high levels of silicate are consumed. They are more likely to develop in coprophagic animals.

- **Cystine uroliths** form in an acid urine and result from an inherited defect in renal tubular reabsorption of the amino acids cystine and lysine.

Management of existing urolithiasis is by surgical removal (after accurate diagnosis) or, in the case of struvite and ammonium urate, by dissolution using an appropriate calculolytic diet.

Dietary dissolution of **struvite uroliths** requires a diet severely restricted in protein, calcium, phosphorus and magnesium and relatively high in sodium. The diet should produce an acid urine (pH < 6). Reducing urinary concentrations of the components of struvite uroliths promotes dissolution over 2–28 weeks. The diet should not be fed to patients requiring sodium-restricted diets nor to growing, lactating or pregnant animals. Appropriate antimicrobial therapy is important if urinary tract infections are present. The concomitant administration of urinary acidifiers (e.g. methionine, ascorbic acid, ethylenediamine or ammonium chloride) or additional salt is contra-indicated.

Recurrence of struvite uroliths may be prevented by controlling infection and by feeding diets low in minerals and protein, while increasing urine production through the addition of salt. In otherwise healthy animals, fed maintenance diets, additional salt may be added to increase urine production.

Ammonium urate uroliths may be dissolved by feeding a protein, and purine restricted diet which produces an alkaline urine (pH > 7). In addition, urinary tract infections should be controlled and the drug allopurinol may be used to decrease endogenous urate production. Foods rich in purines include meat and glandular organs, whereas egg and milk protein are low in purines. Allopurinol is not required if the aim is purely preventative.

Calcium oxalate uroliths must be removed surgically. A diet low in calcium, sodium chloride and oxalate may prevent their recurrence. Endogenous oxalate production is increased in animals given large amounts of vitamin C. Ideally urine pH should be alkaline. Drug therapy with thiazide diuretics and potassium citrate may help prevent urolith formation

Cystine uroliths must be removed surgically. A low protein diet that alkalises urine may prevent their recurrence. The reduction in protein reduces the amount of cystine to be excreted.

Silicate uroliths must be removed surgically. Recurrence is prevented by discouraging coprophagy.

Skeletal and Neuromuscular Diseases

Nutritional skeletal diseases are relatively common (osteochondrosis, cervical spondylomyelopathy), whereas nutritional neuromuscular diseases are uncommon. Almost all nutritionally related skeletal and muscular diseases are diet-induced. The major nutrients concerned with the skeletal system are energy, protein, calcium, phosphorus, copper, iodine, vitamins A and D, and thiamine. Dietary imbalances of each of these nutrients are covered in their relevant sections. However, many skeletal abnormalities are attributable to the stimulation of excessive growth rates by general over feeding. The result is widening and maldevelopment of growth plates and therefore of bones and joints. This is especially relevant in large breeds of dog due to their greater weight. Reducing growth rates allows bones to develop normally and so to reduce the incidence of skeletal abnormalities it is important not to feed for a maximum rate of growth.

The major nutrients of concern in neuromuscular disorders are calcium (post parturient hypocalcemia), thiamine (neurological signs) and potassium (myopathy). Dietary imbalances of these nutrients are discussed under the relevant nutrient.

Obesity

Obesity, probably the most common nutritionally related disorder of dogs and cats, results from metabolic derangements or overfeeding. Obesity is present when an animal's weight exceeds its optimal weight by 15%. Published reports indicate that 25–44% of pet dogs and 6–12% of cats are obese. Obesity can predispose animals to a variety of clinical conditions including orthopaedic, cardiac, hepatic and dermatological diseases. Obesity results from an increase in fat cell size (hypertrophic obesity) in adult animals, or from increased numbers of fat cells (hyperplastic obesity) formed during growth. Prevention of obesity is important in young animals as the management of patients with hyperplastic obesity is extremely difficult. It requires detailed client education on the correct feeding of young animals, particularly during the most active growth phases. Free-choice feeding should be avoided in all growing animals until they have achieved 90% of their adult weight, and should also be avoided in obese prone adults. Risk factors for the development of obesity are listed in Fig. 17.47.

Obese animals should be evaluated for the presence of an underlying primary disease prior to introducing a weight reduction programme. Management of obese animals is hopeless without owner compliance: where the problem is simple obesity, time must be spent talking to owners about the practicalities of weight reduction. The client must be convinced that the animal is overweight and that obesity represents an important health risk. The benefits of successful obesity management and the role that inappropriate feeding behaviour plays in the development of obesity should be explained carefully.

FACTORS THAT MAY LEAD TO OBESITY

Female
Increasing age
Neutering
Breed predisposition, e.g. Labrador retrievers, Cairn terriers,
   Cocker spaniels, Shetland sheepdogs, Basset hounds and
   Beagles
Previous history of obesity
Sedentary lifestyle
Use of home made diets
Increased palatability of foods
Feeding unbalanced diets, particularly where excessive treats
   or supplements are fed
Free choice feeding
Obesity in the owner
Middle-aged to older owners

Fig. 17.47. Risk factors for obesity in animals.

Neither drugs nor surgery are indicated for the management of primary obesity in animals. The aim of any weight reduction programme is to reduce energy intake below energy expenditure until the animal reaches its optimum weight. The loss of 1 kg of adipose tissue requires an energy deficit of 7700 kcal (32217 kJ). This deficit may be produced by decreasing energy intake and/or increasing energy expenditure. Moderate exercise (brisk 1-hour walk) will increase energy expenditure by approximately 10% above the dog's MER and will also increase the energy expenditure at rest. Strenuous exercise increases energy expenditure by a greater amount but may also result in an increased food intake. A greater dependence is placed on restricting food intake in obese cats as it is difficult to increase their energy expenditure.

Energy restriction may be total (i.e. starvation) or partial. Obese cats should never be completely starved as this may induce hepatic lipidosis. There are no known health risks to complete starvation in the dog but there are several disadvantages:

- Loss of adipose tissue in fasted dogs is only 3–4% greater than with moderate calorie restriction.
- Complete fasting requires hospitalisation, which is expensive.
- As there is little client involvement with the fasting method, obesity is more likely to recur than with in-home weight reduction programmes.

The mainstay of any weight reduction programme is the restriction of energy intake to 60–70% of the MER calculated for the animal's estimated optimal weight. This may be achieved in two ways:

- Feeding a smaller amount of the animal's normal diet. This is not ideal, as non-energy nutrients are usually balanced to the energy density, so that the consumption of less energy results in the consumption of inadequate amounts of non-energy nutrients.
- Feeding an energy-restricted, low-fat, high-fibre diet in an amount that the animal is used to eating. There are several advantages to this second approach:

- A **low fat intake** is desirable because, on a weight basis, fat provides more than twice as many calories as carbohydrate or protein and the heat increment (HI) is increased. Up to 50% of the excess energy intake may be lost as a result of the normal meal-induced HI when carbohydrates and protein make up a greater proportion of the diet.
- **Carbohydrates and protein** are more likely to stimulate an increase in the metabolic rate than fat, because they stimulate insulin secretion.
- **Dietary fibre** is needed to provide dietary bulk as the feeling of gastrointestinal fullness is an important satiety factor. Fibre also reduces the digestibility of energy nutrients.

CALCULATION OF THE AMOUNT TO FEED OBESE ANIMALS ON A WEIGHT-REDUCTION PROGRAMME

1. Estimate the MER* for the animals optimal weight:
Cats: MER (kcal ME**/day) = 1.4 x (70 x $BW_{kg}^{0.75}$) or 1.4 x (30xBW_{kg}+70)
Dogs: MER (kcal ME**/day) = 2 x (70 x $BW^{0.75}$) or 2 x (30xBW_{kg}+70)
Multiply by 4.184 to convert to KJ.
Example: Dog obese weight = 24kg
            Estimated optimal weight = 20kg
            MER = 1324kcal [5540KJ]/day

2. Determine the daily energy intake required. Multiply the MER for estimated optimal weight (1) by 60–70%
Example: Energy intake = MER x 0.60
                 = 794kcal [3322KJ]/day

3. Obtain the energy density of the diet eg. 265kcal [1109KJ]/can

4. Calculate the amount of food required each day by dividing the daily energy intake (2) by the energy density of the food (3)
Example: Amount of food = 794kcal [3322KJ] ÷ 265kcal [1109KJ] = 3 cans/day

5. Divide the amount of food (4) into 3 or 4 feeds/day

*MER = maintenance energy requirement
**ME = metabolisable energy

Fig. 17.48. Calculation of the amount to feed obese animals on a weight-reduction programme.

CALCULATION OF TIME SCALE FOR WEIGHT LOSS IN ANIMALS ON A WEIGHT-REDUCTION DIET

1. Obese weight – Ideal weight = Excess body fat
Example*: 24kg - 20kg = 4kg
2. Excess body fat x energy density/kg body fat = Total energy excess
   4g x 7700kcal [32217KJ]/kg fat = 30800kcal [12886KJ]
Estimated MER – energy/day being ingested = Daily energy deficit
1324kcal [5540KJ] - 794kcal [3322KJ] = 530kcal [2218KJ]/day
4. Total energy excess ÷ Daily energy deficit = Days required. to reach optional weight
30800kcal [12886KJ](2) ÷ 530kcal [2218KJ] (3) = 58 days

*The examples are continued from Fig.17.48 MER – metabolisable energy

Fig. 17.49. Calculation of time scale for weight loss in animals on a weight-reducing diet.

Before implementing a weight reduction programme, the animal must be weighed and a target weight chosen. The amount of food required can then be calculated (Fig. 17.48). An estimate of the time required for weight loss through partial energy restriction must also be made (Fig. 17.49) and owners given a goal to aim for, otherwise success will be limited. If a diet provides 60% of the animal's MER at its optimal weight, then weight loss is likely to occur at a steady rate of 3% per week for the first 6 weeks, slowing to 2% per week after 8 weeks. The animal should be fed 3 or 4 times a day and given moderate exercise. All animals on a weight reducing programme should be fed only the prescribed diet and should be weighed weekly.

Further Reading

Kallfelz, F. A. (ed.) *Clinical Nutrition.* Veterinary Clinics of North America Small Animal Practice May 1989. Published by W. B. Saunders.

Lewis, L. D., Morris, M. L. and Hand, M. S. (1987). *Small Animal Clinical Nutrition III.* Mark Morris Associates, Topeka, Kansas.

National Research Council (1986) *Nutrient Requirements of Cats.* National Academy Press, Washington.

National Research Council (1985) *Nutrient Requirements of Dogs.* National Academy Press, Washington.

Simpson, J. W., Anderson, R. S. and Markwell, P. J. (1993) *Clinical Nutrition of the Dog and Cat.* Blackwell Scientific Publications.

Tennant, B. J. and Willoughby, K. (1993) The use of enteral nutrition in small animal medicine. *Compendium on Continuing Education* **15**, 1054

Wills, J. M. and Simpson, K. W. (1994) *The Waltham Book of Clinical Nutrition of the Dog and Cat.* Pergamon, Oxford.

18
Genetics and Animal Breeding

S. E. LONG

Genetics is the science of inheritance, that is, the study of how characteristics are passed on from parents to offspring. These characteristics may be, for example, the colour of the eyes, the length of the fur or the type of enzyme that is produced by a cell. The information for all these factors and many more are located on special structures in the nucleus. These structures are the **chromosomes**.

Chromosomes

Chromosomes are composed of **chromatin fibres**, which are long molecules of **DNA** and associated protein.

DNA (deoxyribonucleic acid) has a unique structure. It consists of two strands, joined together rather like a ladder. The 'steps' of the ladder are formed by two bases, either adenine (A) and thymine (T) or guanine (G) and cytosine (C). A always links with T, and G always links with C. Thus the steps of the ladder are a sequence of **base pairs** and it is this sequence which forms the **genes** (see later). If on one side of the ladder there is a sequence of for example AGTAACGGC, then on the other side of the ladder the sequence *must* be TCATTGCCG (Fig. 18.1). The structure of the base pairs is such that they cause the sides of the ladder to twist, forming a double spiral, or double helix (meaning spiral). The DNA molecule is then very tightly folded and coiled to form the chromatin fibres of the chromosomes.

Each species has a characteristic number of chromosomes. For example, the number of chromosomes in the cell of a cat = 38 (Fig. 18.2), dog = 78, horse = 64. Two of these chromosomes are called the **sex chromosomes** and are designated **X** and **Y**. The female has two X chromosomes (XX), and the male has one of each of the sex chromosomes (XY). The other chromosomes, i.e. those that are not the sex chromosomes, are called **autosomes**. Chromosomes are usually considered in pairs because one of each pair is inherited from each parent. A chromosome pair is alike, one to another, and therefore are said to be **homologous** (meaning 'same'). If you were to weigh all the chromosomes from a cell in each of the different species, you would find that the total weight of the genetic material was more or less the same. In other words, they all have roughly the same amount of genetic material, but it is cut into a different number of pieces.

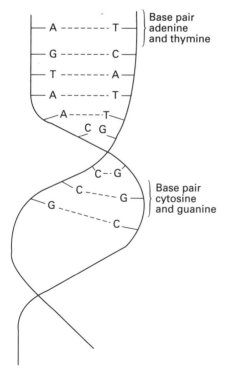

Fig. 18.1. Double helix structure of the DNA molecule.

Base pair adenine and thymine

Base pair cytosine and guanine

Genes

Genes are particular sequences of base pairs along the chain structure of DNA and *it is the genes that code for the characteristic* of the cell and hence the individual. Each gene is located on the chromosome at a particular position, which is called the gene **locus**.

The genes that are located on the sex chromosomes are said to be **sex-linked genes**. There are many more genes on the X chromosome than the Y chromosome so that sex-linked genes are more likely to be on the X than the Y. The orange coat-colour gene in the cat, or the gene for haemophilia A in the dog are examples of sex-linked genes on the X-chromosomes. Genes that can only be expressed in one sex, such as the genes associated with milk quality, are said to be **sex-limited** genes.

Some genes or gene combinations are not compatible with life and are said to be **lethal factors**. If an individual receives such a gene or genes, that individual dies.

If the chromosome is damaged at the site where the gene is located and there is mis-repair, i.e. the

S. E. Long

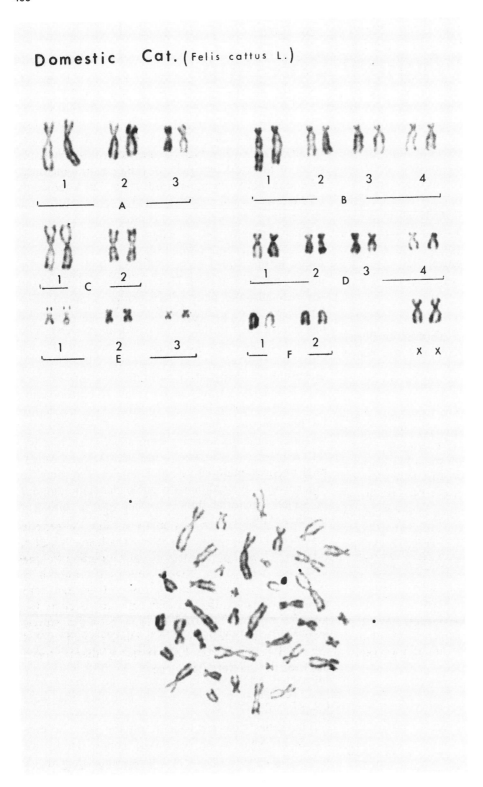

Fig. 18.2. Normal chromosome complement of a female cat. (Top: karyotype; bottom: spread.)

sequence of base pairs is not the same as it was before, then one of two things may happen:

- The sequence is so different that the code no longer exists and so the gene is destroyed.
- The sequence allows coding for the characteristic but in a slightly different way, i.e. there is a **gene mutation**.

Alleles

Two or more genes that occupy the same locus on the chromosome are said to be **alleles**. Alleles arise because of small mutations in genes which make their coded message slightly different from each other. They occupy the same locus because they are just slightly different versions of the same gene. Only one allele can occupy the locus at any one time but, since each animal receives chromosomes from the mother and the father, there will be two loci (one on each homologous chromosome) and thus two alleles in each cell. There can be any number of alleles—in some cases there are literally hundreds—but each cell can have only two because there is only 'space' for two on the chromosomes.

Dominant and Recessive Genes

If there are two different alleles in a cell, it might be expected that both alleles would be expressed. In fact this does happen in many circumstances and the genes are said to be **co-dominant** (e.g. genes coding for blood groups).

However, some alleles are only expressed if there are two copies of the same allele in the cell. These are said to be **recessive** genes. Genes that can be expressed when only one copy is present and which can suppress the other allele are said to be **dominant** genes.

The different actions of genes are symbolised by a capital letter for a dominant gene and a small letter for a recessive gene. For example, the gene for black coat colour in the Labrador is dominant to the gene that codes for brown that produces the chocolate (or liver) coat colour. Therefore, the black gene is designated *B* and the brown gene is designated *b*. A black Labrador can have either *BB* or *Bb* genes, because black is dominant to brown and the *B* gene will suppress the expression of the *b* gene. However, chocolate Labradors must all be *bb* because brown is recessive and can only be expressed if two copies of the allele are present.

If an animal has two copies of the same allele it is said to be **homozygous** for that allele. If an animal has two different alleles, it is said to be **heterozygous** ('hetero' implies 'different').

Epistasis

Some genes can suppress the expression of other genes that are not their alleles, i.e. they suppress the effect of genes on a different locus (e.g. the albino gene blocks the expression of all the coat-colour genes). These genes are said to show **epistasis**.

Genotype and Phenotype

It can been seen, from what has been discussed above, that two animals may look alike but have different genes. What the animal looks like is said to be its **phenotype**, whilst its genetic make-up is said to be its **genotype**.

Cell Cycle

When a cell is carrying out its normal functions, it is said to be in **interphase**. In order to replicate itself, it must first synthesise new genetic material and this is called the **synthesis** (or **S**) phase. This is followed by a resting stage called **G$_2$** (G stands for 'gap') and then there is separation of the new genetic material into the two new cells. This is the nuclear division **M** phase. The two new cells can then get on with their jobs and they are again said to be in interphase. There is thus a **cell cycle** (Fig. 18.3).

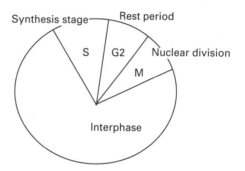

Fig. 18.3. The cell cycle.

Cell Replication

Mitosis

When a cell replicates, it is important that the genetic material (i.e. the chromosomes) replicates exactly, otherwise the new cells would not be coding for the same characteristics. Many cells are continually replicating (e.g. cells from the lining of the intestine) and it is important that the new cells can carry on the job of the old. The actual separation of the genetic material to the new cells is a dynamic process called mitotic division but for the purposes of description it has been divided into four stages:

(1) Prophase
(2) Metaphase
(3) Anaphase
(4) Telophase.

Prophase (Fig. 18.4)—This is the beginning of the division. The nuclear membrane breaks down and the chromatin contracts so that the chromosomes appear as separate objects. Synthesis of the new chromosomes has already taken place (in the S phase of the cell cycle) but they have not separated and appear held together at the **centromere**. Since they have not separated, the two identical chromosomes are called **chromatids**.

Metaphase (Fig. 18.5)—Once contracted down, the chromosomes line up in the middle of the cell and the two chromatids begin to repel each other. This is the stage at which the chromosomes are most easily seen under the light microscope.

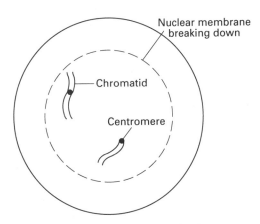

Fig. 18.4. Prophase in mitosis.

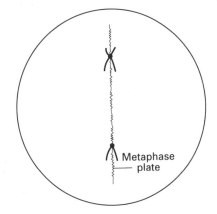

Fig. 18.5. Metaphase.

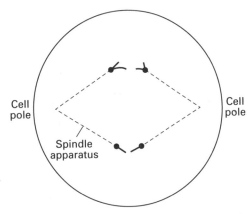

Fig. 18.6. Anaphase.

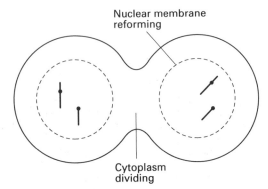

Fig. 18.7. Telophase.

Anaphase (Fig. 18.6)—The chromosomes become attached to the cell spindle, which is a series of fibres. As these fibres contract, the chromatids are pulled apart and the new chromosomes move towards the two poles of the cell.

Telophase (Fig. 18.7)—Once the chromosomes have reached the poles new nuclear membranes are formed, surrounding each set, and the cytoplasm begins to divide. The resulting two new cells are genetically identical to each other and to the cell from which they originated.

Meiosis

Whereas mitosis is the type of cell division that is undertaken by most cells in the body, a different type of cell division is necessary for those cells (the oogonia and spermatogonia) that are going to develop into gametes (ova and sperm). This is called **meiotic** division and its stages are similar to those of mitotic division. However, it is a longer and more complicated process because the chromosomes have to be separated into different gametes in such a way that the total number is reduced by half and yet there is still one copy of each pair of alleles that was present in the parent cell. In this way, when two gametes fuse to form a zygote, the new individual has the right number of chromosomes for the species and the right combination of genes in order that each cell can do its job. Each individual receives half its chromosomes (and thus half the genes) from one parent and half from the other.

During the stages of meiotic division, new DNA is synthesised in the S phase of the cell cycle, as with mitosis, and the new chromosomes are held together at the centromeres. However, the prophase in meiosis is much longer than in mitosis.

Prophase (Fig. 18.8)—The nuclear membrane disappears, the chromosomes contract down and the homologous pairs line up side by side. (*In mitosis, the homologous chromosomes do not lie side by side.*) Effectively, there are four chromosomes lying together (i.e. the homologous pair each comprised of two chromatids held together at the centromere).

The four chromatids become entwined and exchange segments. This is called **crossing over**. The homologous chromosomes then begin to try to pull apart. (Because this is such a long procedure, meiotic prophase is subdivided into five stages: leptotene, zygotene, pachytene, diplotene and diakinesis.)

Metaphase (I) (Fig. 18.9)—The homologous pairs of chromosomes line up in the centre of the cell and start to attach to the spindle apparatus.

Anaphase (I) (Fig. 18.10)—The spindle fibres contract and the homologous chromosomes are separated and move to the opposite poles of the cell. (*In mitosis, this is the stage where the two chromatids separate.*)

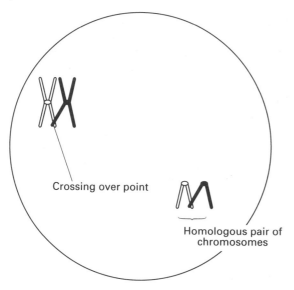

Fig. 18.8. Diplotene of meiotic prophase.

Telophase (I) (Fig. 18.11)—The cytoplasm begins to divide but there is no reconstitution of the nuclear membrane. (*In mitosis, the nuclear membrane reforms at this stage.*) In some cells the cytoplasmic division is completed and in others the cell forms a dumb-bell like structure or **syncytium**.

The cell now immediately goes into a second division which is exactly like a normal mitotic division.

Prophase—This is transitory because the chromosomes have already contracted.

Metaphase (II) (Fig. 18.12)—The chromosomes line up in the centre of the cell and attach to the spindle apparatus. The chromatids begin to repel each other.

Anaphase (II) (Fig. 18.13)—The spindle fibres contract; the chromatids pull apart at the centromeres and move towards opposite poles of the cells.

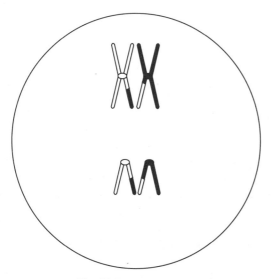

Fig. 18.9. Metaphase I.

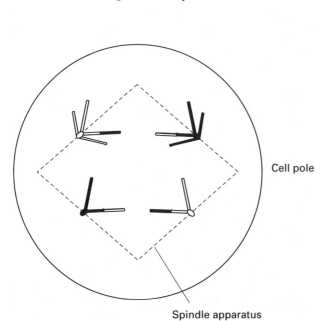

Fig. 18.10. Anaphase I.

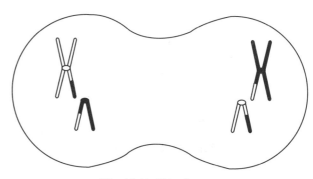

Fig. 18.11. Telophase I.

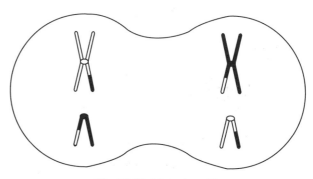

Fig. 18.12. Metaphase II.

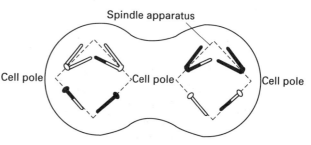

Fig. 18.13. Anaphase II.

S. E. Long

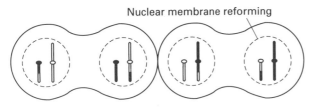

Fig. 18.14. Telophase II.

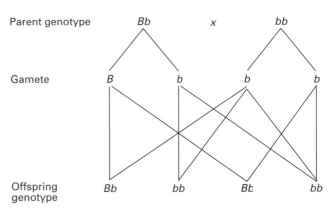

Fig. 18.15. Backcross to the recessive homozygous animal.

Telophase (II) (Fig. 18.14)—The cytoplasm begins to divide and the nuclear membrane reforms.

Thus from one original cell, four new cells are formed which contain half the original number of chromosomes. The new individual inherits the genetic material from each parent but with some variation because of the crossing over.

Mendel's First Law

Mendel's first law describes the outcome of meiosis. Mendel (1822–1884) was an Austrian monk and a biologist. He did not know anything about chromosomes or the mechanism of cell division but he knew that the process was orderly and organised such that the outcome of different matings could be predicted.

> Mendel's first law states: **Alleles separate to different gametes.**

Identification of Animals Carrying a Recessive Gene

Animals homozygous for a particular gene will always breed true when bred together but heterozygous animals will sometimes produce offspring which are homozygous for the recessive gene. Usually (but not always), the recessive gene is unwanted so that breeders would like to be able to identify those animals that are heterozygous for a recessive gene and avoid breeding from them. Identification of the recessive carrier can be done by test mating to either a homozygous recessive animal or to a known heterozygous recessive carrier.

Crossing to a Homozygous Recessive Animal

If you have a black Labrador and you want to know whether its genotype is *BB* or *Bb*, you can cross it with a chocolate or liver pigment (*bb*) Labrador (Fig. 18.15):

- If the black Labrador is *BB*, then all the offspring will be black (although with the genotype of *Bb*).
- If the black Labrador is *Bb*, it will still produce black puppies, but it will also produce chocolate (*bb*) puppies.

Instead of drawing the diagram as in Fig. 18.15, it could be written as a checkerboard (Figure 18.16).

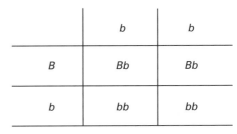

Fig. 18.16. Checkerboard illustrating the genotype of the offspring when heterozygous black (*Bb*) is mated to the homozygous brown (*bb*).

It can be calculated mathematically that if the black Labrador produces *seven* black puppies when mated to a chocolate Labrador, you can be 99% sure that its genotype is *BB*. The more black puppies that are produced, the more sure you can be that the genotype is *BB*. If even one chocolate puppy is produced, irrespective of the number of black, then you *know* that the black Labrador must be *Bb*. You do not have to mate your black Labrador to the same chocolate Labrador to get the offspring—it is the number of offspring that is important.

Crossing to a Known Heterozygous Animal

If there are no homozygous recessive animals available, it is possible to carry out the test mating with a known carrier of the recessive gene. For example, if a second black Labrador has previously produced a chocolate puppy, it must be *Bb*. The first black Labrador (which could be either *BB* or *Bb*) can be mated to the second (*Bb*) black Labrador (Fig. 18.17). The checkerboard for this mating would be as in Fig. 18.18.

This time *sixteen* black puppies would have to be produced before you could be 99% sure that the animal was *BB*. Again, these puppies do not have to be produced from one single mating and the birth of only one chocolate puppy in any litter by the same mating will prove that the dog was *Bb*.

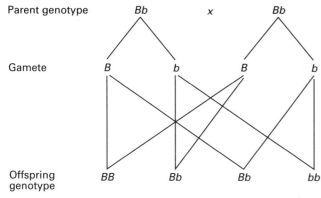

Parent genotype   Bb   x   Bb

Gamete   B   b   B   b

Offspring genotype   BB   Bb   Bb   bb

Fig. 18.17. Backcross to the recessive heterozygous animal.

	B	b
B	BB	Bb
b	Bb	bb

Fig. 18.18. Checkerboard illustrating the genotype of the offspring when a heterozygous black (*Bb*) is mated to a heterozygous black (*Bb*).

Both these matings (i.e. to a homozygous recessive animal or to a known heterozygous animal) are called the **backcross to the recessive**. The animals that are mated are the **parent** generation and the offspring are the **filial** or F_1 generation. If the offspring were to be mated they would produce the F_2 generation and so on.

Inheritance of More Than One Pair of Genes

Animals have a large number of genes but each is inherited without being influenced by the presence of other genes. This is Mendel's second law.

> Mendel's second law states: **Each pair of alleles separates independently of every other pair of alleles.**

There are exceptions to this law due to **linkage**. Genes separate independently because of the processes during meiosis, in particular because of the phenomenon of crossing over. This causes genes on the same chromosome to be separated. However, the closer that two genes lie on the chromosome, the less likely it is that the crossing over will separate them. Therefore, genes lying close to each other on a chromosome are said to be **linked** and if an animal inherits one of the linked genes it is very likely that it will inherit the other gene as well. This is an advantage if both genes are desirable but a big disadvantage if a breeder is trying to retain one gene and eradicate the other.

Multifactorial Inheritance and the Influence of Environment

Some characteristics are governed by single genes but many others are controlled by the combination of a number of genes. Such characteristics are said to be **polygenic** (meaning many genes). Variation in the genes controlling these polygenic traits will cause a variation in the characteristic. Furthermore, the degree to which these genes can be expressed may be influenced by the environment. In other words the final production of a characteristic is **multifactorial** (meaning having many causes). For example, the size of a dog will depend upon its genes but also on the amount of food that is available. There is great scope for variation but polygenic characteristics are difficult to control by selective breeding because of the number of different factors that are involved.

Breeding Strategies

When breeders wish to ensure that animals breed true, they try to make them homozygous for the genes governing the desirable characteristics. One method is by **inbreeding**, which is the breeding of two individuals more closely related than the population as a whole.

Related individuals are more likely to have the same alleles and so more likely to produce offspring that will be homozygous for the genes. The more closely they are related, the more likely it is that they will have the same alleles. Therefore, the closer the inbreeding, the more likely it is that the offspring will be homozygous. Inbreeding is a very good way of 'fixing' a characteristic (i.e. creating homozygosity) but *inbreeding will fix the 'bad' alleles as well as the good*. This is why inbreeding is generally regarded as dangerous.

Line breeding is a form of inbreeding. It involves mating within a certain family or line and aims to maintain a relationship with a particular ancestor (e.g. a show champion). In general, although the animals that are mated are related, they are not as closely related as, for example, father and daughter or brother and sister. They are more likely to be grandparents and grandchildren or cousins. In this way it is hoped that the 'bad' alleles will be different in the two animals to be mated and so not be homozygous in the offspring.

If breeders wish to mask the effects of recessive genes that are considered to be 'bad' then the simplest method is outcrossing or **outbreeding**—the mating of two individuals less closely related than the population as a whole.

The rationale behind this is that such individuals are unlikely to have the same alleles and so the offspring will be heterozygous. Outbreeding masks the effects of recessive genes and results in **hybrid vigour** or **heterosis**. The offspring of an outcross seem to be 'bigger and better' than their parents because they are heterozygous for 'bad' recessive genes which therefore are not expressed. Unfortunately, such individuals will not breed true because they are heterozygous and not homozygous for their alleles.

COMMON INHERITED GENETIC DEFECTS

Inherited defects in the dog

Hip dysplasia	An abnormality of the hip joint. Multifactorial. Eradication scheme: the BVA/KC hip dysplasia scheme. Minimum age of dog entering scheme is one year. Hips are X-rayed by client's own veterinary surgeon and plates are sent to BVA. Panel of scrutineers scores each hip, minimum score 0 to maximum of 53. Mean score for any breed represents overall hip status of that breed. All breeders wishing to control hip dysplasia should breed only from animals with scores well below the breed mean. BVA informs Kennel Club of registered dogs with a score of 8 or less, or not more than 6 on one hip.
Eye defects	Many different defects with different genetic origins. BVA/Kennel Club/International Sheepdog Society eye scheme to monitor inherited ocular disease. Conditions considered are: Central progressive retinal atrophy (CPRA) Generalised progressive retinal atrophy (GPRA) Hereditary cataract (HC) Primary lens luxation (PLL) Gonodysgenesis/primary glaucoma Collie eye anomaly (CEA) Retinal dysplasia (RD) Persistent pupillary membrane (PPM) Congenital cataract (CHC) Persistent hyperplastic primary vitreous (PHPV). Different conditions seen in different breeds at different ages. Animals examined by member of eye scheme panel (not by client's own veterinary surgeon) to whom they are referred by client's veterinary surgeon. Recommended that examination be carried out each year. Result is sent to BVA and also (in case of KC registered dogs) to KC and/or ISDS for publication.
Entropion	Inward turning of the eyelid. Polygenic.
Ectropion	Outward turning of the eyelid. Polygenic.
Cryptorchidism	Failure of one testis (unilateral) or both testes (bilateral) to descend into the scrotum. Mode of inheritance unknown but possibly polygenic.
Umbilical hernia	Protrusion of tissue through the umbilical ring. Probably polygenic.
Merle	Incomplete dominant gene. Homozygotes have white coats, blue eyes which are smaller than normal, with a lack of tapetum, and predisposition to glaucoma. Also often deaf. Heterozygotes have white markings on the head and shoulders and dappled coat or normal and dilute markings. Only matings of Merle with normal are to be recommended in order to avoid producing abnormal homozygote.
Scottie cramp	Rigidity of muscles brought on by excitement or strenuous exercise. Autosomal recessive.
Progressive axonopathy	Axon degeneration of motor nerve fibres. Condition confined to boxers. Due to an autosomal recessive gene.
Haemophilia	Failure in the clotting mechanism of blood. At least nine different types of haemophilia due to different abnormalities of complex cascade of reactions necessary to achieve normal clotting of blood. Haemophilia A (factor VIII deficiency) is most common and is sex-linked.

Some common inherited abnormalities in the cat

Manx	Taillessness. Associated with other abnormalities of conformation of vertebral column. Autosomal dominant. Homozygous is lethal.
Deafness	Due to dominant White gene. Affected cats white with blue eyes.
Polydactyly	Extra toes on front feet. Autosomal dominant.
Flat-chested kitten syndrome	Seen in Burmese breed. Affected kittens show breathing difficulties and do poorly. Probably autosomal recessive.
Folded-ears	Incomplete dominant. Heterozygote has folded ears but homozygote also has abnormalities of the epiphyses leading to a thickened tail, swollen feet and disinclination to move.

Fig. 18.19. Inherited defects in the dog and cat.

Breed Variation

Selection for various characteristics has resulted in a number of different breeds. This has been more extensive with dogs than with cats. Dogs can be divided into six breed groups recognised by the English Kennel Club:

- Hounds
- Gundogs
- Terriers
- Utility dogs
- Working dogs
- Toys.

Cats have not undergone such intensive selection for such a long period and are usually just divided simply into long- and short-hair breeds. However, there is considerable variation in the body size, length of head and coat colour.

The breeds of dogs and cats are listed on pages 177–185.

Deformities and Malformations

Any deviation from the normal anatomy is described as a malformation or deformity. This can arise during foetal development or be acquired during life.

Congenital Abnormalities

When a malformation is present at birth it is said to be **congenital**. Congenital abnormalities may or may not be genetic in origin. The term simply means that it was present at birth. Sometimes, congenital abnormalities that are not caused by a genetic defect look exactly like inherited abnormalities and are said to be **phenocopies** (meaning copies of what the animal looks like). It can be extremely difficult to determine whether or not an abnormality is genetic in origin.

Inherited Defects

Inherited defects are caused by the genes acquired from the parents. Some common inherited genetic defects are shown in Fig. 18.19.

Further Reading

Nicholas, F. W. (1987) *Veterinary Genetics.* Clarendon, Oxford.

Robinson, R. (1990) *Genetics for Dog Breeders.* 2nd ed. Pergamon, Oxford.

Robinson, R. (1991) *Genetics for Cat Breeders.* 3rd ed. Pergamon, Oxford.

19

Obstetric and Paediatric Nursing of the Dog and Cat

G. C. W. ENGLAND

Breeding from a dog or cat should not be undertaken lightly; both the male and female should be carefully assessed and should be clinically sound, free from hereditary diseases, have excellent temperaments, be good examples of the breed and should be free from infectious disease. Many animals which are used at stud do not meet these criteria.

There are both moral and legal responsibilities (under the Sale of Goods Act) for breeders of animals to ensure that the offspring are clinically healthy and have a sound temperament. There are many hereditary defects which should preclude animals from breeding including the presence of congenital cardiac disease, congenital cleft palate, bleeding disorders and disorders of other systems proven to be hereditary in nature. In the case of cryptorchidism the affected dog and both parents should be considered to be carriers and should not be used for breeding.

Two schemes created in collaboration with the Kennel Club and the British Veterinary Association aim to control the incidence of hereditary diseases in pedigree dogs. The BVA/Kennel Club/International Sheepdog Society **Eye Scheme** is designed for the control of specific known inherited conditions such as central and generalised progressive retinal atrophy, hereditary cataract, primary glaucoma, primary lens luxation, collie eye anomaly, retinal dysplasia, persistent pupillary membrane and persistent hyperplastic primary vitreous (other conditions are under investigation). Dogs should be examined every 12 months to ensure that they remain clear from the hereditary condition. This is very important for certain diseases (such as hereditary cataracts and certain retinopathies) which are not evident at birth. However in practice examination generally ceases when the dog exceeds the age at which the disease is commonly identified.

The BVA/Kennel Club **Hip Dysplasia Scheme** is designed to help control hip dysplasia in pedigree dogs. Dogs are usually radiographed on one occasion after they reach 12 months of age. The radiographs are assessed on 9 detailed points and are scored for abnormality; radiographically normal hips score zero (0:0) and the maximum score is 106. Breed averages are regularly published, and it is hoped that breeding from animals with scores less than the average will result in improved quality of hips in subsequent generations.

Other schemes have been adopted by certain breed societies to monitor the level of specific diseases. One example is the monitoring of Dobermann pinscher dogs for cervical spondylopathy. Certain breed societies have established codes of conduct which aim to control the number of litters bred per bitch and the age of first mating. The Kennel Club will not register pups born from bitches over the age of 7 years.

Potential breeders should take advice from many sources before breeding from any male or female animal.

The Male

Male dogs and tom cats are sexually active throughout the year, although a minor seasonal effect may be noted in some countries. The testes are descended into the scrotum at birth in the cat, and are descended into the scrotum 10 days after birth in the dog. Both pups and kittens may show sexual activity from several weeks of age, but puberty does not occur until 6 to 12 months in the dog and 8 to 12 months in the cat. For both species **spermatogenesis** (the production of spermatozoa) commences at approximately 5 months of age.

It is preferable not to use a male at stud until he is at least 12 months of age, since it is not possible to evaluate his qualities fully until this time, and even then the occurrence of certain hereditary diseases may not be apparent. It is advisable that the first mating attempts should be with an experienced female.

The fertile lifespan of a male varies considerably, and is probably related to the longevity of that particular breed. It is certain, however, that seminal quality of male stud dogs is reduced from 7 years of age onwards.

Endocrinology

The interstitial (**Leydig**) cells are the source of **testosterone** production from the testes. The production of this hormone is stimulated by **luteinising hormone** (LH), a gonadotrophin hormone released from the pituitary gland. A second pituitary gonadotrophin called **follicle-stimulating hormone** (FSH) appears to increase the process of sperm production directly via the **Sertoli cells**. Testosterone has a negative feedback effect upon the release of FSH and LH which is mediated by **gonadotrophin releasing hormone** (GnRH).

Control of Reproduction

The majority of male dogs do not cause problems if they remain entire but there are situations where control of 'antisocial' behaviour may necessitate the control of male hormone release. The situation in the entire tom cat is rather different because the problems of territory marking, roaming and aggression are greater than in the dog.

Chemical control of reproductive function can be achieved in both species on a short-term basis with exogenous hormones which suppress the normal release of testosterone. The most commonly used agents include the **progestogens** (drugs with progesterone-like activity) which may be administered orally on a daily basis (e.g. megestrol acetate), or as a depot injection (e.g. proligestone or delmadinone acetate). These drugs reduce libido but do not produce infertility. No single drug is commercially available as a male contraceptive agent; complicated drug regimes are required for this effect.

The most common method for the regulation of sexual activity is **castration** which is not reversible. Castration before puberty may result in failure of development of the secondary sexual characteristics. In some males a change in metabolic rate may result in increased body weight. Castration after puberty and correct dietary control eliminate the majority of problems associated with castration.

Diseases of the Reproductive Tract

A variety of conditions may affect the reproductive organs of the tom cat and the male dog.

Endocrinological abnormalities

Primary abnormalities in the secretion of pituitary hormones may result in the poor development of gonadal tissue—a condition called **hypogonadism**. This is rare but has been reported in both species.

Diseases of the testes

An absence of the testes (**anorchia**) is very rare. More often, the testes fail to descend and are retained within the abdomen. This condition is known as **cryptorchidism**, which literally means 'hidden testicle'. Often the condition is unilateral with one testicle present within the scrotum and the other retained within the abdomen. These cases are often wrongly called monorchids; true **monorchidism** refers to an animal with a single testicle. Some cryptorchid animals are bilaterally affected and testes are not seen within the scrotum. The treatment for all cryptorchids is removal of both testes, because of the

high incidence of neoplasia within the abdominal testis, and the fact that the condition is likely to be inherited.

Inflammation of the testes (**orchitis**) is rare but may follow trauma or ascending bacterial infection.

Testicular tumours are the second most common tumour affecting the male dog but are rare in the tom cat. There are three common tumour types. Some of these may be endocrinologically active and secrete female hormones which produce signs of feminisation.

Diseases of the accessory glands

The prostate gland in the male dog is the only accessory sex gland. The tom cat has both prostate and bulbourethral glands but disease of either is rare.

Prostate abnormalities in the dog are common and include benign enlargement (**hyperplasia**), bacterial prostatitis, prostatic cysts and prostatic tumours. The clinical signs of these diseases may be similar; they include difficulty in urinating and defecating, and the presence of blood within urine and/or semen.

Diseases of the penis and prepuce

It is common for there to be a purulent discharge from the prepuce of the male dog which should be considered normal unless it is excessive. It is not seen in the tom cat.

Phimosis is a condition where there is inability to extrude the penis due to an abnormally small preputial orifice. This may occur either congenitally or as a result of trauma or inflammation, and may result in pain during erection. **Paraphimosis** is a failure to retract the penis into the prepuce and may also be due to a small preputial orifice. The penis becomes dry and necrotic and urethral obstruction may result. **Priapism** refers to the persistent enlargement of the penis in the absence of sexual excitement.

Antisocial behaviour

In many cases behaviour which may be normal for a male animal is considered to be antisocial by man. These problems include territory marking, mounting inappropriate objects and aggression towards other males. They often necessitate treatment, which may include behavioural modification therapy in conjunction with drugs that inhibit male hormone production such as progestogens. Castration may be required in certain cases.

Normal Mating

The sexual behaviour of the tom cat and male dog are considerably different from each other and from other species. It is important that the events of natural mating are known so that abnormalities can be recognised whilst remembering that the modern mating environment is often artificial. On the 'day of mating', bitches and queens are frequently transported long distances, are introduced to the male briefly and then expected to mate immediately. This situation eliminates the normal courtship phase associated with proestrus behaviour and may result in mating problems. In addition, many females are presented to the male at an inappropriate time, either because this is convenient for the owner or because of inexact assessment of the stage of the oestrous cycle. In these events sexual behaviour of both the male and female may not be optimal.

The domestic dog

The dog and bitch normally exhibit play behaviour when first introduced. The bitch will then usually settle and stand with her tail deviated to one side to allow mating. This is not always the case and it may be necessary to steady the bitch by holding her at the head. The dog may ejaculate a small volume of clear fluid before mounting; this does not contain sperm and is termed the **first fraction**. It originates from the prostate gland and probably flushes urine and cellular debris from the urethra. After mounting the dog commences slow thrusting movements until the penile tip enters the vulva. At this stage thrusting movements become rapid and the penis enters the vagina (**intromission**) and the dog achieves a full erection. The **second fraction** (which contains sperm) is then ejaculated, following which the dog turns through 180° and dismounts from the bitch whilst the penis is still within the vagina. This is called the **tie**. It is associated with ejaculation of the **third fraction** of the ejaculate, the function of which is to flush sperm forwards through the cervix into the uterus. This stage may last for 20 minutes or longer in some dogs.

The domestic tom

The period of sexual introduction and play is variable in the cat depending upon the experience and aggression of the male. The normal sequence of events occurs rapidly compared with the dog. The male usually approaches the female from the side or back and grasps her neck in his mouth. Whilst maintaining this grasp he mounts the female and positions himself to align the genital regions. The queen normally lowers her chest and elevates the pelvic region whilst deviating her tail. Pelvic thrusting and ejaculation occur rapidly. During intromission the queen often emits a cry and attempts to end mating by rolling, turning and striking at the male. The female then exhibits a marked postcoital reaction consisting of violent rolling and excessive licking. She will not allow further mating at this time.

Assessment of Fertility

Male fertility may be assessed by the evaluation of semen quality. Semen may be collected by stimulating the male dog to ejaculate by hand; artificial vaginas are no longer used for this purpose. Semen collection is more difficult in the tom cat, and may require general anaesthesia and electroejaculation. A special artificial vagina may be used to collect from trained tom cats. Collection equipment should be warmed before use.

Semen, once collected, should be placed into a water bath at body temperature to prevent damage to the sperm. The second fraction of the dog ejaculate and the entire cat ejaculate should be used for evaluation.

(1) The volume should be measured and the colour recorded.
(2) After gently mixing the sample, a drop should be placed upon a warmed microscope slide and a subjective assessment made of the percentage of sperm with vigorous forward progression.
(3) The spermatozoal concentration should be measured using a haemocytometer counting chamber and the total sperm output should be calculated by multiplying this value with the volume of the sample.
(4) A portion of the sample should then be stained to allow the differentiation of live and dead sperm and the assessment of spermatozoal morphology. A combination of the two stains nigrosin and eosin is suitable for this purpose (Fig. 19.1).

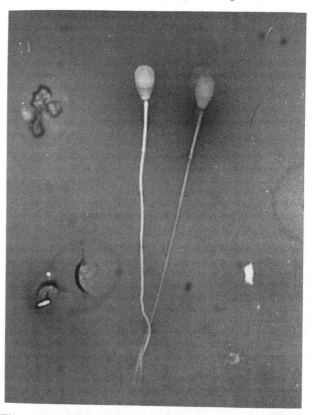

Fig. 19.1. Photomicrograph of a live normal dog spermatozoon (left) and a dead dog spermatozoon with a detached acrosome (right). The specimen has been stained with nigrosin and eosin; the dead sperm appears pink (grey in the black-and-white photograph) whilst the live sperm remains unstained (white).

The semen characteristics of fertile dogs is given in Fig. 19.2.

The Female

The domestic bitch

Bitches generally have one or two oestrous cycles per year followed by a variable period of acyclicity. The bitch is **polytocous** (produces numerous offspring in each litter) and the oestrous periods are non-seasonal and terminate in spontaneous ovulation. The interval between each cycle can vary between 5 and 13 months, the average being 7 months.

The domestic queen

Queens have multiple oestrous cycles each year. They are **seasonally polyoestrus**, and typically cycle from February to September. Ovulation is induced by coitus and the interval between each oestrous cycle varies depending upon whether the queen has ovulated, or fails to ovulate either because she is not mated or because there is insufficient hormone release at mating. Unmated queens return to oestrus at intervals of 14 to 21 days.

Puberty

The domestic bitch

In the bitch the onset of cyclical activity (puberty) is normally between 6 and 23 months of age, with most bitches having their first oestrus by the age of 12 to 14 months. Bitches that do not exhibit oestrous behaviour by the anticipated age are considered to have delayed puberty but it should be remembered that many normal bitches will not cycle until they are 2 years old. The majority of bitches start to cycle about 6 months after they have reached adult height and weight, which may explain some of the variations exhibited between breeds.

The domestic queen

Female cats generally exhibit their first oestrus at 6 to 9 months of age, but this is dependent upon the **photoperiod** (day length). Those which are born in the summer frequently commence cycling at the first spring; those which are born in the winter may not cycle until they are least 12 months of age.

The Oestrous Cycle

The domestic bitch

The stages of the oestrous cycle in the bitch are proestrus, oestrus, metoestrus (dioestrus) and anoestrus. The terms **in season** or **in heat** are used to indicate the stage of the cycle when the bitch is receptive to the male dog, i.e. oestrus.

During **proestrus** the bitch is receptive to the dog but will not allow mating. **Oestrus** commences when the bitch will accept the male and it is during this stage that the eggs are released from the ovaries, a process known as **ovulation**. Ovulation in the bitch occurs spontaneously towards the end of oestrus. Each egg is contained within a fluid-filled structure called a **follicle**. Many follicles are present in each ovary. After ovulation the follicle develops into a solid structure called a **corpus luteum**. One corpus luteum forms from each follicle that has ovulated and the corpus luteum produces a hormone called **progesterone**.

In many species the phase of progesterone production (the **luteal phase**) is divided into two: the early luteal phase is termed **metoestrus** and the mature luteal phase is termed **dioestrus**. However, in the bitch the early luteal phase occurs during **standing oestrus** (i.e. when the bitch will stand to be mated), making this terminology difficult to adopt (since metoestrus would then be occurring during oestrus). In the bitch the terms metoestrus and dioestrus are therefore often used synonymously to reflect the luteal phase of the cycle after the end of standing oestrus. This phase is therefore characterised by the presence of corpora lutea within the ovaries and the presence of the hormone progesterone in the blood.

The bitch is unusual compared with other species in that the duration of metoestrus is similar whether the bitch is pregnant or not (Fig. 19.3). This explains why the condition known as false or **pseudopregnancy** is common in the bitch (see later). Metoestrus is followed by a period of quiescence termed **anoestrus**.

The hormonal changes of the oestrous cycle are shown in Fig. 19.4.

Late anoestrus. During late anoestrus two hormones are released from the pituitary gland: **follicle

THE MEAN SEMINAL CHARACTERISTICS FROM 30 FERTILE STUD DOGS				
	Motility (%)	**Volume (ml)**	**Concentration** $(10^6$ml)	**Total sperm Output** (10^6)
Mean	85	1.3	310	400
Range	42–92	0.4–3.4	50–560	36–620
	Live Normal (%)	**Dead Normal (%)**	**Primary Abnormal (%)**	**Secondary Abnormal (%)**
Mean	75	10	2	10
Range	52–90	2–26	0–12	2–24

There is a wide range of normal values associated with fertility.

Fig. 19.2. Mean seminal characteristics in 30 stud dogs.

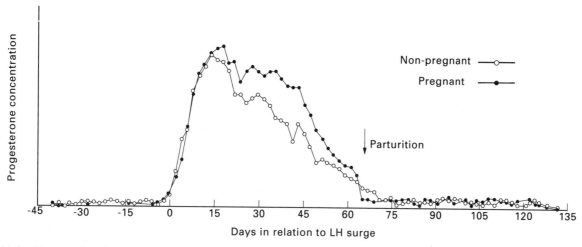

Fig. 19.3. Changes in plasma progesterone concentration in the pregnant and non-pregnant cycle of the bitch. The pregnant cycle demonstrates a more rapid decline in progesterone concentration immediately prior to parturition. Progesterone concentrations cannot be used as a method of pregnancy diagnosis in the bitch.

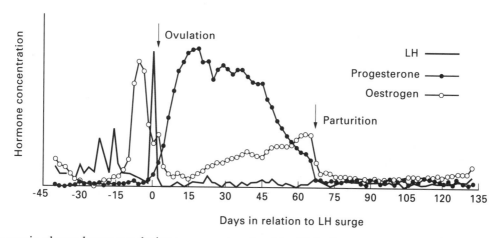

Fig. 19.4. Changes in plasma hormones during a pregnant cycle of the bitch. Oestrogen concentrations are elevated during proestrus, oestrus and late pregnancy. The LH surge stimulates ovulation which occurs within 36–48 hours of its peak. Progesterone is released before ovulation from luteinisation of follicles and subsequently from the corpora lutea.

stimulating hormone (FSH) and **luteinising hormone** (LH). These initiate the growth of follicles within the ovaries and cause the follicles to produce the hormone **oestrogen**.

Proestrus. Proestrus is characterised by increased plasma concentrations of oestrogen which cause swelling of the vulva and the development of a serosanguineous vulval discharge. Oestrogens also induce the release of specific pheromones which are responsible for attracting male dogs. During proestrus the bitch will not allow mating but may show increased receptivity to the male. This period lasts for approximately 7 days. Oestrogens also cause thickening of the vaginal wall and an increase in the number of epithelial cell layers. During proestrus the elevated concentrations of oestrogen have a negative feedback effect upon the release of the gonadotrophin hormones from the pituitary gland, and the

concentrations of FSH and LH are reduced compared with late anoestrus.

Oestrus. During oestrus the bitch demonstrates characteristic behaviour towards the male dog including deviation of the tail and presentation of the vulva and perineum. The bitch will stand to be mated. This period lasts for approximately 7 days. The onset of oestrus is related to a decline in the concentration of plasma oestrogen and at the same time the production of progesterone. The bitch is unusual in that progesterone is produced in low concentrations by luteinisation of the follicle, a process which occurs before ovulation. In many species progesterone is only produced after ovulation. This decline in the concentration of oestrogen and the slight increase in the concentration of progesterone are responsible for stimulating a surge of both FSH and LH. This surge is the trigger for ovulation which occurs approximately 2 days later. It can therefore be seen that the hormonal stimulus for ovulation occurs during standing oestrus and that the release of eggs also occurs during this period. Corpora lutea form after ovulation and produce greater amounts of progesterone. The end of standing oestrus is associated with relatively high concentrations of progesterone in the blood.

Metoestrus (dioestrus). The period of metoestrus lasts whilst the corpora lutea continue to produce progesterone and is approximately 55 days in length. In the pregnant bitch the period of metoestrus is synonymous with pregnancy, for the birth of pups occurs when progesterone secretion is terminated. In the non-pregnant bitch the corpora lutea persist for a similar period.

Towards the end of metoestrus a hormone called **prolactin** is released from the pituitary gland. This is responsible for the development of mammary tissue and the onset of lactation. Prolactin is produced in both the pregnant and the non-pregnant bitch, and is the reason why pseudopregnancy is a common event in the bitch.

Anoestrus. Metoestrus is followed by a period of quiescence, during which time there is effectively no hormonal activity. In the nonpregnant bitch there is no sudden decline in the concentration of progesterone but values gradually reduce and the transition to anoestrus is smooth. The situation is slightly different at the end of pregnancy because progesterone concentrations rapidly decline, and it is this event which stimulates the onset of parturition. The length of anoestrus varies considerably between bitches, but it is 4 months on average.

The domestic queen

The stages of the oestrous cycle in the queen are anoestrus, proestrus, oestrus and interoestrus. The terms 'in season' or 'in heat' are used to indicate the stage of the cycle when the cat is receptive to the male, i.e. **oestrus**. During winter there is effectively no hormone activity; the queen is in **anoestrus**. In springtime cyclical activity commences and in the unmated queen periods of sexual activity (proestrus and oestrus) are interrupted by periods of non-receptivity (**interoestrus**). If the queen is mated and ovulation is induced the queen enters either metoestrus or pregnancy. **Pregnancy** follows a fertile mating; **metoestrus** (also called pseudopregnancy) follows a sterile mating and its duration in the queen is shorter than that of pregnancy (Fig. 19.5), unlike the situation in the bitch.

Proestrus. Follicular development occurs during this phase due to the release of LH and FSH. This causes the secretion of oestrogen which is responsible for the development of the signs of proestrus, including attraction of the male and the changes in the vaginal epithelium similar to those seen in the bitch. Proestrus in the queen is often poorly recognised unless a male is present, but during this stage the queen will not accept mating. Proestrus lasts for 2 to 3 days.

Oestrus. The exact hormonal changes which cause the onset of standing oestrus are uncertain, although this may be associated with declining concentrations of oestrogen similar to that seen in the bitch.

The clinical signs of oestrus (also termed **calling**) include persistent vocalisation, rolling and rubbing against inanimate objects. In the presence of the male the queen may show persistent treading of the hind feet, lateral deviation of the tail and lordosis of the spine. Oestrus lasts between 2 and 10 days.

Interoestrus. In the absence of mating, or when mating does not result in ovulation, the signs of oestrus gradually decline and the queen enters a

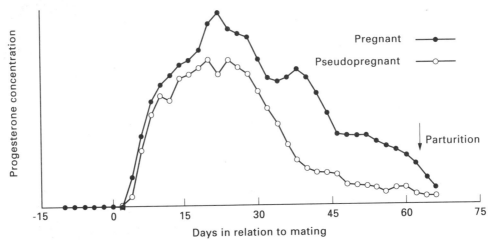

Fig. 19.5. Changes in plasma progesterone concentration in the pregnant and pseudopregnant (ovulation but without conception) cycle of the domestic queen. The pseudopregnant queen returns to cyclical activity 40–45 days after oestrus when progesterone concentrations return to basal values.

stage of nonreceptivity. This period may last for between 3 and 14 days. After this time the queen returns to proestrus and oestrus.

Pregnancy. Ovulation in the queen is caused by the release of LH which is stimulated by mating. Each mating results in a surge of LH, but there appears to be a threshold value below which ovulation will not be induced. Multiple matings are therefore more likely to result in ovulation than are single matings.

Ovulation is followed by an increase in the plasma concentration of progesterone released from the newly formed corpora lutea. Peak progesterone concentrations are reached approximately one month after mating and are maintained for the duration of pregnancy, which varies between 64 and 68 days. It is not uncommon for queens to have an absence of cyclical activity during lactation. This has been called **lactational anoestrus**.

Metoestrus (pseudopregnancy). Non-fertile matings result in ovulation without conception. Ovulation may also occur following stimulation of the vagina (e.g. following collection of a vaginal smear) or of the perineum (which may be self-induced), or it may occur spontaneously in some queens. Ovulation results in the formation of corpora lutea and the production of progesterone in a similar manner to early pregnancy. After approximately 40 days progesterone concentrations decline and the queen returns to cyclical activity. Should pseudopregnancy occur late in the year (autumn) the queen may not return to cyclical activity but may enter anoestrus.

Determination of the Optimum Time for Mating

The domestic bitch

The determination of the time of ovulation is important because the bitch is monoestrous and the mean interoestrus interval is 31 weeks. The clinical signs of oestrus are not always reliable indicators of the time of ovulation; in many bitches the behavioural signs do not correlate well with the changes in hormone concentration. There are, however, two natural methods which increase the likelihood of conception despite these potential problems. The first is the relatively long fertile period of eggs and the second is the relatively long survival of spermatozoa within the female reproductive tract.

There are several methods by which the optimum time for mating can be detected and these include clinical assessments, measurement of plasma hormone concentrations and vaginal cytology.

Clinical assessments. The clinical signs of oestrus do not correlate well with the underlying hormonal events. The 'average bitch' ovulates 12 days after the onset of proestrus and should be mated from day 14 onwards when oocytes have matured. In some bitches ovulation may occur as early as day 8 or as late as day 26 after the onset of proestrus and these animals would be unlikely to become pregnant if mated on the 12th and 14th day (which is common breeding practice).

Studies on laboratory-kept dogs has shown that the LH surge often occurs around the same time as the onset of standing oestrus. Although there is some variation of this event, mating 4 days after the onset of standing oestrus may be a suitable time in many bitches.

One clinical assessment that may be useful in the bitch is the timing of **vulval softening** (Fig. 19.6). This often occurs during the LH surge when there is a switch from oestrogen dominance to progesterone dominance of the reproductive tract.

If only clinical assessments are available, the combination of the onset of standing oestrus and the timing of distinct vulval softening may be useful in the prediction of the best mating time, since each event occurs on average 2 days before ovulation.

Measurement of plasma hormone concentration. The three relevant plasma hormones are LH, oestrogen and progesterone.

The measurement of plasma concentrations of LH would indicate impending ovulation (the fertile period is between 4 and 7 days after the LH surge) but there is no simple method by which such a measurement can readily be made.

There is little value in the measurement of plasma oestrogen concentrations because the oestrogen plateau is not predictive of the timing of ovulation.

However, plasma progesterone concentrations are very useful since this hormone is absent during proestrus and begins to increase coincidentally with

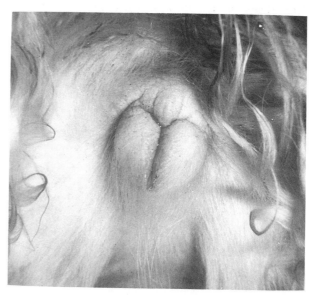

Fig. 19.6. Bitch's vulva during oestrus at the time of distinct softening. This is usually coincidental with the surge of plasma LH and therefore precedes ovulation by 2 days.

the plasma surge of LH, so that a rise in the concentration of plasma progesterone is predictive of ovulation. Progesterone can be measured easily in the practice laboratory within 1 hour of sample collection using a commercial enzyme-linked immunosorbent assay test-kit.

Vaginal cytology. The changes in the concentration of plasma hormones have a marked effect upon the vaginal mucosa.

When the bitch is not cycling, there are approximately 2 or 3 layers of cells lining the vagina.

During oestrus, the vagina develops many cell layers in order to protect itself during mating. The cells within these layers differ from each other in their shape and size. When cells are collected from the vagina (**vaginal smear**), only the cells on the surface of the vagina are removed. Different cell types are therefore collected at the various stages of the reproductive cycle. Staining of these cells and subsequent microscopic examination allows an assessment of the underlying hormone changes to be made. Cells can be collected either by aspirating vaginal fluid with a pipette, or by using a cotton swab. The collected cells are placed on a glass microscope slide, spread into a thin film and stained so that they can be individually examined (Fig. 19.7).

During anoestrus, the vaginal wall is only a few cells in thickness. These cells, which are small and spherical, are called **parabasal cells** because they are positioned close to the basement membrane. Their presence characterises the anoestrus vaginal smear. There are also normally a few white blood cells (**neutrophils**) which remove cell debris and bacteria.

During proestrus the vaginal mucosa increases in thickness under the influence of oestrogen. The mucosa may be up to 5 or 6 cells thick. The cells further away from the basement membrane are larger in diameter than those nearer to the membrane and have a large area of cytoplasm surrounding the cell nucleus. They are called **small intermediate cells**. When surface cells are collected during proestrus they are predominantly these small intermediate cells, with a small number of parabasal cells. White blood cells are also present during proestrus but their numbers are reduced compared with anoestrus because the increased thickness of the vaginal mucosa prevents movement of the white blood cells into the lumen of the vagina. Red blood cells are also present in the vaginal smear during proestrus; they originate from the uterus and pass into the vagina via the cervix.

During oestrus the vaginal mucosa continues to thicken and the number of cell layers increases. There may be up to 12 cell layers during oestrus. Surface cells are large and irregular in shape and are called **large intermediate cells**. Cells of this size may accumulate the material keratin and are then termed **keratinised**. The nucleus of these large keratinised cells often disappears and the cells are then called **anuclear**. White blood cells are not found in the vaginal smear during oestrus because the thick vaginal wall does not allow them to penetrate, but red blood cells are present in large numbers.

During metoestrus there is sloughing of much of the vaginal mucosal epithelium. This is caused by the increasing concentrations of the hormone progesterone. The number of cell layers is reduced and the surface cells are again small intermediate epithelial cells or parabasal cells. Several of the epithelia' cells may have vacuoles within the cytoplasm, giving the cell a 'foamy' appearance. **Foam cells** and epithelial cells with cytoplasmic inclusion bodies are characteristic of metoestrus. Because of the large amount of degenerate cellular material within the vaginal lumen there is a rapid influx of white blood cells as soon as the mucosa is thin enough to allow their penetration. Large numbers of white blood cells are therefore found in the metoestrus vaginal smear. Few red blood cells are present during metoestrus.

The bitch should first be mated when the percentage of anuclear cells is maximal—usually 80% or above (Fig. 19.8). There are variations from the normal: some bitches may have two peaks of anuclear cells and some have a low percentage of anuclear cells during the fertile period.

The domestic queen

In the queen, ovulation is induced by coitus. After mating (assuming that a sufficient release of LH has occurred), follicles increase in size and ovulation follows 24 to 36 hours later. Mating is best planned during the peak of oestrus. Vaginal cytology may be used to assess this time but collection of the smear may induce ovulation. Multiple copulations should be permitted to ensure an adequate release of LH and therefore ovulation.

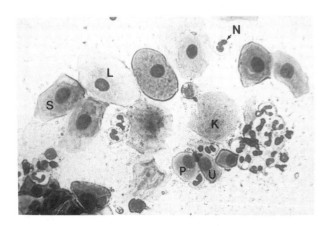

Fig. 19.7. Photomicrograph of the vaginal smear from a bitch in metoestrus demonstrating the range of epithelial cell types (P, parabasal cell; S, small intermediate cell; L, large intermediate cell; K, keratinised anuclear cell). In addition uterine cells (U) and neutrophils (N) are present.

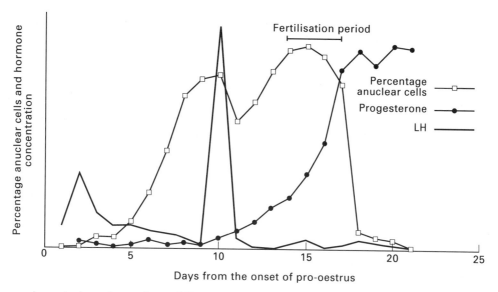

Fig. 19.8. Changes in vaginal cytology, plasma LH and plasma progesterone concentrations during proestrus, oestrus and early metoestrus of the domestic bitch. Eggs may be fertilised from 4 to 7 days after the LH peak. The fertilisation period therefore occurs during increasing concentrations of plasma progesterone whilst there are maximum numbers of anuclear epithelial cells. It is not uncommon for two well-defined peaks of anuclear cells to be identified. Regular collection of vaginal smears is important for the correct interpretation; single smears are of limited value.

Assisted Reproduction

The domestic bitch

There are several techniques that may be used to assist reproduction in the bitch, the most common being **artificial insemination**—the technique of collecting semen from a male animal, and placing it into the reproductive tract of the female.

Artificial insemination (AI) may involve the use of freshly collected semen, semen that has been diluted and chilled, or semen that has been frozen and then thawed. The technique has several advantages over natural mating:

- It reduces the requirement to transport animals.
- It is an acceptable way of overcoming, to some extent, the quarantine restrictions that prevent the movement of animals from one country to another.
- It increases the genetic pool available to an individual breed within a country.
- It reduces the disease risk which is always present when unknown animals enter a kennel for mating. In some countries the use of AI may reduce the spread of infectious diseases.
- In certain circumstances, artificial insemination may be useful when natural mating is difficult—for example bitches that ovulate when they are not in standing oestrus or bitches that have hyperplasia of the vaginal floor.
- Semen may also be collected from male animals which are unable to achieve a natural mating due to age, debility, back pain or premature ejaculation.

The greatest area of interest is probably the storage of genetic material by freezing semen for insemination at a future date. This may be necessary in male animals that are likely to become infertile due to castration or to medical treatments with certain hormones. The more common reason, however, is the preservation of semen from superior animals for use in future generations.

Collected semen may be deposited into the bitch's vagina by means of a long inseminating pipette which is gently introduced near to the cervix. When semen is placed in this position the spermatozoa must swim through the cervix, into the uterus and up the uterine horns. During a natural mating contractions of the vagina and uterus help in transporting semen but these contractions generally do not occur during artificial insemination, although some may be produced by stimulating the vagina. Vaginal insemination is therefore not ideal, but when fresh or chilled semen is used the spermatozoa will usually live long enough to fertilise the eggs. However, in the case of frozen semen the spermatozoa do not live for long after thawing and so vaginal inseminations are not very satisfactory.

The chance of pregnancy can be improved if the semen is placed directly into the uterus rather than into the vagina. It is very difficult to place a catheter through the bitch's cervix into the uterus (a technique that is simple in many other animals) because the vagina is long and narrow and because the cervical opening is small and at an angle to the vagina. A special insemination pipette has been developed for this purpose and recently some research workers have been able to catheterise the cervix using an endoscope. In certain countries the most common way of performing uterine insemination is surgically via a laparotomy.

Because of the short life-span of the preserved sperm, it is most important that inseminations are accurately timed in relation to ovulation. The ideal time is between 2 and 5 days after ovulation, and this is best assessed by the measurement of plasma progesterone concentration and the study of vaginal cytology.

In the U.K., pups which are the result of AI can only be registered if the Kennel Club has given prior permission. The permission of the Kennel Club is not required before semen is imported or exported but there are specific regulations set by the Ministry of Agriculture Fisheries and Food (and by similar organisations in other countries) which aim to prevent the introduction of infectious diseases. Import regulations vary between countries but are particularly stringent for the UK. Import permit requirements usually include: health certification before and a set time period after semen collection; quarantine of semen until the second health examination; and various serological tests.

The domestic queen

Whilst artificial insemination has been widely practised in the domestic cat as a research model for wild cats, the technique is not commonly used in the UK. Techniques are further advanced than for the dog and include the induction of ovulation, *in vitro* fertilisation and embryo transfer.

Control of Reproduction

There have been many methods employed to control the reproductive cycle of the bitch and queen. These involve surgical methods and medical control of cyclical activity. More recently advances have been made in the induction of oestrus and in the termination of pregnancy.

The domestic bitch

Surgical prevention of cyclical activity. **Ovario-hysterectomy** is the removal of both ovaries and the uterus to the level of the cervix. The term **spaying** is commonly used to describe this procedure although by definition this refers to removal of the ovaries only. Ovariohysterectomy should be considered in any bitch that is not required for breeding since it has several advantages to the bitch, including a reduction in the incidence of mammary tumours, elimination of the problems of false pregnancy and of pyometra, as well the obvious advantages of absence of oestrous behaviour and inability to produce offspring. There are also several claimed adverse effects, including an increased incidence of urinary incontinence, changes in coat texture and a tendency to gain weight. Whilst little can be done to prevent the former two conditions, the latter may easily be controlled by correct dietary management.

There is considerable discussion concerning the correct time to perform the procedure on a bitch. Surgery is technically easier and recovery is more rapid in young animals, and some veterinary surgeons perform surgery as early as 4 months of age. However, it has been suggested that when performed before puberty (the first oestrus) there is an increased tendency for underdevelopment of the secondary sexual characteristics and there may also be effects on the closure time of an animal's growth plates. On the other hand, waiting until after the first oestrus carries the risk of pregnancy and false pregnancy.

Medical inhibition of cyclical activity. There are a variety of compounds which may be used to inhibit cyclical activity including progesterone or progester-one-like compounds (**progestogens**), testosterone or other male hormones (**androgens**) and gonadotrophin releasing hormone agonists and antagonists. Drugs may either be administered during anoestrus to prevent the occurrence of an oestrus (the term **prevention** is used), or may be given during proestrus or oestrus to abolish the signs of that particular oestrus (the term **suppression** is used). The most commonly used compounds are the progestogens, which are formulated as **depot injections** for prevention (during anoestrus) or as **oral tablets,** The depot injections may be used during anoestrus to prevent the occurence of the next anticipated heat. The oral tablets may be used either during anoestrus for oestus prevention, or during proestrus to suppress the signs of that oestrus. A normal oestrus often occurs between 4 and 6 months after the administration of these hormones.

These drugs are not recommended for use before the first oestrus or in an animal that is required for breeding. Side effects include increased appetite, weight gain, lethargy, mammary enlargement, coat and temperament changes and the risk of inducing pyometra.

Induction of oestrus. With the development of new drugs and new drug regimes it has become possible to induce an oestrous cycle in the bitch. In many cases the success rate in terms of the birth of live pups is poor and the administration of the drugs is complicated. However, these methods may be useful in bitches which have longer than average inter-oestrus intervals or which are slow to reach puberty and also those which do not exhibit behavioural signs of oestrus.

Termination of pregnancy. Unwanted matings are commonly seen in general practice. The term **mis-alliance** is often used to describe these cases but is best avoided because by definition it means 'an unsuitable or improper marriage'. There are several treatment options should pregnancy termination be necessary. If the bitch is not required for breeding an ovariohysterectomy may be performed early in metoestrus, approximately 2 weeks after the end of oestrus. Medical therapy using oestrogens within 5 days of mating is often successful in preventing conception but there is the risk of inducing pyometra and the disadvantage that oestrus will be prolonged. In later pregnancy it is possible to use various drugs (e.g. cabergoline) which lower the concentration of progesterone in the blood and therefore induce resorption or abortion. These are not commonly used in the UK.

The domestic queen

Surgical prevention of cyclical activity. The indications and potential adverse effects of ovariohysterectomy in the cat are similar to those in the bitch. The procedure is usually performed when the queen is 5 to 6 months of age, regardless of the onset of puberty; poor development of the external genitalia does not cause problems. In the U.K. the surgical procedure is frequently performed through a flank incision. This approach should be avoided in oriental breeds where coat colour is a temperature-dependent effect, and clipping the coat may result in the growth of dark coloured hairs.

Medical inhibition of cyclical activity. The drugs available for use in the queen are similar to those described for the domestic bitch. Long-term drug therapy is less commonly used because queens not wanted for breeding are usually surgically neutered.

Induction of oestrus and termination of pregnancy. Various drugs may be used to induce oestrus or terminate pregnancy. In general the guidelines given for the bitch may be followed.

Diseases of the Reproductive Tract

The domestic bitch

There are several abnormalities of the reproductive tract in the domestic bitch and these may be considered under the general headings of endocrinological, ovarian, uterine or external genital abnormalities.

Endocrinological abnormalities. The common endocrinological abnormalities of the bitch include:

- Delayed onset of puberty (cyclical activity is not present at 24 months of age).
- Prolonged anoestrus (failure of return to cyclical activity resulting in a prolonged interoestrus interval).
- Silent oestrous cycles (normal cyclical activity, including ovulation, but without the external signs of oestrus).
- Split oestrus (signs of proestrus but this does not terminate in ovulation and is followed 2 to 12 weeks later by a normal cycle).

- Ovulation failure (apparently normal oestrous periods with an absence of ovulation—these bitches often return to oestrus with shorter than normal intervals).

One specific endocrinological condition frequently seen in the bitch is **pseudopregnancy** (false pregnancy, phantom pregnancy or **pseudocyesis**). The signs of the condition include anorexia, abdominal enlargement, nest-making, nursing of inanimate objects, mammary development and lactation. False pregnancy should be considered normal in the bitch because the changes in plasma hormones are similar in both pregnant and non-pregnant individuals. It has been wrongly thought that pseudopregnancy is produced by either an overproduction of progesterone or abnormal persistence of the corpus luteum. The actual mechanism is related to the decline in plasma progesterone concentration during late metoestrus which is associated with an increase in plasma concentrations of prolactin. In many cases therapy is not required because the signs will gradually decline, but in certain cases it may be necessary to use hormonal therapy to reduce the plasma concentrations of prolactin.

Diseases of the ovary. There are few abnormalities of the ovary. An absence of ovarian development (**agenesis**) may occur: it usually affects one side only and may affect fertility. **Ovarian cysts** are rare; they may be associated with signs of persistent oestrus, but most cysts originate from the ovarian bursa and are not endocrinologically active. **Ovarian tumours** are also rare.

Occasionally bitches with both ovarian and testicular tissue are seen. These animals are termed **intersex** and may be recognised because of the appearance of their external genitalia. The vulva may be cranially positioned and an *os clitoris* may develop. The gonads may be found in a normal ovarian position or within the scrotum. These animals are usually sterile.

Diseases of the uterus. Developmental problems of the uterus include **aplasia** (abnormal development) or agenesis (failure of development); in these cases reproductive cyclicity will be normal but the bitch may fail to become pregnant. Intersex animals may have the presence of both uterine tissue and vasa deferentia.

The most common uterine disease of the bitch is **cystic endometrial hyperplasia** (CEH) which may develop into pyometra. Hyperplasia of the endometrium occurs in response to progesterone during normal metoestrus. In young animals the hyperplasia resolves at the end of the luteal phase. This is not the case in older bitches and small cystic regions develop within the glandular tissue. The uterus in this state is probably more prone to infection than the normal uterus, and should bacteria enter during oestrus (when the cervix is open) they may proliferate. The accumulation of pus within the uterus (**pyometra**) leads to the bitch to becoming unwell. Clinical signs may include the presence of a malodorous vaginal discharge, lethargy, inappetence, pyrexia, vomiting, polydipsia and polyuria. In some cases the cervix is not open and a vaginal discharge is absent; these cases are called 'closed' pyometra. In all cases of pyometra the treatment of choice is ovario-hysterectomy following stabilisation of the patient by appropriate fluid therapy. Medical treatment has been advocated but the success rate is not high.

Treatment of bitches with progestogens for the prevention or suppression of oestrus, or oestrogens for the treatment of unwanted matings, may predispose to the development of pyometra.

Diseases of the vagina and vestibule. Congenital abnormalities of the caudal reproductive tract include segmental aplasia and hymenal or vestibular constrictions.

Vaginitis (inflammation of the vagina) is sometimes seen in prepubertal bitches and usually resolves after the first oestrus. Specific infectious causes of vaginitis include *Brucella canis* (not present in the UK) and herpes virus. Many bacteria are found within the vagina as normal commensal organisms including beta-haemolytic streptococci which many dog breeders wrongly consider to be venereal pathogens. There is little value in routine bacteriological swabbing of the vagina before breeding, since usually only these commensal bacteria are isolated.

Diseases of the external genitalia. Congenital abnormalities such as vulval atresia and agenesis are rare. Clitoral hypertrophy may occur associated with intersexuality.

The domestic queen

Endocrinological abnormalities. Delayed puberty may be difficult to assess in the queen since the onset of cyclical activity is related to the season of the year at birth. Delayed puberty and prolonged anoestrus have been seen although they are rare.

The most common abnormality is **ovulation failure** which often results from insufficient reflex release of LH at mating. The majority of queens will ovulate if 4 to 12 matings are allowed in a 4-hour period.

Pseudopregnancy also occurs in the queen although this condition is dissimilar to that seen in the bitch and usually follows a sterile mating (or occasionally spontaneous ovulation). After ovulation there is an increase in plasma progesterone, which does not occur in the absence of mating, and no return to oestrus for a further 35 to 40 days. The clinical signs are an absence of oestrus; treatment is not required (see Fig. 19.5).

Diseases of the ovary. Congenital diseases of the ovary such as ovarian agenesis and ovarian hypoplasia are rare. Ovarian cysts and neoplasms, similar to those seen in the bitch, are also rare.

Premature ovarian failure may be seen in queens aged 8 years and above; these animals stop cycling for an unknown reason.

Diseases of the uterus. The range of uterine abnormalities seen in the cat are similar to those of the bitch. Pyometra may be less common because in the absence of mating ovulation does not occur and the luteal phase is therefore absent. However, spontaneous ovulations or the common use of progestogens may cause the development of cystic endometrial hyperplasia and pyometra.

Diseases of the vagina, vestibule and external genitalia. Congenital abnormalities of the vagina, vestibule and external genitalia are rare but include vaginal and vulval aplasia and defects associated with intersexuality. Vaginitis is uncommon.

Pregnancy

The domestic bitch

The *length of pregnancy* in the bitch is relatively consistent at 64, 65 or 66 days from the preovulatory LH surge. However, the apparent length of pregnancy, assessed from the time of mating, may vary between 56 and 72 days since both early and late matings may be fertile:

- Early matings require sperm survival within the female reproductive tract until ovulation and egg maturation; such matings produce an apparently longer pregnancy.
- Late matings occur when eggs are waiting to be fertilised for some time after ovulation; such matings produce an apparently shorter pregnancy.

The *clinical signs* of pregnancy might include:

- Increased body weight and abdominal enlargement (but these signs may not be obvious if the number of pups is small).
- A reduced food intake and a vaginal discharge, common approximately one month into the pregnancy.
- Enlargement and reddening of the mammary glands, especially from 40 days after mating (these signs may also be present in bitches with pseudopregnancy).
- The production of milk—a variable finding: some bitches producing serous fluid from day 40 and milk from day 55 onwards, whilst in others this may not occur until just before parturition.

Certain *physiological changes* occur during pregnancy and include the development of a normochromic, normocytic anaemia and a reduction of the packed cell volume; these changes are normal.

Food intake does not increase during the first 30 days of pregnancy. After this time the absolute requirement for carbohydrate and protein increases. During the last half of pregnancy, food consumption may be doubled. Provided that diet is well-balanced and contains suitable amounts of vitamins and minerals it is not necessary to provide extra supplementation, although it may be necessary to divide the food into 2 or 3 meals during the day. Supplementation with calcium and vitamin D should be avoided: it does not prevent eclampsia and can be dangerous.

Regular exercise should be provided throughout pregnancy, limited by the amount the bitch is willing to undertake.

For the control of ascarid infections (*Toxocara*) it is necessary to administer medication during pregnancy to reduce or prevent perinatal transmission. Various drugs (benzimidazoles) and treatment regimes have been advocated for the treatment of pregnant bitches.

It is advisable to ensure that *routine vaccination* has been performed before mating. Vaccination during pregnancy is unlikely to be damaging to the foetus and therefore may be undertaken if necessary, but no live vaccine is licensed for this purpose.

Pregnancy diagnosis. As well as observation of the clinical signs already described (noting that mammary development, increased weight and abdominal enlargement may be present in pseudo-pregnancy as well as in pregnancy), there are several methods for pregnancy diagnosis in the bitch.

Pregnancy diagnosis in the bitch:

Abdominal palpation.

This is best performed approximately 1 month after mating when the conceptual swellings are approximately 2.0 cm in diameter. The technique can be highly accurate but may be difficult in obese or nervous animals, and may be inaccurate if the bitch was mated early such that pregnancy is not as advanced as anticipated. After day 35, individual conceptuses cannot easily be palpated and diagnosis becomes more difficult.

Identification of foetal heart beats.

In late pregnancy it is possible to auscultate the foetal heart beats using a stethoscope, or to record a foetal ECG. Both of these methods are diagnostic of pregnancy; foetal heart rate is more rapid than that of the dam.

Radiography.

From day 30 it is possible to detect uterine enlargement with good quality radiographs. However, this is not diagnostic of pregnancy since pyometra may have a similar appearance. Pregnancy diagnosis is not possible until after day 45, when mineralisation of the foetal skeleton is detectable radiographically. Although it is unlikely that there will be radiation damage to the foetus at this stage, sedation or anaesthesia of the dam may be required and is a potential risk. In late pregnancy the number of pups can be reliably estimated by counting the number of foetal skulls.

Hormone tests.

Plasma concentrations of progesterone are not useful for the detection of pregnancy in the bitch. Measurement of the hormone relaxin is diagnostic of pregnancy but there is no commercial assay for this hormone in the U.K.

Acute phase protein.

The rise in the concentration of acute phase proteins has been used as the basis of a commercial pregnancy test in the bitch. Concentrations of these proteins increase from approximately 30 days onwards. The test is reliable although these proteins are also released in inflammatory conditions such as pyometra.

Ultrasound examination.

Diagnostic B-mode ultrasound is now commonly used for pregnancy diagnosis (Fig. 19.9). The technique is non-invasive and without risk to the pups, dam or veterinary surgeon. The bitch can be examined in the standing position with minimal restraint.

With ultrasound it is possible to diagnose pregnancy as early as 16 days after ovulation, although because in most cases this time is not known it is prudent to wait until 28 days after mating. At this time the fluid filled conceptuses can easily be imaged, and embryonic tissue can be identified. It is possible to assess the number of conceptuses but this can be inaccurate, especially when the litter size is large. Movement of the foetal heart can be seen ultrasonographically and this confirms foetal viability. It is possible to examine the bitch at any time after day 28 to diagnose pregnancy

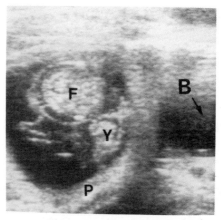

Fig. 19.9. Ultrasound image of pregnant bitch 32 days after the LH surge. A single conceptus is positioned adjacent to the bladder (B). Within the conceptus the foetus (F) can be seen in transverse section, and the collapsing yolk sac (Y) is positioned adjacent to the placenta (P).

and to confirm foetal viability and growth. With later examinations it is less easy to estimate the number of pups.

The domestic queen

The average *length of pregnancy* in the queen is 65 days with a range of 64 to 68 days.

The *clinical signs* of pregnancy include increased body weight and abdominal enlargement (these signs are often apparent in all but young queens) and mammary development which is obvious from approximately day 40. These changes are usually diagnostic for pregnancy since pseudopregnancy is not common, nor is it usually associated with clinical signs.

During the second half of pregnancy there is an increase in *food intake* and in the requirement for both carbohydrate and protein. Provided that diet is well balanced and contains suitable amounts of vitamins and minerals it is not necessary to provide extra supplementation.

Many queens continue to be active during pregnancy, the amount of *exercise* is best limited by the individual cat.

It is advisable to ensure that routine *vaccination* has been performed prior to mating.

Pregnancy diagnosis. As well as observation of clinical signs (mammary development, increased weight and abdominal enlargement may be present from mid-pregnancy onwards and it is unlikely that pseudopregnancy will produce similar signs) various methods may be used for pregnancy diagnosis of the queen.

Pregnancy diagnosis in the queen:

Abdominal palpation.

Conceptual swellings can be palpated from approximately 21 days after mating. These are discrete until 30 days after mating but thereafter become more difficult to palpate.

Identification of foetal heart beats.

In late pregnancy the foetal heart beats may be auscultated using a stethoscope, but at this stage it is usually possible to palpate the foetus in all but the most obese cats.

Radiography.

From day 30 it is possible to detect uterine enlargement with good quality radiographs. Mineralisation of the foetal skeleton is detectable radiographically from 40 days after mating.

Hormone tests.

Plasma concentrations of progesterone are elevated in both pregnancy and pseudopregnancy, therefore measurement of this hormone is not diagnostic. Plasma relaxin concentrations are elevated from day 25; this hormone is diagnostic of pregnancy but there is no commercial assay available.

Ultrasound examination.

Diagnostic B-mode ultrasound may be used for pregnancy diagnosis in the cat. The pregnancy length can be assessed from mating time (unlike the bitch). Conceptuses can be imaged from 12 days after mating, and embryonic tissue can usually be seen from day 14. From this time onwards it is possible to identify pregnancy, confirm foetal viability and assess foetal growth. It is more difficult to assess the number of kittens in later pregnancy.

Abnormalities of Pregnancy

A great concern for owners is the risk of resorption or abortion during pregnancy. To understand the differences in these processes it is necessary to define the stages of development. In general the term **embryo** is used when the characteristics of the pup are not discernible. From approximately 35 days after ovulation the characteristics of the pup become obvious and the term **foetus** is used. **Resorption** refers to the resorption of the entire conceptus and occurs during the embryonic stage of development. **Abortion** refers to the expulsion of the foetus and the foetal membranes before term (i.e. before 58 days after ovulation). A **stillbirth** is the expulsion of the foetus and foetal membranes after day 58 (i.e. close to term).

The incidence of resorption or abortion of the entire litter is not known, although it is certain that up to 5% of bitches suffer isolated resorption of one or two conceptuses with continuation of the remaining pregnancy.

The many potential causes of resorption and abortion include infectious agents, trauma, foetal defects and maternal environment. In the dog the infectious agents *Brucella canis* (not present in the U.K.), canine distemper virus, canine herpes virus and *Toxoplasma gondii* have all been implicated as causes of abortion and resorption. In the cat feline herpesvirus I, feline panleukopaenia virus, feline leukaemia virus, feline infections peritonitis virus and *Toxoplasma gondii* infection may produce abortion, resorption or stillbirths.

In many cases embryonic death and pregnancy loss is best assessed using real-time diagnostic B-mode ultrasound. Resorption may be unrecognised by the owner unless it is associated with a period of illness. Abortion of foetal tissue may be obvious but may not be noticed should the dam eat the aborted material. In the face of an abortion there is little except supportive therapy that can be administered to the patient.

Pregnancy hypoglycaemia has been reported in the bitch and is associated with reduced blood glucose concentrations during late pregnancy. The clinical signs include weakness which may progress to coma.

The condition may be confused with **hypocalcaemia**, which occurs at a similar time (see later).

Parturition

In the last few weeks of pregnancy the bitch or queen should be encouraged to accept a nest in a suitable place—ideally a warm and clean room isolated from the rest of the household into which a whelping or kittening box may be placed.

The box should be large enough to allow the dam to stretch and have sufficient room for a large litter. The sides of the box should be high enough to prevent the pups or kittens from escaping up to about 4 weeks of age. The provision of a ledge around the box sides may be useful to prevent the dam from crushing her offspring. The bedding material should be easy to remove when it becomes soiled. The environmental temperature should be approximately 25–30°C and the avoidance of draughts is most important.

Before parturition, the hair from around the mammary glands and the perineum may be clipped to make the nipples more accessible and to allow cleaning of the dam after parturition.

In the last week of pregnancy it is prudent to record a bitch's rectal temperature at least twice daily in order to detect the **prepartum hypothermia** which precedes the onset of parturition by 24 to 36 hours. This decline in body temperature is mediated by a sudden reduction in the plasma concentration of progesterone. The rectal temperature usually changes from approximately 39°C to below 37°C.

There are five stage of parturition:

(1) Stage of preparation.
(2) First stage parturition (onset of contractions).
(3) Second stage parturition.
(4) Third stage parturition.
(5) Puerperium (after parturition).

The stage of preparation

The stage of preparation for parturition encompasses the decline in plasma progesterone concentration (and subsequent prepartum hypothermia of the bitch) and relaxation of the vaginal and perineal tissue. However, the dam may show few overt signs.

First stage parturition

The first stage of parturition commences with the onset of uterine contractions. First stage parturition averages 1 to 12 hours in duration, although this is variable. Milk is usually present within the mammary glands or appears during this stage.

Contraction of the uterus may cause discomfort and the dam may be restless and pant and may exhibit classical nesting behaviour. In addition anorexia, shivering and vomiting may be observed. Most cats seek seclusion during this time.

The uterine contractions push the first foetus against the cervix, which is starting to dilate. The **allantochorion** (placenta) may rupture and allantoic fluid may be produced from the vulva.

Second stage parturition

The second stage of parturition is characterised by increased uterine contractions and propulsion of the foetus through the cervix into the vagina. As the first foetus enters the pelvic canal, forceful abdominal straining commences. Bitches and queens are often in lateral recumbency during delivery although some bitches will remain standing.

The delivery of the foetal head is often most difficult and this may be associated with some pain; after this the foetus is usually produced rapidly.

The **amnion** (which surrounds each foetus) is often seen at the vulva during straining. This may either rupture spontaneously, be broken by the dam or is unruptured and the foetus is born within it. The dam will normally break the sac if the foetus is born within it but this should be done quickly if she fails to do so.

The time between the onset of straining and the birth of the first foetus is variable; it may be as short as 10 to 30 minutes, but it may take longer in young animals. Non-productive straining for more than 60 minutes may indicate **dystocia**.

The birth of a foetus is usually followed by the expulsion of the allantochorion (placenta) usually within 20 minutes.

The subsequent foetuses may be delivered quickly although the interval between foetuses may be up to 6 hours. The time taken from the birth of the first to the last foetus is variable and may be as long as 24 to 36 hours.

After the delivery of the foetus the dam usually commences vigorous licking, removing membranes and fluid away from the neonate's face and promoting respiration. If she fails to do this, it may be done for her with a clean, soft towel. Usually the dam will sever the umbilical cord with her teeth, and eat the placenta when it is expelled. It is important to ensure that the dam does not excessively chew the umbilicus since this may damage the foetus. If the umbilicus is not severed this can be achieved using scissors.

Pups and kittens are best left with the dam during the remainder of delivery. If they are removed this may be distressing and may inhibit further straining.

Third stage parturition

The third stage of parturition is classically associated with passage of the allantochorion (placenta). However, in the bitch and queen this occurs during second stage parturition and cannot be defined as a separate period. Occasionally one or more foetuses are delivered without their placentae, which are expelled at a later stage or may be delivered together with a subsequent foetus.

There is commonly a dark-coloured vulval discharge after parturition which contains a green pigment originating from the placenta. The discharge declines in volume but may persist for 1 week after parturition.

The puerperium

The puerperium is the period after parturition during which the reproductive tract returns to its normal non-pregnant state. This includes the period of **uterine involution**, which may take 4 to 6 weeks. A mucoid vulvar discharge may be present during this period.

Dystocia

The term dystocia literally means difficult birth and it is used to indicate any problem that interferes with normal birth. Dystocia is rare in the queen but problems are not uncommon in the bitch, especially in brachycephalic breeds such as the bulldog and Boston terrier. The two main causes of dystocia are maternal factors and foetal factors.

Maternal dystocia

Maternal dystocia may be caused by either poor straining efforts by the dam or constriction of the birth canal.

Poor straining efforts of the dam. Poor straining may be the result of nervousness or pain which inhibit normal parturition, but it is more commonly the result of poor myometrial contractions, a condition that has been termed **uterine inertia**. Inertia may be primary, in which case parturition does not commence, or may be secondary to some other factor occurring during parturition.

Primary uterine inertia is rare in the cat but is not uncommon in young bitches with only one or two pups, or in older overweight bitches with large litters. The cause of the condition is unknown but it may relate to poor condition of the uterine musculature in fat or debilitated animals, overstretching of the uterus when the litter size is large, poor stimulus for parturition when there are only a few foetuses or low plasma calcium concentrations.

The endocrinological events of parturition are usually normal but subsequent uterine contractions are not fully initiated and parturition does not follow. A green vulval discharge, which indicates placental separation, may be seen some days after the expected date of parturition. In some cases the owner may have observed initial weak uterine contractions or have noted the decline in body temperature. At this stage the administration of the hormone oxytocin may stimulate uterine contractions but it should only be given if it is certain that there is no obstruction to the birth canal. (However, it is not possible to assess the patency of the cervix in the bitch by digital palpation: the vagina of an average 20 kg bitch is 20 cm long.) Repeated doses of oxytocin may be necessary. Some cases may respond to the intravenous administration of calcium borogluconate; others may require Caesarean operation.

Primary uterine inertia may be anticipated in some bitches because of a previous history of this problem or because of their age, physical condition or the number of pups. The best assessment of the bitch is to monitor the rectal temperature twice daily during the last 7 to 10 days of pregnancy.

Secondary uterine inertia is the cessation of uterine contractions after they have started. It is usually the result of uterine exhaustion following obstructive dystocia but may occur spontaneously during second stage parturition, presumably because of factors similar to those seen with primary uterine inertia. If the cause of the dystocia can be relieved, the administration of oxytocin and calcium may be suitable treatments. In some cases Caesarean operation may be necessary.

Obstruction of the birth canal. Obstruction may be the result of abnormalities of the birth canal, such as:

* Deformity of the pelvic bones. These may be congenital malformations, developmental abnormalities or the result of previous trauma, commonly following a road accident.
* Soft tissue abnormalities within the pelvis which press against the reproductive tract. They might include pelvic neoplasms, although these are rare in animals of breeding age.
* Abnormality of the reproductive tract itself—for example, torsion of the uterus or congenital vaginal or uterine constrictions.

Foetal dystocia

Foetal oversize. Oversize of the foetus relative to the birth canal may be the result of:

* Breed conformation – dystocia may be considered almost 'normal' for certain breeds with exaggerated physical characteristics such as a large head size.
* Actual foetal oversize, when the litter size is small and large foetuses develop within the uterus.
* Foetal abnormalities, including foetal monsters, resulting in relative oversize and dystocia.

In the majority of these cases Caesarean operation is necessary for the delivery of the foetuses, whether normal or abnormal.

Abnormalities of foetal alignment. The orientation of the foetus during delivery is conventionally described by noting the presentation, position and posture of the foetus with respect to the dam (Fig. 19.10). Variation from the normal disposition may result in dystocia, which may be corrected in certain cases by manipulation per vaginum but in others Caesarean operation may be necessary.

(a)

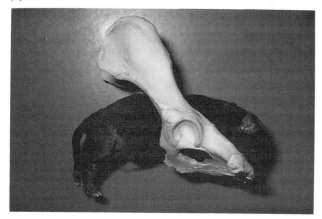

(b)

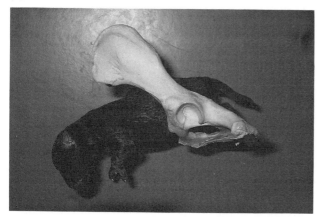

(c)

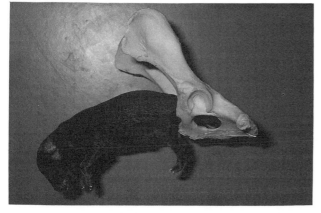

Fig. 19.10. Presentations: (a) lateral view of a pelvis demonstrating anterior longitudinal presentation of a pup in dorsal position with the head and forelegs extended (normal orientation); (b) lateral view of a pelvis demonstrating posterior longitudinal presentation of a pup in dorsal position with the hindlegs extended (normal orientation); (c) lateral view of a pelvis demonstrating posterior longitudinal presentation of a pup in dorsal position with hindlegs flexed cranially (breech orientation).

Orientation of the foetus

The **presentation** of a foetus is a description of the direction of its long axis in relation to the long axis of the dam. Pups and kittens can only be delivered in longitudinal presentation (i.e. the long axis of the foetus is parallel to the long axis of the dam) but may have either anterior (foetal head delivered first) or posterior (foetus delivered backwards) presentation. A posterior presentation is not necessarily a breech presentation (see below).

The **position** of a foetus is a description of its dorsal axis with respect to the dorsum of the dam; this describes the degree of rotation of the foetus. Most species are normally born in dorsal position, i.e. the back of the foetus is uppermost in the same orientation as the dam.

The **posture** of a foetus is a description of the orientation of the head and legs which may be extended or flexed. For anterior presentation the head must be extended, and this occurs naturally during a posterior presentation.

A **breech birth** refers to a foetus delivered in posterior longitudinal presentation, usually in dorsal position with the hindlimbs flexed. This means that the foetus is presented 'bottom first' with its hindlegs directed towards the dam's head (Fig. 19.10). A foetus delivered in posterior presentation with the legs extended is not a breech presentation.

Recognition of dystocia

The normal events of parturition should be clearly understood so that recognition of dystocia can be achieved rapidly, allowing prompt intervention.

Collection of a relevant history is essential in the evaluation of a potential case of dystocia. This includes the estimation of the stage of pregnancy. Determining the mating time is most helpful in establishing the stage of pregnancy of the cat but this is not very useful in the bitch, where pregnancy length can vary between 56 and 72 days from mating. Regular monitoring of rectal temperature is therefore essential in the bitch. It should be established whether this has been done by the owner, and if so what changes were observed.

Of particular importance is the time-course of events from the onset of parturition, e.g. the onset of behavioural changes such as restlessness, nest-making and panting. The time when straining first occurred and the character of the straining efforts may also be useful as an indicator of dystocia, as will the times that any foetuses were produced.

It is not possible to give definite guidelines regarding potential cases of dystocia but examination of the patient is warranted in certain situations:

- A bitch that has exceeded 70 days from the last mating and has no signs of impending parturition.
- A cat that has exceeded 65 days from from the last mating and has no signs of impending parturition.
- The dam is unsettled and strains forcefully but infrequently.
- There are signs of straining which then cease.
- There is a black/green vulval discharge with no signs of parturition.

- Parturition has not commenced within 48 hours of a decline in rectal temperature.
- There has been ineffectual straining for 1 hour or more.
- Several foetuses have been produced, the last more than 2 hours ago, and the dam is restless.
- Several foetuses have been produced, the last more than 2 hours ago, and a larger litter is expected (may not be known by the owner).

Investigation of potential cases of dystocia. In most cases it is necessary to ensure that the animal is pregnant and/or that viable foetuses remain within the uterus. This can be achieved by transabdominal palpation, auscultation of foetal heart beats, real-time ultrasonography and radiography, as described earlier for pregnancy diagnosis.

Further investigation involves digital examination of the vagina by a skilled person to assess whether a foetus is present and to establish foetal alignment. This should only be performed after cleaning the vulvar area thoroughly with an antiseptic solution and scrubbing the hands or wearing surgical gloves. A water-soluble lubricant should be applied to the fingers, and the vestibule and vagina should be carefully examined. The presence of bone or soft tissue abnormalities of the pelvis should be noted. The presentation, position and posture of the foetus should be established before any further intervention is contemplated.

For normal presentations (Fig. 19.10) delivery can be assisted using the thumb and forefinger to cradle the foetal head (anterior presentation) or pelvis (posterior presentation). Traction should only be applied during the straining effort of the bitch; however, pressure may be applied with a finger on the roof of the vagina to stimulate straining. Traction should be applied downwards through the vulva, rather than directly caudally. Traction should never be applied to the feet as these are easily damaged and deformed. Sterile gauze or similar fabric may help the nurse to grip the puppy.

Caesarean Operation

There are many reasons for performing a Caesarean operation. Often this may be for the relief of dystocia, and occasionally it is an elective procedure when there is concern over feto-maternal disproportion.

Anaesthesia

It is important to remember that there are several marked physiological changes during pregnancy which may affect the requirements for anaesthesia. These physiological changes result in decreased minimum alveolar concentrations of anaesthetic gases, an increased oxygen requirement and, commonly, hypoventilation and subsequent hypoxia and hypercarbia. In addition, in cases of dystocia the animal may be debilitated and may have recently been fed. The general aims are to:

- ensure adequate oxygenation (intubation and oxygen administration);
- maintain blood volume and prevent hypotension (intravenous fluid therapy);
- minimise depression of the foetus and dam during and after surgery (reduce the dose of anaesthetic agents used).

There are many anaesthetic regimes suitable for this procedure, including the use of volatile agents for induction and maintenance of anaesthesia and the use of rapid-acting intravenous induction agents (such as propofol) followed by maintenance of anaesthesia using a volatile inhalational anaesthetic.

Complications

There are several complications of Caesarean operation in both species. These include:

- anaesthetic risks in the dam and the neonate;
- risks during surgery of uterine rupture and haemorrhage, resulting in hypovolaemia;
- post-operative risks including wound infection and wound breakdown;
- interference with the wound by neonates trying to suck;
- problems in the young dam of accepting the litter.

Some veterinary surgeons prefer to perform the operation via a flank incision to avoid the problem of wound interference when the neonates try to suck.

The problem of rejection of the litter by a young dam after a Caesarean operation may be overcome by placing the offspring with the dam as soon as possible after surgery. The mother's milk should be squeezed on to the newborn's head if rejection is a problem. The dam should be carefully observed until she is able to coordinate sufficiently enough to not damage them and she must not be left unattended until successful sucking has been noted.

Post-parturient Care

Care and Management of the Neonate

The first essential steps after birth are:

(1) Establish a clear airway and stimulate respiration.
(2) Cut the umblicus.
(3) Keep the neonate warm until active.
(4) Encourage the neonate to suck.

It is essential that a clear airway is established as soon as a foetus has been born (or delivered via a Caesarean operation). This involves removal of the surrounding foetal membranes and clearing of the mouth and nose of foetal fluid using either a dry towel or a small pipette. Gentle compression of the chest usually results in the establishment of respiratory effort. If this is not the case but the heart is beating, respiratory stimulation should be continued by rubbing the thorax; further fluid should be removed by gently swinging the neonate in a small arc—but this should be avoided unless absolutely necessary, because of the risk of brain trauma.

In certain cases the administration of respiratory stimulant agents such as doxopram hydrochloride may be efficacious, as may the administration of oxygen. If respiration does not commence then artificial respiration can be attempted by blowing gently into the nose and mouth of the neonate. This should be done carefully to induce only slight lung expansion without overinflating the lungs. *If the heart is not beating* external cardiac massage combined with artificial respiration may be attempted.

The umbilicus should be cut approximately 3cm from the foetal abdomen. Excessive bleeding can be prevented by the application of a ligature.

Once regular respiratory efforts are maintained the neonate may be placed into a prewarmed box or incubator until it is active, when it should be returned to the dam and encouraged to suck. Sucking normally occurs immediately after birth and at intervals of 2 to 3 hours for the first few days.

Environment

Hypothermia is a major cause of neonatal morality and so the environmental temperature is critical. Recommended temperatures (25–30°C) are only necessary for the first few days; they are often unbearable for the dam and can be safely reduced to 22°C as long as draughts are avoided. One method of reducing heat exposure of the dam is to heat only half of the box.

Underfloor heating is ideal but properly protected hot-waterbottles or circulating water blankets provide good alternatives. Heat lamps suspended above the nest should be used with caution, since the environment may become too hot.

Examination

Pups and kittens should be carefully examined after birth:

- Body weight should be recorded. Normal neonates increase in body weight by 5–10% per day; a failure to achieve this rate may indicate ill health.
- The umbilicus should be clean and there should be no evidence of herniation.
- Respiration should be regular and without excessive noise. The normal respiratory rate is 15–40 breaths per minutes.
- There should be no discharge from the eyes or ears.
- The neonate should be examined for the presence of congenital diseases (described later).

- The rectal temperature need not be recorded but the normal range in the first week after birth is 32–34°C.

Neonatal characteristics

Neonatal pups and kittens are unable to stand at birth but they should be quite mobile, using their limbs to crawl. They should be assessed for their general strength; the weakest should be observed carefully, since these often do not feed adequately and may fail to thrive. Standing may be seen from 10 days after the birth and most neonates should be able to walk at 3 weeks of age.

Pups and kittens are born with their eyes closed. Separation of the upper and lower lids and opening of the eyes occurs approximately 10–14 days after birth. The cornea at this stage may appear slightly cloudy but this will disappear over the first 4 weeks. Many kittens are born with strabismus (squint) which persists until they are 8 weeks old.

Care of the litter

In the first few weeks of life the dam will provide all the care for her offspring, as long as the environment is kept clean and dry. The choice of bedding material includes shredded paper, newspaper with blankets, or newspaper with synthetic rugs. Materials should be washable or easily disposed of, and soiled material should be removed frequently.

The dam normally licks the perineal region of each neonate to stimulate urination and defecation and she continues to do so for the first 2–3 weeks after birth. Pups and kittens defecate and urinate voluntarily at 3 weeks of age and at this time soiling of the bedding increases, so that regular changing of the bedding is necessary. Pups and kittens should ideally be encouraged to soil an area away from the nest as early as possible, to facilitate cleaning and to hasten toilet training.

Care of the Dam

Immediately after parturition or surgery, the perineum of the dam should be cleaned. She should then be allowed to settle during suckling and given the opportunity to exercise shortly afterwards. The bedding may then be cleaned and the dam can be given food. It is likely that in the first few days she will develop diarrhoea, especially if the placentae were eaten. The bitch and queen will spend much of their time with their offspring during the first 2 weeks but should be encouraged to leave the nest as weaning is attempted.

The food intake during lactation may increase up to three times the normal and it is necessary to provide frequent small meals. These may be balanced diets or commercial preparations formulated for lactating animals. It is important not to change food intake dramatically since this may worsen the gastrointestinal disturbances that are normally seen.

Periparturient abnormalities

There are several conditions which may occur during late pregnancy or soon after parturition in bitches and queens. Certain conditions are emergencies and prompt recognition of the clinical signs is essential to allow successful treatment.

Hypocalcaemia (eclampsia, puerperal tetany). Low plasma concentrations of calcium are related to calcium loss in the milk and poor availability of dietary calcium. The condition is most commonly seen during late pregnancy or early lactation. It is rare in the cat. The clinical signs include restlessness, panting, increased salivation and a stiff gait which may progress to muscle fasciculations, pyrexia and tachycardia. If untreated, tetany and death result. The slow administration of calcium borogluconate by intravenous injection produces a rapid resolution of the clinical signs. During administration cardiac rate and rhythm should be monitored. Calcium supplementation may then be given orally or by subcutaneous injection to prevent recurrence of the condition.

Placental retention. The retention of placental tissue is uncommon in both the bitch and the queen but it causes great concern for many owners. Placentae are normally delivered following each pup or kitten and may be quickly eaten by the dam. If a placenta is retained the clinical signs are a persistent green vulval discharge. This should be differentiated from the normal haemorrhagic discharge which may persist for 1 week after parturition (a mucoid discharge may be present for up to 6 weeks). If a retained placenta is diagnosed by either ultrasound examination or palpation, the administration of oxytocin is usually curative.

Post-partum metritis. Infection and inflammation of the uterus may occur following prolonged parturition, abortion, foetal and/or placental retention or obstetrical manipulation. The clinical signs commonly include a persistent purulent vulval discharge, lethargy and pyrexia. Treatment with broad spectrum antimicrobial agents should be instituted immediately. Fluid replacement therapy may be required.

Mastitis. Inflammation of the mammary gland is not common in the bitch or queen but it may have disastrous results should the dam reject the litter because of pain on suckling. It is usually the result of bacterial infection following trauma (sucking). The mammary glands are tender, warm and firm upon palpation and the milk may be contaminated with blood and inflammatory cells so that it becomes yellow, pink or brown in colour. The dam may become lethargic and anorexic if the condition is not treated. Bathing and massaging the gland with warm water and gently removing the infected fluid may be helpful. Antimicrobial agents are usually required but it should be remembered that these agents will be excreted in the milk and ingested by the neonates.

Artificial Rearing of Neonates

Hand-rearing of neonates may be necessary if the dam is unable to nurse the litter or dies. In many cases the litter may be too large or the dam may produce inadequate volumes of milk. It may be necessary either to cull some of the litter or for them to go to a foster home. A bitch in pseudopregnancy or a bitch who has lost her litter may prove to be a suitable foster mother. If these alternatives are not acceptable, the litter can be divided and rotated between the bitch and artificial rearing. It has been suggested that some neonates should be reared entirely artificially rather than alternating the whole litter; however, all neonates should remain with the dam to ensure a normal social development.

It is essential that all neonates receive **colostrum** from the dam during in first few hours after birth to ensure an adequate uptake of maternal immunoglobulins. Colostrum is a yellow viscous material that represents the accumulated secretions of the mammary gland over the last few weeks of pregnancy. It contains high concentrations of immunoglobulins which are necessary for the passive transfer of immunity to the neonate. Should the dam have died, it may still be possible to milk some colostrum from the mammary glands as long as it is not contaminated with high concentrations of drugs or toxins.

After the first day it is possible to commence **supplementary feeding**. There are several commercially available milk substitutes that are useful for feeding pups and kittens. It is important that a correctly formulated diet is utilised. Neither cow's milk nor goat's milk is suitable since their compositions are markedly different from the milk of bitches and queens. It is possible to use home-made milk substitutes but these are often inappropriate in lactose, fat and protein concentration. The milk replacer should be warmed to body temperature (39°C) before feeding, and then fed to the manufacturer's instructions, depending upon body weight.

Normally neonates feed every 2–4 hours for the first 5 days of life and it is best to mimic this regime with artificial feeding. The interval can be reduced to every 4 hours after day 5.

Artificial feeding is time-consuming and demanding, particularly if the litter is being reared without the dam. Milk substitutes may be administered using syringe feeders, eye droppers, sucking devices or stomach tube. In most cases it is easiest to feed from a small syringe (2 ml) for the first 2–5 days. After this time a small bottle with a nipple may be used;

this encourages normal sucking but takes more time. The aperture of these devices must be large enough to prevent wind-sucking but small enough to prevent excessive volumes being administered, since this may result in aspiration.

The technique of feeding using a stomach tube (**orogastric intubation**) is relatively simple. It may be useful in the first few days of life for the rapid feeding particularly of sick neonates. A soft polythene tube (2mm diameter) is measured against the neonate from the mouth to a level with the 9th rib and this distance is marked on the tube. The outside of the tube is lubricated with a little water. The neonate's head is held in the normal position (if the head is extended or flexed, accidental passage of the tube into the trachea is more likely) and the mouth is held just open with a finger and thumb. The tube is directed gently over the tongue into the back of the throat. Swallowing greatly assists passage into the oesophagus, but this is not essential. The tube can usually be seen on the left side of the neck as it passes down the oesophagus. There is little resistance as the tube is introduced into the stomach; the length of tube introduced is the best guide. Once in position the syringe can be attached and its contents slowly injected into the stomach. The tube is then gently removed.

Orphaned pups and kittens should be maintained at the recommended environmental temperature of approximately 25–30°C. Normally the dam would lick the anogenital region after feeding to stimulate urination and defecation and in her absence this stimulation needs to be performed manually, using a moistened soft cloth or cotton wool, every 2–4 hours during the first few days of life.

Weaning

Pups and kittens generally receive all of their nutritional requirements from the dam until 3 weeks of age. (This must be provided artificially if they are hand-reared.) Signs associated with undernutrition include failure to gain weight, crying and inactivity.

Small volumes of meat fed on a finger can be introduced from $2\frac{1}{2}$ weeks of age, and lapping of semi-solids can be introduced from 3 weeks of age by encouraging sucking and licking of a finger and gradually placing the finger in contact with the solution. This is the start of the weaning process, which may last between 3 and 5 weeks. The volume and range of foods fed during this stage may be increased. It is common for semi-solids such as rice pudding and finely chopped meats to be used initially, although there are several proprietary brands of foods designed for this purpose. Neonates generally have twice an adult's energy and nutrient requirement per unit body weight.

For neonates weaned from the dam, the volume of food provided is increased and they usually receive five or six meals during the day at 5 weeks of age. As their food intake increases the dam should be removed from the nest for longer periods. Usually by 5 weeks of age the dam spends very little time in the nest during the day, but returns at night. There is discussion concerning the best time for removing the neonates from the dam. When neonates are introduced into a home environment, weaning can be safely accomplished by 6 weeks of age.

For hand-reared neonates, the volume of bottled milk is reduced in a similar manner to weaning from the bitch.

Abnormalities of the Neonatal Period

A number of diseases may affect pups and kittens early in life. A certain proportion of neonates die before weaning and it has been suggested that this can be as high as 15–20%. However, with good management systems—including the avoidance of hypothermia—the number of offspring lost should not be greater than 5%.

Fading puppy and kitten syndrome

The condition known as fading puppy or kitten syndrome is a true syndrome in that there are multiple potential causes, including: poor maternally derived immunity; viral, bacterial and parasitic infections; and genetic abnormalities. An accurate diagnosis cannot be established in all cases. The clinical signs are often unhelpful because they are similar regardless of cause: the neonates become lethargic, do not feed and usually die before 14 days of age.

Congenital abnormalities

Congenital abnormalities are those which are present at birth. Common problems include **cleft palate**, where there is failure of the normal fusion of the palatine arches. The defect may occur anywhere along the length of the hard or soft palate, although usually it arises caudal to the incisor ridge. It is common in certain breeds and it has been suggested that it is a trait inherited in either a recessive or a polygenic manner. In most of these cases euthanasia of the abnormal neonate is advisable because of the problems of sucking and aspiration of milk.

There are many other congenital abnormalities which may affect each organ system, such as hernias, foetal monsters, hydrocephalus, microphthalmus, flat puppies (swimmers), congenital heart disease and atresia of the terminal rectum. A thorough clinical examination of each pup after birth should allow these abnormalities to be readily detected.

Further Reading

Allen, W. E. (1992) *Fertility and Obstetrics in the Dog.* Blackwell Scientific Publications, London.

Concannon, P. W. (1991) Reproduction in the dog and cat. In *Reproduction in Domestic Animals*, 4th ed. Academic Press Ltd, New York. pp. 517–554.

Hoskins, J. D. (1990) *Veterinary Pediatrics: Dogs and Cats from Birth to Six Months*, 1st edition. W. B. Saunders Ltd, Philadelphia.

20
General Nursing

S. CHANDLER

Artificial Feeding

The importance of maintaining nutrition during recovery of patients from surgery or disease cannot be overemphasised, though in the past it has been sorely neglected. Convalescent periods can be radically reduced when adequate nutrition is provided. As relatively cheap feeding tubes are now readily available, tube feeding should be used more frequently when natural nutrition is impossible or contraindicated. It is important that the veterinary nurse be familiar with their management.

Artificial feeding which is (sometimes referred to as forced feeding) should only be instigated when all attempts to induce the animal to eat voluntarily have failed.

Anorexic patients may be tempted to eat by:

- warming the food;
- hand-feeding;
- offering highly odorous foods;
- offering favourite food (liaise with owners);
- smearing food on their lips;
- liquidising food.

Reasons for forced feeding are:

- failure to entice voluntary eating;
- physical inability (e.g. fractured jaw);
- following injury or surgery to oral cavity, or where feeding is contraindicated (e.g. oesophageal trauma).

Methods of Artificial Feeding

Methods include:

- Placing food on back of tongue and encouraging the animal to swallow (Fig. 20.1), as in per os administration of medicines.
- Syringe feeding of liquid food.
- Tube feeding.

> WARNING
> Aspiration pneumonia is a real risk with syringe feeding. Ensure that the patient's head is in a natural position—*not* raised—and that the animal swallows between the administration of each bolus. Give 0.5–5 ml at a time, depending on the size of the patient.

Tube Feeding

- Pharyngostomy tube (Fig. 20.2)
- Naso-oesophageal tube
- Naso-gastric tube
- Gastrostomy tube, surgically placed in the stomach (Fig. 20.3)
- Enterostomy tube (either duodenostomy or jejunostomy tube).

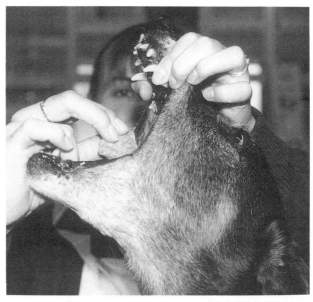

Fig. 20.1. Placing food, by hand, directly into the oral cavity may encourage animals to begin eating after a period of illness or major surgery.

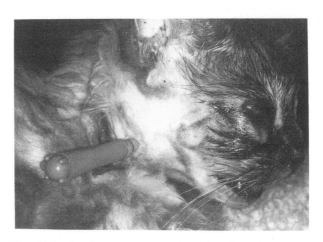

Fig. 20.2. A pharyngostomy tube (placed under general anaesthesia) in a cat with a fractured jaw.

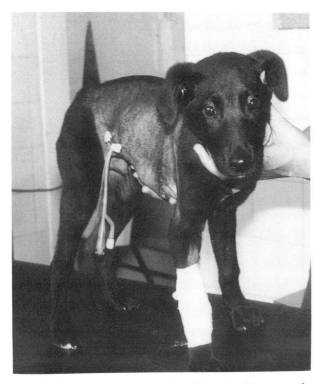

Fig. 20.3. A gastrostomy tube in a 12-week-old puppy after removal of an oesophageal foreign body. Partial thickness oesophageal damage necessitated tube placement. Tube feeding (including all water requirements) were maintained for 5 days. Antibiotics were also given by this route.

Management of these tubes is basically the same. All are indwelling and, with the exception of the naso-oesophageal and naso-gastric tubes, all are placed surgically under general anaesthesia.

Stomach tubing is not recommended for artificial feeding due to its repetitive nature and the stress caused to the patient.

Management of a Pharyngostomy Tube

This is a soft rubber or plastic tube. The tip of the tube usually lies in the caudal oesophagus, passing through the pharynx, and exits just caudal to the angle of the jaw. The tube is stitched in place and is bunged when not in use. It is bandaged to the patient's neck to prevent both patient interference and contamination of the tube.

Pharyngostomy tubes are frequently used for cats with fractured jaws. If the injury is at, or caudal to, the pharynx, there is no indication for the use of a pharyngostomy tube. One of the other tubes would be more appropriate.

Equipment

- Use only liquid food (Fig. 20.4).
- Generally an adapter is required to attach the syringe to the tube, e.g. a spigot or a nozzled syringe (Fig. 20.5).
- Water for flushing the tube (either sterile or, in some cases, tap water).

Method of feeding using a pharyngostomy tube

(1) Restrain patient.
(2) Remove the bung and flush the tube with 2–10 ml of water to ensure patency.
(3) Administer liquid diet. Initially, in the cat, 5–10 ml per feed. This may be increased up to 30 ml after the first 24 hours.
(4) Flush with a further 5–10 ml of water to clean the tube of food and ensure blockage does not occur before next feed.
(5) Replace bung, clean skin and re-bandage.

This procedure should be repeated at regular intervals. It is bad practice to administer the patient's total food requirement at one time since in many cases this would induce vomiting. Avoid this by feeding little and often.

Diets should be balanced so that they supply the correct amount of all nutrients (including water) and meet the patient's calorific requirement (see later).

FOODS SUITABLE FOR TUBE FEEDING	
Food	**Manufacturer**
Concentrated liquidised tinned food	Various:- Hills p/d Waltham concentration diet
Semi-solid foods (need liquidising)	Hills a/d
Liquid complete foods: Reanimyl Concentrated milk powder Clinifeed Liquivite	 Virbac Waltham Roussel Creg Petfoods UK

Fig. 20.4. Foods suitable for tube feeding.

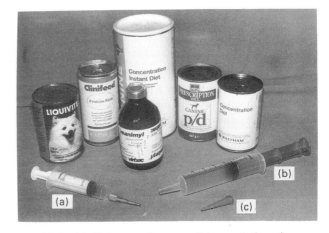

Fig. 20.5. (a) Spigot syringe or (b) nozzled syringe are available for attachment to feeding tubes; (c) solid spigots can be used to keep the lumen of tubes clean and prevent food leakage.

For all tube feeding, it is very important to keep the tube free from blockage. In practice the complete milks cause the fewest problems, having the added advantage of less preparation time, less mess and higher digestibility.

All liquidised foods should be the consistency of whole-fat milk to ensure easy passage down the tubes. Most tinned foods require a large amount of water added to them.

All the diets in Fig. 20.4 are concentrated and easily digested. This is important because normal dog and cat food when liquidised becomes bulk limiting, i.e. the amount of fluid food that needs to be fed to reach the patient's daily kilocalorie (kcal) requirement is enormous and cannot physically be administered over a 24-hour period without the risk of vomiting.

Calculation of Kilocalorie Requirements

This should be carried out for all tube fed patients. The basic energy requirement (BER) is measured in metabolisable kcals per day (see Chapter 17, Nutrition) and calculations depend on the patient's body weight (in kg):

- Patients over 5kg:
  $$BER = 30 \times \text{body weight} + 70.$$
- Patients under 5kg:
  $$BER = 60 \times \text{body weight}.$$

Taking disease factors into the calculation:
$$BER \times \text{disease factor} = \text{kcal requirement}.$$
The factors are:

- Cage rest: 1.2
- Surgery/trauma: 1.3
- Multiple surgery: 1.5
- Sepsis/cancer: 1.7
- Burns: 2.0

Geriatric Nursing

Geriatric nursing involves nursing the ageing animal in both health and disease. Geriatric patients must be treated with extra care, for whatever reason they are admitted. They are less able to adapt to change and recover from medical or surgical interference more slowly (for each 5 years of a pet's age, allow 24 hours longer to recover).

The keys to nursing the geriatric patient are good information (history, drugs), the provision of security (own blanket etc.), comfort (soft bedding), the correct type of food and an adequate source of water.

The changes of old age can be physical or mental (Fig. 20.6). Many of the mental alterations are related to physical change—e.g. disorientation is made worse when the patient is blind or deaf. Ageing changes and the accumulation of any injuries the patient may have sustained result in a loss of functional reserve, i.e. organs of the body become

PHYSICAL AND MENTAL CHANGES THAT MAY OCCUR IN THE GERIATRIC PATIENT	
Physical	**Mental**
Greying of muzzle etc.	Lowered response to
Thickening of the skin	stimuli
Coarse coat	Less adaptable
Loss of musculature	Fussy about food
Loss of stamina and	More likely to develop
strength	food preferences
Weakening of bone	Lower sensitivity to pain
Lowered tolerance to	(questionable)
change	Less interested in activity
Loss of sight	Less obedient
Loss of hearing	Disorientation
Poor tolerance to lack of	
fluid intake	
Impaired temperature	
regulation	
Arthritis and joint	
stiffness	
Higher susceptibility to	
infection	

Fig. 20.6. Physical and mental changes in geriatric animals.

less capable of dealing with extra demands placed on them for repair of tissue, assimilation of substances etc.

Disease

Changes due to disease must be carefully distinguished from those of old age, although disease can become more obvious or affect a patient more rapidly when they become old. Very few sick, elderly patients suffer from a single disease. Many conditions are subtle and multiple. Commonly found disorders of geriatric animals include:

- Cancer
- Chronic renal disease
- Cardiac disease (cardiomyopathy)
- Osteoarthritis (degenerative joint disease—DJD)
- Cataracts
- Dental disease
- Constipation
- Incontinence.

Incontinence is not always truly incontinence but rather where patients lose bladder muscle/sphincter tone. These patients cannot be left alone for long periods without an opportunity to urinate. They urinate in the house or while asleep and may appear incontinent to their owners.

Nursing Considerations

Ensure that the patient's history is known. This includes any current treatment, the preferred food, and conditions they suffer from. Remember that they may be suffering from diseases other than those for which they have been admitted. Specific conditions are dealt with in Chapter 23 (Medical Disorders and their Nursing). The following points are general guidelines.

Drugs

All patients should be weighed but it is particularly important to weigh the geriatric patient so that accurate drug dose calculations can be made. Drug dosage is the veterinary surgeon's responsibility but anaesthetic drugs may well be prepared by nursing staff and accurate calculations are essential. Young patients may have the capacity to survive mild anaesthetic overdosage; **geriatrics do not**.

Feeding

Geriatric patients generally need fewer calories but simply feeding them less can result in a lowered intake of protein, vitamins and minerals.

In the absence of any disease that requires dietary management, it is best to feed a highly digestible, well-balanced proprietary food. There are many available and some companies produce diets specifically formulated for the older dog. Cats tend to stay more active for longer and special diets are less available. To avoid digestive upsets, any changes in diet should be introduced gradually. Lack of interest in food is rarely due to true anorexia in the hospitalised geriatric patient. It is more likely that the patient finds the amount offered too great, has dental disease resulting in pain or has difficulty in standing when eating. All can be simply resolved. Split total intake into two or three small meals, check teeth and assist food intake by hand-feeding or supporting the patient.

Obesity

This is common in the geriatric patient and its treatment is usually a case of client education. Stress to the owners that excess weight is potentially *dangerous* to their pet because extra strain is placed on the heart, kidneys, liver and musculoskeletal system in obese patients. Try to persuade owners that their pet would be happier and healthier if it lost weight. Give them target weights to aim for but be careful to check all diets with a veterinary surgeon to ensure that increased exercise (if possible) and diet changes are not contra-indicated.

Water

> WARNING
> *Do not restrict water intake in the geriatric patient unless they are vomiting.* This is particularly important in relation to the withdrawal of fluids prior to surgery.

No patient should be deprived of water for more than an hour before induction of anaesthesia. Water does *not* need to be withdrawn the night before; this can be extremely dangerous. Younger patients will tolerate the insult but geriatric patients can be pushed over the fine dividing line of renal compromise and may well suffer irreparable damage to renal function that will only be noticeable weeks later.

If vomiting is present, ensure that intravenous fluids are administered.

Exercise

Little and often is recommended. Elderly dogs enjoy 'pottering'. Even hospitalised dogs should be given time to wander, maybe in an outside run. Frequent walks will help to exercise stiff joints and ensure plenty of opportunities to urinate (which might save time on cleaning out kennels).

Take special care if the patient is blind or deaf.

Defecation and urination

Check frequency of defecation. Constipation is more common in the elderly dog and cat.

Observe urination to ensure adequate production of urine, with normal colour and passage (i.e. no straining). Report any difficulty in urination and defecation to a veterinary surgeon as well as any concern about urine production in relation to water intake (e.g. lots being drunk with little urine excreted).

Bedding and kennelling

Blankets and soft bedding should be provided, along with foam mattresses for those with osteoarthritis. Keep geriatrics out of draughts and if possible somewhere not too noisy.

Geriatrics may become cold easily, especially their extremities. If in doubt, check their rectal temperature.

Grooming

Groom elderly patients regularly, as they are less likely to keep themselves clean. It helps to give a feeling of well-being and provides an opportunity to check the coat, skin and to clean discharges from eyes and nose. The human contact is also beneficial.

If the patient has lost its sight or hearing, move slowly and talk reassuringly at all times. This will help to prevent the bite of surprise that elderly dogs so often attempt when suddenly touched or frightened.

Vaccination

Geriatric animals are less responsive to vaccination—they probably have sufficient acquired immunity. However, annual boosters are still advisable.

Convalescence

This will take more time and effort than in younger patients. Have patience and allow a longer period for convalescence.

Maintenance of normal body temperature is especially important pre-, intra- and post-operatively. Thermoregulation in geriatrics is often compromised.

If patients are discharged before they have fully recovered, inform the owners that it will take some time for a pet to complete its recovery. Adequate water intake is very important; ensure that patients can reach water bowls and add water to food if necessary. Exercise should be gentle. Physiotherapy, especially massage, may be used to improve circulation to the extremities.

Care of the Vomiting Patient

Vomiting (**emesis**) is the forcible ejection of contents of the *stomach* through the mouth. It should not be confused with regurgitation, which is the return of undigested food from the *oesophagus.*

Nursing of the vomiting patient can be very straightforward (e.g. in the case of scavenging) or much more complex (e.g. as a result of metabolic imbalances). Some of the common causes of vomiting are shown in Fig. 20.7.

Mechanical and Functional Disorders

Patients suffering from mechanical or functional disorders are usually admitted for surgical correction of the condition. Dietary management is usually simple.

Foreign bodies

Food is generally withheld until surgery has been carried out. If water induces vomiting, it too should be withheld but replaced by intravenous fluids. Most vomiting patients have some degree of dehydration and in these cases an intravenous drip is set up to provide fluid.

The re-introduction of food and water after surgery will vary in each individual case but the following are basic guidelines.

In some cases nothing will be allowed by mouth for 24–48 hours. Intravenous fluid therapy must be continued to supply calculated daily requirements.

Feeding during this time should not be neglected and hopefully some form of enteral feeding will be available, e.g. gastrostomy tube (Fig. 20.3), naso-oesophageal tube or jejunostomy tube (surgically placed into the the small intestine).

Tube feeding allows the surgical site a chance to heal whilst still providing a route for nutrition, which is essential to rapid recovery.

If fluids by mouth are allowed, initially offer small amounts frequently (50–100 ml every hour). If these are not vomited, then the amounts can be increased slowly over the next 8 hours. Intravenous fluids may be continued during this time as total fluid requirements will not be achieved initially.

Reintroduction of food begins once fluids are retained, usually over 24–72 hours. Food offered will vary: usually it will be a bland diet of liquidised or semi-moist chunks of food, offered little and often. Bland foods include chicken, fish or a commercially prepared diet.

Similar protocol is used in the management of pyloric stenosis. In this case food will initially be very well liquidised.

Megaoesophagus

Patients with megaoesophagus regurgitate rather than vomit. Food becomes lodged in the oesophagus cranial to a stricture or narrowing, so that only a limited amount of food reaches the stomach.

Dietary management (even after surgery, if performed) will involve liquidised/semi-solid food fed from a height (Fig. 20.8). Feeding from a height helps to prevent regurgitation and the possible development of aspiration pneumonia—gravity helps the passage of food to the stomach. Passage of food can also be aided after feeding by gentle coupage whilst the patient is in an upright position (see p. 441).

Metabolic Disorders

Patients that vomit due to metabolic disorders are generally more challenging to the nurse. If vomiting has been prolonged, they will be dehydrated and require fluid therapy in combination with other

CAUSES OF VOMITING		
Mechanical/functional disorders	**Metabolic disorders**	**Miscellaneous**
Pyloric stenosis Pyloric stricture Gastric foreign bodies Other gastro-intestinal foreign bodies Intussusception	Kidney disease (nephritis) Liver disease Metabolic alkalosis Electrolyte imbalances e.g. hyponatraemia, hypokalaemia Diabetes mellitus Toxaemia Poisoning	Motion sickness Scavenging Pain Drug reactions Neurological disorders Food allergies Distasteful smells

Fig. 20.7. Causes of vomiting.

treatment. The percentage of dehydration can be estimated clinically (Fig. 20.9).

It is pleasant for the patient to have moist cotton wool wiped around the mucous membranes of the mouth, especially if water has been withdrawn. This not only freshens the mouth but also removes excess saliva.

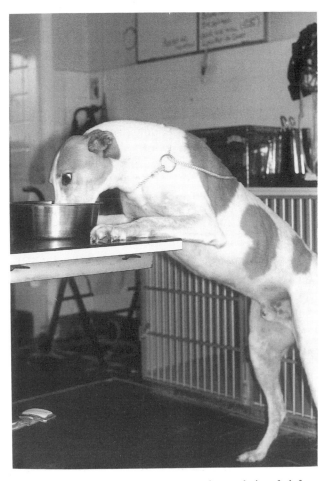

Fig. 20.8. Patient with a megaoesophagus being fed from table-height to aid passage of food to the stomach.

If water is not vomited, oral electrolyte fluids may be useful (Chapter 21 gives more details about fluid therapy).

Anti-emetic drugs, such as metochlopramide, are frequently prescribed. They must be administered by a route other than per os in these situations. Intravenous administration is usually the best route. For continuous effect, the veterinary surgeon may request drugs to be placed in the drip fluid.

When vomiting ceases, water and then food can be re-introduced.

Reintroduction of Food

The following is a general plan for the re-introduction of food to a patient that has been vomiting. It assumes that water does not cause vomiting. *If at any stage vomiting reoccurs, return to the previous day's protocol.*

- **Day 1**: Offer small amounts of bland food 3–4 times daily. Total amount offered should equal one-quarter to one-half of normal daily requirement.
- **Day 2**: Offer small amounts of bland food frequently, to total one-half to three-quarters of daily requirement.
- **Day 3**: As for days 1 and 2 but total amount offered should be equal to normal requirement.
- **Days 7–14**: Reintroduce normal diet by mixing increasing amounts with the bland diet.

Patients that have had a single acute vomiting episode due to scavenging, will need to be starved for 24–48 hours before the reintroduction of food. In these cases the above regime can be followed and can be given as advice to owners over the 'phone. For any other reason it is only a guideline. Specific types of food may be required, or longer periods of starvation may be necessary. A veterinary surgeon will give instructions on the course to be followed.

RECOGNITION OF DEHYDRATION		
Grade	**% Dehydration**	**Clinical signs**
Slight	less than 5%	Not detectable
Mild	5–6%	Slight decrease in skin turgor
Mild	6–8%	Delay in skin fold return Slight increase in capillary refill time (CRT) Dry mucous membranes Sunken eyes
Moderate	10–12%	Tenting of the skin Sunken eyes Increased CRT Tachycardia Cold extremities Early signs of shock
Severe	12–15%	Clinical signs of shock, i.e. tachycardia, weak pulse, pale mucous membranes and cold extremities. These may lead to coma and death.

Fig. 20.9. Recognition of dehydration.

General Points to Remember

- Nausea is an unpleasant feeling. It can be identified in dogs and cats by:
  —restlessness;
  —salivation;
  —repeated swallowing;
  —retching.
  Bring these signs to the attention of the veterinary surgeon.
- Clean away any excess vomitus and clean the mouth. If not contra-indicated, offer small amounts of cool, fresh water (10–15 ml) to allow rinsing of the mouth.
- Handle gently. Lift only if absolutely necessary, ensuring that no pressure is placed on the patient's abdomen.
- Hand-feeding and encouragement may be required during the recovery period.
- If syringe feeding of fluids is instituted at any time, remember the potential for the development of aspiration pneumonia. It is surprisingly easy to cause pneumonia, especially in smaller dogs and cats.
- When patients are discharged, give the owners **written** instructions regarding the type of food, the amounts to be offered, its consistency and the method of feeding.

The Soiled Patient

Many hospitalised patients become soiled at some time during their stay. It is the nurse's responsibility to ensure that all soiling is cleaned efficiently, effectively and quickly.

Regular walking of inpatients may seem time consuming but it may conserve time spent in cleaning kennels and soiled patients. Cats must be supplied with litter trays; check with owners regarding types of litter used as some cats are fussy.

Animals may become soiled by:

- Urine
- Faeces
- Blood
- Vomit
- Food
- Other body fluids.

Reasons for soiling include:

- Confinement to a small area.
- Disturbed routine.
- Medical or surgical condition.
- Untrained puppies.
- Recumbency.

Action when Soiling Occurs

(1) Clean as quickly as possible.
(2) Choose shampoos carefully. Take into consideration patient's coat length, reason for hospitalisation and area to be cleaned or bathed. Chlorhexidine gluconate or povidone iodine are preferable if the patient has any surgical or open wounds. Dry dog shampoos are available, but they are inadequate if soiling has occurred.
(3) Once the area has been cleaned, dry it thoroughly. Most patients will tolerate a hair dryer after a towel rub down. All knots in the coat should be removed since they frequently harbour faeces. Conditioners will make the process much less tiresome for nursing staff and the patient, especially in long-coated breeds.
(4) Whilst grooming, check for any area of soreness, especially if the patient is recumbent. If necessary, clip hair away from these areas.
(5) It is best to clip heavily contaminated areas, especially if further contamination is expected (e.g. under drainage tubes). Ensure that client permission has been given. White petroleum jelly can be applied around these areas after clipping, to prevent soreness and make cleaning easier.
(6) Cats generally keep themselves very clean. If bathing is necessary, use mild shampoos and avoid products based on coal tar (phenol is poisonous to cats). Regular grooming of long-haired cats whilst hospitalised is essential.
(7) Cats with oral lesions or fractured jaws are unable to clean themselves and regular cleaning of the lips, chin and paws will be required.

Enemata

An enema is a liquid substance placed into the rectum and colon of a patient. The enema is not intended to flush colonic contents but to distend the rectum and distal colon gently, initiating normal expulsive reflexes.

Reasons for performing an enema include:

- to empty the rectum;
- as a diagnostic aid;
- to administer drugs.

Emptying the rectum

- To relieve constipation or impaction.
- As preparation for radiographic studies. The colon and rectum overlie abdominal structures and will obscure them if they are not emptied.
- As part of a radiographic contrast study.
- To enable the administration of drugs.

As a diagnostic aid

Barium sulphate enemata can be given to outline the rectal and colonic walls. Remember that the patient needs to evacuate the barium after radiography—a quick retreat to the outside is strongly advised!

Administering drugs

The colon has a large capacity for absorbtion. For this reason it is a good route for the administration of soluble drugs. Although, it is rarely used in veterinary medicine due to lack of patient co-operation.

Solutions used for Enema Administration

The choice of solution depends on the purpose of the enema.

Water

Warm tap water is the preferred solution. It is cheap, readily available, non-toxic and non-irritant. In addition, any cleaning of the perianal area is reasonably straightforward.

Liquid paraffin

This is readily available and quite cheap. Cleaning the patient after the enema can be difficult since liquid paraffin is oil-based and not water-soluble. The patient needs to be bathed with shampoo to remove this substance.

Mineral oil

This suffers the same disadvantages as liquid paraffin and is more expensive. However, oil-based substances are an advantage when treating a constipated patient. The oil helps to soften and lubricate the faecal masses and allows easier evacuation of the bowel.

Saline

This is usually available as manufactured sachets with phosphate included. They promote defaecation by being osmotically active, promoting water retention in the colon. These enemata should be used with care in small and young patients because their excessive use can result in unwanted absorption of certain ions resulting in system toxicity.

Ready-to-use mini-enemata

A proprietary brand of miniature enema is introduced into the rectum by an attached nozzle. It is extremely useful in cats: the procedure is no more stressful than using a rectal thermometer.

Miscellaneous substances

- Glycerine and water.
- Olive oil and water.
- Obstetrical lubricant.

These variations are all more expensive and have no advantages over solutions already mentioned.

Equipment

The basic equipment is shown in Fig. 20.10. It includes enema solution, gloves, lubricant (e.g. KY jelly) and any of the following: can and tubing, Higginson syringe, prepared barium bag, syringe and catheter.

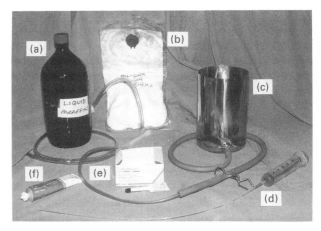

Fig. 20.10. Basic range of equipment and products for carrying out an enema: (a) liquid paraffin; (b) prepared barium; (c) can and tubing; (d) syringe and catheter; (e) microlax; (f) lubricating jelly.

ADMINISTRATION OF AN ENEMA

Figure 20.11 gives guidance on the volumes of solution. The method, for dogs which requires two people, is as follows.

(1) Prepare all equipment.
(2) The assistant restrains the patient in a suitable area, preferably outside where cleaning will be easier.
(3) Lubricate the end of the tube or nozzle.
(4) Elevate the patient's tail and place the tube into the anus. Twist gently until access to the rectum is achieved (this is easy in the dog but occasionally more difficult in the cat).
(5) Advance the tube into the rectum.
(6) Stand to the side of the patient and allow fluid to run into the rectum by gravity.
(7) Allow the patient free exercise to evacuate bowels.

The Recumbent Patient

An animal that is lying down and unable to rise is described as recumbent. A large number of conditions might result in recumbency, the more common being:

- Fractures (e.g. pelvis, limbs).
- Spinal trauma (e.g. disc protrusion).
- Electrolyte imbalances, head injuries, shock.
- Weakness due to medical disease (e.g. Cushing's syndrome, cardiac disease).
- Neurological disease (e.g. coma).

ENEMA SOLUTIONS AND VOLUMES		
Solution	Volume used (ml/kg)	Frequency
Water	5–10	Every 20–30 minutes if necessary
Liquid paraffin	2–3	Every 1–2 hours
Saline solution	1–2	Do not repeat for 12 hours
Barium sulphate	5–10	Not necessary

Fig. 20.11. Enema solutions and volumes.

Kennelling

Bedding

Bed the patient on thick, waterproof (PVC-covered) foam mattresses, with 'Vetbed' or similar on the top. If these are unavailable use thick layers of newspaper with blankets on top. Beanbags, although very comfortable, become soiled very easily and are difficult to clean; they are impractical in the hospital situation.

Size

Previously active animals attempt to drag themselves around (especially fracture and spinal cases in which pain has been relieved). The kennel should be large enough for such a patient to lie in lateral recumbency comfortably, but not so big that it can drag itself around.

Position

Most recumbent patients benefit from being nursed in a kennel sited in an area of activity. This stimulates them and relieves boredom since nursing staff inevitably talk to them more frequently. Ensure kennels are not in direct sunlight, since these patients may be unable to move to a shady area.

Food and Water

Ensure that both food and water are within easy reach. Patients who are recumbent due to a medical condition may well be depressed and hand-feeding may be necessary.

Patients who fail to drink sufficiently can have water added to their food or be encouraged to drink by syringing water into the side of their mouths.

Most recumbent patients require a concentrated, highly digestible diet to meet the extra nutritional needs of stress due to kennelling or continuing tissue repair. Highly digestible diets have the added advantage of producing less faecal material. The energy requirement supplied by carbohydrates is generally lower during recumbency and the amount of carbohydrates offered may need reducing. Note, however, that ill animals may have an *increased* nutrient requirement, since these are necessary for tissue repair.

If a recumbent patient fails to eat, seek advice from the owner regarding preferences and favourite foods.

Obesity may be an existing problem or weight may be gained during the period of recumbency due to less energy being used. It may be necessary to introduce reducing diets, but only in consultation with the veterinary surgeon.

Urination and Defecation

If possible, recumbent patients should be taken outside. The change of environment and fresh air are beneficial to their mental attitude. In addition natural urination and defecation are always preferable to catheterisation and enemata. Help patients to stand since many are unwilling to urinate lying down. Towel support is useful (Fig. 20.12); even tetraplegics can be managed in this way, using crossed towels to support the chest. When an animal is supported, apply gentle pressure to the bladder to encourage urination (Fig. 20.13).

Indwelling catheters can be used. They are beneficial in keeping the patient dry by preventing soiling from urine overflow 24 hours a day.

In bitches, Foley catheters with a bag attached have the added advantage of enabling urine output to be measured. Dog catheters can be sutured to the prepuce in the male dog or catheterisation can be carried out 2–3 times daily.

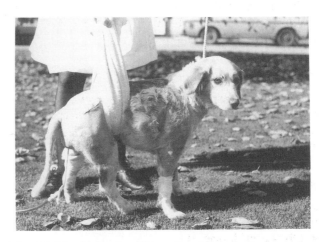

Fig. 20.12. Assisted walking for the recumbent patient supported by a towel. The method can be adapted using crossed towels over the chest when tetraplegia is present.

Cats' bladders can generally be manually expressed although catheterisation may also be performed.

Ensure a record of defecation is kept. It is easy for 3–5 days of non-production to go unnoticed. If the patient becomes constipated, a laxative may be required.

Any diarrhoea in the recumbent patient increases the risk of sores, infection in any wounds, fly-strike in the summer and discomfort to the patient. Inform the veterinary surgeon. Clip excess hair in the perianal/anal area.

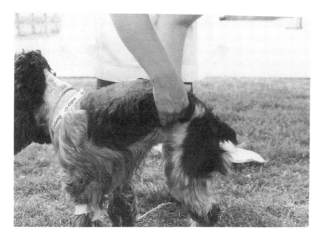

Fig. 20.13. Manual bladder expression whilst supporting a recumbent patient.

Decubitus Ulcers and Urine Scalding

Prevention

It is better to prevent both decubitus ulcers (bed sores, Fig. 20.14) and urine scalding, rather than treat them after they have occurred.

- The use of soft bedding with absorbable blankets (e.g. 'Vetbed') together with regular turning of the patient (every 4 hours) will help to lessen the occurrence of sores.

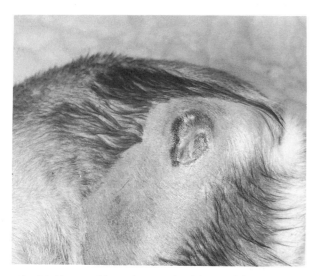

Fig. 20.14. Decubitus ulcer on the skin overlying the ilium.

- Bony prominences are most likely to suffer (e.g. elbows and ischial wings). These areas can be padded with foam rings from the top of tablet pots (Fig. 20.15) or the patient can be encouraged to lie laterally for *short* periods (a balance between lateral and sternal recumbency needs to be found—see hypostatic pneumonia, below).
- Massage is beneficial and can be performed while the patient is recumbent.
- Slings to raise patients for longer periods are used in the United States but rarely in the UK (Fig. 20.16).
- Catheterisation (indwelling or repeated) enables bladder drainage without soiling. Otherwise assisted walking is essential to provide opportunities for urination.
- Waterbeds may be useful but are rarely used in the UK.

Action

Any patients which are dirtied by urine should be checked for the presence of urine scalds. They begin as innocent-looking red patches and if treated at this stage, are very easily managed. There is no excuse for them getting worse if nursing care is adequate.

Urine scalding is relieved by:

- Regular washing with a mild antiseptic shampoo (e.g. dilute chlorhexidine gluconate or povidone iodine). Both must be rinsed off thoroughly.
- Catheterisation.
- Clipping of hair and the application of soothing healing or barrier creams.

Decubitus ulcers are far more serious and can be extremely difficult to resolve.

Treatment:

(1) Clip the area around the sore.
(2) Clean with a mild antiseptic solution (e.g. dilute povidone iodine or chlorhexidine gluconate).
(3) Dry thoroughly.
(4) Apply an appropriate cream.
(5) If it is summer, and the position of the ulcer allows, cover with a dressing to prevent fly strike and contamination.

WARNING

Hardening of areas prone to decubitus ulcers with spirit is *not* to be recommended.

Hypostatic Pneumonia

Hypostatic pneumonia is caused by the pooling of blood and a consequent decrease in viability of the dependent lung. It is more likely to occur in an old, sick and debilitated animal that has been in lateral recumbency for a long period. Turning the patient at least every 4 hours—24 hours a day—is essential nursing. Encourage sternal recumbency by using

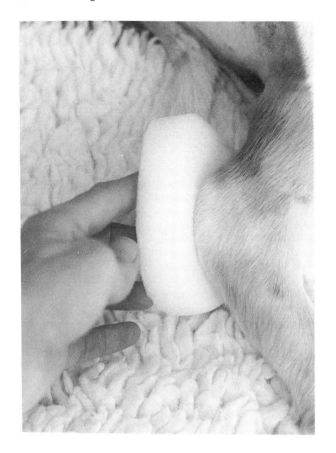

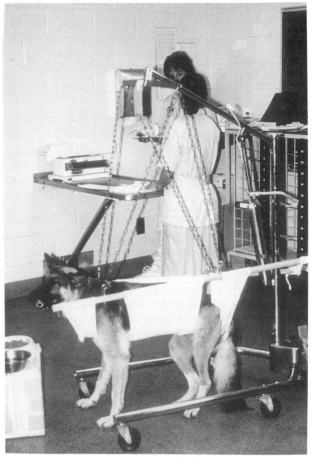

Fig. 20.16. Wheeled 'total support' sling systems are frequently employed in the United States.

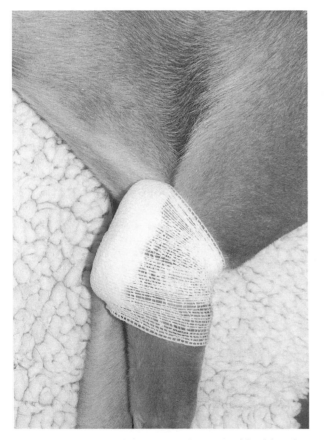

Fig. 20.15. Padding of bony prominences with either foam or cotton wool can help to prevent occurrence of decubitus ulcers.

sandbags, water/sand-filled containers or X-ray cradles, and remember to support the head.

Regular **coupage** (the external slapping of the thorax with cupped hands) 4–5 times daily for 5 minutes will improve thoracic circulation; by promoting coughing it also aids removal of secretions that build up in the bronchial tree. *Check with a veterinary surgeon before using coupage* to ensure that there are no contraindications such as fractured ribs.

WARNING
It is important to realise that serious secondary chest infections may result if hypostatic pneumonia is allowed to develop. This alone can cause *death.*

If hypostatic pneumonia with a secondary infection is present, continue all the above guidelines for prevention. In addition treatment (e.g. antibiotics) will probably be prescribed.

Signs of hypostatic pneumonia are:

- Fast/frequent shallow breathing.
- Increased respiratory effort.
- Moist noises when breathing, possibly even gurgling.
- Depressed attitude.

If you suspect hypostatic pneumonia inform a veterinary surgeon immediately. Experienced auscultation of the lung fields and radiography may be required to confirm the diagnosis.

Passive Physiotherapy

Physiotherapy helps to maintain and improve peripheral circulation. It is of benefit to all recumbent patients, even if only for the extra human contact and attention.

Massage

This is particularly useful for the limbs. Massage from the toes towards the body to encourage venous return to the heart.

Supported exercise

Towel-walking is the most common (and cheapest) method. Make sure that adequate staff are available, as both the patient and the staff member can be injured if the patient is heavy.

Hydrotherapy

Swimming is very useful physiotherapy for dogs (cats generally do not appreciate it!). Small dogs can be swum in large sinks and baths in the hospital; larger patients need pools. Swimming enables patients to move their limbs freely without weight-bearing forces.

Check the temperature of the water before immersing the patient. *Constant* support and observation are essential to prevent panic and possible drowning.

Passive joint movement

Manually moving joints within their normal range helps to prevent stiffness and improves circulation.

Coupage—as previously described

Body Temperature

Recumbent patients expend very little energy, therefore heat production is lower than normal. Body temperature will frequently fall to a subnormal level. Blankets to cover the patient may be sufficient. Other heating methods include:

- Veterinary duvet-type covers with reflective filling.
- Veterinary instant heat pads, which should be wrapped initially: when activated, they heat to 52°C.
- Hot water-bottles, which should be wrapped to prevent burning of the patient.
- Heated water beds—use only if the patient is very debilitated and will not bite or scratch. They are expensive pieces of equipment.
- Bubble packing—cheap and effective.

- Silver foil is good for extremities. Remove if patients become active, especially young ones (it is 'edible').
- Infra-red lamps.

> WARNING
> Electrically heated beds are *not* recommended unless the patient is under *constant supervision*. Some varieties have been implicated in causing serious burns when patients were placed directly on top of them. A blanket should always be between the heated pad and the patient.

Home Nursing

Recumbent patients are generally managed in a hospital environment. Some will inevitably be recumbent for a longer period and may be nursed at home. Most owners are quite capable of learning how to nurse their own pet but remember that tasks which come automatically to a nurse need to be pointed out to an owner. It is helpful to write clear instructions to which owners can refer once they are home. Reassure owners that they can phone at any time if they are worried. Arrange weekly checks at the surgery to check for signs of decubitus ulcers, urine scalding or hypostatic pneumonia.

Comatosed Patient

In this context, 'comatosed' is interpreted as a long-term coma rather than simple recovery from anaesthesia. This may occur in conditions such as tetanus, neurological disease or after major convulsions. In reality these patients are rarely nursed in general practice—they really need an intensive care unit and a large number of personnel.

The nursing of a comatosed patient is essentially similar to that for a recumbent one and all the nursing points made for the care of the recumbent patient can be implemented for the comatosed patient—with the exception of eating, drinking and exercise. In addition, the following points should be considered when nursing the comatosed patient:

- Keep a patent airway—pull the tongue forward and consider endotracheal intubation.
- Clean any secretions from the oral cavity—use a sucker or swabs or lower the head to encourage drainage by gravity.
- Monitor at 15-minute intervals:
  —temperature, pulse and respiratory rate and rhythm;
  —mucous membrane colour;
  —capillary refill time;
  —urine output;
  —drip rates;
  —drug administration.

> *Constant* 24-hour observation is essential for the comatosed patient.

Urinary Catheterisation

A **catheter** is a tubular, usually flexible instrument passed through body channels for the withdrawal of fluids from (or the introduction of fluids into) a body cavity.

Reasons for urinary catheterisation:

- To obtain a (sterile) urine sample when:
  - a patient will not micturate when required (this may be because the patient is only at the surgery for short periods, e.g. at consultation, or timed urine samples are required, e.g. water deprivation test);
  - obtaining a midstream urine sample (MUS) is impossible because the amount produced during exercise is little (e.g. the male dog that squirts 2 ml at every tree);
  - a culture and sensitivity examination is requested (it is essential that urine is collected in a sterile manner for this examination: MUS samples become contaminated at the prepuce and vulva and provide meaningless results).
- To empty the urinary bladder:
  - before abdominal, vaginal and urethral surgery;
  - before a pneumocystogram;
  - when there is a partial obstruction or inability to urinate but a catheter can be passed into the bladder (e.g. due to prostatic enlargement).
- To introduce contrast agents for radiographic procedures.
- To maintain constant, controlled bladder drainage (indwelling catheters):
  - in the recumbent or incontinent patient to prevent soiling;
  - after bladder surgery, to avoid over distension of the bladder, thereby reducing tension on the suture line and helping to provide optimum healing conditions for the operative site.
- In **hydropropulsion** (the use of water pressure to dislodge particles causing an obstruction: a urinary catheter is placed caudal to the particle and water pressure is used to dislodge the calculi from the urethra back into the bladder). Hydropropulsion can be used to relieve a partial blockage in an emergency situation. It is nearly always followed by surgery (e.g. cystotomy or urethrostomy).
- To maintain a patent urethra:
  - in male cats suffering from feline urological syndrome (a catheter may be placed to maintain bladder drainage whilst treatment or diet is initiated; catheter placement also allows flushing of the bladder with solutions which may dissolve struvite crystals, e.g. Walpole's solution);
  - where dysuria or anuria is present but surgery is delayed due to the patient being in a poor condition for surgery (e.g. raised blood urea levels, electrolyte imbalance etc.).
- To monitor urine output:
  - where a patient with renal compromise is on large volumes of intravenous fluids;
  - if the patient is in intensive care;
  - after renal surgery to ensure adequate production of urine.

Minimum urine output =
1 ml/kg body weight/hour.

- Introduction of drugs.

Complications Associated with Catheterisation

Complications which might arise include infective cystitis, reactive cystitis, urethral damage, failure to catheterise the urethra, resistance by the patient, blockage of indwelling catheters or removal of indwelling catheters by the patient. Reasons for these complications are described below, and Fig. 20.17 outlines methods of preventing them and the action to be taken should they arise.

Infection

Urinary tract infection (UTI) can result from catheterisation fairly easily if bacteria present in the urethra are pushed into the bladder by the catheter. In most circumstances the bacteria will be eliminated and cause no further concern. The risk of infection is increased when:

- the bladder is traumatised;
- a prepucial or vaginal discharge is present;
- indwelling catheters are used;
- the patient is immunosuppressed, i.e. its immune system is compromised in some way and the body's natural defences are not operating correctly.

> WARNING
> Any urinary tract infection is potentially serious. Prevention is better than cure!

Cystitis after catheterisation

This is associated with indwelling catheters. It is rarely seen otherwise, unless repeated catheterisation has been carried out.

Urethral damage

This is most likely to occur in the male dog, due to the ischial curve of the urethra—some epithelial damage is inevitable as the catheter is passed around the curve. (This is why a small amount of blood may be present in the tip of the catheter on removal from the urethra.)

COMPLICATIONS ASSOCIATED WITH CATHETERISATION: PREVENTION AND ACTION		
	Prevention	**Action**
Infection	Use only new or re-sterilised catheters. Plastic catheters should only be re-sterilised once. Use sterile gloves to handle catheters or employ the 'no touch' technique desribed for dog catheterisation. Use sterile lubricants. Clean penis or vulva thoroughly before catherisation; clip surrounding hair if necessary. Catheterisation should be carried out in a clean environment, not in the patient's kennel. Ensure that sytemic antibiotics are prescribed by the veterinary surgeon. A single (long-acting) dose may be sufficient after just one catheterisation of a healthy patient. Patients with indwelling catheters should receive systemic antibiotics whilst catheterised and continue the course for 5–10 days after removal.	If infection becomes evident, treatment will consist of systemic antibiotics and, in some cases, soluble antibiotics flushed directly into the bladder.

Cystitis after catheterisation	Gentle introduction of the catheter – no force should be necessary.
	Use of lubricants is beneficial – they help to limit the epithelial damage to the urethral mucosa, thereby reducing inflammation.
	Trauma is less likely if an experienced person catheterises debilitated patients.
		With indwelling catheters there is inevibility some degree of cystitis after removal of the catheter. If it is significant:
		  * Encourage the patient to increase its fluid intake, either as water or by adding water to the food.
		  * Walk the patient frequently to allow urination; observe colour and amount of urine passed.

Urethral damage	*Never* use force. Use adequate lubrication. If an obstruction or difficulty occurs, stop, and inform a senior member of staff.	If trauma caused by catheterisation is suspected, a veterinary surgeon will have to decide what further action is to be taken. Minor trauma will be treated with a course of antibiotics.
Failure to catheterise the urethra in the bitch	The only prevention is to gain experience in bitch catheterisation, which can only be achieved with practice. The easiest way for the student nurse to appreciate the position of the urethral orifice is the use of a lighted speculum to provide viewed introduction of the catheter.	If catheterisation of the cervix does occur, remove the catheter and begin again with a new one.
Patient resistance		Sedate or, in extreme cases, anaesthetise the patient.
Blockage of indwelling catheters	General hygiene and cleaning. Encourage increased water intake (this helps to maintain a continuous flow of urine through the catheter). If bags are attached, check regularly to ensure that urine is able to drain freely.	Flush with sterile saline or water.

Fig. 20.17. Complications associated with catheterisation.

Failure to catheterise the urethra

Failure to catheterise the urethra may occur in the bitch if the urethral orifice is passed and the catheter cannot be advanced because it meets the cervix. Catheterisation of the cervix is a rare occurrence and is easily identified:

- by viewing the urethral orifice with a lighted speculum;
- because no urine flows through the catheter—but note that catheters can be placed correctly and still not produce urine, due to either an empty bladder or an obstruction to urine flow (e.g. excessive lubricant blocking the drainage holes).

Patient resistance

This is common in bitches and female cats.

Blockage of indwelling catheters

Urine will cease to flow from the catheter.

Removal of indwelling catheters by patients

Adequate suturing (tom cat, dog) and the application of Elizabethan collars should prevent catheter removal by the patient.

Types of urinary catheter

All catheters (Fig. 20.18) manufactured for the veterinary market, excepting metal bitch catheters, are supplied individually, double wrapped, with an inner nylon and outer paper or plastic sleeve. The catheters are ready for use, having been sterilised by either ethylene oxide gas or gamma radiation.

Urinary catheters are designed for *single use only*. The cleaning and re-use of these catheters is not recommended, though single re-use might be acceptable if thorough cleaning and proper sterilisation techniques are employed.

Re-sterilisation often costs *more* in respect of nursing time (cleaning and packing) and money (cost of packaging, running an autoclave or an ethylene oxide system acceptable to the COSHH regulations) than it would to use a *new* catheter.

Dog catheters

Dog catheters (Fig. 20.19(a)) have a rounded tip behind which are two oval drainage holes (one at each side). They are designed for single use in the male dog and can be used as indwelling catheters.

Choose the largest gauge appropriate for patient size. If too small a catheter is used, the tip of the catheter has a tendency to 'catch' in the urethral epithelium and bend. This may cause significant urethral trauma.

The only exception is where the urethra is narrowed due to a partial obstruction such as enlarged prostate, or a stricture. In these cases, there is no option other than to use a catheter that would otherwise be too small for the patient.

A second disadvantage of using small catheters in large patients is that the patient is stimulated to urinate when the catheter is introduced into the urethra, and urine will flow around the catheter as well as down the lumen.

In recent years, dog catheters have been used to catheterise bitches. They have no curved tip but are much firmer, providing more control for insertion into the urethral orifice, particularly when digital catheterisation is used. This extra rigidity far outweighs the advantage of the Tieman's catheter curved tip.

All lubricants are compatible with these catheters.

Bitch catheters

Tieman's catheter. Designed for catheterisation of the human male, these catheters (Fig. 20.19(b)) became popular for use in the bitch due to their curved tip. The moulded tip was found to be advantageous when placing it into the urethral orifice. However, the rest of the catheter is so soft and flexible that the amount of control over the tip is negligible. This makes placing the catheter into the urethral orifice a very difficult task. The excessive length of the catheter is a further disadvantage.

Foley indwelling bitch catheter. Foley catheters (Fig. 20.19(c)) incorporate an inflatable balloon behind the drainage holes at the tip of the catheter.

TYPES OF URINARY CATHETER							
Type	Species	Sex	Material	Indwelling	Sizes	Length	Luer fitting
Dog catheter	Dog	Male (or female)	Flexible grade of nylon (Polyamide)	No but can be adapted to be indwelling	6–10 FG	50–60cm	Yes
Tieman's	Dog	Female	PVC (Polyvinyl chloride)	No	8–12 FG	43cm	Yes
Foley	Dog	Female	Teflon coated latex	Yes	8–16 FG	30–40cm	No
Cat catheter	Cat	Male and female	Flexible grade of nylon	No	3 and 4 FG	30.5cm	Yes
Jackson cat catheter	Cat	Male and female	Flexible grade of nylon	Yes	3 and 4 FG	11cm	Yes
Metal	Dog	Female	Plated brass	No	Various	20–25cm	No

FG = French gauge. Each unit on this gauge is one third of a millimetre and refers to the external diameter of the catheter.

Fig. 20.18. Types of urinary catheter.

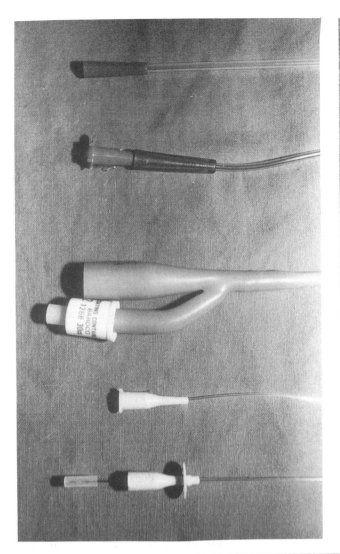

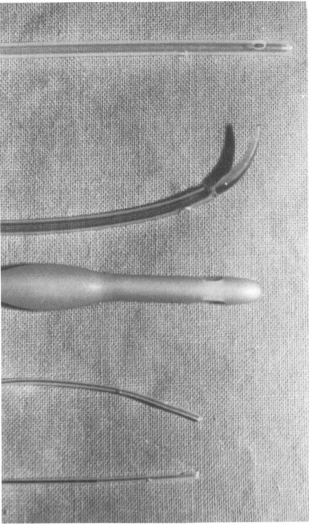

Fig. 20.19. Types of catheter: dog; Tieman's; Foley; conventional cat; Jackson cat; metal bitch catheter.

The balloon is inflated after placement of the catheter into the bladder, making it an indwelling catheter.

Foley catheters are produced for the human market, but suitable sizes are available for use in most bitches except very tiny puppies. They cannot be used in cats or the male dog (unless in conjuction with a urethrostomy). The balloon is inflated (usually with sterile water or saline) via a channel built into the wall of the catheter which ends in a side arm and a one-way valve. The catheter is removed by deflating the balloon through the same side arm.

These catheters *must not be re-used*: the balloon is weakened after use and cannot be relied upon to function correctly if re-used.

Foley catheters are very flexible—this provides maximum patient comfort but causes a problem when introducing them. Placement is achieved by the use of a rigid metal stylet or probe laid beside the

catheter with the point secured in one of the drainage holes at the catheter's tip. The stylet is removed once the balloon is inflated.

> WARNING
> The stylet is *not* placed up the middle of the catheter (Fig. 20.20).

Foley catheters must not be lubricated with petroleum-based ointments or lubricants, which will damage the latex rubber so that the balloon may burst on inflation.

The absence of a luer mount in this catheter may cause problems for continuous collection of urine but urine collection bags with appropriate connectors are available from medical suppliers. If these bags cannot be supplied, the catheter must have an adapter placed so that drip bags can be used for urine collection (Fig. 20.21). Unless 3-litre drip bags are

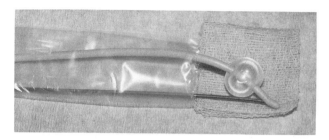

Fig. 20.20. Correct placement of the stylet in the tip of the Foley catheter. The balloon is inflating correctly and therefore the catheter is ready for use.

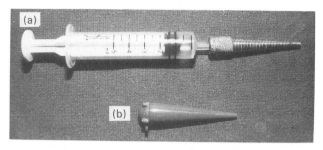

Fig. 20.21. (a) Spigot: to provide a Leur connection for the Foley catheter to enable empty drip-bag attachment (to collect urine) or to allow bladder drainage with a syringe. (b) Bung: to prevent continuous drainage and therefore soiling of the patient, when a urine collection bag is not in use.

employed, frequent emptying will be required in most dogs. It would be unwise to leave a large dog with only a litre collection bag attached overnight.

An alternative is to bung the catheter and drain the bladder at regular intervals with a spigot (Fig. 20.21). This method may be acceptable for a recumbent patient but not, for example, after bladder surgery.

Metal. Metal catheters (Fig. 20.19(f)) are rather outdated and are rarely used in modern veterinary establishments. Their rigid construction may result in considerable trauma unless the operator is very experienced. Even then some urethral damage is inevitable. The use of metal catheters is not recommended.

Cat catheters

Conventional. These straight catheters (Fig. 20.19(d)), with a leur connection and compatible with all lubricants, are for single use. They are basically a small version of the dog catheter.

Jackson. Jackson catheters (Fig. 20.19(e)) were designed primarily for use in male cats suffering from feline urological syndrome (Walpole's solution may be used to flush the bladders of male cats suffering from FUS). They can be used in any male or female cat.

A fine metal stylet, lying in the lumen of the catheter, gives extra rigidity and provides better control for insertion into the urinary bladder. It also helps to displace any loose obstruction (e.g. protein plugs or struvite crystals in the urethra). A normal catheter would be too flexible to achieve this. The stylet is removed once the catheter is in place.

The Jackson is much shorter than the other cat catheters, in order to allow suturing to the prepuce. Sutures are placed in the circular plastic flange which is present just behind the leur fitting of the catheter. In this way the catheter becomes indwelling.

All lubricants are compatible. Re-use is not recommended.

Equipment

Specula

A speculum is an instrument which assists cavities to be viewed. Specula assist catheterisation of bitches by holding back the vaginal tissue and allowing good visualisation of the urethral orifice. This is of great aid to the student nurse: digital catheterisation can be difficult without a visual knowledge of the urethral position.

It is preferable for all specula to be sterile and it is often cheaper in the long run to invest in a metal speculum that can be autoclaved, rather than using the home-made variety that needs gas sterilisation. If no specula are available, bitch catheterisation is still possible digitally.

There are several varieties of speculum, most of which are not specifically designed for catheterisation.

Nasal speculum. There are many slight variations, the adult size being the most appropriate. All have two flat blades which separate when the handles are closed together (Fig. 20.22(a)). Some have a retaining device; others have to be held open. A light source may be attached to one of the blades to illuminate the vagina. If this is not available, a pen torch held by an assistant is an effective alternative.

Rectal speculum. This is used rarely, mainly due to expense. Rectal specula (Fig. 20.22(b)) are conical in shape and, once in place, a section of the conical arm slides out to allow viewing of the urethral orifice. The main problem is to align the removable section with the urethral orifice—easy in theory, but difficult in practice.

Auriscope. This is a normal auriscope handle and light but the attachment used has a section removed from its wall (Fig. 20.22(c)).

Home-made speculum. Monoject syringe packing cases are ideal rigid plastic specula and they are cheap. Simply remove one section of the cover, file

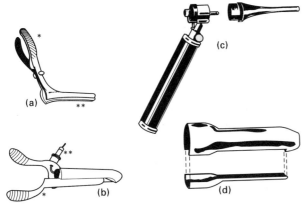

Fig. 20.22. (a) Nasal speculum, suitable for use as a bitch vaginal speculum. Pressing together the handles* causes the blades** to move apart and open the vestibule. (b) Rectal speculum, suitable for use as a bitch speculum. The lower sliding panel* is removed after insertion into the vestibule to expose the urethral opening. The lighting attachment**, which is connected to a battery, provides a self-contained light source. (c) Catheterisation speculum for attachment to an auriscope resembles an ear speculum except that a segment of its wall is absent. (d) A speculum made from the container of a Monoject disposable syringe by cutting away a segment of the plastic.

the edges and use an external light source (Fig. 20.22(d)).

Batteries and transformers

Ensure that these are electrically tested and working correctly. Spare batteries should always be in stock. Transformers are usually away from the vulva and do not require sterilisation.

Speculum bulbs

These are best stored separately as they break easily. They cannot be sterilised in the autoclave and therefore need gas or, more realistically, chemical sterilisation.

Stylets

Stylets can be made or bought. Ensure that they are long enough for easy use—they need to be at least the length of the longest Foley catheter stocked (approximately 40 cm). Stylets can be packed and autoclaved or chemically sterilised.

Urine collection bags

Manufactured varieties come pre-packed and sterile; they are designed for single use.

Previously used drip bags can be used with a giving set attached. Ensure that the end of the giving set is thoroughly cleaned and chemically sterilised before being attached to the urinary catheter. Attach a needle to the end of the giving set during storage to keep it clean from dust and dirt.

Bungs and spigots

Plastic bungs come pre-packed but are rarely sterile. They are best sterilised chemically. Metal spigots can be autoclaved or placed in chemical sterilising solution until needed.

Three-way taps

These are invaluable when draining bladders via a catheter. They avoid mess by controlling urine flow whilst syringes are emptied.

Catheter Storage and Checking

Catheters should be stored in a dry environment and laid flat without any pressure on top of them. Unless a suitably long drawer is available, urinary catheters are best left in their boxes and removed only when required.

All catheters have a shelf life, after which sterility is no longer guaranteed by the manufacturer. Make regular checks, especially if the practice's use of catheters is infrequent. If catheters are resterilised, it is advisable to re-use them as quickly as possible—prolonged storage can result in further degradation. Check that:

- there are no splits, tears, holes etc. in the packing;
- no kinks are visible;
- the balloon inflates before placement of a Foley catheter;
- the stylet moves freely in the lumen before using a Jackson cat catheter.

Cleaning and Sterilisation of Catheters

Practice policy regarding re-use of catheters is rarely the nurse's decision, however, the process of cleaning and sterilisation is time-consuming and is *not* recommended for urinary catheters.

Cleaning

(1) Flush, with force, copious amounts of cold water through the catheter immediately after use. This is usually done with a syringe. Cold water prevents coagulation of any protein that may be present.
(2) Remove any blockage with a wire stylet and repeat step (1).
(3) Wash the exterior and interior of the catheter with a mild detergent. Rinse thoroughly, as in (1).
(4) Check catheter for kinks, holes etc. If any damage is found the catheter *must* be discarded.
(5) Dry in a warm, dust-free atmosphere.

Sterilisation

Pack appropriately (autoclave bags or ethylene oxide). Autoclaving is the best method for nylon catheters. The COSHH Regulations have made the use of ethylene oxide in most practices difficult andexpensive. There are no short cuts and therefore it is unlikely that any but the largest of veterinary establishments will continue to sterilise equipment by this method on their own premises.

WARNING
Boiling is not acceptable—it is *not* a method of sterilisation.

Methods for Urinary Catheterisation

Actual procedures for urinary catheterisation of dogs, bitches (three methods), tom cats and queens are set out in Fig. 20.23. Several general points apply to all methods.

Physical restraint

Most patients will allow urinary catheterisation under gentle physical restraint without resistance. If necessary, use a muzzle on a dog. Ensure that the patient is at a comfortable working height.

- Dogs and cats can be restrained in a standing position or in lateral recumbency.
- Bitches can be restrained in dorsal recumbency.

Chemical restraint

Sedation.
- Dog: rarely required unless the patient is aggressive or very nervous.
- Bitch: most bitches will accept catheterisation more readily if lightly sedated, especially if dorsal recumbency is chosen. Standing catheterisation is best done without sedation, otherwise the patient tends to keep sitting down—which can be tiring for the assistant.
- Cat: catheterisation of the cat is generally less stressful for all concerned if the cat is sedated.

General anaesthesia (GA). This is rarely indicated or necessary unless the patient has sustained other trauma which makes catheterisation under sedation humanely unacceptable (e.g. fractured pelvis, vaginal mass). It is sensible to catheterise during general anaesthesia if this is required for other treatment (e.g. catheterise a tetraplegic patient whilst under GA for a myelogram).

Equipment preparation

Prepare all equipment *before* restraining the patient. Patient co-operation will be greater if prolonged restraint is avoided.

Lubricants

There is some debate over the necessity for the use of lubricants. Urinary catheterisation can be done without but lubricants aid passage of the catheter and help to avoid abrasive trauma.

- Check contents of lubricants before using them with Foley catheters, most are water-based and are compatible with commonly used catheters.
- Make sure that lubricants are sterile. Xylocaine gel (Astra) and KY jelly (Johnson and Johnson) are ideal choices. Xylocaine gel has the added advantage of desensitising the urethra, penis or vestibule.

Cleaning

- Clean the area with an antiseptic solution to remove any discharges and surface dirt.
- Clip around the area if necessary, especially in long-haired breeds. (Remember to check that permission for this has been obtained from the owner.)

Gloves

The use of gloves is recommended for health and safety. In general, multiple packs of non-sterile gloves are adequate because the catheter will be fed from its package using a 'no touch' technique. Gloves are therefore used to prevent contamination of staff with urine, rather than protection of the patient from infection.

Sterile gloves will be required when digital catheterisation is performed, as the catheter tip is inevitably touched by the finger.

Length of catheter

Measure a dog or cat catheter against the patient before unpacking the catheter. This measurement gives a rough estimate of the length of catheter to insert into the patient.

Stop inserting once urine flows. Over-insertion can result in the catheter bending and re-entering the urethra or, even worse, knotting in the bladder and requiring surgical removal.

Other Methods of Emptying the Urinary Bladder

Natural micturition

This is non-invasive and usually easy to achieve by nurse or owner. In most circumstances it is the preferred method for emptying the bladder but there are several disadvantages:

- The sample is always contaminated and therefore useless for culture and sensitivity evaluation.

- If the patient is unable to urinate normally, another method has to be employed.
- Patients often refuse to produce urine when convenient and required.

If not required for culture, then collection of samples from the environment may be acceptable in some cases, e.g. urine can be retrieved from litter trays that have been left empty.

URINARY CATHETERISATION		
	Equipment	**Method**
Dog catheterisation	Catheter Lubricant Swabs for cleaning Syringe to assist urine drainage Three-way tap (if required) Sample pot Gloves Urine bag or a bung Kidney dish *If the catheter is to be made indwelling:* Suture material Zinc oxide tape	1. Wash hands and put on gloves. 2. Clean prepuce. 3. Extrude penis; if not experienced, get an assistant to do this two-handed (Figure 20.24). 4. Clean prepuce. 5. Remove catheter from the outer wrapping and cut a feeding sleeve from the inner sterile packaging (Figure 20.25). This allows easy feeding of the catheter from the packaging into the urethra using a no touch technique. 6. Lubricate the catheter and insert the tip into the urethra (Figure 20.24). 7. Advance the catheter up the urethra. Resistance may be met at the os penis, where there is a slight narrowing of the urethra, at the ischial arch and area of the prostrate gland if enlarged. Steady but gentle pressure should overcome this resistance. If the catheter cannot be passed, re-evaluate catheter size. 8. Proceed according to reason for catheterisation (e.g. drain bladder, collect sample, hydropropulsion). To provide an indwelling dog catheter (Figure 20.26): 1. Place zinc tape around catheter near to prepuce. 2. Stitch to prepuce; or 3. Stick to prepuce. Neither of these options is ideal because dog catheters are not designed to be indwelling.
Bitch catheterisation Method 1: Urethra viewed in dorsal recumbency	Speculum (with or without light source) Alternative light source if required Catheter Lubricant Swabs for cleaning Gloves *If a Foley catheter is being placed (Figure 20.20):* Stylet Sterile water/saline to inflate cuff Urine bag Syringe	1. Wash hands and put on gloves. 2. Ensure the bitch is in a straight dorsal recumbent position with the hindlimbs flexed and drawn forward (Figure 20.27). The tail needs to be under control too. 3. Clean vulva. 4. Remove catheter from outer wrapping and expose tip only from inner sleeve. 5. If a Foley catheter is being used, insert the stylet. 6. Place speculum blades between the vulval lips as caudally as possible to avoid the clitoral fossa (Figure 20.28). 7. Insert *vertically* into the vestibule and turn handles cranially (Figure 20.28). 8. Open the blades of the speculum. The urethral opening will be visible on the cranial side of the vertically oriented vestibule, approximately half way between the vulva and cervix (Figure 20.29). 9. Insert the tip of the catheter into the urethral orifice (Figure 20.29). **Draw the hindlimbs backwards.** This straightens the urethra, making it easier to push the catheter into the bladder.

Table 20.23 continued   *Fig. 20.23.—continued*   ♦

URINARY CATHETERISATION

	Equipment	Method
		10. Proceed depending on reason for catheterisation. If a Foley catheter is being used, inflate balloon, withdraw stylet, attach bag and place Elizabethan collar (Figure 20.30).
Bitch catheterisation Method 2: Urethra viewed standing	As in Method 1. Generally only one assistant is required.	1. Wash hands and put on gloves. 2. Ensure tail is well restrained. 3. Clean vulva. 4. Place speculum between vulval lips and advance at a slight angle towards the spine, then horizontally (Figure 20.31). 5. Open blades and identify urethral orifice. This will be on the ventral floor of the vestibule. 6. Insert catheter at a slightly ventral angle so as to follow the direction of the urethra into the bladder. 7. Proceed as for Method 1.
Bitch catheterisation Method 3: Digital	Sterile gloves Catheter Lubricant Swabs for cleaning Collection pots If a Foley is being placed, additional equipment is as in Method 1.	1. Restrain in preferred position, lateral or standing (standing is generally easiest). 2. Scrub hands and put on sterile gloves in an aseptic manner. 3. Ask an assistant to clean the vulva (gloved member having sterile hands). 4. Assistant removes outer wrapping from catheter and the inner package is removed by the scrubbed member. 5. Holding the sterile part of the packaging, place stylet if necessary. 6. Lubricate first finger of *non-writing* hand. 7. Place finger into vestibule and feel along ventral surface for a raised pimple (Figure 20.32). 8. Place finger just cranial to this raised area, which is the urethral orifice (Figure 20.32). 9. Raising hand and finger dorsally, digitally guide catheter, tipped slightly ventrally (as in Method 2) into the urethral orifice. The catheter will run past the fingertip if the orifice is missed. 10. Proceed as for Method 1.
Tom cat catheterisation	As for dog catheterisation.	1. Wash hands and put on gloves. 2. Restrain patient and have control of the tail. 3. Prepare feeding sleeve as for the dog catheter and lubricate tip. 4. With one hand extrude penis by applying gentle pressure each side of the prepuce with two fingers (Figure 20.33). 5. Introduce catheter into the urethra. 6. Collect sample or drain bladder. 7. If a Jackson catheter is being placed for continuous drainage, stitch flange to prepuce.
Queen catheterisation This is rarely carried out but is quite straightforward if required (e.g. for contrast studies)	As for dog catheterisation.	1. Restrain patient. 2. Wash hands and put on gloves. 3. Remove outer wrapping and cut a feeding sleeve. 4. Lubricate tip of catheter. 5. The catheter is placed between the vulval lips and 'blindly' introduced into the urethra. Angle the catheter ventrally, placing gentle pressure until the catheter slips into the urethra. 6. The catheter is not designed to be indwelling.

Fig. 20.23. Methods for urinary catheterisation.

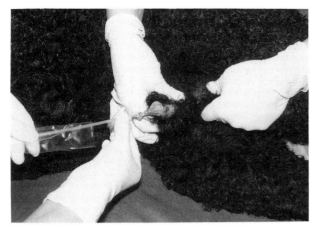

Fig. 20.24. Two-handed method for penis extrusion for introduction of a catheter into the urethra.

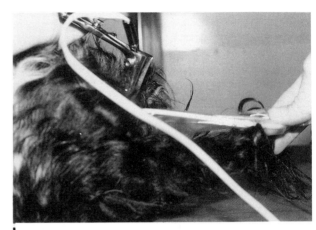

Fig. 20.28. Correct speculum angle in the vestibule and the horizontal position of the Foley catheter as it is advanced into the bladder.

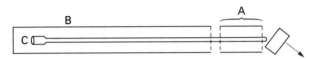

Fig. 20.25. Creating a feeding sleeve for easy introduction of urinary catheters. A: feedings sleeve; B: outer packaging; C: catheter.

Manual expression of the bladder

In cats this is probably the most common method. Dogs, especially recumbent ones, can also be encouraged to urinate in this way.

As long as the bladder is of a reasonable size, this task becomes easier with practice. Pressure should be applied steadily and slowly—do not use sudden pressure as this may cause trauma to the bladder. Generally very little pressure will initiate a free flow of urine. Excessive pressure should never be required.

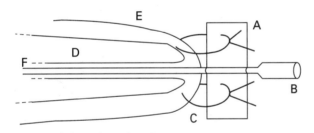

Fig. 20.26. Suturing of catheter to prepuce, to create an indwelling male urinary catheter. A: zinc tape butterfly; B: Leur tip catheter; C: suture; D: penis; E: prepuce; F: catheter in urethra.

Cystocentesis

This should only be carried out when the bladder is of a palpable size (Fig. 20.34). The method is as follows:

(1) The patient is restrained in a position between lateral and dorsal recumbency.
(2) Clip an area about 5 × 5 cm on the midline caudal abdomen.
(3) Prepare the skin aseptically, and manually immobilise the bladder, through the abdoman wall.
(4) Using a syringe (5–20 ml) with a needle attached (23 gauge × 1 inch), insert through the abdominal wall and into the bladder.
(5) Remove urine.
(6) Apply gentle pressure at the injection site as the needle is quickly removed. The use of larger gauge needles is to be discouraged because it increases the possibility of urine leakage from the bladder after needle removal.

> This technique is fairly straightforward and generally without complications, as long as an aseptic technique is used. It may be the only method available for urine drainage in an obstructive emergency.

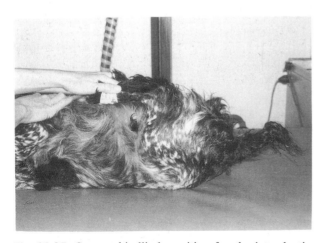

Fig. 20.27. Correct hindlimb position for the introduction of a Foley catheter with the patient in dorsal recumbency.

This procedure must only be carried out by a veterinary surgeon.

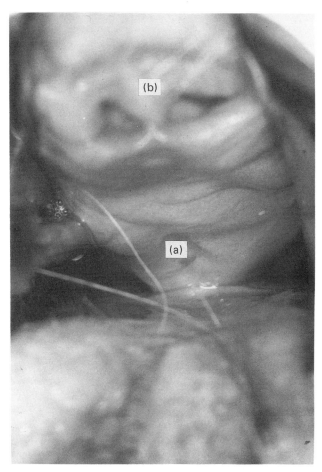

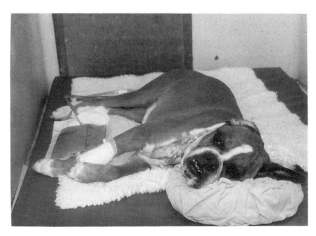

Fig. 20.30. Recumbent patient with Foley catheter in place and urine collection bag attached. (This patient was unable to raise her head; therefore no Elizabethan collar was necessary.)

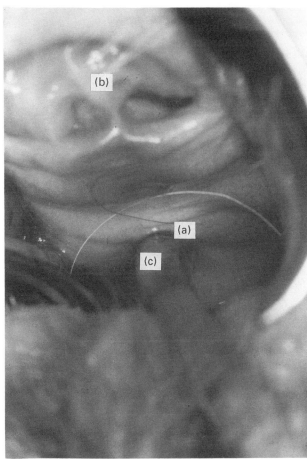

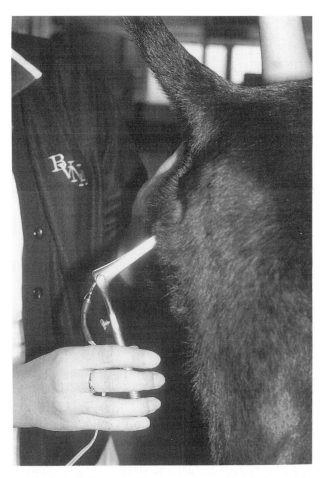

Fig. 20.29. Close-up view of the position of (a) the urethral orifice, (b) clitoral fossa and (c) catheter in position.

Fig. 20.31. Angle of speculum for introduction between lips of vulva in standing bitch. The speculum handle is then raised to insert the blades fully into the vestibule, avoiding painful interference with the clitoral fossa.

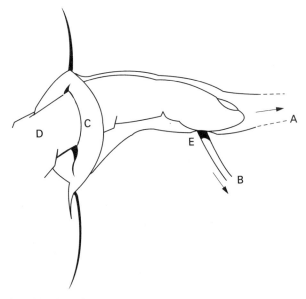

Fig. 20.32. Digital catheterisation: A: to cervix; B: to bladder; C: vulva; D: finger; E: raised area (urethral orifice).

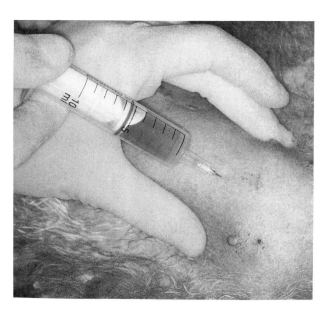

Fig. 20.34. Cystocentesis in a dog.

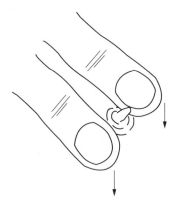

Fig. 20.33. Extrusion of tom cat penis.

21
Fluid Therapy and Shock

E. WELSH

Many medical and surgical conditions and interventions cause disturbances of body fluid, electrolyte and acid–base balance within the body. A knowledge of the homeostatic mechanisms which normally govern these physiological processes is essential if disturbances within this system are to be identified, and subsequently rectified, in a logical and effective manner. This chapter reviews briefly the physiology of body fluid, electrolyte and acid–base balance and then examines how to determine if fluid therapy is required, what the most appropriate fluids and routes of administration are and how to assess the patient's response to treatment.

Units and Definitions

It is important to be familiar with the various methods of measurement of fluids and electrolytes within the body, and to understand the units which describe them.

A **solution** consists of a solute dissolved in a solvent. Saline solution is comprised of sodium chloride (a solute) dissolved in water (a solvent). In the body, water is the main solvent.

An **electrolyte** is a substance which yields ions when dissolved in water.

An **ion** is a small water-soluble particle of atomic or molecular size which carries one or more positive or negative charges. Sodium chloride (NaCl) is an electrolyte which, in solution in water, dissociates into sodium ions and chloride ions. The sodium ion loses one electron (Na^+); in contrast, the chloride ion gains an electron (Cl^-). Both sodium and chloride ions are referred to as **univalent** ions, whereas ions which lose or gain two electrons are referred to as **divalent** ions (e.g. O^{2-}, Ca^{2+}).

Cations are ions carrying one or more positive charges (e.g. Na^+, Ca^{2+}).

Anions are ions carrying one or more negative charges (e.g. Cl^-, O^{2-}).

Frequently, the strengths of biological solutions are measured in terms of their molecular, electrostatic or osmotic composition.

Molecular composition is described by the **molar concentration** measured in the number of moles per litre. However, since biological fluids are very dilute, it is more convenient to measure concentrations in millimoles per litre (mmol/l), that is one thousandth of a mole (1 mmol = 1/1000 mol, or 1 mol = 1000 mmol). Molar concentration is determined as follows:

$$\text{Molar concentration (mmol/l)} = \frac{\text{Concentration (g\%)} \times 10\,000}{\text{Molecular weight}}$$

For example, a 0.9% solution of sodium chloride (molecular weight 58.5) contains approximately 154 mmol/l. The **equivalence** system is an older system of measurement which is still often used in physiology and in clinical practice, as it gives an indication of the ionic composition of a fluid. It is related to the molecular weight and the valence (see above).

$$\text{Equivalent weight} = \frac{\text{Molecular weight}}{\text{Valence}}$$

When the valence is 1, the equivalent concentration in milliequivalents per litre (mEq/l) is the same as the molar concentration in millimoles per litre. Where the valence is 2, the equivalent concentration is twice the molar concentration. In a solution, the sum of the equivalent weights of the cations must be balanced by the anions to ensure electroneutrality.

The **concentration of a solution** is measured by the mass of solute which is dissolved in a volume of solvent. The gram per cent (gram % or g/dl) unit describes the number of grams of solute in 100 ml of solvent. Therefore, 5% dextrose has 5g dextrose in 100 ml of water (or 50 g/l).

Osmosis is the process by which pure solvent (water) moves from a region of low solute concentration to a region of high solute concentration when separated by a **semi-permeable membrane**, to equalise or at least minimise, the difference in concentrations. Semi-permeable membranes are very common in the body and are effectively permeable to solvents but not to solutes.

The **osmotic pressure** of a solution is the pressure needed to prevent osmosis from happening and it is proportional to the **number of particles** (not the size of the particles), both ions and undissociated molecules, in the solution.

- **Isotonic** solutions exert equal osmotic pressures to body fluid.
- **Hypertonic** solutions exert a higher osmotic pressure than body fluid.
- **Hypotonic** solutions exert a lower osmotic pressure than body fluid.

In general, when choosing fluids for parenteral administration isotonic solutions should be used, although hypertonic solutions are occasionally administered (e.g. hypertonic saline; 10% glucose) When fluids are administered to an animal, by whatever route, they initially enter the extracellular fluid (ECF). If hypertonic solutions are added to the ECF, water will be drawn out of the cells into the ECF resulting in cellular dehydration. Conversely, if hypotonic solutions are added to the ECF, water may move into the cells resulting in cellular overhydration and possible lysis of the cells, although excess water is readily excreted if the kidneys are working normally.

Protein molecules contribute to the osmotic pressure of certain body fluids, because in general proteins are large molecules which cannot diffuse freely across cell membranes. In contrast, both water and salts can move freely across biological membranes by diffusion. Consequently, the proteins exert a steady osmotic pressure which is referred to as the **effective osmotic pressure** (colloid osmotic pressure or oncotic pressure). The osmotic pressure exerted by the blood proteins—primarily albumin—maintains the difference between the osmotic pressure of the plasma and the interstitial fluid. This difference is important in maintaining an adequate volume of fluid within the blood vessels. Similarly, non-diffusable proteins within the cells contribute to the intracellular osmotic pressure.

Distribution of Body Water

It is generally accepted that, on average, the water content of the body is 60% by weight, ranging from 50% to 70% in normal healthy animals. It varies with age, sex and nutritional status. For example, the water content of the body of young animals may be as much as 70–80%, while in older animals it may be as little as 50–55% of body weight. Such details highlight the importance of prompt and adequate fluid therapy in neonatal and young animals suffering from excessive fluid losses, especially as their kidneys are less efficient at producing concentrated urine. The body water content is also affected by the proportion of fat to lean tissue in the body, since fatty tissue contains a much smaller amount of water than do other organs and tissues. Therefore, to avoid the danger of overhydration, fluid therapy in obese animals should be based on the requirement of their ideal body weight as they will have a slightly lower requirement than that calculated from their actual body weight.

Almost two-thirds of the total body water is located inside the cells of the tissues (**intracellular fluid**, ICF), while the remaining one-third is located outside the cells (**extracellular fluid**, ECF). The ECF may be further divided into: **plasma water** (PW), which is the water contained within the vascular compartment; **interstitial fluid** (ISF), which is present in the spaces between the cells; and **transcellular fluids** (TCF), which are specialised fluids formed by active secretory mechanisms but comprising only a very small proportion of the ECF (e.g. cerebrospinal fluid, gastrointestinal secretions). The distribution of body water into its principal compartments is shown in Fig. 21.1.

The Composition of Body Fluids

The intracellular and extracellular fluids differ in both composition and function; the interstitial fluid and the plasma water are similar in composition (Fig. 21.2). The composition of transcellular fluid reflects its specialised function and may bear no resemblance to any other body fluid.

Plasma contains sodium as the main cation, with smaller amounts of potassium (K^+), calcium (Ca^{2+}) and magnesium (Mg^{2+}). Chloride and bicarbonate (HCO_3^-) are the main anions with small amounts of phosphate (PO_4^{2-}) and protein. In all body fluids the number of positive charges must equal the number of negative charges so that an electrical gradient does not exist. Normal blood capillaries have only a limited permeability and the large protein molecules cannot pass easily through this barrier. Therefore, ISF is an **ultrafiltrate** of plasma and contains everything found in plasma except proteins. In the ECF, sodium is the main cation with chloride and bicarbonate as its neutralising anions.

The intracellular fluid has potassium and magnesium as its main cations and relatively small amounts of sodium. The major neutralising anions are phosphate and protein. There is also some bicarbonate and chloride in the ICF.

Sodium is sometimes referred to as the 'osmotic skeleton' of the ECF, maintaining the volume of the ECF against the osmotic pull of the ICF. Protein (primarily albumin) acts in a similar manner within

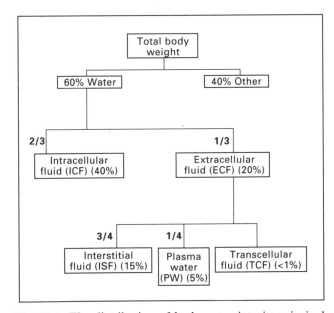

Fig. 21.1. The distribution of body water into its principal compartments.

THE APPROXIMATE COMPOSITION OF PLASMA WATER, INTERSTITIAL FLUID AND INTRACELLULAR FLUID (mmol/l)		
	Plasma Water	Interstitial fluid	Intracellular fluid
Cations			
	138	130	10
Sodium	4	4	110
	2.5	1.5	–
Potassium	1	1	15
Calcium	102	110	10
	27	27	10
Magnesium	17	–	50
Anions	1	1	26

Fig. 21.2. Composition of body fluids.

the vascular compartment. Blood pressure tends to force fluid out of the vascular compartment and into the ISF, while the protein within the plasma acts to pull this fluid back into the vessels.

Body Water and Electrolyte Balance

The normal healthy animal is able to match the intake and output of water and principal electrolytes. It obtains water from two main sources:

- Ingestion (fluids and food)
- Metabolism (fats and carbohydrates).

Metabolism of ingested fats and carbohydrates provides about 10% of the animal's water requirement.

Animals lose water by four main routes:

- Kidney (this is the only route by which water loss can be regulated within certain limits by varying the urinary water content to compensate for changes in water availability).
- Gastrointestinal tract (loss of water occurs in the faeces and abnormal losses occur during vomiting and diarrhoea).
- Respiratory tract (water is lost from the respiratory tract during breathing and panting because air is humidified as it passes along the tracheobronchial tree and nasal passages).
- Skin (water is lost from the surface of the skin (pores in paws) by evaporation and this loss is influenced by ambient temperature and humidity).

The water loss via the respiratory tract and the skin is known as **inevitable** or **insensible** because it cannot be regulated by the body and continues even at times of water deprivation.

Water loss (in terms of body weight) over 24 hours is as follows:

- Respiratory/cutaneous losses: 20 ml/kg
- Faecal loss (normal faeces): 10–20 ml/kg
- Urinary loss (normal range): 20 ml/kg.

Therefore to maintain a normal water balance in a healthy dog or cat, a total of approximately 50–60 ml/kg/day of water is required. Although the inevitable water losses from the respiratory tract and skin cannot be regulated, within the body the kidneys play an important role in the regulation of not only water and electrolytes but also acid–base balance. At times of reduced intake or increased loss of water and electrolytes the osmotic concentration of the body fluids increases and the volume of the ECF (more specifically the plasma water) is depleted. This has two effects. Firstly, the animal will become thirsty because of stimulation of thirst centres within the hypothalamus. Secondly, the increase in plasma osmotic concentration will be detected by **osmoreceptors** (cells which are sensitive to osmotic changes in the plasma water) which stimulate the release of **antidiuretic hormone (ADH)**, which is stored in the posterior pituitary. Release of ADH promotes the reabsorption of water from the renal tubules and this will increase the concentration of the urine that is voided. (Conversely, if the osmotic concentration of the plasma is reduced, less ADH will be released; therefore less water will be reabsorbed within the kidney and the urine will become more dilute.) In addition, a reduction in plasma water will be detected directly by the kidneys as a reduction in renal perfusion. This stimulates the release of a renal hormone, **renin**, which causes generation of **angiotensin** in the blood. In turn, angiotensin stimulates the release of another hormone from the adrenal cortex, **aldosterone**. Aldosterone acts on the kidney to increase the reabsorption of sodium within the distal tubule, and thence water, resulting in more concentrated urine (Fig. 21.3).

The urine **specific gravity** reflects the solute concentration and may be measured with a urinometer,

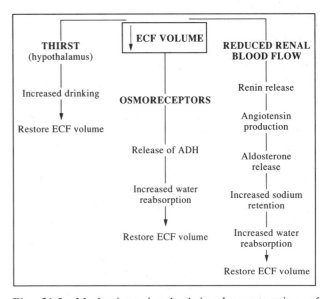

Fig. 21.3. Mechanisms involved in the restoration of extracellular fluid volume.

refractometer or dip-stick test. The normal range for urine specific gravity is:

- Dog: 1.015–1.045
- Cat: 1.020–1.060.

If an animal is dehydrated the specific gravity of the urine will generally increase because the urine becomes more concentrated, e.g. in the dog the specific gravity may increase to 1.060 and in the cat to 1.080.

The management of water balance is probably more important than the regulation of electrolyte status. However, electrolytes too are delicately balanced within the body, and the balance of sodium, potassium, chloride and bicarbonate is the most important. In general, conditions resulting in increased loss of water also cause loss of electrolytes. In the normal animal the daily requirement for sodium is 1mEq/kg/day and for potassium 2mEq/kg/day, but these requirements will change where abnormal losses or retention of body fluids are occurring.

Thus the recording of the daily intake and loss of fluid in veterinary patients is an important part of patient care, especially in animals suffering from water and electrolyte imbalances. Recording ranges from the simple monitoring of the drinking and urinary habits of elective surgical patients to the accurate observation of volumes of fluid consumed orally and administered parenterally, measurement of urine and faecal output and recording of abnormal losses. Ideally water balance should be recorded on a chart detailing route of administration, type and volume of fluid given and details of fluid losses. Each page would represent a 24-hour period and a glance at the chart would then be a useful guide to each animal's fluid status.

Disturbances of Water and/or Electrolyte Balance

Many medical conditions and surgical interventions can disrupt the body's water and/or electrolyte status. Such conditions arise through altered intake or output of water and/or electrolytes. The term **dehydration** describes a reduction in the total body water and the signs and symptoms associated with such a loss.

Dehydration can be caused by a loss of water only which is known as **primary water depletion**. This is common where water intake is reduced or absent because of continued inevitable water losses, e.g. during excessive panting or when an animal is deprived of drinking water. In addition, certain disease states (such as diabetes insipidus) can cause a primary water depletion. More commonly, water losses are accompanied by electrolyte losses, especially sodium which is the main cation of the

ECF, and this is referred to as a **mixed water/electrolyte depletion**. The losses which are incurred during vomiting and diarrhoea include water, sodium, chloride and bicarbonate depletion. If diarrhoea is prolonged, potassium is also lost. In haemorrhage, protein, haemoglobin, platelets and clotting factors are lost in addition to water and electrolytes.

In conditions where urinary output has failed (e.g. blocked urethra, ruptured urinary bladder and acute renal failure), metabolites and electrolytes which are normally excreted in the urine accumulate within the body. In addition, insensible losses lead to water depletion. Therefore, the fluid imbalance which is present is very complicated and relates mainly to water loss, elevated serum potassium levels and acidosis.

Common diseases and the principal fluid disorders they cause are given in Fig. 21.4

Assessing Fluid Requirements

It is important to assess the degree of dehydration and the state of the circulation prior to initiating fluid therapy. There are a number of clinical and laboratory methods which may be used to establish the amount of fluid which is required by an individual animal.

History

A good history enables accurate assessment of fluid deficits. The owner should be asked questions about the animal's food and water consumption (anorexia, polydipsia), any gastrointestinal losses (vomiting,

---

CAUSES OF THE PRINCIPAL FLUID ABNORMALITIES

1. **Primary water depletion**
   Prolonged inappetence (fractured jaw, head or neck injury etc.)
   Water unavailable (forgetful/neglectful owners)
   Unconsciousness (coma)
   Fever or excessive panting
   Diabetes insipidus
2. **Water and electrolyte depletion**
   Vomiting
   Diarrhoea
   'Third space' losses (intestinal obstruction, peritonitis)
   Pyometra
   Wound drainage
3. **Potassium depletion**
   Prolonged inappetence (starvation)
   Vomiting
   Prolonged diarrhoea
   Prolonged diuretic therapy
4. **Potassium accumulation**
   Ruptured urinary bladder
   Urethral obstruction
   Acute renal failure
   Addison's disease

Fig. 21.4. Causes of fluid abnormalities.

diarrhoea), urinary losses (polyuria, oliguria), abnormal discharges (open pyometra) and traumatic losses (blood loss, burns).

EXAMPLE

Consider a 20 kg dog which has been off food and water for three days and vomiting about three times daily for the last 2 days.

- 3 days' inevitable water losses (20 ml/kg/day): 1200 ml
- 1 day's urinary water loss (20 ml/kg/day): 400 ml
- 2 days' vomiting 3 times/day (4 ml/kg/vomit): 480 ml

Total water deficit: 2080 ml

Physical Examination

Clinical signs are a useful, but not always accurate, means of assessing dehydration. Signs such as loss of skin elasticity, sunken eye and prolonged capillary refill time do not start to appear until the animal is 5% dehydrated, and 15% dehydrated animals are moribund. When assessing the elasticity of the skin it is important to remember that it is generally reduced in cachectic animals, even when they are not dehydrated, while fat animals will lose their skin elasticity when more severely dehydrated than an animal of normal weight. Intermediate changes are described in Fig. 21.5.

The animal's fluid requirement is calculated by multiplying the percentage dehydration by the bodyweight in kilograms.

EXAMPLE

10% dehydration in a 20 kg dog represents a fluid deficit of 2000 ml ($0.1 \times 20 \times 1000$).

CLINICAL SIGNS ASSOCIATED WITH DEHYDRATION	
Percentage Dehydration	**Clinical signs**
<5%	Not detectable
5–6%	Subtle loss of skin elasticity
6–8%	Marked loss of skin elasticity
	Slightly prolonged capillary refill time
	Slightly sunken eyes
	Dry mucous membranes
10–12%	Tented skin stands in place
	Prolonged capillary refill time (>2 sec)
	Sunken eyes
	Dry mucous membranes
12–15%	Early shock
	Moribund
	Death imminent

Fig. 21.5. Dehydration: clinical signs.

Laboratory Analyses

There are some simple laboratory tests which can be helpful in estimating losses:

- Packed cell volume (PCV)
- Haemoglobin
- Total plasma protein (TPP)
- Blood urea and creatinine
- Plasma electrolytes
- Acid–base estimations.

Packed cell volume

The PCV is an inexpensive but revealing parameter. For each 1% increase in the PCV, a fluid loss of approximately 10 ml/kg body weight has occurred. Rarely will the normal PGV of the patient be known, and therefore an estimate of 45% is made in dogs and 35% in cats.

EXAMPLE

If a 20 kg dog was found to have a PCV of 55%, the deficit should be calculated thus:

$$20 \text{ kg} \times 10 \text{ ml/kg/\%} \times (55-45\%) = 2000 \text{ ml.}$$

The equation is unreliable where pre-existing anaemia is present unless the PCV prior to fluid loss is known. Similarly acute blood loss cannot be evaluated by the PCV unless compensation has taken place or fluid has already been administered to replace the loss.

Haemoglobin

Dehydration will also result in an increase in the haemoglobin concentration of the blood but care must be taken when interpreting results from an anaemic animal.

Total plasma protein

Dehydration will cause a rise in TPP, but care must be taken because a dehydrated hypoproteinaemic animal may present with an apparently normal TPP. It is useful to assess both the TPP and PCV in an animal which has been diagnosed clinically as dehydrated because only rarely will pre-existing disease result in an elevation of both these parameters.

Blood urea and creatinine

Blood urea and creatinine levels will rise in the dehydrated animal but it is important to consider the possibility of renal disease, which can also result in an elevation in these two parameters.

Plasma electrolytes

Estimation of the plasma electrolyte level (e.g. Na^+, K^+, Cl^-) is possible but is frequently of limited value as recorded values are not always an accurate reflection of the total body content of the individual ion. However, determination of serum potassium concentration is of value because a marked deficit of this ion can result in severe muscle weakness and cardiac disturbances and equally an excess of this ion can result in fatal cardiac dysrhythmias.

Clinical Measurement

The following measurements can be used to estimate fluid deficits but are more frequently used to monitor progress of fluid therapy and response to treatment in intensive care patients.

Body weight

Body weight is easily measured and acute losses may be due to fluid loss or catabolism. Acute increases in body weight are nearly always caused by increased fluid content. However, the usefulness of body weight in the initial estimation of fluid loss is limited because few owners know the weight of their pet.

Central venous pressure (CVP)

The CVP is a useful means of estimating the need for fluids in any situation but especially where congestive cardiac failure is present or where circulatory overload may be a problem (acute renal failure). Following severe, acute haemorrhage, CVP is invaluable in determining the adequacy of replacement therapy. Measurement of the CVP will be discussed more fully later.

Urinary output

Measuring the urinary output is a useful means of assessing the adequacy of fluid replacement. As already discussed, urine output is low during dehydration (oliguria), and the return of normal urine output signifies that replacement is adequate. Urine output can be monitored casually by observation, but placing an indwelling urinary catheter allows accurate measurement. Normal urine output is 1–2 ml/kg/hour. A urine output of less than 0.5 ml/kg/hour is defined as oliguria. If fluid therapy fails to improve the urine output in an oliguric animal, the possibility of acute renal failure should be considered.

Acid–Base Balance

In a similar way to water and electrolyte balance, the acid–base balance is a closely guarded parameter which can be upset at times of disease. Hydrogen ions within the body are produced as a result of normal metabolic activity, and the body's acid–base status is a measure of the hydrogen ion concentration within its tissues. Hydrogen ions are measured according to the pH scale. The **pH** is defined as the negative logarithm (to the base 10) of the hydrogen ion concentration. The pH scale has a range of 1 to 14. A pH of 7 is regarded as neutral; a pH of greater than 7 is alkaline (bases) and a pH less than 7 is acidic (acids).

In the normal animal, blood is slightly alkaline—it has a normal range of pH 7.35–7.45. When the pH of the blood falls below 7.35 a state of **acidaemia** is said to exist, whereas when the pH of the blood greater than 7.45 a state of **alkalaemia** is said to exist.

Acidosis and **alkalosis** describe abnormal processes and conditions which would cause acidaemia or alkalaemia respectively if there were no secondary (compensatory) changes in response to them. Acidosis and alkalosis can exist without producing acidaemia/alkalaemia because of the body's secondary compensatory mechanisms. Acidosis and alkalosis may be either **metabolic** or **respiratory**, depending on their origin.

It is essential for proper cellular function that the blood pH is kept within the normal range. Large changes in pH may result in the animal becoming depressed and may ultimately lead to its death. Therefore the body has efficient mechanisms for dealing with the hydrogen ions which are produced within the body to prevent dramatic fluctuations of pH. There are three principal means of dealing with hydrogen ions, and these systems work in sequence to try to limit the effects of changes in hydrogen ion concentration. **Buffers** are the first to respond to alterations in the pH, followed by a **respiratory response** and finally a **renal response**.

Buffering

Buffers are able to react with acids and bases and reduce the extent of the pH change which they would normally produce. Buffers act by trapping the H^+ ions rather than eliminating them from the body, but are required to keep the pH within narrow limits until the H^+ ions can be delivered to either the lungs or the kidneys, where they can be removed from the body. In general, buffers are weak acids or proteins. Because weak acids do not dissociate completely in water (unlike strong acids such as hydrochloric acid, HCl) they restrict the number of H^+ ions in solution, whereas proteins (such as haemoglobin) act as anions and have many sites to which cations such as H^+ ions may bind. Most buffering that takes place within the body occurs within the cell, and proteins are among the most important intracellular buffers.

Extracellular buffers include bicarbonate and phosphate (Fig. 21.6). The reaction which converts bicarbonate (HCO_3^-) to carbonic acid (H_2CO_3) does not become saturated in the same way as the phosphate (HPO_4^{2-}) reaction because the action of the enzyme carbonic anhydrase upon the carbonic acid results in the formation of carbon dioxide and water, both of which can be expelled from the body (or in the case of water incorporated in the body water).

Respiratory System

The respiratory system controls the level of carbon dioxide within the body. The carbon dioxide is in equilibrium with the carbonic acid in solution in the body fluids which is a source of H^+ ions (see above). Increasing respiration will remove carbon dioxide from the body and therefore reduce acidity. Decreasing respiration will retain carbon dioxide and therefore increase acidity.

It has already been noted that the reaction which converts bicarbonate (HCO_3^-) to carbonic acid (H_2CO_3) does not become saturated because of a build-up of water and carbon dioxide (see above); however, the reaction may be limited by the amount of available bicarbonate.

Renal System

Bicarbonate can be generated within the cells of the kidney by a reversal of the reaction which results in the formation of water and carbon dioxide (Fig. 21.7). The bicarbonate which is generated enters the ECF pool while the H^+ ions that are generated are excreted.

Thus, it is apparent that the pH of the body fluids is dependent upon the concentration of carbon dioxide and bicarbonate ions within the body:

$$pH = [HCO_3] \div pCO_2.$$

Therefore, the pH will fall if there is an increase in the concentration of carbon dioxide within the body, a fall of bicarbonate ions within the body or if H^+ ions are added to the system. Conversely, reducing the concentration of carbon dioxide within the body, adding bicarbonate ions to the system or removing H^+ ions will cause an increase in the pH.

Acid–Base Abnormalities

To obtain an estimate of the acid–base balance of an animal it is necessary to obtain an arterial blood sample, although venous blood samples can provide useful information if an arterial sample cannot be taken. In dogs and cats, arterial blood is generally taken from either the main femoral artery, or a superficial branch of the femoral artery. The anti-coagulant which is used is heparin, and the sample should be drawn anaerobically. If the arterial blood is not analysed immediately, it should be stored on ice, or at 4°C, until analysis. Analysis of the blood will provide the pH of the sample, the bicarbonate ion concentration and the carbon dioxide tension (a measure of the amount of carbon dioxide within the sample), and from this information the clinician will be able to establish what deficits the animal is suffering.

Acid–base abnormalities are not uncommon during disease and Fig. 21.8 shows the four major disturbances that can occur and the situations in which they are likely to arise. **Respiratory acidosis** arises through inadequate ventilation, or a failure of the respiratory system to respond to the increased levels of carbon dioxide which are characteristic of rebreathing or increased production. The buffers will lessen the pH disturbance but renal compensation will only occur when the condition becomes long-standing. **Respiratory alkalosis** occurs much less frequently than respiratory acidosis in veterinary practice.

(a) bicarbonate

$$H^+ + HCO_3^- \rightleftharpoons \underset{\substack{\text{carbonic}\\\text{acid}}}{H_2CO_3} \underset{\substack{\text{carbonic}\\\text{anhydrase}}}{\rightleftharpoons} CO_2 + H_2O$$

(b) phosphate

$$H^+ + HPO_4^{2-} \rightleftharpoons H_2PO_4^-$$

Fig. 21.6. Buffers: (a) bicarbonate reaction; (b) phosphate reaction.

$$CO_2 + H_2O \rightleftharpoons H_2O_3 \rightleftharpoons H^+ + HCO_3^-$$

Fig. 21.7. Bicarbonate in kidney cells.

CAUSES OF ACID–BASE ABNORMALITIES	
Metabolic acidosis	
Accumulation of H⁺	Shock
	Ruptured bladder/blocked urethra
	Diabetic keto-acidosis
	Aspirin/ethylene glycol poisoning
Loss of base	Chronic renal failure
	Chronic diarrhoea
Metabolic alkalosis	
Loss of H⁺	Prepyloric vomiting
Accumulation of base	Over-administration of bicarbonate
Respiratory acidosis	
Impaired ventilation	General anaesthesia
	CNS injuries (cerebral oedema)
	Severe lung damage
	Certain nerve/muscle diseases
Inspired carbon dioxide	Anaesthetic equipment
Increased carbon dioxide production	Malignant hyperthermia
Respiratory alkalosis	
Overventilation	Mechanical/manual ventilation
	Apprehension/pain/fear

Fig. 21.8. Causes of acid–base abnormalities.

Metabolic acidosis arises when acid metabolites are retained within the body or when the loss of buffer is marked. Respiratory compensation is rapid but incomplete, and ultimately the kidneys must restore the balance, either by excreting hydrogen ions or by retaining bicarbonate, or both. **Metabolic alkalosis** again occurs much less frequently.

The treatment of the various acid–base abnormalities should be directed initially at the source of the problem. Respiratory acidosis and alkalosis require therapy aimed at curing the ventilatory disturbance. Metabolic acidosis can be ameliorated by providing extra buffer in the form of sodium bicarbonate (usually 1–2mEq/kg i/v is adequate). Often reduced renal perfusion is the cause of a metabolic acidosis and using fluid therapy to restore renal perfusion will be sufficient to correct the abnormality.

Objectives of Fluid Therapy

The purpose of fluid therapy is to replace deficits from previous losses, improve and maintain renal function and supply maintenance requirements.

The most important initial treatment is to restore an adequate circulating volume, as severely dehydrated animals may be showing signs of shock. After this, the remaining deficit can be replaced more slowly. In general, existing deficits should be replaced within the first 24 hours after admission. Thereafter it is important to remember that, while the animal is undergoing treatment, provision must be made to replace the continued inevitable and urinary losses as well as any continuing abnormal losses, e.g. diarrhoea.

Routes of Administration of Fluids

Oral Fluid Administration

If an animal is willing to drink, is not vomiting and does not have an intestinal obstruction, the oral route of fluid (and food) administration is a simple, cheap and painless method to treat an animal with mild dehydration. In addition, it is an ideal route by which to supply daily maintenance requirements after initial deficits have been replaced. Moreover, the animal does not need to be hospitalised and so the owner may take the animal home.

The intestine acts as a barrier for selective absorption of water and electrolytes, providing a wide margin of safety. However, there are a number of disadvantages and the oral route is not the route of choice if an animal is severely dehydrated. Although administering fluid orally does not require absolute sterility, only a limited range of fluids can be given (it is inappropriate for whole blood or plasma expanders such as dextrans), and it can be time-consuming.

Oral therapy is not ruled out where prehension is limited or impossible: fluid may be administered by either nasogastric tube, pharyngostomy tube or gastrostomy tube.

- A **nasogastric tube**, lubricated with a local anaesthetic gel, may be passed via the nostril to the stomach, and fluids given directly into the stomach. The tube should not remain in place if the animal is to be left unattended, and animals may resent repeated tubing.
- A **pharyngostomy tube** must be placed under anaesthesia via an incision in the skin of the neck. The tube is introduced via the pharynx into the oesophagus and stomach, allowing fluid and food to be administered.
- A **gastrostomy tube** again must be positioned under anaesthesia, and is placed directly into the stomach via an incision in the left flank. Again, fluid and food may be administered through this tube. In general, pharyngostomy tubes and gastrostomy tubes are well tolerated by the animals.

Hypotonic fluids are recommended for oral administration to prevent the movement of water out of the ECF and into the bowel. However, it has been demonstrated that 120 mmol/l sodium chloride in 2% glucose will produce enhanced absorption of sodium and increased uptake of water. This can be prepared by mixing a teaspoonful of salt and a dessertspoon of glucose in two pints of water. There are many commercially available oral rehydration solutions available, and in general they use a similar principle to that described, although some include glycine for further promotion of electrolyte and water absorption.

Subcutaneous Administration

Subcutaneous administration of fluids is practical in small animals, where the animal is only mildly dehydrated and fluids cannot be administered orally. Because absorption from this route tends to be slow, especially where peripheral vasoconstriction is present, it is unsuitable for severely dehydrated animals. Only isotonic electrolyte solutions (e.g. Hartmann's), should be administered subcutaneously, and only small volumes should be given at one time. Repeated administration can be painful, and in addition there is a risk of skin infection or skin slough.

Intraperitoneal Administration

The intraperitoneal route of fluid administration shares many of the advantages and disadvantages of the subcutaneous route, and should only be used where the animal is mildly dehydrated and fluids cannot be administered orally. Hypotonic or isotonic electrolyte solutions may be administered intraperitoneally. The large adsorptive capacity of the peritoneum makes it a more efficient route of administration, but absorption is reduced during shock. Because of the risk of infection it is important that all manipulations are carried out aseptically. Great care must also be taken not to puncture any of the abdominal organs.

When fluids are administered intraperitoneally, the animal is held almost vertically with its hindlimbs on the ground. A second person introduces a short needle or catheter into the abdomen, just behind the umbilicus and in a cranial direction.

Intravenous Fluid Therapy

The advantages and disadvantages of intravenous administration of fluids are shown in Fig. 21.9.

When the intravenous route of fluid administration is going to be used, one of the first considerations is the selection of an appropriate vein. The cephalic or recurrent tarsal veins are used for short-term therapy in dogs. However, the jugular is more appropriate where long-term therapy is anticipated, or where hypertonic solutions have to be given. In cats the cephalic vein is used commonly, although the jugular is often a better choice. Fluids should be warmed to 37°C prior to administration.

Needles and catheters

There are a number of different ways of administering fluids intravenously.

- **Needles** are inexpensive but are unsuitable for intravenous fluid administration. They are dislodged easily, and the sharp point can irritate the wall of the vein and can also penetrate the other side of the vein, thus delivering the fluid perivenously (extravasation).
- **Butterfly needles** (scalp vein sets) are safer because they can be secured to the limb more easily and are less likely to become dislodged. However, the sharp point of the needle may still irritate the wall of the vein.

- **Over-the-needle catheters** or cannulae are extremely useful in peripheral veins although they can also be used in the jugular vein of small dogs and cats. Catheters are plastic and may be tefloncoated for ease of placement. They can be secured to the limb and are less likely to become dislodged than needles. Moreover, the smooth tip of the catheter is less likely to cause phlebitis than needles or butterfly needles.
- **Through-the-needle catheters** or cannulae are longer and are therefore more appropriate for use in the jugular vein. They are the only catheters suitable for monitoring central venous pressure. Unfortunately they may leave haematomas at the site of needle insertion in some animals. In other respects they are similar to over-the-needle catheters.

Rules for reducing the incidence of thrombophlebitis:

(1) Select a suitable catheter and vein (generally the largest vein).
(2) Prepare the site by carefully clipping and cleansing as if for surgery.
(3) Avoid touching the barrel of the catheter or the site of insertion.
(4) Discard any catheters which develop flared tips (after repeated attempt of cannulation).
(5) Secure the catheter firmly to the leg so that it does not move.
(6) Use only sterile fluid administration sets and change them daily.
(7) Cover catheter with sterile bandage. Change at least once daily or if it becomes contaminated. Some people recommend that antibiotic or antiseptic cream should be applied to the site of insertion of the catheter.
(8) Check the vein and monitor the animal's temperature 3 or 4 times daily.
(9) Do not leave a catheter in a vein for more than 48 hours.
(10) If fluid therapy is discontinued, flush with saline containing 5–10iu heparin/ml and properly seal the catheter (with an injection cap or a three-way tap).

Drip sets and pumps

There are three main types of drip set (**giving set**) available. A normal administration set gives approximately 15–20 drops/ml. For smaller patients, a mini-drip fluid administration set (paediatric set) giving 60 drops/ml is useful because it allows more accurate administration of small volumes. A burette often is incorporated into this type of set which again is useful when only small volumes of fluid are

---

INTRAVENOUS ADMINISTRATION OF FLUIDS

Advantages	Disadvantages
Rapid administration of fluid directly into the vascular space. Large volumes of fluid may be administered. Hypertonic solutions may be administered, in addition to plasma expanders and blood products. No contraindications – may be used where intravenous access is possible.	Greater risk of side effects (phlebitis, thrombophlebitis, bacteraemia, septicaemia). Specialised equipment. Time-consuming. Animal requires constant monitoring (to ensure catheter remains within vein and fluid not being administered perivenously). Risk of overhydration.

Fig. 21.9. Intravenous administration of fluids: advantages and disadvantages.

required, helping to prevent accidental overhydration. Giving sets are supplied in sterile packaging and the number of drops per ml that they deliver is written on the packaging and should be checked prior to calculating the drip rate. A variety of automated infusion pumps are available for delivering a set amount of fluid over a defined period. These pumps are usually fitted with an alarm system which will alert the nurse or clinician when the fluid line is obstructed, or when the fluid bag is empty. If infusion pumps are used, it is important to remember that they are not a substitute for careful patient monitoring.

When blood is to be administered, a special blood administration set is required, which incorporates a nylon net filter to remove any aggregated red blood cells or other coagulation debris.

EXAMPLE

A 3 kg cat requires a total of 60 ml of fluid. The fluid is to be administered at 5 ml/kg/hour. A paediatric giving set which delivers 60 drops/ml is available. What flow rate (drops per minute) will be required?

$$\frac{60 \text{ drops/ml}}{60 \text{ minutes}} \times 5 \text{ ml} \times 3 \text{ kg} = 15 \text{ drops/minute}$$

Various other pieces of equipment are useful when fluids are being administered via the intravenous route (Fig. 21.10). **Injection caps** and **stopcocks** are useful means of plugging catheters when fluids are not being administered, whilst allowing the catheter to be flushed periodically with heparinised saline. Simple **stylets** are also available which may be used to maintain the patency of indwelling catheters when they are not in use, and are designed to remove the requirement for periodic heparinisation to maintain patency. **Blood collection sets** containing an anticoagulant are the simplest means by which blood may be collected from a dog.

Other Methods of Fluid Administration

Rectal administration

This route of administration should not be used if an animal is suffering from diarrhoea, nor is it suitable in severely dehydrated patients. Both isotonic and hypotonic fluids may be administered via this route. Sterility of fluid and equipment is not essential. It is important that the fluid is instilled into the colon and not into the rectum or an evacuent enema will result.

Intraosseous administration

Where it is difficult to place indwelling intravenous catheters (e.g. puppies, kittens, birds, adults with

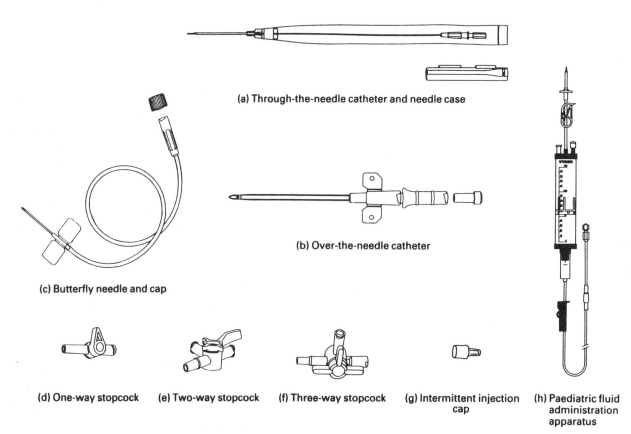

(a) Through-the-needle catheter and needle case

(b) Over-the-needle catheter

(c) Butterfly needle and cap

(d) One-way stopcock   (e) Two-way stopcock   (f) Three-way stopcock   (g) Intermittent injection cap   (h) Paediatric fluid administration apparatus

Fig. 21.10. Equipment for intravenous administration of fluids.

inaccessible veins), indwelling intraosseous catheters—femur via intratrochanteric fossa—may be used. Fluid generally is administered by gravity flow. The risk of severe infection must be considered.

Solutions Commonly Used in Fluid Therapy

Whole Blood

Blood for transfusion should be collected only from fit, healthy adult animals (cats should be FeLV, FIV and Haemobartonella negative), which have not previously been transfused themselves. Approximately 10–20 ml/kg of blood may be collected from a donor dog, and a total of 40 ml from a cat. Animals should not be bled more than once in every 3–4 weeks. It is important that strict asepsis is observed when collecting the blood. Blood from a donor animal may be collected in commercially available collection sets containing an anticoagulant (either acid citrate dextrose (ACD) or citrate phosphate dextrose (CPD)) to prevent the blood from clotting. However, if the blood is to be used immediately, heparin or EDTA may be used as an anticoagulant. In cats, blood is generally collected into a syringe containing anticoagulant.

Before infusion into the recipient animal, a cross-matching test should be carried out in the laboratory to ensure that the blood is compatible for transfusion. The A antigen is the most important factor in canine blood typing and ideally donor dogs should be A negative (or DEA 1.1 or DEA 1.2 negative). Blood typing is not generally carried out in cats. However, most cats are type A, and there is < 40% chance of an incompatible reaction occurring if the blood is not typed prior to transfusion. Blood samples can be taken from both the donor and the recipient animal for cross-matching to ensure compatibility before obtaining a large volume of blood from the donor.

Commercially available blood collection units contain sufficient anticoagulant for 500 ml of blood, and blood may be stored in these bags in the refrigerator until required. When ACD is used as the anticoagulant the blood may be stored at 4°C for a period of 3 weeks; when CPD is used the blood may be stored for 4 weeks. Blood in which EDTA or heparin has been used as the anticoagulant should not be stored. If blood has been stored in the refrigerator, it should be warmed gently to a temperature of 37°C (and not greater than 40°C), prior to transfusion. Blood which has been stored in this manner is useful for replacement of red blood cells. However, where platelets are required (e.g. clotting abnormalities) blood must be given to the recipient immediately after collection.

Where an animal has lost only a small amount of blood, other less potentially harmful fluids may be used to restore fluid balance.

Indications for transfusion

- Haemorrhage (acute and chronic)
- Anaemia (acute and chronic)
- Specific deficiencies (e.g. platelets, clotting factors).

Dangers associated with transfusion

- **Incompatibility reaction.** This usually occurs after a second transfusion of blood which has not been cross-matched and is incompatible. Mild cases show jaundice and anaemia due to haemolysis. Severe cases may show salivation, vomiting, tachycardia, muscle tremors, prostration, haemoglobinuria and bleeding.
- **Pyrogenic reactions**. Fever due to pyrogens or bacteria in the blood or transfusion equipment. It is also possible to transfer viral and other agents, especially in cats.
- **Acidosis** (metabolic) after administration of stored blood.
- **Over-administration** resulting in circulatory overload.
- **Air emboli**. This occurs infrequently when plastic blood collection bags are used, but is possible when blood is withdrawn using a syringe.

Blood Products

Plasma

If fresh blood can be obtained from donors, plasma may be extracted and stored. Blood should be centrifuged immediately after collection and the plasma separated from the red blood cells. The plasma may be frozen, and can be stored for 6 months at −70°C. Prior to use, the plasma should be thawed and warmed. Remember to maintain sterility when transferring and decanting the plasma. Plasma is a useful replacement fluid in hypovolaemic animals and is suitable for animals which are hypoproteinaemic. Because it does not contain any red blood cells there is less risk of incompatibility reactions.

Packed red blood cells

Separated red cells may be kept in the refrigerator for 3 weeks and can be given to animals which require red cell replacement. The red cells should be resuspended in an isotonic replacement fluid which does not contain calcium (e.g. 0.9% NaCl) because calcium reacts with the citrate used to prevent clotting.

Plasma Replacement Fluids/Colloids

When whole blood or plasma are unavailable, commercial plasma replacement fluids (colloids, plasma substitutes, plasma volume expanders) may be used. These fluids contain large molecules that will remain within the circulation thus increasing the plasma's effective osmotic pressure and expanding plasma volume. They may be used where there has been haemorrhage (although they will not replace red blood cells), or where the plasma volume is reduced for other reasons, e.g. fluid and electrolyte depletion. The two most commonly used products are gelatins and dextrans.

Gelatins

These solutions (e.g. Haemaccel, Gelofusin) are derived from gelatin and are isotonic with plasma. They are non-antigenic, and do not interfere with cross-matching tests for blood. The solution will remain in the circulation for about 5 hours and most of it will be excreted within 24 hours.

Dextrans

These solutions contain high molecular weight (MW) glucose polymers in either 0.9% NaCl or 5% dextrose. The solutions are classified by the MW of the glucose polymer; for example, the MW of dextran 70 is 70,000 and that of dextran 40 is 40,000. They remain in the circulation for times ranging from 2 to 24 hours, depending on their MW. Unfortunately, these solutions tend to interfere with the red cells: some solutions promote clumping of cells and others produce haemolysis. In addition, they interfere with the interpretation of cross-matching reactions. The raised plasma osmotic pressure caused by the dextrans tends to draw water from the cells and ISF space into the vascular compartment. Therefore crystalloids should be administered at the same time as dextrans to avoid cellular dehydration.

Crystalloids

In contrast to the plasma volume expanders, crystalloids are noncolloidal substances which pass readily through cell membranes. This means that they will not remain within the ECF compartment but will equilibrate with the ICF compartment, and will be excreted in the urine if renal function is normal. Figure 21.11 summarises the principal constituents and some of the major indications for the most commonly used solutions in general practice, which are as follows:

- **0.9% sodium chloride (NaCl).** Useful for replacing water and electrolyte losses, especially in vomiting patients.
- **5% dextrose in water.** The dextrose in the solution is rapidly metabolised; therefore these solutions effectively provide free water which can be used to replace primary water deficits.
- **0.18% sodium chloride in 4% dextrose.** Used to replace primary water deficits, and to replace the inevitable losses of sodium and water occurring on a daily basis (maintenance requirements). Potassium will also be required during long-term administration.
- **Hartmann's solution.** Useful for replacing water and electrolyte losses, especially where the losses are post-gastric (e.g. diarrhoea).
- **Potassium chloride (KCl).** Can be used when potassium supplementation is needed. Ten millilitres 10% KCl contains 13.4 mmol. This can be added to each 500 ml of maintenance fluids to prevent further depletion. There is already adequate potassium in Hartmann's or Ringer's solution to prevent depletion. If supplementary potassium is added to a crystalloid solution, it is important that the bag is clearly labelled to avoid possible over-administration (relative or absolute).
- **Sodium bicarbonate 8.4%** Should be available to treat severe acidosis. This solution may be used intravenously as an injection but frequently it is added to intravenous infusions. However, do not add bicarbonate to any fluids which contain calcium (Fig. 21.11), as a precipitate will be formed. If sodium bicarbonate is added to a crystalloid solution, it is important that the bag is clearly labelled to avoid possible over-administration (relative or absolute).

Parenteral Nutrition

Caloric balance is difficult to achieve by any route other than by mouth, and provision of enteral nutrition is the most effective way to provide the calories and proteins which are required by animals. However, animals that are unable to eat or drink for prolonged periods, and cannot be given enteral nutrition (gastrointestinal disease), not only require parenteral fluids but also need calories and proteins to prevent excessive breakdown of body tissues. During acute illness, provision of these needs is less important because the animal will be able to correct any deficits accrued in the convalescence period. However, in chronic illness, fluids containing electrolytes, amino acids and dextrose may be given parenterally in an attempt to correct some of these deficits. Requirements for replacement and maintenance are calculated in a similar manner to fluid replacement. Several commercial solutions containing amino acids and calories are now available. Fat emulsions may also be given intravenously and provide an excellent source of calories in dogs but may be dangerous in cats. These more complex fluids are not isotonic: they therefore need to be administered via a jugular catheter to ensure adequate mixing with blood and to minimise damage to the blood vessels. Manufacturers' recommendations about rates of administration should always be followed to avoid side effects associated with over-rapid administration.

CONSTITUENTS OF USEFUL REPLACEMENT FLUIDS (mmol/l)							
Solution		Na+	K+	Ca2+	Cl-	Others	Indications
Haemacoel	Isotonic	143	5	3	154	gelatins	Restore circulating volume
Dextrans	Hypertonic	154	–	–	154	–	Restore circulating volume
	Hypertonic	–	–	–	–	5% dextrose	
0.9% NaCl	Isotonic	154	–	–	154	–	Replace ECF. Gastric losses from vomiting
Hartmann's solution (Ringer's lactate)	Isotonic	131	5	2	111	lactate	Replace ECF. Especially from diarrhoea and post gastric losses
Ringer's solution	Isotonic	147	4	2.5	156	–	Replace ECF. Gastric losses from vomiting
5% dextrose	Isotonic	–	–	–	–	5% dextrose	Primary water deficit replacement
0.18% NaCl + 4% dextrose	Isotonic	30	–	–	30	4% dextrose	Maintenance requirements. Primary water deficit replacement. Neonatal ECF replacement

Fig. 21.11. Constituents of replacement fluids.

Volume and Rate of Infusion

Volume

The replacement volume can be calculated from the history, clinical signs and simple laboratory tests described earlier. Usually, this volume can be replaced within the first 24 hours of treatment, with half of the replacement being made in the first 6–8 hours. Priority should be given to replacing the circulating blood volume and so therapy usually starts with a plasma volume expander. One-twelfth of the total deficit should be replaced with a plasma substitute; the remainder of the deficit should be replaced by one of the fluids of choice. The animal also has maintenance requirements for fluids which must be met in addition to replacing existing deficits, and approximately 50ml/kg/day of 0.18% NaCl with 4% dextrose should be given to replace normal losses of sodium and water.

EXAMPLE
Consider a 20 kg dog which has been off food and water for 3 days and has been vomiting about 3 times daily for the last 2 days.

Replacement:
Inevitable water losses (20 ml/kg/day × 3 days) 1200 ml
Urinary water loss (20 ml/kg/day × 1 day) 400 ml
Vomiting 3 times/day for 2 days (4 ml/kg/vomit × 6) 480 ml
Total water deficit 2080 ml
ECF deficit (one-third of total water deficit) 693 ml

Plasma deficit (one-quarter of ECF, 173 ml i.e. one-twelfth of total loss)

Maintenance
50 ml/kg/day × 20 1000 ml

Contemporary losses
Fluids should be administered to replace losses incurred due to ongoing vomiting, diarrhoea, haemorrhage etc.

Because the animal in this example is suffering from a mixed water and electrolyte deficit, the fluid loss will be primarily from the ECF and a larger proportion of the total deficit will be from the plasma water. Consequently, up to one-third of the replacement fluid could be provided as plasma volume expander. This is in contrast to a primary water deficit, where fluid loss is shared between all body compartments, and only one-twelfth of the total deficit should be replaced by a plasma volume expander.

Rate of Fluid Replacement

The rate of fluid replacement often poses problems. A large number of factors govern how fast fluids can be given:

- Rate of loss.
- Health of patient.
- Type of fluid administered.
- Presence of ongoing losses.

During active severe haemorrhage, fluids have to be administered as rapidly as they are being lost from the circulation. Otherwise, in mild to severely dehydrated animals the **maximum** rate of infusion of crystalloids should be limited to **90 ml/kg/hour**. Slower rates of **20–30 ml/kg/hour** are satisfactory in situations where dehydration is not severe or where colloidal substances are being given. It is important that **potassium** should not be given at a rate greater than **0.5 mmol/kg/hour**.

Overzealous fluid administration may result in the circulatory system becoming overloaded, or the body overhydrated. This is particularly a problem in smaller cats and dogs. Typically, excess of a **colloid** leads to circulatory overload with right-sided heart failure (indicated by an elevated CVP), and ultimately congestive cardiac failure. Too much **crystalloid** on the other hand, will initially stimulate diuresis (via inhibition of ADH release), but as the electrolyte solution moves from the circulation into the remainder of the extracellular space, signs of oedema may develop. i.e. fluid will accumulate in the ISF space. Most seriously, pulmonary oedema may develop which will initially impair oxygenation and can ultimately result in the death of the patient.

Overinfusion is most likely to occur with:

- Reduced cardiac output (e.g. congestive heart failure).
- Renal/urinary conditions (e.g. acute renal failure, ruptured bladder, where urine output is prevented).
- Fluid administration to normovolaemic animals (e.g. blood given in chronic anaemia).

When any of the above conditions are present, fluid should be administered slowly and the animal should be very closely monitored.

Monitoring During Fluid Therapy

Monitoring during fluid administration should include:

- Cardiovascular system
  —Pulse (rate, rhythm, strength).
  —Mucous membrane colour.
  —Capillary refill time.
  —Jugular distention.
  —Central venous pressure (CVP).
  —Chest auscultation (cardiac arrhythmias, pulmonary oedema).
- Respiratory system
  —Respiratory rate and depth.
  —Chest auscultation (pulmonary oedema).
  —Mean arterial blood pressure.
- Temperature
  —Core body and limb.

- Urine output
- General checks
  —Peripheral oedema.
  —Body weight.
  —Skin turgor.

Central Venous Pressure (CVP)

In critical patients, invasive monitoring of CVP is useful. The CVP is a measurement of the pressure in the right atrium, i.e. the chamber of the heart to which all the venous blood is returned. A long catheter is placed aseptically in a jugular vein, and advanced until the tip of the catheter lies within the chest. Note that measurements will be less sensitive if a very long catheter is used. Ideally, the catheter should lie in the right atrium itself but it is often located within the anterior vena cava, which will reflect changes in the right atrial pressure. Extension tubing is attached to the catheter (a threeway tap is helpful but not essential), and a three-way tap is attached to the other end of the tubing. A water manometer tube (marked in centimetres) and a drip set attached to a bag of crystalloids are also attached to the three-way tap (Fig. 21.12). Before the monitoring equipment is attached to the jugular catheter, the three-way tap should be adjusted fill (a) the manometer line and (b) the extension tubing. This will prevent air emboli. To measure CVP, turn the three-way tap so that the catheter is connected directly to the manometer and read the height (cm) of the column of fluid. The zero line of the scale should be level with the right atrium, i.e. at approximately the level of the sternum when the animal is lying on its side (Fig. 21.12).

If the tip of the catheter is in the correct place, the meniscus in the manometer will fall and rise with inspiration and expiration, reflecting the changes in intrathoracic pressure that accompany respiration.

If this is not seen, either the catheter is blocked or the catheter tip is not in the chest.

Blood is returned from the great veins (anterior and posterior vena cava) to the right atrium; from there it enters the right ventricle, which pumps blood to the lungs. The CVP therefore measures the filling of the great veins, which is a balance between the central blood volume, the vascular tone and the heart's contractile ability. The normal range is 3–7 cm of water. An isolated measurement of CVP may be used to indicate the need for fluids, but repeated measurements are far more useful. As fluids are administered, they will fill the vascular compartment, improve venous return and increase CVP.

- If fluids are stopped and the CVP falls, more fluids need to be administered.
- If the CVP remains elevated, fluid administration can be reduced or terminated.

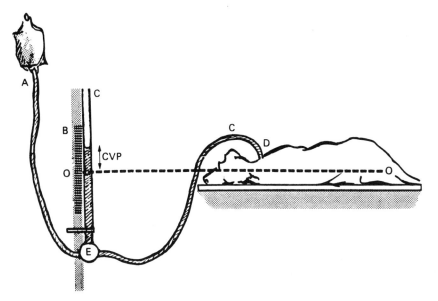

Fig. 21.12. Measurement of central venous pressure. A—Infusion fluid and administration set; B—centimetre scale; C—extension tubing; D—connection to jugular catheter; E—3-way tap.

• If the administration of modest amounts of fluid produce a high CVP which only declines slowly, circulatory overload or congestive cardiac failure should be suspected.

Provided that the CVP does not rise significantly during fluid administration, the infusion may be continued safely at its current rate.

High CVP:
• Occlusion of catheter.
• Over-administration of fluid.
• Right ventricular heart failure.

Low CVP:
• Reduced blood volume.

Shock (Acute Circulatory Failure)

Shock is a clinical term used to describe a clinical syndrome generally characterised by a fall in cardiac output which results in inadequate capillary perfusion of the peripheral tissues, i.e. acute circulatory failure. Insufficient capillary perfusion to meet the needs of the body tissues for oxygen and nutrients, along with inadequate removal of metabolic waste products from the tissues results in abnormal cell function and, ultimately, tissue devitalisation. Shock is a progressive condition which may be life-threatening if it is not reversed. Its clinical signs are described in Fig. 21.13.

Causes of Shock

Although there are many recognised causes of shock, it is frequently categorised as follows:

• Hypovolaemic

• Vasculogenic
 —Neurogenic
 —Anaphylactic
 —Endotoxic (septic)
• Cardiogenic

Hypovolaemic shock

Hypovolaemic shock occurs when there is an inadequate circulating blood volume, e.g. haemorrhage (external, internal), loss of plasma, severe water and electrolyte depletion (prolonged vomiting or diarrhoea which has not been treated).

CLINICAL SIGNS OF SHOCK	
Clinical signs	**Due to**
1. Weak rapid pulse.	
2. Increased heart rate (tachycardia) with quiet heart sounds.	Poor cardiac filling Vasoconstriction
3. Pale mucous membranes.	Vasoconstriction
4. Prolonged capillary refill time (>2 seconds).	
5. Increased ventilation.	Metabolic acidosis / pain
6. Slow jugular refill and "poor" peripheral veins.	
7. Hypothermia and cold extremities.	Reduced metabolic rate and Vasoconstriction
8. Depressed level of consciousness.	Reduced blood flow to brain
9. Muscle weakness.	Hypoxia, vasoconstriction, etc.
10. Reduced renal output (oliguria, anuria).	Reduced blood flow to kidneys
11. Low CVP and low mean arterial blood pressure.	
12. Elevated PCV, Hb (haemoglobin), TP, urea and creatinine (a blood sample should be obtained prior to fluid administration).	

Fig. 21.13. Clinical signs of shock.

Vasculogenic shock

Vasculogenic shock occurs where the blood volume is normal but the capacity of the blood vessels (primarily the veins) is increased, i.e. vasodilation. Administration of drugs which have an effect on the capacity of the blood vessels (e.g. acetylpromazine) can induce vasculogenic shock after absolute or relative overdose.

Neurogenic shock. Neurogenic shock occurs where neurological phenomena—such as CNS trauma—result in acute vasodilation (increased capacitance).

Anaphylactic shock. Anaphylactic shock may be classified as vasculogenic shock because many endogenous vasoactive substances (substances which affect venous capacitance and/or total peripheral resistance) are released. This occurs in association with a generalised increase in vascular permeability.

Endotoxic shock (septic shock). Endotoxic shock occurs when endotoxins, formed from the cell walls of principally Gram-negative bacteria, act to release endogenous vasoactive substances. An initial rise in cardiac output may occur, but it does not compensate for the disturbance of the distribution of blood to the tissues and the increased vascular permeability.

Cardiogenic shock

Cardiogenic shock is not common in animals. It occurs when the cardiac output is severely reduced as a result of either:

- reduced cardiac filling (e.g. pericarditis, an accumulation of the fluid in the sac surrounding the heart); or
- reduced cardiac emptying (e.g. dilated cardiomyopathy—the heart muscle is not strong enough to force the blood out of the ventricles and round the circulatory system).

Pathophysiology of Shock

Hypovolaemic shock, the most common form in veterinary practice, provides a simple model (cause, effect and result) of the course of developing shock in an animal.

Cause. Loss of blood, or effective circulating volume, ultimately reduces the venous return to the right side of the heart, and subsequently there is a fall in the output from the left side of the heart (i.e. cardiac output falls).

Effect. Pressure-sensitive baroreceptors in the aorta and carotid artery perceive the drop in blood pressure (hypotension) secondary to the fall in cardiac output. Consequently, centres within the

medulla of the brain are stimulated to initiate compensatory mechanisms to restore blood pressure to normal. These compensatory mechanisms mainly involve the sympathetic nervous system and stimulation of the adrenal medulla. Adrenaline and noradrenaline are released and cause the blood vessels of the skin, intestine, kidneys and muscles to constrict, i.e. there is an increase in peripheral vasoconstriction (increase in **total peripheral resistance (TPR)**). This causes a direct increase in blood pressure and thus promotes increased venous return to the heart. At this stage, blood flow to the vital organs (heart and brain) is maintained. In association with these changes the heart rate increases and there is an increase in the force of contraction of the myocardium (heart muscle). *The overall result of the compensatory mechanisms so far is to increase the cardiac output.*

The pressure changes within the vascular system cause a net movement of water from the ISF into the blood vessels. Release of the hormones aldosterone and ADH promote salt and water retention by the kidneys. *These mechanisms act to restore the circulating blood volume to normal.*

Result. In cases of mild shock, all of the compensatory mechanisms mentioned will come into play and often are sufficient to protect the vital organs (brain and heart) by providing an effective cardiac output. Thus, *in mild shock, homeostatic mechanisms will allow a gradual return of the circulation towards normal.*

Summary:

- Loss of effective circulating volume.
- Fall in cardiac output and mean arterial blood pressure.
- Sympathetic nervous system stimulation.
- Increase in TPR, heart rate, myocardial contractility.
- Increased cardiac output.
- Blood flow maintained to heart and brain.
- Blood flow reduced to gut, skin, kidney.

This occurs in association with:

(a) • Movement of fluid from ISF space to vascular space.
    • Increase in circulating volume.
(b) • Aldosterone and ADH release.
    • Water and salt (Na^+, Cl^-) retained by kidney.
    • Increase in circulating volume.

Worst case. If the haemorrhage or volume depletion is severe, then these mechanisms, which are normally life-saving, can lead to the animal's death. Prolonged vasoconstriction and low perfusion cause tissue hypoxia, anaerobic metabolism and acidosis. Consequently, the peripheral vessels dilate and become engorged with blood. Moreover, cells in the capillary wall become nonfunctional and fluid is lost from the capillaries into the ISF space. Both of these mechanisms act to reduce the blood returning to the heart even further. The blood soon becomes viscous and slow-moving; platelets may start to aggregate and ultimately the blood will clot within the vessels. This effectively blocks the capillaries. If it is widespread, all the clotting factors will be used up, resulting in a bleeding state known as **disseminated intravascular coagulation (DIC)**.

These changes have severe effects on the various organs of the body. Blood flow to the kidneys is reduced and urine output falls. Hypoxia causes the renal tubules to become damaged. In the gut, mucosal damage allows the invasion of bacteria and bacterial toxins are absorbed. In the lungs, although there is an initial increase in ventilation, eventually, microthrombi and other factors cause the lung to become very inefficient, and '**shock lung**' may occur during recovery. The heart is depressed by the prevailing hypoxia, acidosis and the presence of the toxins. In due course, a state of multiple organ failure develops and the animal dies.

Treatment of Shock

The clinical signs of shock are given in Fig. 21.13. Treatments might include:

- Fluid therapy.
- General measures.
- Oxygenation.
- Corticosteroids.
- Sodium bicarbonate.
- Reduction of blood viscosity.
- Vasodilation.
- Myocardial stimulation.
- Antibiotics.
- Other treatments.

Fluid therapy

Adequate volume replacement is the single most important measure in the treatment of peripheral circulatory failure. However, fluids should be administered with care in cardiogenic shock, which is primarily a failure of the heart to pump fluid effectively around the body rather than a volume depletion.

After clinical assessment of the animal when a 'diagnosis' of shock has been made (Fig. 21.13), at least one intravenous catheter should be inserted. If the peripheral veins are collapsed and difficult to catheterise, a jugular catheter should be used. To facilitate administration of large volumes of fluid over a short period of time, large gauge catheters are required, or more than one intravenous line should

be established. In general, the fluid used should resemble the fluid which has been lost; for example, whole blood would be appropriate in severe acute haemorrhage. However, the speed of fluid replacement is probably the most important factor initially. A balanced electrolyte infusion can be used in almost any circumstance of peripheral circulatory failure, while the need for other fluids is assessed by the clinician.

Blood will provide red blood cells, haemoglobin, platelets, clotting factors and protein, whereas plasma will only provide clotting factors and protein. Blood, plasma and the plasma volume expanders will all increase the effective osmotic pressure of the plasma and so are very useful.

All fluids are given to effect. The volumes required may be very large, because of vasodilation or because of contraction of the ISF, which also must be replaced. Frequently, fluid replacement will be the only treatment required to promote recovery.

General measures

If there is an obvious source of blood loss, this should be stemmed if possible. Frequently, animals which are in shock will be (or will become) hypothermic. Although it is inadvisable to warm a hypothermic animal rapidly (because vasodilation will occur), further loss of body heat can be prevented by ensuring a reasonable ambient temperature, avoiding draughts, lying the animal on an insulated surface, covering the animal and warming fluids to body temperature prior to administration.

Oxygenation

If hypoxia is suspected, oxygen should be provided by either face mask, nasal insufflation (via nasal catheter) or endotracheal tube. In general, animals in shock will not object to the use of a face mask, but a nasal catheter may be more suitable if the animal struggles.

Corticosteroids

The early use of corticosteroids is advocated in the treatment of shock. When they are used, it is important that they are administered in high doses and repeated at regular intervals. It is generally the aqueous soluble salts of glucocorticoids (corticosteroids) that are administered, e.g. methylprednisolone sodium succinate. There has been much debate about the effectiveness of corticosteroids in established shock but they still are used widely. They are *not* a substitute for adequate volume replacement but should be used in association with fluid therapy.

Sodium bicarbonate

Sodium bicarbonate should be administered intravenously to correct the metabolic acidosis. If the animal's exact requirement cannot be established, 1–2mEq/kg of sodium bicarbonate may be administered initially (8.4% sodium bicarbonate contains 1mEq/ml).

Reducing blood viscosity

The viscosity of blood increases in shock and reducing the viscosity of the blood will aid tissue perfusion. Fluid therapy will help to reduce the blood viscosity, but dextran 40 may be used specifically for this purpose.

Vasodilators

Once adequate volume replacement has occurred, vasodilators (e.g. acetylpromazine) may be used in an attempt to improve tissue perfusion. However, they are contraindicated in hypovolaemic shock as they will exacerbate the existing problem.

Myocardial stimulants

These agents (e.g. dopamine, dobutamine, isoprenaline) are useful in cardiogenic shock and in advanced shock where myocardial depression is possible. They are frequently administered as infusions because of their short half-lives within the circulation. Dopamine will also act to increase renal blood flow.

Antibiotics

Broad spectrum antibiotics are indicated because shocked animals are susceptible to infection. Antibiotics should be administered intravenously in high doses.

Other treatments

Hypertonic saline. Small volumes (4 ml/kg) of hypertonic saline (e.g. 7.0%) have been used to improve cardiac output and peripheral perfusion in shocked animals.

Anticoagulants. Heparin may be used in advanced shock where DIC (disseminated intravascular coagulation) is developing. However, care must be taken as this drug may exacerbate bleeding during subsequent surgery or where the animal has suffered trauma.

Vasoconstrictors. There is little room for the use of these agents in the treatment of shock because they will act to reduce further tissue perfusion. However, adrenaline may be used in anaphylactic shock.

Monitoring during shock

The same monitoring procedures that are used in fluid therapy also apply to animals that are in shock. Perhaps one of the most useful parameters which can be monitored is the CVP. This gives the nurse and the clinician an indication of the adequacy of fluid replacement and also serves as a useful indicator of the animal's continuing fluid requirements.

22
Diagnostic Tests

P. A. BLOXHAM

Collection of Specimens

Quality laboratory results start with the collection of quality samples (remember the old adage: rubbish in means rubbish out). It is essential to collect the correct sample and that it should be in a suitable condition.

Blood

To collect blood by means of venipuncture, using a needle and syringe, first ensure that the animal is safely and securely restrained (Chapter 1). Next, select a suitable vein. In the dog this is likely to be the cephalic vein in the foreleg; in the cat the jugular may be more suitable. Part the hair (or clip the site) and clean and swab with a topical alcohol wipe.

For the **cephalic**, raise the vein with the left hand under the leg and the thumb on top, or apply a quick-release tourniquet, and approach the vein from the side, using a 1 inch 22 gauge needle. Penetrate into the lumen and up the inside of the vein. Slowly pull back on the syringe and let the blood flow into it. It is important not to apply too much pressure and to ensure that the needle remains in the lumen of the vein. For most practical purposes a 10 ml syringe is preferred but a 5 ml syringe may be used if the correct volume anticoagulant tubes are available.

When sufficient blood has been collected release the pressure on the vein and remove the needle from it. Place a swab of cotton wool on the venipuncture site and apply direct light pressure. Tape the swab in place to stem any bleeding.

Collection from the **jugular** is best achieved with the cat on its side or back and the head extended. The vein is raised by pressure below the point of venipuncture and the pressure should be removed before removing the needle from the vein.

Vacutainer systems

A 'vacutainer' is an evacuated tube (i.e. with a vacuum) as part of a complete system incorporating a double-ended needle screwed into a holder. The small vacutainers have a 3 ml volume but only a 2 ml draw, in order to minimise the amount of pressure put on the red cells. It is important to collect blood with the complete vacutainer system.

If the sample is collected with syringe and needle, remove the needle before slowly allowing the blood to be discharged gently from the syringe into the sample tube. If this happens to be a vacutainer, remove its bung. Do not inject blood from a syringe into a vacutainer.

It is also possible to insert a needle into the vein and collect the blood directly into a container drop by drop. In this case the animal should ideally be standing and the collection tube is held beneath the shank of the needle.

Type and condition of blood

When blood clots and clot retraction takes place, the fluid is referred to as **serum**. **Plasma** is that fluid separated from non-clotted blood. To prevent clotting **anticoagulants** are used, the most common being heparin, EDTA, oxalate fluoride and sodium citrate.

Haemolysis. If the red cells become broken or lysed they release their contents into serum or plasma. This is referred to as haemolysis. If serum or plasma is reddish in colour after separation, then haemolysis has occurred. This might result from:

- excess pressure when pulling back the syringe plunger;
- too vigorous mixing of samples;
- osmotic pressure because the skin or the needle/syringe has water on or in it;
- the use of too fine a needle, damaging red cells;
- leaving the plasma unseparated in transit.

Lipaemia. Lipaemia is the presence of lipids/fats in the blood. This is often a physiological condition which occurs after feeding (especially ingestion of fatty foods) and so it is advisable to sample fasted animals, not ones just fed. Lipaemia may also be a pathological condition associated with metabolic conditions.

Icteric samples. Icteric samples are those with significant amounts of bilirubin in the blood. The level of 'normal range' bilirubin varies between species: equine serum, for example, will always appear more icteric than feline because of the much higher level of bilirubin in the horse due to the lack of gall bladder.

Chromatins. Chromatins are colour agents and they may interfere with colorimetric or spectrometric biochemical determinations by influencing the colour of serum and plasma. They include the carotene intake in the diet: the serum or plasma colour of grazing animals ingesting high carotene levels, such as dairy cattle, is more yellow than in other species.

Coagulants and colour codes

Figure 22.1 shows the colour codes used in vacutainers and the appropriate anticoagulants for

VACUTAINER COLOUR CODES, THEIR ANTICOAGULANTS AND APPLICATIONS			
Colour	Anticoagulant	Type of sample	Application
Red	None	Clotted blood/serum	Biochemistry, Serology
Green or yellow/green	Heparin	Whole blood Plasma	Biochemistry, Lead, GSHPx and Transketolase Biochemistry
Lavender	EDTA	Whole blood	Haematology
Grey	Oxalate fluoride	Whole blood	Glucose
Light blue	Sodium citrate	Whole blood/plasma	Coagulation tests
Dark blue	None	Clotted blood/serum	Trace elements

Fig. 22.1. Vacutainer colour codes, their anticoagulants and applications.

specific tests. The general principle is that ethylene diamine tetra-acetic acid (**EDTA**) whole blood is used for haematology. **Oxalates** are usually used as either sodium, potassium, ammonium or lithium salts, but currently the only useful routine salt is the potassium oxalate salt with sodium fluoride (**OXF**) which is used for glucose determination. **Heparin whole blood** is used for lead determination, while **sodium citrate** is used for clotting times and special coagulation studies. **Clotted blood with serum taken off** is used for most routine biochemistry or serology but **heparin plasma** may be used in many (but not all) cases, as an alternative to serum.

COLLECTION OF SERUM

(1) Using the vacutainer system, select the red-topped tube to collect blood which, because no anticoagulant is added, will clot.

(2) Leave these tubes upright (out of the sun) and undisturbed until clotting and clot retraction occur.

(3) Centrifuge the sample at 2500 RPM for 5 minutes in a swing-head centrifuge.

(4) When this has switched off, carefully remove the tube without shaking and place upright in a test-tube rack.

(5) Take Pasteur pipette (Chapter 12), squeeze its bulb and insert the fine tip into the serum near but above the surface of the clot. Do not touch the clot with the tip.

(6) Gently release the pressure on the bulb and suck up the serum into the Pasteur pipette.

(7) Transfer the serum into a suitable plastic or glass tube by gently applying pressure on the bulb again.

(8) Immediately label this tube (or do so in advance).

(9) If the serum is to be sent away, the type of tube or container for the sample must be suitable for postage and have a secure top to prevent leakage, as well as being clearly labelled with the owner's name, the animal's name or identification and the date and time of collection.

COLLECTION OF HEPARIN PLASMA

(1) Take a blood sample into a heparin vacutainer and gently roll and invert the sample to ensure adequate mixing. The benefit of vacutainer systems is that better mixing is easily achieved.

(2) Centrifuge the heparin sample as soon as possible after collection.

(3) The supernatant is plasma and may then be removed with a Pasteur pipette (as for serum) but do not insert the fine tip of the pipette so far down.

(4) Be careful to avoid disturbing the sedimented red and white blood cells as the pressure is carefully reduced by releasing the bulb.

(5) On withdrawing the pipette, ensure that fluid is not dispensed back into the tube.

(6) It is always better to transfer a little plasma and then go back for more rather than trying to collect all at once and sucking up some red cells at the same time.

Storage of serum and plasma

If serum or plasma is to be stored rather than immediately tested or posted to a laboratory, label the sample clearly with indelible marker and then store at $-20°C$ in a suitable deep-freeze. Do not keep at room temperature for any length of time, but samples can often be retained in a reasonably stable state for a few hours at $+4°C$ in a refrigerator.

Serum and plasma should never be exposed to extremes of heat. If frozen, samples that have been thawed should not be frozen again: they should only be frozen and thawed once.

Urine

Collection of urine should be a routine procedure, as the simple examination of urine is a practical and valuable diagnostic tool. Use a sterile universal container to collect voided urine or urine that is expressed by means of gentle pressure on the bladder. It is important to allow the initial urine to pass out (and with it any surface/skin bacteria) before collecting a reasonably sterile **mid-stream** sample. Mid-stream sampling is also more representative of the urine in the bladder, rather than the first few drops which may contain mucoid material from the other parts of the urinogenital tract.

Animals may be put into special 'metabolic' cages in order to collect all urine voided over a 24-hour period but these are not usually found in general practice.

Collection of sterile sample by means of a **urethral catheter** (Chapter 20) may require sedation of the animal. A suitable sterile catheter should be selected. It is passed up the urethra slowly and gently into the bladder and urine is collected aseptically as it flows out of the catheter into a sterile universal container.

Figure 22.2 lists the preservatives used in urine and details the reasons for using them. However, in a practice laboratory it is better to test a urine sample immediately rather than use any preservative. Urine should not be stored frozen but kept at refrigerator temperature, unless some specific analytic requirement calls for freezing.

Spun-down (centrifuged) sediment should be examined as soon as possible, but formalin may be used to preserve the material.

Faeces

Use a wide-mouthed universal container or faeces pot, which must be sterile, and bear the following points in mind.

- It is preferable to collect fresh faeces per rectum with a gloved finger or hand rather than use a stale defecated sample picked up from the ground or litter tray.
- Ensure that the animal is securely restrained so that it is unable to bite, scratch or wriggle while the procedure is carried out.
- It is best to collect urine before collecting faeces, as collection per rectum may cause voiding of urine.
- Long fingernails may damage the mucosa.
- Do not use force to collect from the rectum.
- It is important that the area around the anus is cleaned and lubricated to prevent skin flora being introduced into the faeces sample, and to prevent damage to the anal/rectal mucosa.

URINE PRESERVATIVES AND THEIR APPLICATION	
Hydrochloric acid	Biochemical analysis of the urea, ammonia, calcium, total nitrogens and uric acid (mix well before testing, as deposits form).
Acetic acid	For ascorbic acid determination.
Boric acid	Similar to HCL.
Chloroform	Cannot use for glucose, is a COSHH risk.
Toluene	Is a COSHH risk.
Thymol	For most biochemistry.
Formalin	As above but not glucose.
Sodium bicarbonate	For porphyrins.
Refrigeration	The most satisfactory method.

All urine preservatives are used to prevent bacterial action or chemical decomposition, or to stabilize constituents.

Fig. 22.2. Urine preservatives and their applications.

- The faeces should fill the pot, to prevent too much air getting into the sample (which may kill off any anaerobic bacteria or lead to desiccation of the faeces and any parasites present).

Faeces should be kept at room temperature for only a short period before being examined, and should be kept out of sunlight. If examination of the faeces has to be delayed for a few hours, take a transport swab of the sample for bacteriology and place the labelled pot, with its lid screwed on securely, in the refrigerator. Do not freeze it. Be aware that stored faeces may ferment in the pots: lids may blow off if not secured.

To summarise:

- Collect fresh rectal samples.
- Fill sterile screw-top universal containers.
- Examine immediately.

Skin

Collection of **plucked hairs** for examination for ringworm infection should be made at the active edge of the lesions. Pluck individual hairs, including the root.

A **tape technique** may be used to examine an area of skin for surface mites:

(1) Take a section of clear adhesive tape.
(2) With the sticky face down, press the tape against the hair and skin.
(3) Pull off and repeat over the area to be investigated.
(4) Place the tape on to a microscope slide for examination.

To obtain samples of **coat brushing** for mite examination, use a toothbrush or similar small bristle brush (this method is unlikely to identify ringworm, which affects the root shaft):

(1) Work a small area at a time in the one direction, brushing the coat.
(2) Tap the brush into a petri dish or on to a glass slide.
(3) Use forceps or tweezers to pick out the hairs.
(4) Do not put hair samples into plastic bags, as static electricity builds up and the samples are then very difficult to handle and examine.

For **skin scrapes**, use a scalpel blade to remove the surface layer of skin. It is important to go sufficiently deep to achieve **petechial** blood oozing (pinpoint clusters of surface capillary bleeding) (see Chapter 16, Elementary Mycology and Parasitology).

(1) Place a drop of paraffin oil on the clipped skin area to be examined.
(2) Gently squeeze the skin into a fold to bring any bacteria or parasites nearer to the surface.
(3) Scrape with the scalpel blade.
(4) Carefully scrape the scalpel on to a microscope slide for examination.

If the sample is to be submitted to a laboratory, put a clear warning that a scalpel blade is included (especially if it is unprotected).

To prevent desiccation, if a sample is to be looked at later:

(1) Place some filter or blotting paper in the lid of a Petri dish and wet it with sterile water.
(2) Place two stick applicators or match sticks on top.
(3) Suspend the slide on the sticks.
(4) Put the base on as a lid, seal with tape and label the dish.
(5) Place in a cool, dark place.

Some refrigerators may be suitable for storage but be warned that some of them extract moisture as they cool and therefore the period of storage should not be too long (as the seal on the dish is not totally airtight).

For longer storage, use airtight jars with a moist bed—but all must be prepared aseptically. For material under a cover slip on a slide, the area may be protected from desiccation by sealing the edges with nail varnish or epoxy resin.

Pustules may be sampled with a sterile needle on a small 1 ml or 2 ml syringe:

(1) Suck the contents of the pustule into the needle.
(2) Express on to a glass slide.
(3) Make either a **squash preparation** (by placing a second slide on top at right angles to the first and squashing) or a **smear** (by use of a spreader).
(4) Samples may then be examined fresh under low power or stained and examined under high power.

Cerebrospinal Fluid (CSF)

The examination of CSF may be very useful in diagnosing some neurological conditions. The animal must be anaesthetised before the fluid is collected. The area of the spine that is tapped is normally either the atlanto-occipital or the lumbosacral space.

(1) Prepare the selected area by shaving and full sterile/aseptic precautions, as for any surgical procedure.
(2) Insert a suitable spinal tap needle into the sub-arachnoid space of the spinal column, taking care not to advance the needle too far (which could damage the spinal cord).
(3) Normally the animal is placed in lateral recumbency and the fluid is collected into an EDTA tube for cytology, by means of free flow.
(4) Do not aspirate the fluid.
(5) It is also possible to collect a second, plain tube sample (with no anticoagulant added) for bio-chemical tests after the sample has been centrifuged to spin down any cellular material.

Synovial Fluid

Synovial fluid is collected by means of **arthrocentesis** from the joint in order to investigate a particular joint problem such as arthritis or in some cases of shifting lameness. Collection may be made on an unanaesthe-tised animal or following anaesthesia, depending on the animal and the joint. Arthrocentesis is made aseptically with a syringe and needle after the site has been prepared as for any surgical procedure.

Thoracic Fluid

The pleural cavity contains only enough fluid for adequate lubrication of the intrathoracic organs and the cavity lining. The main reason for collection and examination of thoracic fluid (by means of **thora-centesis**) is to find the cause of an increase in fluid volume. Collection is performed aseptically into EDTA tubes and plain tubes.

Abdominal Fluid

The amount of peritoneal fluid in the abdominal cavity is only sufficient to provide lubrication of the abdominal organs and peritoneum. Any increase in volume may be investigated by means of **abdomino-centesis**. Aseptic collection is usually performed via the most dependent part of the ventral midline in the standing animal following normal skin surgical preparation. Some of the fluid sample is transferred into EDTA for cytology while the rest should be transferred into plain tubes or sterile containers for biochemistry and perhaps bacteriology.

Tissue Samples, Tumours and Abdominal Organ Biopsy

Biopsy techniques relate to the sampling of a section of tissue, tumour or organ for cytological or histo-pathalogical examination.

FORMALIN

Formalin is a strong antiseptic and disinfectant that has the ability to preserve tissue samples by 'fixing' or hardening them. It is commercially pre-pared from a pungent gas, formaldehyde, as a solution of 40% strength in water, i.e. a **40% formal-dehyde** solution. Formalin is a hazardous substance (it gives off a gas that irritates eyes and nose) and it is important that local COSHH and Health and Safety rules are understood and adhered to.

Containers or pots for formalin-fixed tissues should be wide-mouthed and screw-topped: the fixing process hardens the tissue, so that its removal from a narrow-mouthed container becomes awkward or impossible.

For routine cases, tissues for histopathology are fixed in **10% formal saline**, which is made by diluting formalin in a buffered saline solution so that it contains 10% formalin (Fig. 22.3). This buffered solution is preferred but it is possible to use normal saline (sodium chloride in sterile distilled water), though the specimen is likely to be affected by cellular and histochemical changes because, with the lack of a buffer, there is no control of pH.

BUFFERED 10% FORMAL SALINE: TO MAKE ONE LITRE	
Formalin (40% formaldehyde solution)	100 ml
$NaH_2PO_4.2H_2O$	4.5 g
Na_2HPO_4	6.5 g
Distilled water	900 ml

Fig. 22.3. Buffered 10% formal saline: to make one litre.

Fresh tissues need to be transferred immediately into the fixative, as the process of **necrosis** (cell death and lysis) can occur very rapidly. The container should be of an adequate size to allow a minimum of 10 parts fluid to one part tissue, by volume, which will ensure sufficient formalin penetration into the tissue for rapid fixation.

When submitting tissue to a laboratory, ensure that the container is labelled and securely sealed, and that there is an indication of the original location of the tissue.

Toxicology Specimens

- All specimens should be collected free from any extraneous contamination. They should not be washed.
- Each sample must be collected and submitted in separate leak-proof, airtight, sterile and chemically clean plastic or glass containers.
- Each container must be labelled with the owner's name, animal identification, type of sample, date of collection and the name and address of the practice.
- All samples must then be placed together in one large container.
- Unless tissues are to be examined histologically, samples are best collected fresh and then frozen. They should then be dispatched to the toxicology laboratory on ice. Consult the laboratory prior to packing and submitting as they may have special requirements in certain cases.
- In cases of poisoning, it is essential that accurate records are kept at all stages as evidence may be needed for possible litigation.

Submission of Pathological Samples to Laboratories

In order to maximise the potential for diagnostic information, the intention is that material should arrive at the laboratory in a condition as similar as possible to that when it was actually collected. Correct preservation, properly completed paperwork, clear labelling and good packaging are all essential.

Preservation for Transit

Tissue, once it has been removed from an animal, immediately starts to die. Cell membranes break down, leading to destruction or lysis of cells, and this process of **autolysis** is hastened by increased temperatures and humidity. 'Fixing' and freezing are methods of preventing or reducing autolysis. Tissues for standard histological examination should *not* be frozen.

Haemolysis is a form of cell degeneration in blood cells. Red blood cells are likely to be damaged if exposed to heat, cold or violent shaking. If possible, separate serum from the clot by centrifugation before dispatch. Whole-blood samples should be gently but adequately mixed with the correct amount of anti-coagulant to avoid clotting (which would make them unsuitable for examination). Pack whole-blood samples and serum in a way that minimises temperature variation and physical damage in transit.

Labelling and Paperwork

If samples are being sent away, the name of the veterinary surgeon and the practice's name and address should be recorded. All request forms should also contain:

- name of owner;
- name of animal (or some reference number relating to that animal);
- animal's species, breed, age, sex, and whether intact or neutered;
- date of sampling and time of collection;
- list of samples collected, including type of anti-coagulants used (if applicable);
- clinical history, including any specific presenting signs and any current treatment;
- details of site or sites (if swabs, skin scrapings or biopsy material are submitted) with a schematic diagram to show the position;
- indication of tests or examinations required.

Submit the completed forms in plastic envelopes to protect them from possible contamination. Each sample relating to the case should be individually and clearly labelled with the name of the owner and the animal, and should be in agreement with details on the submission form.

Packaging

Most commercial laboratories supply special postal packs for submitted samples. All samples must be packed in compliance with postal regulations (Figure 22.4).

Always assume that if something can be broken in transit, it will be. Packing should be such that:

- sample material is not damaged;
- containers do not break or leak;
- samples do not contaminate each other or the accompanying paperwork, or anybody who handles the package in transit or on receipt.

POSTING PATHOLOGICAL SPECIMENS

1) Use First Class or Datapost. DO NOT USE PARCEL POST.
2) Label the outside with the words: PATHOLOGICAL SPECIMEN – FRAGILE. WITH CARE.
   As well as the laboratory address it must show the name, address and telephone number of the sender who will be contacted in case of leakage or damage.
3) Every specimen must be in a primary container which is securely sealed. Maximum of 50 ml volume unless Post Office approved multi-specimen packs.
4) Primary container must be wrapped in sufficient absorbent material to absorb all of the sample if leakage or breakage occurs.
5) The container and absorbent material must be sealed in a leak-proof plastic bag.
6) The plastic bag must then be placed in one of the following:
   a) Plastic clip-down container.
   b) Cylindrical lightweight metal container.
   c) Strong cardboard box with full depth lid.
   d) Two-piece polystyrene box with special grooved join.
7) It is recommended that this complete package is placed in a padded (Jiffy) bag.
8) Other packaging systems must be Post Office approved.

Fig. 22.4. Postal regulations for pathological specimens.

Containers should be secure, leakproof and protected from breaking but not so bound up in clingfilm, cotton wool, bubblepack and sticky tape that the laboratory staff are unable to open them on receipt.

Transport swabs should be used with the correct media in them to prevent desiccation of microbial material. Fixed tissue should be in secure formal saline containers.

Haematology

Blood Smears

Clean, washed, oil-free glass microscope slides are required for the preparation of blood smears (Fig. 22.5). The most useful slides have a frosted area at one end on which sample identification can be recorded.

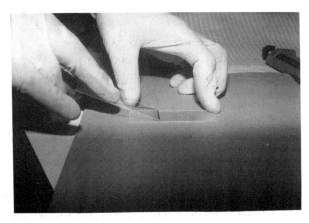

Fig. 22.5. Making a blood smear.

(1) Place a drop (10µl) of well-mixed EDTA whole blood at one end.
(2) Place a spreader slide just in front of the drop of blood and angle the slide at about 25–30° with the surface of the first slide.
(3) Draw the spreader slide back into the drop of blood, causing the blood to run along the interface between the two slides.
(4) Push the spreader slide steadily with an even, rapid motion towards the far end of the other slide. This will draw the blood along behind the spreader slide and make a thin, even blood film.
(5) Allow to air dry.
(6) Clean the edge of the spreader slide.
(7) Once the film is air-dried, it may be stained using Romanowsky stains (various alkaline methylene blue stains combined with eosin) such as Wright's, a modified Wright's/Giemsa, or Leishman's stains. Figure 22.6 shows the staining protocol.

Examination of Blood Films

The blood film is used to perform a **differential white blood cell count (WBC Diff.)**. The aim of this important procedure is to estimate the relevant proportions (as percentages) of the different types of white cells in a sample.

(1) The film should be scanned under low power to note the quality of the film and stain and the cell numbers.
(2) Then scan the far end of the film for platelet clumps and large abnormal cells.
(3) Finally, under low power, select an area of the film at least one third from the end of the film at the side edge which is to be examined under high power oil immersion for cell counting.

GIEMSA STAINING PROTOCOL FOR DIFFERENTIAL BLOOD FILMS

Solution 1:	Methyl alcohol, absolute (Analar)
Solution 2:	Giemsa stain consisting of:
	Azure 11-eosin.............................3 g
	Azure 11.......................................0.8 g
	Glycerol.......................................200 ml
	Solution 1...................................300 ml
Solution 3:	Buffer solution (pH 7.0) consisting of: Disodium hydrogen orthophosphate ....9.47 g Potassium dihydrogen orthophosphate ....9.08 g Distilled water...............................1 litre
Protocol	1) Air-dried films fixed in solution 2 for three minutes. 2) Dilute one volume of solution 2 with nine volumes of solution 3. Flood slide and stain for 15 minutes. 3) Wash and differentiate with solution 3, until cells are identifiable microscopically. 4) Drain and air dry.

Fig. 22.6. Giemsa staining protocol for differential blood films.

(4) Swing out the low power objective, place a drop of oil on the area and then swing in the oil immersion lens; focus; and count using the battlement technique.

Battlement technique

Rather than count each cell of each type (though the greater the number counted, the greater the accuracy), technicians often use the battlement technique (Fig. 22.7) to cover a reasonable area of the sample and to counteract distribution bias.

(1) Move 2 fields along the edge of the field, 2 fields up, 2 fields along and 2 fields down.
(2) Continue the sequence until 100 cells have been counted.
(3) Record the numbers of each type of cell.
(4) Express these as percentages of the total WBC count or in absolute numbers.

The total WBC count is determined by means of an automated haematology analyser or a microscopic counting chamber. Many manual types of commercial differential counters are available to keep tally of the differential cells and there are also several electronic systems. Figure 22.8 shows the normal reference haematology data for a number of species.

Poor quality films—either too thick (so that it is impossible to identify the cells due to poor separation) or too thin (so that insufficient cells are found) or of uneven thickness due to poor spreading technique—need to be remade. The stains should be filtered, as often debris and deposits prevent adequate staining and cellular differentiation. Production of good quality smears requires practice. Uniform staining may best be achieved by use of autostaining machines.

When examining the WBCs seen in a blood film, it is important to remember that red cells are also present and that they too should be looked at and commented upon. Figure 22.9 shows the various aspects of red cell development and morphology.

Red cells: morphology and terminology

Erythrocytes (red blood cells, RBCs) are non-nucleated biconcave discs that are pale greenish-yellow when unstained. They take up eosin when stained by Romanowsky stains, and become pinkish.

Proerythroblasts are the first stem cells of **erythropoiesis** or red cell production. They have a large nucleus with nucleoli and a rim of blue-stained cytoplasm. Haemoglobin synthesis commences on cell division within the cytoplasm and the cells become smaller. These are referred to as **nucleated RBCs (NRBCs)**.

NRBC cytoplasm changes from purple to greyish pink as the cells get smaller through stages of cell division (**normoblasts**). When the cell is completely haemoglobinised, the small dense nucleus is extruded leaving a greyish-blue or polychromatic cell with a reticular structure which stains blue with supravital stains such as brilliant cresyl blue or new methylene blue. These cells have no nucleus and are referred to as **reticulocytes**. Within normally 12 days in the peripheral blood stream, these lose their polychromasia and are adult red cells.

Crenation is a term applied to cells showing irregular margins and prickly points due to shrinkage. It is usually found in association with too slow airdrying of blood films.

Howell Jolly bodies are basophilic nuclear remnants seen as the NRBCs change to young erythrocytes. They are found in response to anaemia and splenic disorders or after splenectomy.

Target cells are RBCs with a central rounded area of haemoglobin surrounded by a clear zone, with a dense ring of haemoglobin around the perimeter of the cell due to increased membrane or decreased volume. They are often found in non-regenerative anaemia.

Rouleaux is a type of red cell arrangement used to describe grouping of RBCs in stacks. This is common in healthy horses but is otherwise associated with increased fibrinogen or globulin concentration in the blood.

Supravital stains are used to detect inclusions and other cellular material such as blood parasites including *Haemobartonella* spp. and *Babesia* spp.

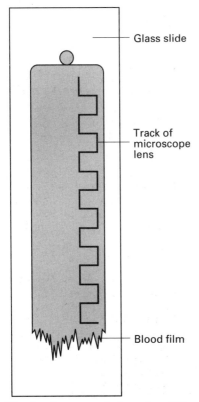

Fig. 22.7. The battlement technique for differential blood films.

HAEMATOLOGY REFERENCE RANGES FOR DOMESTICATED ANIMALS						
Parameter	Units	Canine	Feline	Equine	Thoroughbred	Bovine	Ovine
RBCs	x 10¹²/l	5.0–8.5	5.5–10.0	5.5–9.5	7.0–13	4.5–9.0	5.0–10.0
Haemoglobin	g%(100ml)	12–18	9.0–17	8.0–14	10–18	9.5–14.5	8.0–14
PCV	%(1/1)	37–57	27–50	24–44	32–55	30–40	22–38
MCV	fl	60–77	40–55	39–52	37–50	40–60	23–48
MCH	pg	19–23	13–17	15.2–18.6	13.3–18	14.4–18.6	9–13
MCHC	g%(100ml)	31–34	31–34	30–35	31–38	26–34	29–35
WBCs	x10⁹/l	6–15	4–15	6–12	7–14	3.5–10	4–10
Lymphocytes	x10⁹/l	1–4.8	1.5–6.5	1–6	1.7–9.8	1.4–6	2.6–7.2
	%	12–30	25–33	15–50	25–70	40–60	65–72
Mature	x10⁹/l	3.6–10.5	2.5–12.5	2.1–9	2.1–9.1	0.7–4.9	0.7–3.2
Neutrophils	%	60–70	45–75	35–75	30–65	21–49	18–32
Band	x10⁹/l	0–0.3	0–0.45	0–0.24	0–0.28	0–0.2	0–0.1
Neutrophils	%	0–2	0–3	0–2	0–2	0–2	0–1
Eosinophils	x10⁹/l	0.1–1.5	0.1–1.8	0.1–1.4	0–1.5	0–1.6	0–1.0
	%	2–10	4–12	2–12	1–11	0–16	0–10
Monocytes	x10⁹/l	0.18–1.5	0.0.6	0.12–1.2	0–1	0–1	0–1
	%	3–10	0–4	2–10	0.5–7.0	2–10	0–10
Basophils	x10⁹/l	0	0	0–0.3	0–0.4	0	0–0.2
	%	rare	rare	0–3	0–3	rare	0–2
Platelets	x10⁹/l	200–500	200–600	90–500	100–300	200–300	200–700

(source Bloxham Laboratories Ltd, Teignmouth, Devon)

Fig. 22.8. Haematology reference ranges for domesticated animals.

White blood cells (leucocytes)

WBCs are nucleated cells consisting of various types (Fig. 22.10) which may be classified into three morphological forms: polymorphonuclear (PMNL) granulocytes, lymphocytes and monocytes.

Polymorphonuclear granulocytes. PMNL granulocytes have a single nucleus consisting of a number of lobes. They have granular cytoplasm and can be differentiated by the staining reaction of these granules into neutrophils, eosinophils and basophils.

The nucleus of a **neutrophil** will stain purple-violet. The immature or juvenile cell is shaped first like a kidney-bean and then like a horse-shoe, at which stage it is often termed a **metamyelocyte**. As the cell matures it forms lobes, the number of which increases with increasing maturity. The cytoplasm stains a light pink; the granules are violet.

Neutrophilia is an increase in neutrophils and is found in infectious inflammatory conditions and under 'stress' or conditions induced by steroids.

Eosinophils are similar to neutrophils but they do not usually become as multilobular and their cytoplasmic granules will stain orange-red. In each species of animal, the shape and colour of stained eosinic granules are slightly different: some are small and oval, others are larger (such as in the horse), while cats tend to have large rod-shaped granules.

Eosinophilia is an increase in the number of these cells and is often found in association with allergy and parasitism. **Eosinopenia** is a lack of these cells and is often found in the dog in association with steroid usage and Cushing's disease (hyperadrenocorticism).

Basophils are often slightly smaller than neutrophils (8–10 μm in diameter). The nucleus is usually shaped like a kidney-bean and the cytoplasm contains a mass of large granules that stain deep purple and may obscure the nucleus. They contain histamine and heparin, which are released at the site of inflammation. They are rarely found in normal films for most animal species but may be present in conditions of chronic tissue damage and myeloid leukaemias.

Lymphocytes. Lymphocytes are of two types. The nucleus of the smaller (7–10μm in diameter) is round and will stain deep purple; it occupies most of the cell so that the cytoplasm, which stains a pale blue, is seen only as a rim around the nucleus, often only to one side. This is the most common form. The nucleus of the larger type (12–20μm in diameter) stains slightly lighter and has more light blue cytoplasm, which may contain a few reddish granules.

Lymphocytes play an important protective role and are associated with the production of antibodies and recognition of 'foreign' substances such as bacteria and viruses, or the body itself in autoimmune

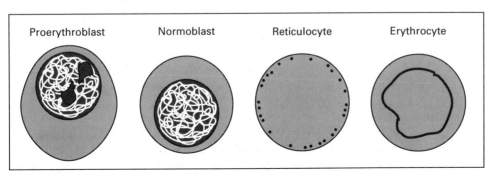

Fig. 22.9. Erythrocyte development and morphology.

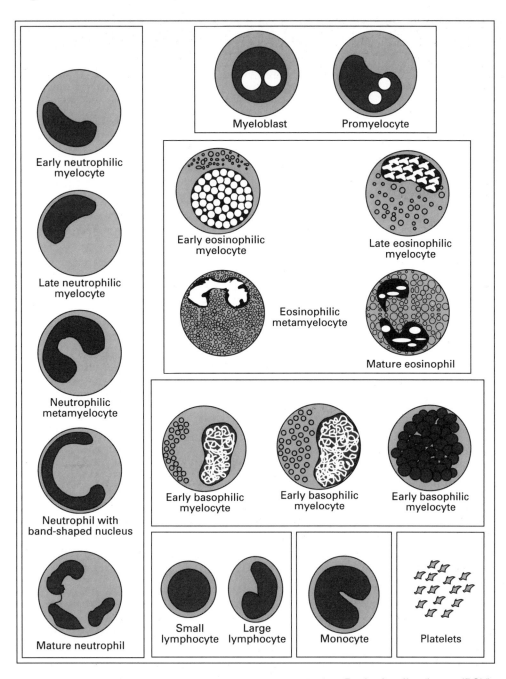

Fig. 22.10. White blood cell development and morphology.

conditions. **Lymphocytosis** is found in some viral conditions and leukaemias. **Lymphopenia** is a decrease in lymphocyte cells that is found in some viral conditions, after steroid use and in some chemotherapy patients. It is important to note that many lymphomas and other neoplastic conditions do not produce a lymphocytosis and may in fact show up as a lymphopenia.

Monocytes. Monocytes are large cells (16–20) and they contain many pink granules. They are involved in the repair of damage to blood vessels: they adhere to the damage and to each other to plug the 'leak' and are then involved in the clotting process (coagulation) to produce fibrin.

Thrombocytopenia, a reduction in the number of platelets, may result in internal or external haemorrhage, while an increase (**thrombocytosis**) may follow haemorrhage or surgery.

Packed cell volume (PCV)

The PCV, also referred to as the **haematocrit**, is that percentage of whole blood composed of red blood cells. For whole blood collected in EDTA vacutainers:

(1) Mix adequately by hand or on a roller mixer.
(2) Fill a plain capillary microhaematocrit tube to about three-quarters full by capillary action.
(3) With a finger on the top, seal or plug the bottom end with a clay or plastic material.
(4) Place in a microhaematocrit centrifuge with the plugged end facing out and resting on the rubber rim cushion. Give 5 minutes centrifugation.

Fresh blood samples, collected directly from the patient by means of a lancet-type puncture or from a drop of blood at the time of venipuncture, contain no anticoagulant and it is necessary to use a **heparinised**

microhaematocrit capillary tube. These tubes are internally coated with heparin: as the blood flows up the tube, the anticoagulant mixes with the blood to prevent clotting.

(5) After centrifugation, place the tubes in a **haematocrit reader**. This has a linear scale: the bottom of the tube contents is at zero and the top of the plasma meniscus is at 100. From the scale, read off the level of the top of the RBCs (the **red supernatant layer**). This percentage is the **PCV**.

(6) A white-to-grey layer sitting on top of the red cells and below the plasma is referred to as the **buffy coat** and consists of white blood cells and platelets.

(7) The clear-to-yellow layer at the top is the **plasma**.

Normal PCV ranges for various species are shown in Fig. 22.8. A decrease in PCV is often found in anaemia, haemorrhage etc., while increases may be found in cases of dehydration.

Total red and white cell counts

Manual or machine total cell counts are an essential part of the haematological examination. Manual cell counting is still required for avian and reptile bloods because their nucleated red cells are not differentiated readily by automated machine counting systems. The procedure for performing manual cell counts involves diluting the blood and counting in a special microscopic chamber, using specific chemical diluents to lyse red cells in order to count the white cells. Refer to standard haematological texts for details of these procedures.

Haemoglobin and calculated RBC parameters

Haemoglobin estimation is a routine part of any haematology examination, generally by colorimetric or spectrophotometric chemical reactions and calculated either manually or by an automated haematology analyser. Calculated values include mean corpuscular volume (MCV), mean corpuscular haemoglobin (MCH) and mean corpuscular haemaglobin concentration (MCHC).

Biochemistry

This section covers the main biochemical tests involved commonly in practice laboratory investigations using simple wet or dry chemistry systems.

Urea and BUN

Urea is a nitrogenous waste product that is formed in the liver from two molecules of ammonia as the end product of amino acid utilisation. It is then transported in the plasma fraction of the blood to the kidneys, where it is excreted in the urine.

The term **blood urea nitrogen (BUN)** expresses the amount of nitrogen atoms in the blood incorporated to urea. Laboratory analysis and measurement of the concentration of BUN and of urea have been used in the evaluation of renal function but are not the same. There is a difference of 2.144 times in magnitude between the weight (in mg/100ml plasma or serum) of urea and that of BUN.

In the international system (SI) of units, these substances are expressed in terms of **molecular** or **molar** concentration, a **mole** (mol) being the unit of amount of the substance. The multiplication factors to convert the old units, expressed in mg/100ml, to the SI units of millimoles per litre (mmol/l) are 0.17 for urea and 0.36 for BUN.

Increased urea may be associated with several conditions:

- High levels of urea in serum or plasma are usually assumed to be due to renal failure but there are other considerations.
- Chronic heart failure combined with poor renal perfusion will reduce the amount of urea taken to the kidney in the circulation and hence lead to an increase of the amount in the blood. Obviously if severe renal hypoxia occurs due to the poor circulation, renal failure will ensue and urea levels will rise even more.
- High-protein diets may increase the level of urea.
- Low-carbohydrate diets may lead to breakdown of body proteins or catabolism and then increase in urea.
- Dehydration may cause an apparent increase in urea.
- Urethral obstruction and ruptured bladder both may lead to increased urea concentrations.
- Other systemic and metabolic conditions may also increase urea.

Figure 22.11 shows the normal reference values for urea and a number of other biochemical parameters.

Blood Glucose

Most laboratories continue to refer to 'blood glucose' but the correct term now is 'plasma glucose'. Modern glucose methods are performed on plasma, whereas in the past whole-blood samples were used. As the level of glucose in RBCs is low, blood glucose values quoted in older texts may be lower than those found by current methods.

The level of glucose in the blood is an indication of carbohydrate metabolism and a measure of the pancreatic endocrine function, as it is controlled by insulin and glucagon:

- **Insulin** increases the cellular utilisation of glucose from blood.
- **Glucagon** production causes an increased production and release of glucose from tissue in the blood.

BIOCHEMICAL REFERENCE RANGES FOR DOMESTICATED ANIMALS

Parameter	Units	Canine	Feline	Equine	Thoroughbred	Bovine	Ovine
Albumin	g/l	25–37	21–39	23–38	21–34	27–37	24–32
T. Protein	g/l	54–77	54–78	57–84	43–67	70–88	65–78
T. Globulin	g/l	23–52	15–57	16–50	22–50	32–56	27–50
Urea	mmol/l	1.7–7.4	6–10	2.5–8.3	2.8–6.1	2–6.6	3–8
Creatinine	μmol/l	0–106	80–180	60–147	106–168	44–165	44–150
T. Bilirubin	μmol/l	<16	<10	10–40	10–40	<9	<8
Glucose	mmol/l	2–2.5	4.3–6.6	2.8–5.5	3.4–5.9	2–3	2–3
Cholesterol	mmol/l	3.8–7	1.9–3.9	2.3–3.6	2.3–3.6	1–3	1–2.6
ALT	U/l@30°C	<25	<20	<25	<25	<40	<50
SAP	U/l@30°C	<80	<60	40–120	40–160	<80	<40
γGT	U/l@30°C	<20	<20	<25	<40	<15	<20
CK	U/l@30°C	<100	<80	<150	<150	<50	<50
AST	U/l@30°C	<25	<35	<130	<212	<100	<50

(source Bloxham Laboratories Ltd, Teignmouth, Devon)

Fig. 22.11. Biochemical reference ranges for domesticated animals.

Figure 22.12 shows some of the conditions that cause increase or decrease in plasma glucose.

In the practice, it is possible to determine glucose by means of reagent strips or dip-stick methods. Newer reagent strips use whole blood: glucose levels can then be reliably measured by means of a small reflectance meter or by comparing the colour change on the pad with reference colours that indicate the relevant concentration. A number of systems are available and the manufacturer's methodology supplied with the system should be followed.

When sending a sample (plasma) to the laboratory by post, the standard anticoagulant to use for glucose is oxalate fluoride (OXF).

Other Biochemical Estimations

Determination of total serum protein, albumin, globulin, creatinine, cholesterol, bilirubin and various enzymes assist in the diagnosis of several common conditions (Fig. 22.13). Various 'dry' or 'wet' chemistry systems are available, and a refractometer might be used to determine total serum protein as well as urine specific gravity.

In determining enzymes, controlled temperature conditions are important: in animal biochemistry a temperature of 30°C is recommended. However, it should be noted that some laboratories and some texts quote enzyme activity at either 25°C or 37°C.

CONDITIONS ASSOCIATED WITH INCREASED AND DECREASED BLOOD GLUCOSE

Increased glucose	Decreased glucose
Post-feeding sample	Hepatic disorders
Increased glucocorticoids	Insulin treatment or
(stress, Cushing's)	Insulinoma
Administration of	Starvation/malabsorption
corticosteroids	Hypothyroid/hypoadrenal
Diabetes mellitus	Severe renal glucosuria
Pancreatitis	Idiopathic in some toy
Glucose treatment	breeds
Use of morphine	Artifact in old sample

Fig. 22.12. Conditions associated with increased and decreased blood glucose.

Examination of the Skin

Examination of samples for external parasites such as insects (fleas and lice) and arachnids (ticks and mites) depends on collection of suitable samples by means of skin-scraping, pustular collection, ear wax collection or hair brushing. The samples are mounted on slides and examined under the microscope.

As the insect may be present in the sample in the form of eggs, larvae, nymphs or adults, or only its faeces may be detected, it is important to understand the parasite's life cycle and to recognise the various stages of development. These are described in Chapter 16. Figure 22.14 gives some of the features to look for in identifying evidence of lice, fleas, Dipteran maggots and mites.

Ringworm

Ultraviolet light from a Wood's lamp may be used to examine hair samples from animals possibly infected by dermatophyte fungi such as *Microsporum* spp. (Chapter 16, Fig. 16.3). Affected material may fluoresce a bright yellow-green. However, only about 60% of cases of *M. canis* show this fluorescence and its lack does not rule out ringworm infection. It should be noted that non-specific bluish-white fluorescence is not due to ringworm but is commonly found due to scales of flaky skin, mud, dirt, nail surfaces and any petroleum-based materials, including many detergents and paraffin oil.

> WARNING
> Ultraviolet light is potentially dangerous and can damage the conjunctiva of the eye. Long exposure burns the skin, rather like sunburn (which of course is due to UV rays). Both the operator and the animal must be protected by careful use of the Wood's lamp.

Microscopic examination should be made of any specific fluorescing hairs by plucking them out. If none are seen:

CONDITIONS ASSOCIATED WITH INCREASED AND DECREASED BLOOD BIOCHEMISTRY VALUES		
Parameter	**Increased values**	**Decreased values**
T. Protein	Dehydration, lactation, infection and neoplasm	Liver disease, renal disease, malabsorption, immunodeficiency
Cholesterol	Hypothyroidism, Cushing's, post-feeding, diabetes mellitus, pancreatitis, nephrotic syndrome	Liver disease, lipoprotein deficiency
Bilirubin	Intra and extra hapatic icterus, pre-hepatic icterus or haemolysis	Of no diagnostic significance
ALT	Hepatic anoxia, metabolic disorders, hepatoxins, hepatitis	Of no diagnostic significance
SAP	Liver and bile duct damage, bone growth in young, steroids (in dogs)	EDTA sample, haemolysis No diagnostic significance
GT	Cholestasis and cirrhosis	No diagnostic significance
CK	Myositosis, muscular trauma, myopathy, haemolysis, myocardial infarct	No diagnostic significance
AST	Myopathies, hepatic damage and haemolysis	No diagnostic significance

Fig. 22.13. Conditions associated with increased and decreased blood chemistry values.

(1) Take hairs plucked from the edge of the lesion, together with a skin scraping, and place on a microscope slide with a few drops of 10% potassium hydroxide (KOH). Place a cover slip over.

(2) Heat the slide over a Bunsen flame, for a few seconds only, to assist in clearing the hairs so that details of the hair shaft may be seen with the microscope under high dry.

In cases of ringworm, the fungal spores or arthrospores will appear as small, spherical, refractile bodies occurring in chains or as a complete sheath around the hair shaft and totally invading the keratinous epithelium. **Hyphae** may be seen as filaments infecting the hair from which the arthrospores are produced. A 20% KOH digest may be used but this is often too strong and damages the hairs too much.

IDENTIFICATION OF ECTOPARASITES				
		Eggs	**Nymphs**	**Larvae**
Lice	Dorsoventrally flattened, wingless Sucking lice — Biting lice Grey to red — Yellower No eyes Membranous abdomen with hair on segments Pincer claws — Clasping or running legs Elongated head — Rounded head Piercing — Mandibular mouthparts — mouthparts	(nits): Oval white, plug/operculum at one end.	Similar to adults but smaller and no reproductive organs.	
Fleas	Small wingless (4–5mm long) Laterally compressed body Large hindlegs Adults have piercing/sucking mouthparts	(cat flea): Oval, white, glistening, 0.5mm long.		White to brown (creamy yellow on hatching); small, maggot-like; very active, light-shy; 2–5mm long; sparse hairs. Pupae: Very sticky.
Flies (Diptera)	Large adults with wings	Small (1mm long), elongated, creamy white.		House fly maggots can grow up to 12mm long in less than one week.
Mites	Almost circular body 4 pairs short legs, perhaps with suckers (only front 2 pairs project beyond body) Adult female 400–600 x 300–400μm *Cheyletiella* larger, less rounded; legs longer; horn-like hooks either side of head.	Oval	4 pairs of legs	3 pairs of legs; 'orange-tawny'

Fig. 22.14. Identification of ectoparasites.

MORPHOLOGICAL IDENTIFICATION OF DERMATOPHYTES		
Dermatophyte	**Colony identification**	**Microscopic identification**
Microsporum canis	Flat, white and silky centre. Bright yellow edge. Reverse of culture yellow.	8–15 celled macroconidia or macroaleurospores, knobby end. Thick-walled.
Microsporum gypseum	Flat powdery irregular fringe. Brown colour with reverse yellow/brown.	Symmetrical thin-walled 3–8 cell macroconidia. Pointed ends. Boat-shaped.
Trichophyton mentagrophytes	Flat, granular, tan coloured, or heaped white cottony. Reverse yellow-red/brown.	Cigar-shaped 2–6 celled. Heaped colonies may have no Macroconidia.
Trichophyton verrucosum	Small velvet white.	Macroconidia seldom seen.

Fig. 22.15. Morphological identification of determatophytes.

Ringworm culture. The standard medium for ringworm culture is Sabouraud's dextrose agar, which is incubated at 25°C for up to 2 weeks. Plucked hairs or skin scrapings are pushed into shallow cuts made in the agar. Dermatophyte identification is based on colony morphology and pigmentation together with microscopic examination of the macroconidia or macroaleuriospores (Fig. 22.15).

There is also a modified commercial Sabouraud's agar with added pH indicator (phenol red): the pathogenic fungi usually grow faster than saprophytes and they produce alkaline metabolites, so that the indicator in the agar turns from yellow to red. Cultures should be examined at 7, 10 and 14 days if an indicator is used.

Faecal Examination

The first stage of any faecal examination is to note:

- consistency (hard, soft, fluid);
- colour (yellow; brown; green; red, due to blood; or black, due to digested blood);
- whether fatty or mucoid;
- presence of any specific obvious material such as worms (round or tape), bones, hair, fur or some other foreign bodies.

Following this macroscopic examination, a direct smear of the faeces may be made for microscopic examination. This enables a rapid assessment of any parasitic burden by looking for worm eggs and protozoan oocysts (Fig. 22.16) and also an initial examination of partially digested or undigested material in the faeces. For **direct wet preparation:**

(1) Place a drop of saline on to a microscope slide.
(2) Add an equal amount of faeces.
(3) To assist in contrast, add stains such as Lugol's iodine (which stains starch granules blue-black) or new methylene blue (which will show up undigested meat fibres).
(4) Mix thoroughly, make a thin smear and place a cover slip on top.
(5) Use low power to examine the field for the presence of worm eggs.
(6) Use medium power to look for protozoa.

Alternatively, instead of putting on a cover slip, allow the slide to dry; then flame-fix and stain for more detailed high-power or perhaps oil immersion examination.

Faecal Flotation

Faecal flotation is based on differences in specific gravity. Water has a specific gravity of 1.000; parasitic eggs are heavier at 1.100–1.200; and many solutions of salts or sugar have a higher specific gravity of 1.200–1.250. Faeces placed in such solutions will partition: heavy debris will sink but the

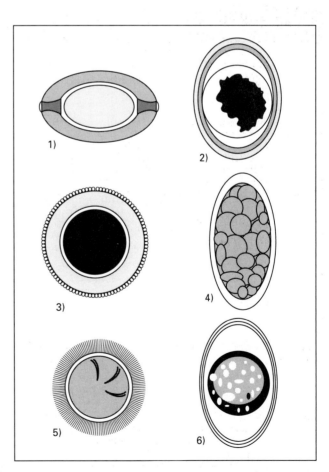

Fig. 22.16. Worm eggs and oocysts: (1) *Trichuris* spp; (2) *Toxascaris* spp.; (3) *Toxocara* spp.; (4) *Uncinaria* spp.; (5) *Taenia* spp.; (6) *Isospora* spp.

lighter eggs will rise to the surface. The most common solutions used for this procedure are sugar solution, zinc sulphate, saturated sodium chloride or sodium nitrate.

The standard flotation method is as follows:

(1) Mix faeces and the solution to break them up.
(2) Push the mixture through a fine sieve or muslin cloth or gauze.
(3) Transfer to a test tube so that the solution fills the tube completely, forming a meniscus at the top.
(4) Place a cover slip on and leave to stand upright, undisturbed for 10–20 minutes.
(5) Carefully lift the cover slip off vertically and place it on to a microscope slide, ensuring that the fluid is trapped between the slide and the coverslip.
(6) Examine the slide under a low-power microscope objective.

Centrifugal flotation is normally performed rather than standard flotation. The tubes are spun at low speed (1000–1500 rpm) in a centrifuge for 3–5 minutes, then the top fluid meniscus is removed and examined.

Commercial kits are based on the standard flotation technique but they consist of a plastic vial containing a filter, so that the sample does not need to be filtered or sieved in advance.

Faecal Sedimentation

Faecal sedimentation concentrates eggs by centrifugation in water but microscopic detection is difficult because of the presence of faecal debris.

(1) Mix about 2 g of faeces with tap water and then strain.
(2) Half-fill a centrifuge tube with the strained fluid.
(3) Spin for about 5 minutes at 1500 rpm.
(4) Pour off the supernatant.
(5) With a Pasteur pipette, transfer some of the sediment on to a microscope slide and put on a cover slip.
(6) Lugol's iodine may be mixed with the sediment prior to examination under low power.

McMaster Technique

The standard quantitative technique used to determine the number of eggs per gram of faeces is the McMaster technique, which requires a special counting chamber. Figure 22.17 describes one of several modified methods based on this technique (See Chapter 16, for various parasite ova found in dog and cat faeces).

Occult Blood

Occult ('hidden') blood is evidence of insidious chronic bleeding from ulcers, neoplastic lesions or

---

MODIFIED McMASTER'S PROTOCOL FOR WORM EGG COUNT

1) Weigh 3 g faeces. Put into 120 ml wide-mouthed glass-stoppered bottle with glass beads. Add 42 ml tap water and shake well.
2) Pour faeces suspension through wire mesh screen, collecting filtrate in clean bowl.
3) Mix and transfer to 10 ml centrifuge tube. Fill to within 10 mm of top.
4) Centrifuge for 2 mins at 1000 rpm (800g).
5) Discard supernatant and emulsify packed sediment.
6) Fill to within 10 mm of top with saturated NaCl.
7) Invert tube several times until even suspension.
8) Centrifuge for 2 minutes at 1000 rpm (800g).
9) Fill both McMaster counting chambers.
10) Count oocysts and worm eggs under 10x objective and 10x eye piece.
11) Count/gram of faeces = total number from both chambers x 50.

Fig. 22.17. Modified McMaster's protocol.

parasitism in the digestive tract. Dramatic bleeding is usually obvious: faeces are either black (melaena), containing partially digested blood, or they show frank blood (haematochezia). Confirmation of the presence of occult blood requires biochemical detection. The reagents orthotoluidine or benzidine react with haemoglobin peroxidase in faeces with occult blood to yield a colour change which is detected visually. However, both reagents are so sensitive that they will react with any dietary haemoglobin or myoglobin; hence the animal must be placed on a totally meat-free diet for 3 days before its faeces are collected for occult blood testing. Commercial test kits are available.

Other procedures that may also be carried out as part of a faecal examination include:

- faecal trypsin (protease) tests to determine presence or absence of pancreatic trypsin faecal activity;
- special stains such as Sudan IV to detect undigested fats.

Urine Examination

Gross examination should start with the amount produced. The normal dog will produce 25–60 ml/kg body weight while a cat normally voids 10–20 ml/kg body weight every 24 hours. **Polyuria** is production of excess urine; **oliguria** is a reduction in the amount voided. Other factors to be checked include colour, turbidity, odour and specific gravity.

Colour

The colour of urine is normally yellow. The intensity of the colour may give some indication as to the specific gravity or concentration of the urine: the darker it is, the more concentrated.

- If the urine is browny-yellow and on shaking a slight greenish foam appears on the surface, then bile pigments are likely to be present.
- Red or red-brown coloration is likely to indicate the presence of red blood cells, haemoglobin or myoglobin.
- Drugs may alter the colour of the urine and so will some foods, such as beetroot.

Turbidity

Normal urine should be clear. If it is cloudy or turbid, sediment is likely to be present and this should be harvested by centrifugation for microscopic examination.

Red and white blood cells, crystals, epithelial cells, casts, bacteria, yeasts and fungi may cause increased turbidity of urine and can be identified microscopically.

Odours

Ammonia is produced in stale urine, due to bacterial activity, and an odour is given off.

- This same odour in freshly voided urine may be due to urease-producing bacteria involved in cystitis.
- Male cats tend to produce a strong odour—the males of many species similarly produce strong urine odours to mark their territory.
- The typical sweet acetone smell of peardrops is found in urine from ketotic animals.

Specific Gravity

Specific gravity is the density or weight of a known volume of a fluid compared with an equal amount of distilled water. Water has a specific gravity of 1.000.

Refractometer

The specific gravity of urine may be determined by using a refractometer to assess the fluid's refractive index: the higher the concentration, the higher the refractive index. Density is also influenced by temperature and the determination should be made at a constant temperature, or the refractometer should be corrected to compensate for the operating temperature.

Only a few drops of urine are required for determination using a refractometer. They are placed on the glass of the chamber and the lid is closed. The refractometer is held up to the light and the specific gravity is read from the scale. If the reading goes off the top end of the scale, the urine is very concentrated: dilute it with an equal volume of distilled water and measure again. In this case multiply the actual scale reading after the decimal point by 2 to give the correct final specific gravity of the urine.

Hydrometer

Specific gravity may also be determined by means of a hydrometer, which floats in water. The bottom of the meniscus reads zero on the scale of the stalk. The urine volume required may be 10–15 ml and the accuracy is not as good as that of the refractometer. Temperature is much more critical using a hydrometer.

Factors affecting specific gravity

Dehydration increases the specific gravity of urine, as does fluid loss. Other causes of increase include reduced water intake, acute renal failure and shock.

Excess water intake (**polydipsia**), diabetes insipidus, pyometra and some liver and chronic renal conditions exhibit reduced urine specific gravity.

Chemical Determination

Reagent urine dip-stick methods have been developed and are commercially available, but they are not reliable for specific gravity measurement of animal urine. They may have limited value for human use but the variations in pH and other chemical constituents in all types of dog and cat urine produce inconsistencies that make dip-sticks unacceptable for reliable determination.

Commercial reagents strips are plastic strips mounted with a variable number of test reagent pads. For example, a 10-determination urine stick can be used for determination of pH, specific gravity, blood, protein, glucose, bilirubin, ketone (acetoacetic acid), urobilinogen, nitrate and leucocytes. These sticks are best used on fresh urine and should never be used on preserved samples. Stale samples are likely to have bacteria growth from the environment or skin or faecal contamination which may affect glucose pH and blood determination. The older the sample, the more any ketones, bilirubin or urobilinogen present will decrease in the urine. Some strip systems enable a reflectometer determination of the end result rather than relying on visual determination.

Figure 22.18 gives reference values for pH and specific gravity in the urine of domestic animals.

NORMAL RANGES IN URINE		
Species	pH	Specific gravity
Canine	5.2–6.8	1.018–1.045
Feline	6–7	1.020–1.040
Equine	7–8.5	1.020–1.050
Bovine	7–8.5	1.005–1.040
Ovine	7–8.5	1.020–1.040

Fig. 22.18. Reference ranges for urine pH and specific gravity.

Determination of pH

The pH of a solution is the expression of its hydrogen ion concentration. A pH above 7.0 is alkaline, while below 7.0 is acidic. Stored samples tend to become more acid as CO_2 is lost to the air and false results may occur if the samples are not kept cool and covered.

- Urine pH is affected by diet: vegetarian diets produce more alkaline urine, while carnivorous animals have acid urines.
- Acidic urines (decrease in pH) may be due to pyrexia (fever), starvation, acidosis, high-protein diets, muscle catabolism or some drugs.
- Alkaline urines (increase in pH) may be due to high vegetational content of the diet, urinary retention, urinary tract infections, alkalosis or certain drugs.

The pH may be determined simply by means of pH papers or with multi-reagent dip-sticks/strips. It is important to realise that the colour of urine may itself colour the detection strip and cause an artifact in the visual determination. Electrode pH meters are available as small stick-type instruments with digital read-out: they are inexpensive and should be considered as a more reliable method.

Blood in urine

Blood in urine is detected by means of a similar principle to the detection of occult blood in faeces. Red blood cells, haemoglobin and myoglobin cause oxidation of the reagents, turning them from yellow-orange to green and then to dark blue as the amount of haemoglobin or myoglobin increases. Spots of green are likely to indicate whole RBCs, while solid colour suggests the presence of haemolysed blood. Ascorbic acid may inhibit the detection, giving false negatives, and high specific gravity and high protein levels in the urine may reduce the reactivity. Oxidising agents such as hypochlorites and bacterially produced peroxidases may give false positives. Myoglobin from muscle breakdown will also yield a positive reaction. Any positives found on dip-sticks should be examined microscopically to confirm the presence of blood.

Haematuria is the presence of whole blood in the urine. The presence of lysed blood is referred to as **haemoglobinuria**; and **myoglobinuria** indicates the presence of myoglobin in the urine.

- The most common causes of haematuria are cystitis and associated infection or inflammation of the urinary tract, urolithiasis, acute nephritis, thrombocytopenia and various coagulopathies which cause bleeding.
- Haemoglobinuria is associated with haemolysis of blood in the blood stream or haemoglobinaemia. Conditions such as autoimmune haemolytic anaemia (AIHA), systemic lupus erythematosus (SLE), *Leptospira haemorrhagica* infection, babesiosis and poisoning should be considered as causes.

- Myoglobinuria occurs due to muscle breakdown in cases such as azoturia (rhabdomyolysis) in horses.
- If no haemoglobinaemia is detected in blood but the urine is red-brown and the dip-stick indicates the presence of blood in the urine, then it is more likely to indicate myoglobinuria than haemoglobinuria. Haemoglobin precipitates in ammonium sulphate while myoglobin does not and so confirmatory testing is possible.

Protein in the urine

Protein in the urine is normally present in only very small amounts but collection methods associated with free collection or expressing of the bladder are likely to contain more due to production of secretions from the urinogenital tract. The main cause of increased proteins, however, is associated with decreased re-absorption of proteins by the tubules and leakage from the glomerular part of the kidney. The dip-stick protein reagent primarily detects albumin, not total proteins, and is less sensitive to globulins, mucoproteins and monoclonal proteins. Alkaline urines, and those contaminated with some antiseptic or detergents, may show up as false positive for protein.

True **proteinuria** is found in acute and chronic nephritis, congestive heart failure, other causes of renal damage or nephrosis, cystitis, urethral inflammation, vaginitis and other conditions of the genital tract and traumatic catheterisation. Following parturition or during oestrus the level of protein may rise and be detected but normally any protein detected by the dip-stick is suggestive of **urogenital damage**.

Glucose in the urine

Glucose in the urine is referred to as **glucosuria** and the amount present depends on the amount in the blood and the ability of renal filtration and reabsorption. The so-called **renal threshold** is the blood level of glucose above which the normal kidney cannot filter or reabsorb (Chapter 23).

- Strip-test reagents use a double enzyme reaction system to detect glucose and the test is very specific.
- Tablet reagent systems use a copper reduction method, which is less specific and detects any sugars.

The normal minimum detection level is around 5.0 mmol/l. Ascorbic acid may give false negative results and the presence of ketouria may reduce the detectable level of glucose in such urine. Stale or bacterially contaminated urine may also have false negative glucose due to the presence of glucose-using organisms.

Glucosuria may occur in diabetes mellitus and occasionally in cases of adrenal hyperplasia (Cushing's disease), hyperthyroidism, chronic liver damage, stress, general anaesthesia and in a specific renal conditions in which the tubules are unable to resorb glucose.

Ketones in the urine (ketouria)

Ketones are detected by means of dip-stick or reagent tablets, but these primarily detect one ketone body—that of acetoacetic acid—and are less sensitive to acetone, while they do not detect betahydroxybutyric acid (BHB).

Ketouria may indicate liver damage, diabetes mellitus or ruminant ketosis.

Bile pigments

Bilirubinuria is the presence of bile pigments (urobilinogen and conjugated bilirubin) in the urine. It is found in a number of conditions including obstruction of bile flow into the intestine, bowel changes, cholangitis, bile duct obstruction, liver damage due to release of conjugated bilirubin from hepatocytes and in cases of haemolytic anaemia. Bilirubin may be detected by the multi-strip dip-stick but this is not as sensitive as reagent tablets which incorporate a diazo reagent:

(1) Urine is placed on a supplied pad.
(2) A tablet is placed on the pad.
(3) Two drops of water are placed on top of the tablet so that they run down on to the pad.
(4) If the area of the mat around the tablet turns blue, bilirubin is present in the urine.

Urobilinogen is an intestinal bacterial breakdown product of bilirubin. Some of it is absorbed from the intestine into the blood stream and then small amounts are excreted from the kidney into the urine. It is therefore normal to find some urobilinogen in the urine (urobilinogenuria) and a lack of it may indicate bile duct obstruction. However, oxidation occurs rapidly and the oxidised form is not detected. It is essential to test fresh samples of urine. Increased amounts occur in haemolysis and some cases of hepatocyte damage.

Microscopic Examination of Urine

Normal urine does not contain much sediment, but a few epithelium cells, some mucus and blood cells may be found. Bacteria may be present due to contamination at the time of collection or during subsequent storage. Reagent sticks provide some information but examination of spun-down sediment in urine is potentially a very useful diagnostic aid.

(1) Place 5ml of fresh mixed urine into a conical centrifuge tube and spin at 1500 rpm (around 100g) for 5 minutes.
(2) Pour off the supernatant, leaving the sediment with a little urine in the bottom of the tube.
(3) Flick the base of the tube to resuspend the sediment and withdraw some by Pasteur pipette.
(4) Make an unstained wet preparation by placing a drop on a slide and placing a cover slip on top.
(5) Examine by microscope with the condenser down and the iris diaphragm partially closed so that only a little light passes through.

It is possible to add a stain such as 0.5% new methylene blue to aid examination prior to putting on the cover slip. If high-power oil immersion examination is required, make a smear similar to a blood film; air-dry and then stain by Gram stain for bacterial examination, or by Giemsa or modified Wright's stain for cellular study.

Commercial urine microscopic analysis chambers similar to McMaster worm-egg slides and manual blood cell counting chambers are available and these maybe used instead of the standard microscope slide and cover slip method.

- **Pyuria** is the presence of large numbers of WBCs (usually neutrophils) in urine and suggests inflammation in the urinogenital tract.

- **Haematuria** is the presence of large numbers of RBCs in urine and indicates bleeding into the urinogenital tract. In concentrated urine the cells shrivel up and are crenated. In dilute urine they swell and lyse, leading to haemoglobinuria—the empty cells are referred to as ghosts and must be distinguished from yeasts, fat globules or crystals.

- **Epithelial cells** are flat, irregular squamous cells with a small nucleus. They are shed from the surface of the urethra, vagina or vulva in naturally voided urine.

- **Transitional cells** are rounder and smaller; they come from further up the tract and in voided urine they indicate cystitis or pyelonephritis. Catheterised samples are likely to have higher numbers than voided urine.

- **Tubular epithelial cells** are the same size as WBCs and are easily confused with them. They tend to be round with a large nucleus and their presence is suggestive of tubular damage.

- **Casts** are formed in the tubules and consist of precipitated proteins due to the acidic condition of the lower (distal) collecting tubules of the kidney. They are defined into various types depending on the other material incorporated with the protein. They dissolve in alkaline urine and should be looked for in fresh urine. High speed centrifugation may break them up and so it is important to prepare the sediment carefully.

- **Hyaline casts** are clear, cylindrical, colourless and refractile and they rapidly dissolve in alkaline urine. An increased number is found with mild tubular inflammation, pyrexia and poor circulation.

- **Cellular casts** may contain RBCs, WBCs, epithelial cell, or a mixture of cell types.

- **Granular casts** are hyaline casts with granules in them. These granules are remnants of epithelial cells and WBCs. They are associated with significant inflammatory change.

- **Waxy casts** are more opaque than hyaline casts and usually wider with square rather than round ends. They are often found in more chronic degenerative renal tubular changes.

- **Mucus threads** are thinner, without definite walls, and are usually twisted strands or ribbons. They are not casts and are normal products of the lower urinogenital tract.
- **Spermatozoa** may be found in entire male urine and are of no diagnostic significance.
- **Bacteria**, **fungi** and **yeasts** may be found as contaminants of urine but their presence is only likely to be significant if accompanied by large numbers of leucocytes and if the sample was collected aseptically by catheterisation or mid-stream void and examined fresh. Yeasts in particular are likely to be urine contaminants from the external genitalia.

Crystals

Crystals in urine may be associated with clinical conditions such as cystitis, urolithiasis and haematuria, but may also be found in apparently normal animals.

Alkaline urines tend to contain phosphates and calcium carbonates, which dissolve in acid urine. Acid urine may contain urates, oxalates, cystine, leucine and tyrosine crystals.

Crystals are more likely to be found if freshly collected urine is allowed to stand and cool. Figure 22.19 shows the typical morphological pattern of some common crystals seen microscopically in urines.

Uroliths are calculi composed of crystals in the urine and they may cause blockage or damage to the urinary tract. The condition is referred to as **urolithiasis** and chemical analysis of the 'stones' may be performed to identify the materials involved and to assist in the treatment and control of them.

Bacteriological Examination

Bacteria may be examined by means of microscopic study using stains. They may be grown on culture

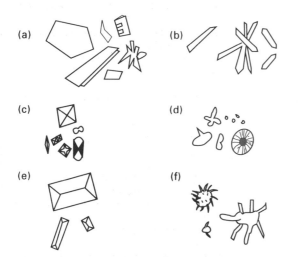

Fig. 22.19. Urine crystals: (a) urates; (b) hippuric acid; (c) calcium oxalate; (d) calcium carbonate; (e) struvite; (f) ammonium urate.

media plates (usually a mixture of nutrients and blood in agar): their colony growth may assist in identification and their particular fermentation ability may be used alone or in conjunction with serological tests to confirm their identity.

Sampling

The first stage in any bacterial examination is to obtain suitable samples. Swabs from open wounds, pus or orifices such as the buccal cavity, vagina and ears may be obtained using commercial sterile cotton-tipped swabs.

- If these are to be posted to a laboratory, it is essential that they are placed into **transport media**. Most commercial laboratories supply the transport media and swabs for postal submission.
- For use in the practice, dry swabs maybe perfectly acceptable, especially in the preparation of smears.

The collection of body fluids has been described earlier in this chapter. **Vesicles** and **abcesses** are best sampled by means of a needle and syringe. Sampling of **post-mortem organs** is best achieved by heat-searing the surface with a spatula that has been flamed over a Bunsen and placed on the surface to sterilise it. The surface is then cut with a sterile scalpel and a swab of the cut internal surface is taken.

In all cases, it is important to ensure aseptic collection of microbiological samples.

Smears

The making of bacterial smears requires only a thin application of material on to a slide.

- For **direct smears from swabs**, lightly roll the end on to the middle of a clean microscope slide.
- For **fluid samples**, a drop of the fluid is transferred aseptically with a Pasteur pipette or by means of a flamed and cooled bacterial wire loop.
- **Colonies from agar plates** may be picked off individually by a wire loop and mixed with a drop of sterile saline on the slide.
- It is also possible to smear directly from tissue or pus.

Heat-fixing

When the sample has air-dried, the smear is passed through a Bunsen flame 2–3 times with the sample side up. This achieves heat-fixing and prevents the sample from being washed off, provided that the smear is not too thick. It kills the bacteria but preserves the cell morphology. It is important not to overheat: the back of the slide should feel warm but should not burn the back of the hand. When the slide has cooled it is ready for staining.

Staining

Methylene blue

Methylene blue is a simple stain which will show up the presence and morphology of bacteria. A specific aged and oxidised version referred to as polychromatic methylene blue is used for staining anthrax bacilli in blood smears and for demonstrating McFadyean's reaction. Freshly made or **new methylene blue** should never be used when polychromatic methylene blue is required.

Gram stain

The Gram stain is the standard staining method that basically separates bacteria into two types: Gram-positive and Gram-negative organisms, based on the structure of the cell wall. This stain consists of a primary stain of crystal violet which is treated with a mordant iodine (1.0 g iodine crystals, 2.0 g potassium iodide and 200 ml of distilled water). The next stage is to decolorise with alcohol and then counterstain with carbol fuchsin.

- **Gram-positive** bacteria resist decolorisation and remain blue-violet in colour.
- **Gram-negative** bacteria are decolorised; they take up the counterstain and become red in colour.

A procedure for performing a Gram stain is illustrated in Figure 22.20.

Lugol's iodine

Lugol's iodine is more concentrated than Gram's iodine: the same amount of stain is combined with only 100 ml of distilled water. Lugol's is used rather than Gram's for a darker colour, giving less chance of excessive decolorisation.

Ziehl–Neelsen stain

This is another commonly used stain, which detects acid-fast bacteria such as mycobacteria (tuberculosis and Johnes' disease). They are stained with carbol fuchsin and heated; they are then resistant to decolorisation with acid alcohol and so retain the red colour when counterstained with methylene blue.

Shape

The other aspect of microscopic examination of bacteria is to define their shape. Round bacteria are **cocci**; they may be single or in pairs (**diplococci**), clusters or bunches (such as staphylococci) or chains (streptococci). Rod-shaped bacteria are termed **bacilli**; some are rods with enlarged round ends (**coccobacilli**) and others may be spiral in shape. Bacteria that have variable shapes are referred to as **pleomorphic**.

Culture Media

Culture media for routine bacteriology are available from various commercial suppliers, as either pre-poured plates, dry powder or dehydrated media. Some of the most commonly used media—blood agar, MacConkey's, selenite broth and Sabouraud's agar—are described in Chapter 15 (Elementary Microbiology) along with simple (basal) and enriched media, and biochemical media.

After a bacterium has been cultivated and identified as a potential pathogen involved in a disease process, antimicrobial treatment of the animal is ideally based upon *in vitro* sensitivity of the bacterium, so that the most relevant antimicrobial agents can be selected. A specific medium is preferred for performing sensitivity testing and is usually an agar-based medium such as Mueller–Hinton or Sentest agar.

(1) The specific bacterium is plated out to cover the agar.

(2) Antimicrobial discs containing various antimicrobial agents are placed on the surface of the agar. The discs may be placed individually by means of sterile tweezers or loaded into commercial cartridge disc dispensers that can dispense up to eight different antimicrobial discs at a time on to the inoculated plate.

(3) Following incubation, zones of inhibition around some discs indicate that the antimicrobial substance has prevented the growth of the bacterium and the isolate is therefore sensitive to that drug.

(4) If the bacteria grow to the edge of the disc, they are resistant to the particular agent on that disc.

GRAM STAINING PROCEDURE	
Solution 1:	Oxalate crystal-violet solution (containing 2% crystal-violet, 20% ethyl alcohol and 0.8% ammonium oxalate).
Solution 2:	Stabilised Lugol–PVP complex (containing 1.3% iodine, 2% potassium iodide and 10% PVP).
Solution 3:	Decolorise (containing 50% alcohol (95%) and 50% acetone).
Solution 4:	safranin solution (containing 0.25% safranin and 10% alcohol (95%)).
Protocol	1) Cover smear with solution 1 for one minute.
	2) Rinse in tap water.
	3) Cover smear with solution 2 for one minute.
	4) Rinse in tap water.
	5) Decolourise with solution 3.
	6) Rinse in tap water.
	7) Cover smear with solution 4 for one minute.
	8) Rinse in tap water.
	9) Dry.
	10) Examine microscopically under oil immersion lens.

Fig. 22.20. Grain-stain protocol.

Inoculation of agar plates

Whatever the origin of the sample, once it has been aseptically collected and put on to a point of the agar near the edge of the dish it must then be spread on the plate and diluted so that individual colonies are produced. The most common procedure is the **streaking method** (Fig. 22.21):

(1) Take a platinum bacterial loop; flame it until it is red-hot and then allow it to cool. Touch it on to the agar to ensure that it has cooled.
(2) From the point of application of the sample on the plate, streak in a zigzag over one-third of the plate.
(3) Remove the loop and flame it again, using a hooded Bunsen to prevent dissemination of bacteria.
(4) Cool, and then place the loop on agar.
(5) Streak through the previous pattern and over a different third of the plate.
(6) Flame again, and repeat the process a third time, commencing the streak from the previous zigzag.
(7) The loop should then be flamed and put away. Place the petri dish lid on top of the inoculated agar dish.

Incubation of cultures

Culture plates should be placed upside down in an incubator to prevent moisture accumulating on the bacteria and agar surface. Most common pathogenic bacteria can be grown aerobically at 37°C. The incubator temperature must be constant and the correct temperature must be maintained at all times.

Following incubation (usually for 18–24 hours) the growing bacteria should be seen as separate colonies at the end of the streak (Fig. 22.22). Any growth that is not associated with the streak lines is likely to be due to contamination of the media, either when being poured or while inoculation was taking place. There may be many airborne yeasts and fungi in the environment and these can become contaminants of the culture plates if sufficient care is not taken.

Identification of bacterial growth on blood agar starts with recording the colony characteristics, such as:

- any zone of haemolysis in the blood agar around the colony (haemolytic or non-haemolytic);
- the size of the colony—pinpoint, medium, large—and the measurement in millimetres (mm);
- the colour of the colony (grey, cream, yellow, white etc.);
- if opaque, translucent or transparent;
- the shape and consistency (either irregular or circular, raised, flat, convex, mucoid, flaky, sticky, hard and crusty);
- the odour (sweet, musty, pungent etc.).

The important subject of disposal of clinical waste, including culture plates, is discussed in Chapter 12.

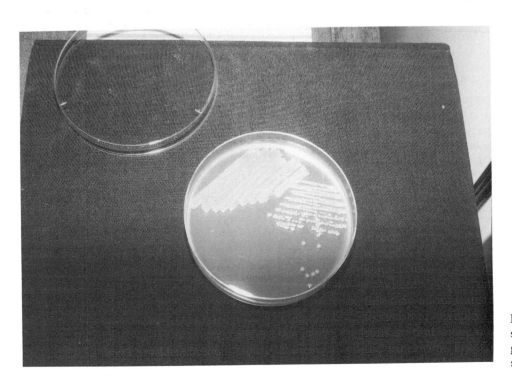

Fig. 22.21. Plating out of a sample: culture plate with growth showing the streaking pattern.

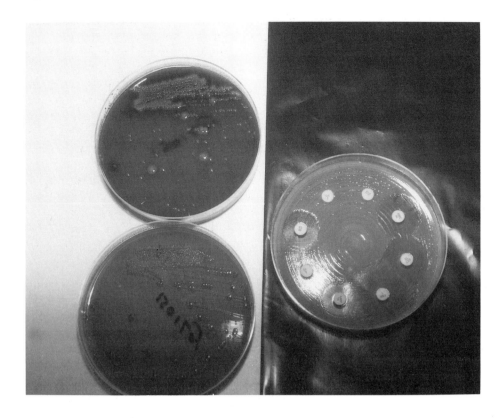

Fig. 22.22. Culture plate growth (left) and sentest plate (right).

Further reading

Baker, F. J. and Silverton, R. E. (1985) *Introduction to Medical Laboratory Technology, 6th ed.* Butterworth & Co.

Benjamin, M. M. (1978) *Outline of Veterinary Clinical Pathology, 3rd ed.* Iowa State University Press.

Cowell, R. L. and Tyler, R. D. (1989) *Diagnostic Cytology of the Dog and Cat.* American Veterinary Publications Inc., Santa Barbara.

Doxey, D. L. and Nathan, M. B. F. (1989) *Manual of Laboratory Techniques.* BSAVA Publications.

Hawkey, C. M. and Dennett, T. B. (1989) *A Colour Atlas of Comparative Veterinary Haematology.* Wolfe Medical Publications Ltd, London.

Jain, N. C. (1993) *Essentials of Veterinary Hematology.* Lea & Febiger, Philadelphia.

Kaneko, J. J. (1989) *Clinical Biochemistry of Domesticated Animals, 4th ed.* Academic Press.

Ministry of Agriculture, Fisheries and Food (1978.) *Manual of Veterinary Investigation Laboratory Techniques, 2nd ed,* Parts 1–8. MAFF Publications.

Pratt, P. W. (1992) *Laboratory Procedures for Veterinary Technicians, 2nd ed.* American Veterinary Publications Inc.

Sloss, M. W. and Kemp, R. L. (1958) *Veterinary Clinical Parasitology, 5th ed.* Iowa State University Press.

Soulsby, E. J. L. (1982) *Helminths, Arthropods and Protozoa of Domesticated Animals, 7th ed.* Baillière Tindall.

Willard, M. D., Tvedten, H. and Turnwald, G. H. (1989) *Small Animal Clinical Diagnosis by Laboratory Methods* W. B. Saunders Company.

23
Medical Disorders and their Nursing

J. W. SIMPSON

Prevention and Spread of Infection

The purpose of this section is to explain how infectious diseases are transmitted from one animal to another. There are basically three steps in the process:

- How the infection may leave the infected animal.
- How the infection may pass from one animal to another.
- How the infection can enter the new host.

The actual mode of transmission varies with each disease as does the speed at which the whole process occurs and examples will be used to illustrate the different stages of transmission. Before considering the transmission of disease, it will be necessary to define some terms commonly used when discussing infectious diseases.

With an understanding of how infectious diseases are transmitted from one animal to another, it is possible to discuss ways in which the spread of disease can be controlled. This is often termed **preventive medicine**. In modern medicine the aim is to try to prevent animals becoming ill in the first place, rather than trying to treat life-threatening conditions. For dogs and cats, prevention involves:

- Vaccination programmes.
- High levels of hygiene.
- Use of isolation/quarantine facilities.
- Improving environmental conditions.

Infectious and Contagious Disease

An **infectious** disease is one that is caused by micro-organisms which can successfully invade, establish and grow within the host's tissues. The most common infectious agents encountered in small animal practice are:

- Bacteria: *Salmonella* spp.; *Campylobacter* spp.
- Viruses: canine parvovirus; cat 'flu (FHV/FCV).
- Fungi: *Aspergillus* spp.
- Protozoa: *Giardia lamblia*; *Toxoplasma gondii*.

A **non-infectious** disease is one that does not involve micro-organisms, e.g. diabetes mellitus, renal failure or warfarin poisoning.

A **contagious** disease is one that is capable of being transmitted by direct or indirect contact from one animal to another. In this category are all the infectious diseases listed above together with internal and external parasitism.

For a contagious disease to spread by **direct contact** it is necessary for the affected animal to come into physical contact with another susceptible animal. This might be achieved by:

- Animals being housed together in the same kennel.
- Sexual contact during mating.
- Licking or grooming behaviour between animals.
- Biting.

Disease spread by **indirect contact** infers that the affected animal and susceptible animal do not come into direct physical contact (Fig. 23.1). In this context 'indirect' refers to the affected animal **contaminating** the environment in some manner, usually by body secretions such as faeces, urine, saliva or other discharges. A contaminated environment might include, for example, bedding, feed bowls, public parks or consulting-room floors.

The contaminating micro-organism must remain viable away from the host until another susceptible animal contacts the contaminated material. The length of time micro-organisms may remain viable off the host varies considerably.

Some of these micro-organisms can live on **inanimate** objects (such as bedding or feed bowls), in which case the contaminated objects are termed **fomites** (sing. fomes). Other micro-organisms are carried by **animate** agents referred to as **vectors**.

Fomites

Examples of the indirect spread of disease by fomites include parvovirus and ringworm. The organisms that cause these diseases are capable of living on inanimate objects for long periods, ready to infect

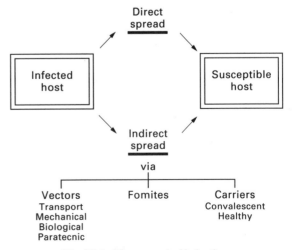

Fig. 23.1. The spread of infection.

any susceptible host that happens to come into contact with the contamination. The vomitus or diarrhoea from a dog with parvovirus can contaminate a public park in this way; the virus is resistant and remains viable off the host for long periods, providing plenty of opportunity for a suitably susceptible dog to become infected.

Ringworm (a fungal infection of dogs and cats) may be spread by direct contact, or by indirect contact following contamination of the animal's environment; again, the fungus can live on inanimate objects for long periods.

Vectors

Another indirect method of spreading disease involves **vectors**, which are animate carriers of disease and include insects (flies), ticks or mites. There are various types of vector:

- Biological vectors, or intermediate hosts.
- Non-biological or mechanical vectors, subdivided into:
      transport hosts;
      paratenic hosts.

Biological vectors act as intermediate hosts in the life cycle of micro-organisms or parasites. Good examples are the fleas, rabbits and sheep which act as intermediate hosts in the life cycle of tapeworms. The biological vector or intermediate host varies with each tapeworm but some of the organism's development must occur within the intermediate host, which is then ingested by the definitive host—in these cases the dog or cat.

Mechanical vectors transmit disease without playing any role as an intermediate host. They simply transfer infection from the affected animal to the susceptible animal.

Transport hosts pass on infection to a susceptible host at any time. The transport host is unaffected by the infectious agent and acts only to maintain the viability of the micro-organism and then to pass it on directly to another animal. Examples include the fleas that carry either feline panleucopenia virus or *Haemobartonella felis*. In each case the infection is passed on when the flea bites a susceptible animal.

Paratenic hosts must be eaten by the host in order to pass on infection because the organism lives within the tissues. There is no development of the micro-organism or parasite in the paratenic host; it simply remains in the host's tissues until consumed. An example of this is *Toxoplasma gondii*: to become infected, a cat must eat raw meat (from hunting mice).

Routes of Transmission

In considering how an infection can be passed from one animal to another, there are three factors to bear in mind:

- the routes by which an organism may leave an animal.
- the routes of transmission from one animal to another.
- the routes of entry into a new host.

Routes by which organisms leave the animal

The most common routes by which micro-organisms leave an animal are via natural body secretions:

- oral, nasal and ocular discharges;
- in urine;
- in faeces;
- in vomitus;
- in blood;
- via the skin;
- in milk;
- venereal contact, semen and parturition;
- from dead animals.

These secretions may contain large numbers of micro-organisms.

Oral, nasal and ocular discharges. An increase in secretion from the nose and eye, together with a change in its character, may result from infections such as cat 'flu, canine distemper and kennel cough. These secretions are rich in micro-organisms, which are released into the environment in the form of an aerosol when the infected animal coughs or sneezes.

In rabies and FIV infection the saliva of infected animals contains large amounts of virus. Aerosols play no major role in the transmission of disease but if these animals bite a susceptible animal the disease will be inoculated into the new host.

In urine. In some infections the kidney is specifically targeted by the micro-organism and consequently the urine may contain large numbers of the micro-organisms concerned. *Leptospira canicola* and infectious canine hepatitis virus are examples of diseases where infection is disseminated via the urine.

In vomit and in faeces. The gastrointestinal tract may be targeted by micro-organisms. This invasion results in dysfunction of the gastrointestinal tract, usually manifest as vomiting and diarrhoea. Both these secretions are heavily laden with micro-organisms which can result in significant contamination of the environment. Examples of this method of spreading disease include canine and feline parvovirus infection.

In blood. Vectors are important in this method of spreading disease. A flea feeds off a cat infected with *Haemobartonella felis*; in so doing picks up the micro-organism and carries it without becoming infected. When the flea moves to a new host it feeds again and passes on the infection.

Via the skin. This is principally associated with the spread of external parasites, including ringworm, lice, fleas and mites. Direct contact is required in order to transmit lice as they cannot live off the host. Fleas and mites, however, are not host specific and may live off the host for some time. Fomites may also be important in the dissemination of parasitism particularly where ringworm and fleas are concerned as they can live off the host on inanimate objects (e.g. grooming equipment).

In milk. The milk produced by a lactating bitch or queen is an excellent medium by which disease can be spread from one generation to the next. Feline leukaemia virus and *Toxocara* larvae may be spread by this method.

Venereal contact, semen and parturition. Disease may be spread during mating, or via the foetal fluid and placenta at parturition. Brucella abortus is an example of a disease which may be spread in this manner.

From dead animals. All dead animals, unless cremated, decompose and may become a source of infection to others. In particular animals which die of anthrax (a notifiable disease) may seriously contaminate the environment unless disposed of carefully. Dead sheep must not be allowed to lie around in fields as they can be a source of tapeworms. Dogs which eat dead contaminated sheep may acquire *Echinococcus granulosus.*

Routes of transmission from one animal to another

These routes include:

- Direct contact.
- Indirect contact.
- Aerosol transmission.
- Contamination of food and water.
- Carriers.

Direct contact. Direct spread requires physical contact between the infected animal and the susceptible animal so that body secretions or ectoparasites may be passed directly from one animal to another.

Indirect contact. Diseases which are spread indirectly from one animal to another require the presence of fomites (e.g. bedding, feed bowls and kennel runs) or vectors (e.g. fleas, mice or sheep).

Wherever environmental contamination occurs this may allow transfer of infection from one animal to another. Hookworms may contaminate kennel runs so that other dogs receive infection when using the same run. The soil is also a source of infection: *Clostridium tetani* spores can cause tetanus in dogs,

and *Toxocara canis* eggs remain viable in soil for a considerable time.

Aerosols. Aerosols are particularly important in the transmission of respiratory disease. When an infected animal coughs or sneezes this creates an aerosol which carries large numbers of water droplets loaded with micro-organisms into the atmosphere. Other susceptible animals within the same air space inhale the aerosol and may become infected.

Contamination of food and water. Ingestion of contaminated food or water is an important method of spreading disease. In addition to the well-recognised organisms associated with food poisoning, such as *Salmonella* and *Campylobacter*, other micro-organisms may also be spread in this way. Urine contamination of food or water is an important method of spreading leptospirosis. Cats may become infected with *Toxoplasma gondii* by eating uncooked meat or catching infected mice. Sewage contamination of water supplies may also be a source of infection.

Carriers. Occasionally an animal that has come into contact with a micro-organism may harbour the disease without showing clinical signs. These animals are called **carriers** and may excrete the micro-organism without showing any evidence of ill health (Fig. 23.1). There are two types of carrier: the convalescent and the healthy.

The **convalescent carrier** is an animal which has recovered from a clinical disease. The animal may shed large numbers of micro-organisms into the environment for variable periods after recovery. There are many good examples of this situation, including cat 'flu (FHV and FCV infection), canine infectious hepatitis and leptospirosis.

A **healthy carrier** is an animal which has been exposed to an infectious disease but has never shown clinical signs of that disease, yet carries the micro-organism and sheds it into the environment. These animals are usually immune to the infection and tolerate the presence of micro-organisms without showing signs of ill health. Examples of diseases harboured by this type of carrier include *Campylobacter* infection and *Haemobartonella felis.*

Both types of carrier may harbour the micro-organism without shedding it into the environment (**closed carriers**) or may continuously shed micro-organisms into the environment (**open carriers**).

Routes of entry into a new host

These routes include:

- Ingestion.
- Inhalation.
- Through the skin.
- Via mucous membranes.
- Congenital route.

Ingestion. Ingestion is one of the most common routes by which infections may establish. Whether clinical disease occurs will depend on the dose of infective agent ingested and the susceptibility of the host. Examples of ways in which micro-organisms may be ingested include:

- Food.
- Water.
- Eating faeces of another animal (**coprophagia**).
- Consuming vectors following grooming (fleas).
- Direct licking and grooming of other animals.
- Fomites (including feed bowls, bedding, chewing sticks or playing with balls).
- Ingestion of other body secretions.

Inhalation. This involves the inhalation of aerosols containing large numbers of water droplets loaded with micro-organisms. In some cases dust or other debris rather than water droplets may be inhaled. Animals housed within the same air space are at risk from both types of medium. The risk is further increased if there is a large number of animals within a small air space or an inadequate air turnover. In such cases the infective load or amount of aerosol present is very high and this increases the chance of disease spreading.

Through the skin. Both primary skin disease and systemic diseases can enter through the skin. The likelihood of disease successfully establishing depends on the type of infection and the physical condition of the skin itself. There are several means of establishing infection by this route:

- Penetration of intact skin by hookworm larvae or sarcoptic mites. (Mercury absorption by this route, which acts systemically, is not an infection but is considered in Chapter 3 under Poisoning.)
- Where the skin is physically damaged and the barrier to infection is destroyed, for example if the animal cuts its foot, undergoes surgery, receives burns, or traumatises itself, then secondary bacterial infection can establish. This may remain localised or become systemic.
- Inoculation following the use of dirty hypodermic needles, insect bites (fleas), bite wounds (rabies) or scratching. In these cases the skin is healthy but the physical barrier is breached and infection establishes itself.
- Transference from one host to another by direct or indirect contact. Lice, mites and fleas may be transferred in this manner.

Via mucous membranes. The importance of the mucous membrane of the digestive and respiratory systems as routes of entry to the body has been discussed. There are other mucous membranes which may also act as points of entry for infection:

- The conjunctiva (*Chlamydia psittaci* infection).
- The vaginal mucous membrane (bacterial and fungal infections).
- The prepuce/penis (balanitis and venereal diseases).

Congenital route. During pregnancy, micro-organisms can pass from the bitch or queen to the fetus via the placenta. This very important method of transmission is often termed **vertical transmission**. Examples include:

- *Toxocara canis.*
- Feline leukaemia virus infection.
- Feline panleucopenia virus causing cerebellar hypoplasia in kittens.
- *Toxoplasma gondi* infection.

In some of these cases the foetus will survive, although clinically infected, but in others transplacental transmission of disease results in stillbirth, abortion or resorption of the foetus.

Modes of Transmission of the Major Organisms

Viruses

In most cases viruses accumulate in large numbers in the secretions produced by the infected animal, particularly in saliva, nasal and ocular discharges, faeces and urine. Aerosols created from respiratory secretions are an effective method of spreading respiratory disease. Urine and faeces often contaminate the environment and may induce disease following ingestion. Saliva plays a special role in the transmission of rabies, where biting inoculates the virus into a new host.

Bacteria

Although bacteria can cause primary infections, they are often associated with secondary infection following initial invasion of the tissues by viruses. For example, cat 'flu is primarily caused by a viral infection but secondary bacterial infection is common.

Some bacteria, called **commensals**, can live in harmony with the host without causing disease but have the potential to become pathogenic under the right conditions. A good example is some of the *Pasteurella* spp.: these are often 'normally' present in the oral cavity of cats but cat bites will inoculate the bacterium into the skin, often resulting in cellulitis. *Pasteurella* spp. can also act as a secondary invader in feline respiratory infections.

Other bacteria are **obligate pathogens** and these always cause ill health. *Clostridium tetani* is a good example: it is never present in animals without causing tetanus.

Ectoparasites

This group includes mites, fleas and lice which are found in or on the skin. They are readily spread by direct and indirect contact between animals. Some ectoparasites (i.e. ticks) must live off the host for a period to complete their life cycle before finding another suitable host. Some ectoparasites of dogs and cats are not host specific—for example fleas and sarcoptic mange mites.

Endoparasites

This category includes tapeworms, roundworms, lungworms and coccidial parasites. The majority of endoparasites enter the new host by ingestion. Hookworms are an exception as they can penetrate intact skin and migrate to the tissues. Some ectoparasites, especially tapeworms, require an intermediate host to complete their life cycle.

Incubation of disease

The **incubation period** is the interval of time between the animal coming into contact with a micro-organism and the development of clinical signs of disease. The actual interval varies with each disease and is normally given as a range of days rather than an exact number, because the speed at which infection establishes depends on several factors:

- The dose of micro-organisms.
- The immune status of the animal.
- The general health of the animal.
- The age of the animal.
- The route of entry.

The incubation periods of the common infectious diseases of dogs and cats are shown in Fig. 23.2.

In the majority of cases an infectious agent will initially invade the mucous membrane of the respiratory and digestive tracts. The mucus and cilia of the respiratory tract and the mechanical movement and secretions of the digestive tract will prevent the micro-organisms from becoming established, unless the animal is susceptible and the dose of micro-organisms is great.

Initially the micro-organism invades the cells of the mucous membrane and possibly the local drainage lymph nodes. It then replicates in these tissues. If the host fails to mount an adequate immune response, the infectious agents will leave the initial site of invasion and spread to other target tissues.

The presence of virus particles in the circulation is called **viraemia**. This is the usual way by which viruses spread to specific target organs that include the intestine, bone marrow and lymphoid tissue, which are all associated with rapidly dividing cells. When these target tissues have been invaded, clinical signs associated with dysfunction of the affected system can be observed (Fig. 23.3).

Methods of Disease Control

With a sound knowledge of how disease is transmitted, it is possible to devise methods of reducing the risk of disease spread. These include:

- avoiding direct contact between animals (isolation or quarantine);
- maintaining very high levels of hygiene to prevent formation of fomites and infestation with insect vectors;
- reducing the number of animals kept within the same air space, or improving the efficiency of air movement;
- providing early and effective treatment of infected animals;
- routine vaccination and routine control of ectoparasites and endoparasites;
- maintaining strict import controls to avoid entry of disease into the country.

Client education

Client education is the key to achieving these goals. The veterinary surgeon and veterinary nurse are ideally qualified to provide information and so help to prevent rather than treat disease. In modern veterinary practice there are many examples of how preventive medicine is being employed to good effect. The veterinary nurse plays a vital role in this process in helping to educate clients by:

- running obesity clinics;
- sending out vaccination reminders;
- providing dietary advice;

AVERAGE INCUBATION PERIODS FOR INFECTIOUS DISEASES OF THE DOG AND CAT			
Dogs	**Incubation period**	**Cats**	**Incubation period**
Canine distemper	7–21 days	Feline enteritis	4–5 days
ICH	5–9 days	Cat 'flu	2–10 days
Leptospirosis	5–7 days	FIP	Months
		Chlamydia psittaci	4–10 days
Kennel cough	5–7 days	FeLV	Months/years
Parvovirus	3–5 days	FIV	Months/years

Fig. 23.2. Incubation periods.

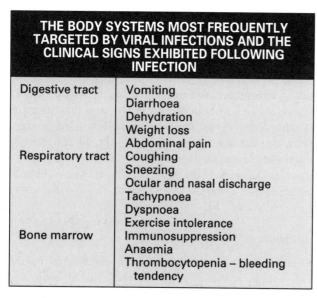

THE BODY SYSTEMS MOST FREQUENTLY TARGETED BY VIRAL INFECTIONS AND THE CLINICAL SIGNS EXHIBITED FOLLOWING INFECTION	
Digestive tract	Vomiting
	Diarrhoea
	Dehydration
	Weight loss
	Abdominal pain
Respiratory tract	Coughing
	Sneezing
	Ocular and nasal discharge
	Tachypnoea
	Dyspnoea
	Exercise intolerance
Bone marrow	Immunosuppression
	Anaemia
	Thrombocytopenia – bleeding tendency

Fig. 23.3. Viral targets and clinical signs.

- advising on worming policy;
- providing general advice, and redirecting to a veterinary surgeon.

Isolation and quarantine facilities

When animals are brought together in a confined space, the risk of introduction of infection and its rapid spread are greatly increased. For this reason animals should be kept physically separate and a close watch kept for early signs of disease. Any animal that shows signs of ill health should be moved to an isolation unit immediately.

Isolation is the the physical separation of animals so that direct and indirect contact become very difficult. Healthy dogs and cats which are hospitalised or kennelled should be kept in separate cages so that direct contact is impossible. This will help to prevent the spread of some infectious diseases. The facilities should ensure not only physical separation but also that as few animals as possible share the same air space. Where large numbers of dogs or cats have to share the same air space, air turnover should be adequate for the removal of infective aerosols. Several important management points are relevant:

- All new arrivals to a breeding unit should be adequately vaccinated before entry.
- They should then be isolated for at least 21–28 days to ensure that they are not incubating disease which could be introduced to the entire group.
- The isolation unit should always have its own equipment so that cross-contamination cannot occur with the main group.
- Special precautions should be taken by staff servicing the isolation unit with regard to protective clothing and personal hygiene.

Quarantine is a term usually reserved for compulsory isolation. At present all dogs and cats imported into the UK must undergo six months quarantine to prevent rabies from entering the country. These animals must not come into contact with other quarantined animals nor with any animal outside the quarantine station. The subject of quarantine and kennel management is covered in greater detail in Chapter 5.

Hygiene

Avoiding primary contact between animals, maintaining small groups to reduce aerosol spread and keeping infected animals in isolation units are all important factors in preventive medicine, but these barriers will be of little value unless very strict levels of hygiene practised. The isolation of an infected animal is ineffective if those who care for it do not wear protective clothing or do not wash themselves after handling the animal, or if equipment used in the isolation unit is not kept separate to ensure that fomites do not spread infection back to the main group of animals.

In any hospital or kennelling facility where any animal might be incubating disease, the risk of its transmission will be reduced if the level of contamination is kept as low as possible by practising the following good hygiene routines:

- All equipment should be thoroughly washed and disinfected as a matter of daily routine.
- All surfaces should be regularly cleaned and disinfected, including work tops, kennel runs, sleeping areas and food preparation areas.
- Do not rely on disinfectants to kill infective agents. Disinfectants are often unable to destroy pathogenic micro-organisms in a physically dirty environment. It is essential to *wash* the premises thoroughly with hot water and soap on a regular basis. This will remove the dirt and many of the micro-organisms at the same time. Those that remain can be destroyed by disinfection.
- All bedding should be either disposable or made of materials that can be thoroughly washed.
- Personal hygiene should be of a high standard and suitable protective clothing should be worn.
- Always prepare food at a different location to the area in which waste is handled. Ideally, all foods used should be commercially produced (home-made diets should be kept to a minimum). Do not use uncooked or raw foods. (If home-made diets are used, ensure that they are thoroughly cooked first.) No food for human consumption should be prepared or stored in the same areas as that for animals.
- Keep all vermin under control. They can act as carriers of infection, especially mice and rats. Insect vectors may also spread disease by transferring infection from waste material to food preparation areas.

Treatment

The veterinary nurse should be vigilant and constantly observing animals for early signs of illness, which may initially present as very subtle changes such as partial anorexia, polydipsia, depression, occasional sneezing or coughing. More obvious signs may then follow such as vomiting, diarrhoea, dehydration or collapse. Keep careful records so that early signs are noted and acted upon before a disease can seriously affect the animal or spread to others.

Quickly remove and isolate any suspect animal. Thoroughly wash and disinfect its kennel, including feed bowls, and dispose of all bedding material.

A veterinary surgeon should then examine, diagnose and treat the affected animal. The diagnosis should predict whether the disease is likely to spread. If so, it may be possible to improve the protection of other animals in the group by vaccination or prophylactic treatment.

Prevention and vaccination

Disease prevention is far more effective than having to treat affected animals. All animals, especially those entering a hospital or kennelling facility, should have up-to-date vaccinations against the common infectious diseases. In addition they should have been recently wormed and treated for ectoparasites. The risk of disease can be greatly reduced by maintaining the animals free from infectious disease and parasites.

Zoonoses

A **zoonosis** is a disease which can be transferred from animals to humans, for whom diseases such as leptospirosis and rabies can have fatal consequences. Many other canine and feline diseases and disease-causing organisms may also infect humans, including:

- Salmonellosis.
- Leptospirosis.
- Toxoplasmosis.
- *Toxocara canis.*
- *Echinococcus granulosus.*
- Ringworm
- Fleas.
- Sarcoptic mange.
- *Chlamydia psittaci.*
- Rabies.

Those working in veterinary practice have a much greater risk of contracting a zoonotic disease than members of the general public and should try to minimise the risk of personal infection by taking the following precautions on behalf of themselves and others:

- Always wash hands thoroughly after handling animals with *any* disease. It might turn out to be zoonotic even if it appears unlikely at first.

- Do not allow animals to lick human faces or mouths. This is especially important when children are playing with animals.
- Never let animals eat or drink off utensils used for serving food to humans.
- Wash all dishes and prepare all food for animals in a separate area from those intended for human use.
- Those who are pregnant must take special care if handling animals.
- Keep gardens and kennel runs clear of faeces. Prevent cats from contaminating children's sand-pits with faeces.
- Ensure that the very young and very old are not exposed to animals with possible zoonotic infections.
- Wear protective clothing at all times. Upgrade the amount of such clothing according to the degree of risk anticipated.
- Seek medical advice quickly if you think you have been exposed to a zoonotic disease.

Canine Infectious Diseases

Five important canine diseases are considered in this section:

- Distemper.
- Infectious canine hepatitis.
- Canine contagious respiratory disease.
- Canine leptospirosis.
- Canine parvovirus.

The clinical signs, diagnosis and control for each disease are given in Fig. 23.4.

Distemper

Canine distemper is a common infectious disease of the dog and other species including fox, badger, mink and ferret. It has a high morbidity rate and a variable mortality rate depending on the body systems affected and how quickly therapy is provided. Distemper is most frequently observed in dogs between 3 and 9 months of age, following the fall in maternal immunity, where acquired immunity has not been established. However, distemper can occur in susceptible dogs of any age.

Most outbreaks of disease occur in cities, housing estates, rescue centres and where dogs are kept in high density populations. The severity of clinical signs depends on:

- The degree of maternal antibody protection present in puppies.
- The nutritional status of the dog.
- Concurrent infections, including parasitism.
- Level of viral challenge.

Both acute and subacute forms of distemper are recognised, with clinical signs of inflammation of the respiratory and gastrointestinal tracts. Dogs may develop nervous signs following recovery from the acute disease; and in a small number of cases, only nervous signs are observed. Distemper virus may also be responsible for the many of cases of **old dog encephalitis (ODE)** observed in middle-aged to old dogs.

CANINE INFECTIOUS DISEASES: CLINICAL SIGNS, DIAGNOSIS AND CONTROL			
	Clinical signs	Diagnosis	Control
Distemper	Incubation period – 7-21 days (a) *Mild* or *sub-acute:* rarely diagnosed, may present simply as transient period of depression, anorexia and mild pyrexia (<40°C). Recovery rapid; secondary bacterial infection rare. Some cases remain subclinical and unreported by owner. (b) *Acute:* typical clinical signs associated with CDV infection. Within 7 days of exposure, dog becomes depressed, anorexic and pyrexic (<40°C) due to viraemia. Within 48 hours temperature may have returned to normal but in susceptible dogs rises again ('diphasic temperature rise' – Figure 23.5) due to epithelial invasion, immunosuppresion and secondary bacterial infection. Clinical signs include some or all of: * Persistent depression, anorexia, pyrexia. * Tonsillitis, pharyngitis with a dry cough. * Conjunctivitis, rhinitis initially associated with serous discharge changing to mucopurulent discharge (secondary bacterial infection). * Exudative pneumonia associated with *Bordetella bronchiseptica* with tachypnoea and dyspnoea. * Vomiting, diarrhoea, dehydration, loss of body condition. * Hyperkeratosis of nose and foot pads (hard pad – – foot pads painful, thickened with irregular fissures and eventually exfoliate). * Mortality can be high but many dogs survive if treatment is provided quickly. * If acute disease developed at less than six months old, may show changes to subsequent permanent dentition: damage to enamel and exposure of dentine (particularly canine teeth) – – 'distemper rings'. (c) *Nervous disease:* approximately 50% with acute disease subsequently develop nervous signs, type and severity of which vary individually (Figure 23.6). Nervous signs occasionally observed without any previous acute disease. In all cases onset of nervous signs leads to grave prognosis but in some, signs are not detected until years after acute infection, when ODE develops in old age due to latent CDV infection in nervous tissue.	History and clinical signs confirmed by: * Presence of eosinophilic inclusion bodies in epithelial cells. * Rising antibody titre of at least four-fold. * Immunofluorescence for virus in lymphoid tissue. * Detection of antibody in CSF. * Post-mortem changes.	Vaccination using modified live vaccine – allows virus to multiply in lymphoid tissues and stimulate good immune response. Measles vaccine also available to provide unweaned puppies with passive immunity without interference with maternal immunity. Puppies safely vaccinated from 6 weeks of age, primary vaccination programme complete by 12 weeks. Boosted annually.
ICH	Incubation period – 5–9 days (a) *Sudden death*, more common in neonatal puppies – most die without showing any clinical signs, other very short period of anorexia, depression, pyrexia (>40°C), collapse and shock before death. Occasionally haemorrhagic diarrhoea, abdominal pain and crying prior to death. (b) *Acute* ICH is most common form – sudden onset of depression, anorexia, pyrexia (>40°C) and shock. Pallor of the mucous membranes followed by jaundice as disease progresses. Tonsilitis, generalised lymphadenopathy, abdominal pain, haemorrhagic diarrhoea and hepatomegaly are common. Most dogs reluctant to move and may appear tucked up	History and clinical signs together with laboratory analysis: * Haematology – leucopenia. * Biochemistry – elevated SALT, bilirubin and blood urea. * Urine analysis – proteinuria. * Rising antibody titre. * Intranuclear inclusion bodies found within hepatocytes. * Virus isolation from tissues such as liver and kidney. * Post-mortem findings.	Maintain high levels of vaccinal protection. Most vaccines now use live CAV-2 virus rather than CAV-1 to avoid risk of blue eye. Primary vaccination can start at 6 weeks of age in combination with distemper vaccination; programme can be completed by 12 weeks. Boosted annually

Fig. 23.4.—continued ♦

CANINE INFECTIOUS DISEASES: CLINICAL SIGNS, DIAGNOSIS AND CONTROL			
	Clinical signs	Diagnosis	Control
	and occasionally assume praying position due to abdominal pain and crying prior to death (c) *Subacute* form – signs may include depression, anorexia, mild pyrexia; occasionally transient corneal oedema. (d) *Complications* – blue eye; – interstitial and glomerular nephritis; – nervous signs.		
CCRD	*Incubation period* 5–7 days following inhalation of micro-organisms Hallmark is dry non-productive cough; coughing often induced by excitement, change of environmental temperature or exercise; paroxysms of coughing frequent, may induce retching and occasionally vomiting. Owners often believe 'something stuck in dog's throat'. Initially serous nasal discharge but may become mucopurulent if significant secondary bacterial infection establishes. Dogs usually remain bright and retain appetite. Lower respiratory disease (bronchopneumonia) rare. Recovery usually uneventful, within 14 days, but a few may be refractory to treatment and infection may persist for months.	History of recent kennelling and clinical signs. Diagnostic tests rarely carried out as patients respond well to symtomatic therapy. Collect pharyngeal swabs for culture or serology to confirm diagnosis.	Vaccines available against *Bordetella bronchiseptica*, CAV and CPIV. Vaccination against CPIV using primary course of 2 injections given 2 weeks apart; a boost annually. Ideally vaccinate 10–14 days prior to kennelling. Live vaccine against *B. bronchiseptica* also available, administered intranasally, gives high level of immunity within 5 days, maintained for up to 6 months. Booster vaccinations every 6 months.

Canine leptospirosis	As the clinical signs observed in Leptospirosis vary it may not be possible to differentiate between the sero-types on clinical signs. However in general the clinical picture with each sero-type may be described as follows;
	 * *L. icterohaemorrhagiae*
	  Peracute: sudden death in young puppies without any previous signs of ill-health.
	  Acute: sudden onset of pyrexia, anorexia, marked depression and jaundice, followed by vomiting, polydipsia, haemorrhagic diarrhoea and petechial haemorrhages on mucous membranes. More generalised bleeding including epistaxis in individual cases. Dehydration, shock and collapse follow rapidly, and can result in death within a few hours even if treatment provided early.
	 * *L. canicola*
	  Acute: sudden onset of pyrexia, depression and polydipsia, followed by vomiting, oligiuria, dehydration together with swelling and pain involving kidneys. Rapidly become azotaemic, develop halitosis and eventaully oral ulceration. In a few cases hepatic involvement results in jaundice.
	  Subacute: Vague illness associated with anorexia, lethargy and pyrexia lasting only a few days; rarely diagnosed.
		Suspected from history and clinical signs and confirmed by:
		 * Serology to detect a rising antibody virus.
		 * Urine or blood culture.
		 * Clinical chemistry
		  – elevated blood urea and creatinine.
		  – hyperphosphataemia.
		  – elevated SALT, bile acids, bilirubin.
		 * Urine analysis
		  – proteinuria, haematuria, granular casts.
		 * Leucocytosis.
		 * Post-mortem changes.
			Good vaccines available containing killed sero-types of *L. canicola* and *L. icterohaemorrhagiae*. Primary course of 2 injections given 2–3 weeks apart, can be completed by 12 weeks of age. Annual boosting essential as immunity is short-lived.

Canine parvovirus	Depend on age of dog, and body system targeted by virus. Sudden deaths or puppies showing signs of heart failure. * *Myocarditis* – now rarely seen due to presence of adequate levels of maternal antibody. Sudden deaths or puppies showing signs of heart failure. * *Gastroenteritis* – depression, anorexia and persistent vomiting; initially vomitus contains food but eventually only bile-stained or bloody fluid. Within 24 hours a profuse liquid diarrhoea, red/brown in colour, foul-smelling; marked dehydration, shock and subnormal temperature. If left untreated, death within short period.	Most are severely immunosuppressed with total white blood cell counts less than $1.0 \times 10g/litre$. Highly susceptible to secondary bacterial infections involving any body system.	Vaccination: live vaccine in some cases given to puppies at high risk of infection as early as 6 weeks of age, repeated at 12 weeks, followed by annual booster. Booster at 16–20 weeks less essential as vaccines improve.

Fig. 23.4. Canine infectious diseases.

Aetiology and pathogenesis

Canine distemper virus (CDV) is caused by a morbillivirus which is related to measles and rinderpest. The virus is labile (unstable) off the host and is very susceptible to ultraviolet light, desiccation, heating and disinfection.

Virus is shed in the urine, vomitus, saliva, nasal and ocular discharge and faeces of infected dogs. Inhalation is thought to be the most important route of entry following either direct dog-to-dog contact or droplet/aerosol spread between dogs in close contact. Ingestion is not thought to be of significance in transmitting the disease because gastric acid and bile salts effectively destroy the virus. Carriers of infection rarely occur but virus may be retained in the central nervous system for long periods.

Distemper virus has an affinity for macrophages and lymphocytes and this is where initial viral replication occurs following exposure to infection. Only after replication in these cells will the virus target epithelial cells of the gastrointestinal and/or respiratory tracts. Whether epithelial cell invasion occurs depends on the immune response of the dog. A good immune response will prevent epithelial invasion while a poor response will allow the virus to invade these cells.

Sites of initial replication include the lymph nodes of the respiratory tract, after which infected macrophages and lymphocytes enter the circulation via lymphatic vessels and invade other lymphoid tissue and the bone marrow. Virus may be found in the central nervous tissues within 10 days of exposure to infection and may remain there for long periods. The virus next invades epithelial cells, resulting in typical clinical signs. In particular the virus targets the following tissues:

- Respiratory system, conjunctiva.
- Gastrointestinal system.
- Nose and pads of the feet.
- Nervous system.

Some degree of **immunosuppression** is associated with distemper and this assists in the establishment of secondary bacterial infection. *Streptococci* spp., *Staphylococci* spp., *Mycoplasma* spp. and *Bordetella* spp. are most often involved and result in a significant increase in the severity of clinical signs. Concurrent infection with infectious canine hepatitis, leptospirosis, parvovirus or toxoplasmosis may also occur.

Treatment

There is no specific therapy for CDV infection and so treatment remains symptomatic:

- Broad-spectrum antibiotics—secondary bacterial infections.
- Intravenous fluid therapy—water and electrolyte losses.
- Anti-emetics and anti-diarrhoeal drugs.
- Anti-convulsants—for nervous signs.
- Hyperimmune serum is of little value in clinical cases.

Nursing care

- Disinfect the consulting room and associated areas with which the patient had contact.
- Change protective clothing and thoroughly wash hands after handling clinical cases.
- Isolate infective patients from other dogs to prevent the spread of infection, especially with regard to public places.
- Advise owners on the nursing care required by the patient:
  (1) Keep patient in a warm but well-ventilated room with washable impervious floors.
  (2) Keep the nose and eyes free of caked discharge.

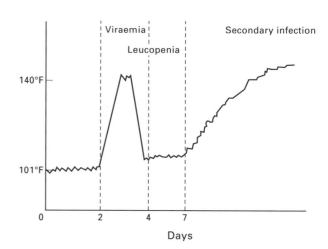

Fig. 23.5. Diphasic increase in temperature in canine distemper.

POSSIBLE NERVOUS SIGNS WHICH MAY OCCUR IN DOGS WITH CANINE DISTEMPER VIRUS INFECTION	
Cranial nerve defects	Poor light reflex. Blindness.
Cerebral	Ataxia. Circling. Pacing. Seizures.
Cerebellar	Ataxia. Dysmetria. Hypermetria. Head tilt. Nystagmus.
Spinal	Weakness. Paresis or occasionally paralysis of hindlimbs. Faecal and/or urinary incontinence. Chorea or twitching associated with any group of muscles, often those of the limbs or flanks.

Fig. 23.6. Possible nervous signs in distemper.

(3) Remove vomit or diarrhoea soiling and clean the patient.

(4) Administer therapy prescribed by veterinary surgeon.

- Advise regarding the examination and vaccination of all in-contact dogs.
- Make future appointments to allow the veterinary surgeon to monitor progress, taking into account the need to ensure minimal contact with other clients during consulting hours.

Infectious Canine Hepatitis (ICH)

Infectious canine hepatitis, also known as **Rubarth's disease**, is a virus disease of dogs and foxes which targets three types of tissue:

- The liver.
- The lymphoid tissue.
- Vascular endothelium.

Complications associated with ICH infection include:

- Nephritis.
- Corneal oedema or 'blue eye'.

Mortality can be high, especially in unweaned puppies where ICH often presents as sudden deaths. The severity of clinical signs declines with the age of dog infected and sudden deaths are rare in dogs over 2 years of age.

Aetiology and pathogenesis

There are two adenoviruses which cause disease in the dog:

- Adenovirus 1 (CAV-1), which is associated with ICH.
- Adenovirus 2 (CAV-2), which is associated with contagious respiratory disease and possibly enteritis in dogs.

Adenoviruses are more resistant than CDV and can survive off the host for up to 10 days. This means that dogs may become infected from a contaminated environment as well as direct dog-to-dog contact. In spite of this increased resistance the virus is readily destroyed by heat, desiccation and disinfection.

Virus is excreted in the saliva, faeces and urine of infected dogs. Dogs that have recovered from infection may continue to excrete virus in their urine for up to 6 months (convalescent carriers). Transmission of infection requires either direct dog-to-dog contact or contact with infected material. Ingestion is the main method of entry for CAV-1 infection, while aerosol spread is more important in CAV-2 infection section on canine contagious respiratory disease).

Following ingestion, the virus replicates in local lymph nodes and possibly intestinal Peyer's patches and mesenteric lymph nodes. A viraemia follows within 5–9 days associated with infected lymphocytes. If the animal fails to mount an immune response the virus targets the bone marrow, liver, other lymphoid tissue and vascular endothelium resulting in typical clinical signs.

When the dog mounts an immune response to acute infection, antigen–antibody complexes form in the circulation and may be deposited in the renal glomeruli leading to glomerular nephritis. At the same time virus invasion of the renal tubular cells can occur, leading to an interstitial nephritis in about 70% of cases.

Following recovery, about 20% of dogs develop unilateral or bilateral corneal oedema or 'blue eye'. This represents a local immune reaction associated with interaction between the virus and corneal endothelium. The corneal changes are transient in the majority of cases but occasionally become permanent, leading to visual impairment.

Although some degree of immunosuppression does occur, it is unlikely to result in significant secondary bacterial infection.

Treatment

There is no specific therapy for ICH and clinical cases are treated symptomatically:

- Intravenous fluid therapy.
- Where bleeding has been severe, whole-blood transfusions can be of great value.
- Antibiotics.
- B-vitamin therapy.

Nursing care

- Check vaccinal status of in-contact dogs.
- Disinfect infected premises.
- Advise owners of the importance of vaccination.
- Assist in therapy devised by the clinician.

Canine Contagious Respiratory Disease (CCRD)

Aetiology and pathogenesis

CCRD, tracheobronchitis or '**kennel cough**' is a highly infectious disease which is particularly prevalent where large numbers of dogs are kept within the same air space—such as in kennels, breeding establishments and rescue centres.

The canine upper respiratory tract normally harbours many micro-organisms, including *Streptococcus* spp., *Staphylococcus* spp., *Klebsiella* spp., *Pasteurella* spp., *Pseudomonas* spp. and *Bordetella bronchiseptica*. Of these only *B. bronchiseptica* is now considered to act as a primary pathogen in the aetiology of kennel cough, together with some viruses including:

- CAV-1 (canine adenovirus 1).
- CAV-2 (canine adenovirus 2).
- CPIV (canine parainfluenza virus).

- CHV (canine herpes virus).
- Reovirus.

Both CAV-1 and CAV-2 can be associated with respiratory disease. However, CAV-1 induces systemic disease while CAV-2 only results in respiratory disease.

CHV and reovirus may cause a mild respiratory infection in adult dogs and are much less important in the aetiology of kennel cough than CPIV, CAV-1 and CAV-2.

CPIV acts in a similar manner to CAV-2 and can induce marked respiratory disease. It is very likely to be implicated in the aetiology of kennel cough and can act together with other agents such as *B. bronchiseptica* in order to induce disease.

Infection follows either direct dog-to-dog contact or aerosol transmission of micro-organisms, especially where dogs are housed within the same air space. It is now clear that kennel cough is not normally caused by one micro-organism but probably by both viral and bacterial agents acting together on the respiratory epithelium. Following inhalation, the micro-organisms rapidly colonise the respiratory epithelium and this leads to an acute inflammatory reaction within 5–7 days of transmission. The severity of the resultant tracheobronchitis depends on which micro-organisms are involved in the process, the most severe being associated with CPIV and *B. bronchiseptica* (Fig. 23.4).

Treatment

Symptomatic treatment is usually provided and helps to reduce the duration of clinical signs:

- Use of antibiotics in order to reduce the risk of secondary bacterial infection.
- Anti-tussants such as codeine and butorphanol.

Nursing care

- Advise owners regarding the need to vaccinate in-contact animals.
- Prevent spread of infection and warn owners of the highly infectious nature of the disease.
- Ensure hospitalised cases are kept in isolation, especially with regard to sharing the same air space as other patients.
- Clean and disinfect consulting rooms and other areas where the dog has been hospitalised.
- Ensure the treatment prescribed by the clinician is carried out.
- Advise owners regarding the factors (sudden changes in air temperature, excitement, exercise) that induce coughing so that they may be avoided.

Canine Leptospirosis

Aetiology and pathogenesis

Leptospira is a Gram-negative bacteria recognised throughout the world as an important zoonotic organism. Although there are many serotypes, only two are of significance in the dog:

- *Leptospira canicola*, associated with acute interstitial nephritis.
- *Leptospira icterohaemorrhagiae*, associated with inflammation of the liver, vascular damage and haemorrhage. This form of leptospirosis in humans is known as Weil's disease or 'the yellows' (because it causes jaundice).

The clear-cut distinction between the two forms of leptospirosis indicated above does not exist in reality as both serotypes can cause hepatic disease and nephritis.

Infected dogs continue to shed leptospiral organisms in their urine for weeks following recovery. Although the acid pH of urine tends to destroy the organisms, urine contamination of water often results in their survival for long periods, though they are readily destroyed by desiccation, disinfection and UV light.

Urine from infected dogs is the main source of infection. Rats may also play an important role in the transmission of disease by harbouring the organism and excreting it in their urine. Routes by which leptospira may infect dogs include:

- Penetrating intact skin.
- Through cuts and abrasions in the skin.
- Transplacental and venereal transmission.
- Through intact mucous membranes of gastrointestinal or respiratory tracts.

Entry via one these routes is followed by a leptospiraemia which persists for about 7 days. At this time the organism invades its target organ: (Fig. 23.4).

- *L. canicola* invades the proximal tubules of the kidney, causing tubular cell death and local inflammatory cellular infiltration. This produces marked swelling of the kidneys.
- *L. icterohaemorrhagiae* invades the liver, resulting in hepatocellular destruction and perivascular haemorrhage. The vascular damage usually involves the lungs and gastrointestinal tract. Occasionally this serotype may target the renal tubules in a similar manner to *L. canicola*.

Treatment

Intravenous fluid therapy is essential in both forms of leptospirosis, although dogs with *L. icterohaemorrhagiae* will benefit from whole-blood transfusions. Antibiotics (especially penicillin, streptomycin and tetracyclines) form an essential part of therapy.

Nursing care

> **WARNING**
> **Remember that this disease is transmissible to humans.** It is therefore extremely important to take great care in handling dogs with leptospirosis. Disinfection of all contaminated areas is essential. *Always* wear gloves and other suitable protective clothing when handling the patient or its body fluids.

- Examination and vaccination of all in-contact dogs.
- Help in the provision of therapy as directed by the veterinary surgeon.
- Inform the owner that the dog has a zoonotic disease and will require careful handling. This is especially true where there are children in the household. Owners should seek medical advice.
- Advise owners regarding disinfection of kennels and home, and the need to control rats, if present on the premises.
- Liaise with veterinary surgeon regarding re-visits outside normal consulting hours to avoid contact with other dogs.

Canine Parvovirus

Canine parvovirus (CPV) infection is a relatively new disease, first recognised in 1978, which is thought to have resulted from a mutation of the feline parvovirus associated with feline panleucopenia. It causes two distinct disease syndromes in dogs:

- Acute myocarditis, which occurs in puppies.
- Acute gastroenteritis, which occurs in weaned puppies and adult dogs.

Aetiology and pathogenesis

There are two canine parvoviruses. CPV 1 has been known for many years and is associated with mild diarrhoea. CPV 2 is antigenically distinct and was not recognised before 1978. In 1981 a second mutation is thought to have occured, making the virus even more host specific for dogs.

The virus is highly resistant to destruction compared with the other canine viruses discussed so far. It can remain viable off the host for up to one year facilitating spread of infection by indirect contact. It resists many of the established disinfectants such as phenols and quaternary ammonium compounds but is destroyed by hypochlorite and formalin. Following the recognition of the disease in 1978, a new series of disinfectants was designed especially to destroy parvoviruses.

Large numbers of virus particles are shed in the faeces of infected dogs and constitute the main source of infection for other dogs. Transmission of disease occurs by either direct or indirect contact between a susceptible dog and an infected dog or faecal contamination.

Following ingestion, the virus replicates in the local lymph nodes and induces a viraemia within 3–5 days following infection. The virus targets rapidly dividing cells in which to replicate, in particular those in the intestine, lymphoid tissue, myocardium and bone marrow, depending on the age of the dog.

Prenatal and neonatal puppies have rapidly dividing myocardial cells and infection at this time results in myocarditis. This myocardial development ceases after 7 weeks of age and so the virus invades the rapidly dividing cells of the intestine. Lympoid tissue and the bone marrow are also targeted in both neonates and adult dogs, resulting in severe immunosuppression.

In 1978 the entire canine population was susceptible to CPV 2 infection. Therefore both myocardial disease and gastroenteritis were commonly observed. However, breeding bitches have now acquired good levels of immunity to CPV 2 and this has been passed on to their puppies, resulting in a marked reduction in the incidence of myocarditis. It is now more common to observe gastroenteritis in weaned puppies following the loss of maternal antibody protection or in adults which have not been adequately vaccinated (Fig. 23.4).

Treatment

Treatment for myocardial CPV is rarely successful and carries a very guarded prognosis. Where cases do show clinical signs, symptomatic therapy should be provided, including cage rest, diuretics and nutritional support.

Treatment for enteric CPV requires intensive intravenous fluid therapy. Where the dog is severely shocked, whole blood or plasma expanders should be considered. Anti-emetics such as metoclopramide will reduce fluid and electrolyte loss and the weakening effects of persistant vomiting. Once vomition ceases, careful introduction of oral fluids may be attempted. If this is tolerated, small amounts of low-fat veterinary diets may be provided. Return to normal diet slowly as these dogs have varying degrees of malabsorption.

Nursing care for enteric CPV

- As the virus is resistant and survives off the host, thorough cleaning of contaminated areas must be carried out using a modern parvocidal disinfectant (see Chapter 5).
- Isolate all clinical cases and ensure strict hygiene to prevent spread of infection to other hospitalised cases. Protective clothing should be used when handling dogs. Individual food and water bowls should be used. Careful disposal of infected material is also required.

- Advise the owner regarding the effects of the virus on the dog, including the need for a good vaccination programme (especially for any in-contact dogs) and the need for careful dietary management through the convalescent period because of the degree of intestinal damage and malabsorption.

Feline Infectious Diseases

The following feline infectious diseases are considered in this section:

- Feline panleucopenia
- Feline upper respiratory disease
- Feline pneumonitis
- Feline infectious anaemia
- Feline infectious peritonitis
- Feline leukaemia virus
- Feline immunodeficiency virus.

Clinical signs, diagnosis and control are outlined in Fig. 23.7.

Feline Panleucopenia

This highly contagious disease of the cat family is also known as feline infectious enteritis, feline distemper and feline parvovirus. Although it is primarily a disease of young kittens, cats of all ages may be infected. The disease has high mortality and morbidity, especially in kittens.

Aetiology and pathogenesis

Feline panleucopenia is caused by a parvovirus similar to canine parvovirus. The virus can survive for many months off the host and is resistant to heating, phenols, acids and alkalis. Modern parvocidal disinfectants are effective in destroying the virus.

Large amounts of virus are shed in the saliva, vomitus, faeces and urine of infected cats and excretion may persist for months after recovery. Transmission is thought to occur by ingestion following direct or indirect contact and may also be spread by fleas. The highest incidence of disease occurs where susceptible cats are intensively housed such as in rescue centres, breeding establishments and boarding catteries.

A viraemia occurs after ingestion of the virus and replication in local lymph nodes. The virus then targets the rapidly dividing cells of the small intestine, lymphoid tissue and bone marrow. Following invasion of these tissues the cat shows signs of severe gastroenteritis and immunosuppression. Unlike canine parvovirus infection, there are *no* cardiac signs associated with feline panleucopenia.

As the virus can cross the placenta, infection during pregnancy results in viral damage to the cerebellum of the growing foetus, leading to cerebellar hypoplasia. As the cerebellum is still developing at birth, infection up to 2 weeks postpartum can also cause cerebellar hypoplasia.

Treatment

There is no specific therapy available so treatment remains supportive:

- Intravenous fluid therapy to reverse dehydration and the electrolyte losses.
- Broad-spectrum antibiotics to protect from secondary bacterial infection due to the immunosuppression.

Once vomition ceases, oral fluids may be provided. Assuming no relapse occurs, a slow return to normal food intake may be made but *care* is required in the speed at which this occurs and the type of food offered. Most cats have severe small intestinal damage (and therefore some degree of malabsorption) and it is essential to provide highly digestible low-fat diets to prevent chronic diarrhoea and weight loss.

Nursing care

- Ensure that treatment prescribed by the clinician is carried out.
- Provide a comfortable environment for clinical cases.
- Careful disposal of clinical waste.
- Discuss with the owner the need to have all in-contact cats examined and vaccinated.
- Ensure strict hygiene when handling infected cats.

Feline Upper Respiratory Disease (FURD)

FURD, or cat 'flu, is a highly contagious disease of the cat and is the traditional scourge of catteries, where a sneezing cat can herald the beginning of a major outbreak of cat 'flu. The morbidity rate is high but the mortality rate is generally low.

Aetiology and pathogenesis

Cat 'flu is caused by two viruses:

- Feline calici virus (FCV), a fragile RNA virus that is easily destroyed once it is off the host.
- Feline herpes virus 1 (FHV-1), a more resistant DNA virus that can survive for up to 8 days off the host; it has also been known by the descriptive name of feline viral rhinotracheitis (FVR) virus.

Reovirus has also been suggested in the primary disease but its role is considered minor compared with FCV and FHV-1. In addition to primary viral infection, secondary bacterial infection can play an important role in the severity of clinical signs and speed of recovery (Fig. 23.7).

Transmission of infection is associated with inhalation of virus aerosols created by sneezing cats.

Chronic carriers of both FHV and FCV may be an important source of infection and each of the viruses behaves differently in this situation. FHV-1 can remain latent with intermittent shedding of virus associated with stress, steroid administration or concurrent infection, whereas FCV carriers excrete virus continuously. Detecting carrier cats can be difficult, especially with regard to FHV-1. The only effective method of detecting these cats is by repeated oropharyngeal swabbing. Ideally this should be carried out once shedding starts as cats often exhibit mild upper respiratory tract signs at these times.

Following inhalation, the viruses replicate in local lymph nodes before invasion of the epithelial cells of the respiratory tract and conjunctiva. FCV has a greater tendency than FHV-1 to cause ulceration of mucous membranes, which may permit secondary bacterial infection to establish. The complications that may follow infection include:

FELINE INFECTIOUS DISEASES: CLINICAL SIGNS, DIAGNOSIS AND CONTROL			
	Clinical signs	Diagnosis	Control
Feline panleuco- penia	Four clinical syndromes associated with feline panleucopenia. (a) *Peracute* – sudden death in young kittens without any obvious signs of ill-health. Owners may suspect kitten has been 'poisoned' because of speed of death. (b) *Acute* more common – sudden onset of marked depression and anorexia, quickly followed by persistent vomiting of food and subsequently bile-stained fluid. Cats often assume pathetic 'hunched up' appearance with nose resting on floor. Often cry in pain when handled or picked up and abdomen may feel distended. No diarrhoea initially but often appears after 2–3 days of clinical disease – often liquid, yellow-brown and may contain blood. (c) *Subacute* usually many of clinical signs observed in acute but less severe. (d) Cerebellar hypoplasia – kittens show dysmetria and hypermetria, muscle tremors, weakness and ataxia.	History of poor vaccinal status, together with typical clinical signs. Definitive diagnosis from: * Routine haematology revealing marked leucopenia. * Detection of virus in the diarrhoea.	Killed and modified live vaccines available. Initial course with injection as early as 6 weeks and a second at 12 weeks of age, then boosted annually. Maintain high levels of hygiene in catteries and isolate all new arrivals.
FURD	Incubation period 2–10 days. Generally acute disease observed but severity varies considerably between individuals. Clinical disease appears more severe in very young or old and in purebred cats, especially Siamese. Paroxysmal sneezing and conjunctivitis with serous ocular and nasal discharge are first clinical signs, followed by anorexia, depression and pyrexia, then signs of nasal and ocular ulceration, hypersalivation, loss of voice and coughing. Secondary bacterial infection results in viscous mucopurulent ocular and nasal discharge – often causes eyelids to stick together (risk of keratitis and corneal ulceration); nasal passage become blocked, loss of olfaction makes it necessary to breathe through mouth. Anorexia and salivation may be due to pyrexia, oral ulceration, loss of olfaction. Clinical signs normally resolve within 7–21 days depending on the breed, age and degree of secondary infection.	From typical clinical picture; can be confirmed by virus isolation from oropharyngeal swabs.	Many cats which recover become carriers and extrete both FCV and FHV-1. FHV-1 is not a resistant virus but FCV remains viable off the host and therefore essential to reduce the level of environmental contamination: * Good hygiene. * Isolation of sick cats and new arrivals. * Keeping the number of cats sharing same air space as low as possible. * Ensure at least 20 air changes/hour in catteries. * Ensure cats unable to come into direct contact. * Establish good vaccination policy: injectable and intranasal vaccines available; modified live vaccine can be used intranasally to provide good local immunity with rapid onset of action (protection usually achieved within 5 days); Occasionally mild signs of upper respiratory disease following this form of vaccination. Dead vaccine useful for pregnant queens. Initial vaccination 2 injections at 9-12 weeks of age, must be boosted annually.

Fig. 23.7.—continued

FELINE INFECTIOUS DISEASES: CLINICAL SIGNS, DIAGNOSIS AND CONTROL

	Clinical signs	Diagnosis	Control
Feline pneumonitis	Initially serious ocular discharge with some degree of blepherospasm, hyperaemia and chemosis, progressing to nasal discharge and sneezing, mucupurulent discharge. Cats initially pyrexic but generally remain bright and continue eating. Improvement expected within 2-3 weeks but persistent infections last many months. May be concurrent FCV and FHV-1 infection.	Confirmation by conjunctiual swabs for culture and blood samples detect rising titre.	*Chlamydia psittaci* very difficult to eliminate if endemic with cattery. If not endemic, all new arrivals should be isolated and carefully observed for evidence of infection. If they have no serological titre to Chlamydia psittaci it is unlikely they have been exposed to infection. Modified live vaccine available for all cats except pregnant queens. Initial course can start at 9 weeks of age: 2 injections 3-4 weeks apart; boost anually.
Feline infectious anaemia	Sudden onset of weakness, lethargy and anorexia. Often pyrexic, marked pallor of mucous membranes; associated tachycardia, tachypnoea and splenomegaly.	Routine haematology reveals high reticuloctye count indicating regenerative anaemia. Definitive diagnosis from examination of Giemsa-stained blood smears to showing the parasites attached to the red blood cells, but several blood smears may have to be examined before the parasite is detected, due to fluctuating parasitaemia.	Flea control. Use of tetracyclines.
FIP	Early signs vague, including pyrexia, anorexia, weight loss, diarrhoea. Failure to grow common in kittens. Possible chronic unresponsive diarrhoea with prolapse of third eyelid. Progresses to more specific signs of two clinical forms within few weeks or may take months: *(a) Effusive FIP* (some 60% of all cases – much shorter duration of ill health): fluid accumulates in the abdomen (and in 25% of cases within the thorax as well); Pericardial effusion not uncommon. *(b) Non-effusive FIP:* No effusions; granulomatous lesions on any abdominal organs, particularly spleen, liver and kidneys; organs often become swollen, palpable; eventually organ failure. In about 50%, only central nervous signs: generalised and progressive neurological defects including ataxia, paresis, paralysis, disorientation and convulsions. Eye lesions associated with retinitis and uveitis; may be unilateral or bilateral.	Difficult interpretation of serology. Biopsy collection and histopathological examination of granulomatous lesions is only method currently definitive Other non-specific findings include: * Examination of ascitic or thoracic fluid – yellow, viscous, sterile and may clot on standing.Protein content usually high (> 35g/l) * Anaemia. * Hyperglobulinaemia. * Jaundice. * Lymphopenia. * Concurrent FeLV and/or FIV infection.	Vaccines available in USA, none at present in the UK.
Feline leukaemia virus	May remain asymptomatic for years. When clinical signs occur, may be associated with either neoplastic disease (20% of cases), or non-neoplastic diseases associated with immunosuppression (80% of cases). Clinical picture with FeLV-related disease varies but may include any of conditions shown in Figure 23.8.	Suspected from the history and clinical picture; Confirmation by examination of serum, and/or white blood cells or bone marrow cells for viral protein. Infected cells produce protein P27, released in large amounts along with new virus particles. ELISA test detects this protein antigen and provides very reliable method of confirming FeLV infection. False positive and negative results rare as long as test procedure carried out carefully.	*Multi-cat households:* testing all cats and isolate those which are positive. Repeated at 3-month intervals, removing any new positive cases, until all cats remain negative on at least two separate occasions. Colony can then be considered FeLV negative; isolate all new arrivals and carefully screen for infection. *Single-cat households:* confining cats to reduce the risk of infection. Genetically engineered vaccine now available in UK. Initial course 2 vaccinations 2-3 weeks apart; annual boosting. Ideally test cats for FeLV before vaccination, no beneficial effect on cats already infected.

Fig. 23.7.—continued

CANINE INFECTIOUS DISEASES: CLINICAL SIGNS, DIAGNOSIS AND CONTROL			
	Clinical signs	**Diagnosis**	**Control**
Feline immuno-deficiency virus	Transient pyrexia and generalised lymphadenopathy after exposure to virus, followed by asymptomatic phase which may last for years before clinically detectable immunodeficiency syndrome develops. Many different clinical conditions associated with immunosuppression and secondary bacterial infections, varying individually. Lethargy, weight loss and anorexia always present; clinical signs associated with either respiratory or digestive tract. Most common forms include: Chronic rhinitis. Lymphadenopathy. Chronic diarrhoea. Chronic gingivitis. Chronic skin disease. Uveitis. Neurological disease (behaviour changes, convulsions). Neoplasia, especially lymphoid tumours. Most of these associated with secondary opportunist organisms which establish because of FIV-induced immunosuppression. History of chronic or recurring infections which respond poorly to treatment, in a lethargic thin cat, strongly suggestive of FIV infection.	Detection of antibodies to viral protein: Commercial ELISA test kits available and generally very reliable.	No vaccines available in UK; prevention involves avoiding situations where cats likely to become infected: * Keep indoors or limit outdoor exposure. * Castrate males to prevent aggression and fighting. * Control free roaming.

Fig. 23.7. Feline infectious diseases.

- Prolonged recovery.
- Keratitis and corneal ulceration.
- Lower respiratory disease – bronchopneumonia.
- Chronic rhinitis – 'snufflers' (chronic FHV-1).
- Latent carrier of FHV-1.
- Persistent excretors of FCV.

Treatment

Treatment of cat 'flu is mainly supportive and includes:

- Correction of dehydration and maintenance of hydration using intravenous fluid therapy.
- Use of broad spectrum antibiotics to control secondary bacterial infection.
- Enteral nutrition.
- Good nursing care.

Nursing care

Nursing care is especially important in cat 'flu as most cats are unable to smell their food and find eating painful because of oral ulceration. They stop eating and drinking, and this leads to dehydration and weight loss.

- Ensure that fluid therapy maintains adequate hydration.
- Bathe the eyes and nose of discharge to aid breathing, improve olfaction and prevent corneal damage.
- Use inhalants prior to feeding.
- Encourage eating by offering highly aromatic, warmed foods.

- Maintain high levels of hygiene to prevent spread of disease.
- Discuss vaccination programmes with the client.
- Advise on examination and vaccination of in-contact cats.

Feline Pneumonitis

Feline pneumonitis is caused by *Chlamydia psittaci* and is one of the most common causes of conjunctivitis in cats. The infection is recognised throughout the world and accounts for over 30% of conjunctivitis in the UK. Kittens appear to be the most severely infected.

The organism targets the conjunctiva of cats. It may also be a cause of infertility: although no cases have been proved, the organism has been isolated from the reproductive tract and abortions have been recorded.

Pathogenesis

The actual method of transmission is not known but direct contact between cats, especially when there is any ocular or nasal discharge, appears to be important. It also seems likely that long-term carriers may exist without evidence of clinical disease and may act as a source of infection. The organism may also be harboured in the gastrointestinal and genital tract. The incubation period last between 4 and 10 days.

Treatment and nursing care

The most effective treatment for *Chlamydia psittaci* infection is local (topical) and systemic use of tetracyclines. Doxycycline is the drug of choice and all cats within the household should be treated at the same time. Treatment should be maintained for 2 weeks after clinical signs have ceased.

Feline infectious anaemia

Aetiology and pathogenesis

Haemobartonellosis or feline infectious anaemia (FIA) is associated with the rickettsial micro-organism *Haemobartonella felis*, an extracellular parasite of red blood cells. FIA can occur in all age groups but appears more common in male cats. Infection may be transmitted by:

- Cat bites.
- Flea infestations.
- Vertical transmission in utero.
- Via the queen's milk.

It is thought that many cats may be exposed to the parasite without showing signs of clinical disease. Some of these cats may become carriers and only develop clinical disease if stressed or immuno-suppressed, or if suffering concurrent disease. In particular, there is an association between FIA and FeLV/FIV infection.

Following infection, cycles of parasitaemia develop and are associated with profound anaemia which can occasionally be fatal (Fig. 23.7). The parasitaemia may be recurrent, interspersed with periods of complete remission, but in spite of these remissions cats may remain chronically infected. This may be due to a complex relationship between the parasite and the cat's immune system.

Treatment

Assuming there is no evidence of concurrent FeLV or FIV infection, tetracyclines are the drugs of choice in the treatment of *Haemobartonella felis*. The use of prednisolone is now thought to be of value, due to the immune-mediated nature of the disease. Cats with severe anaemia may require a blood transfusion. If the cat has a flea infestation, this should also be treated.

Nursing care

- Assist in the administration of treatment directed by the veterinary surgeon.
- Discuss with the owner the need to examine other cats within the household, including treatment for fleas.
- Careful observation and monitoring of hospitalised cats, with particular reference to their cardiac and respiratory function.

- Reduce stress and provide a good environment for recovery.
- Ensure that the cat maintains adequate fluid and nutritional intake.

Feline Infectious Peritonitis (FIP)

This disease was first recognised in the early 1960s and now has a world-wide distribution in both domestic and wild cats. The incidence of infection is low (1–5%) and prognosis is very poor. FIP is more common in multi-cat households and among pedigree cats, especially the Burmese (20% of cases). There is no sex predisposition. Clinical cases can occur in any age group but those less than 2 years of age are most often affected.

Aetiology and pathogenesis

FIP is caused by a coronavirus similar to the enteric coronavirus (FECV) commonly encountered in cats. The virus is labile and readily destroyed by modern disinfectants.

Direct contact between susceptible and infected cats does not seem to be important, while indirect contact with virus shed in urine and faeces appears more likely. However, carriers may be important in the epidemiology of disease and may carry the virus for years. This may have significance with regard to the queen passing on infection to her kittens.

The mode of transmission is not understood and the incubation period appears to be extremely variable. Entry is thought to occur via the oronasal mucosa. When cats are exposed to coronavirus some 90% develop transient gastrointestinal disease and in about 10% of cats viral replication then develops in macrophages. Infected macrophages reach the general circulation and then target vascular beds such as the peritoneum, pleura, eye, meninges or kidneys. The outcome depends on the virulence of the virus, concurrent disease, stress and type of immune response.

A cell-mediated immune response appears to be important in determining the outcome to viral challenge. If this response is good, the cat eliminates the virus (90%) but a poor response leads to FIP infection.

Antibodies to coronavirus are not protective and result in formation of perivascular antigen/antibody complexes, which cause vasculitis, leading to fluid leakage from peritoneal or pleural blood vessels.

Two forms of FIP occur:

- A wet or effusive form, thought to be associated with a very poor immune response.
- A dry form, which may occur following a partial immune response.

Treatment and nursing care

The prognosis remains very guarded and there is no specific treatment for FIP. Concurrent FeLV or FIV results in a further deterioration in the prognosis.

Symptomatic therapy using antibiotics and corticosteroids may result in temporary remission.

Feline Leukaemia Virus (FeLV)

Aetiology and pathogenesis

FeLV is a species specific retrovirus (Fig. 23.8) of world-wide distribution affecting both domestic and wild members of the cat family. It has also been suggested that two out of every three cats have been exposed to infection during their life and it is estimated that 18% of sick cats and 10% of healthy cats are FeLV positive. In multi-cat households up to 30% of cats may be FeLV positive.

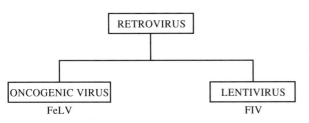

Fig. 23.8. FeLV/FIV in retrovirus family.

Susceptibility to infection appears to depend on the age of the cat. Kittens infected *in utero* will become persistently viraemic and die. Exposure at less than 8 weeks old gives a 70–80% chance of becoming permanently viraemic whilst adults have only a 10% chance of becoming persistently viraemic.

SOME OF THE CLINICAL CONDITIONS WHICH MAY BE ASSOCIATED WITH FELINE LEUKAEMIA VIRUS INFECTION	

Neoplastic disease	Lymphosarcoma
	    Multicentric.
	    Thymic.
	    Alimentary.

Non-neoplastic disease	Myeloproliferative disease.
	Non-regenerative anaemia.
	Immunosuppression
	    FIP.
	    FIV?
	    Cat 'flu.
	    Feline enteritis.
	    Toxoplasmosis.
	    Oral infections.
	Immune diseases
	    Glomerular nephritis
	    Polyarthritis.
	    Polyneuritis.
	Reproductive
	    Stillbirths.
	    Fetal resorption.
	    Abortion.

Fig. 23.9. FeLV-associated clinical conditions.

Infection can be transmitted vertically from the queen to her kittens either *in utero* or via the milk. Horizontal transmission can also occur following direct contact between cats. The virus is present in saliva, mucus, urine, faeces and milk. Saliva contains high levels of virus and so cat bites may be an important method of transmitting infection.

Following oral infection the virus replicates in the local lymph nodes. A viraemia results and disseminates the virus to distant lymphoid tissue. A second viraemic phase leads to dissemination of virus to the bone marrow and other tissues.

Several outcomes are now possible, depending on the cat's immune response to the virus (Fig. 23.10). Some 40% will eliminate the virus completely and recover. In the 30% where the immune response is poor, the virus is likely to invade the following tissues:

- The bone marrow—leading to anaemia, leukaemia, immunosuppression.
- The crypts of Leiberkuhns of the intestine—enteritis.
- Salivary, lacrymal and pancreatic glands—excretion of virus.
- Urogenital system—abortions, stillbirths, infertility.
- Remain viraemic.

In the remaining 30% of cases, FeLV may invade host cells and lie dormant – this is termed **latent infection**. Over a number of months or years this latent infection may be slowly eliminated. However in a small number of cases viral replication may be switched on again, during;

- periods of stress;
- concurrent infection;
- use of corticosteroid therapy.

Treatment and nursing care

There is no specific therapy for FeLV infection. Symptomatic therapy is aimed at reducing the effects of secondary bacterial infection. However, the prognosis remains very guarded.

Feline Immunodeficiency Virus (FIV)

Aetiology and pathogenesis

FIV is an RNA retrovirus which was first recognised in 1986 in the USA, but stored blood samples have revealed that it was present in samples taken as early as 1968. The infection is now known to have a world-wide distribution and affects both domestic and wild cats. Originally FIV was known as feline T lymphotrophic lentivirus (FTLV) but this name is no longer used.

Infection is rare in cats less than one year old but increases with age to a peak at around 8 years old. The disease is 30 times more common in outdoor cats than in housed cats and is 3 times more common

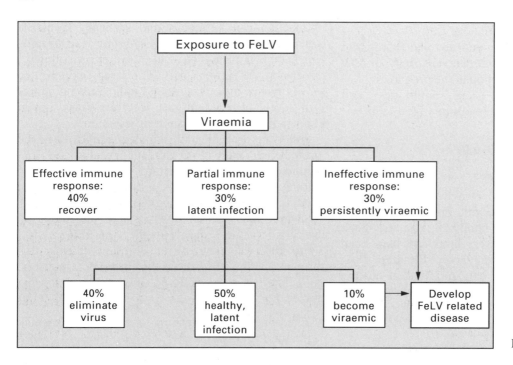

Fig. 23.10 FeLV flow chart.

in males than females. This is probably because cat bites are thought to be the main mode of transmission: saliva contains significant amounts of virus and transmission is by biting. Simple direct contact between cats appears to be unlikely to cause infection but sexual transmission may be important. As the virus is labile, environmental contamination and therefore spread by indirect contact seem highly unlikely.

Recent work suggests that 13% of sick cats and only 4% of healthy cats are positive for FIV. The highest incidence appears to occur in Northern Ireland, Scotland, and the south and south-east of England.

It appears that FIV infection cannot be eliminated by a normal immune response. Within 2 weeks of being bitten, the infected cat will show evidence of antibody production and virus may be detected in circulating lymphocytes. After a further 4 weeks the cat may develop pyrexia and generalised lymphadenopathy which can last for many weeks.

Many cats appear to 'recover' and remain asymptomatic for years before developing a clinically detectable immunodeficiency syndrome.

Treatment and nursing care

There is no treatment for FIV at present but symptomatic treatment can be offered in the form of antibiotics for secondary bacterial infection. However, the prognosis must remain very guarded.

Rabies

Rabies is a disease of the nervous system. It is recognised world-wide, although countries such as the UK, Norway, Sweden, Portugal, Japan, Eire and Iceland have managed to remain free of infection.

The main risk to the UK lies in importation of dogs from Asia, Latin America and Africa. Foxes appear to be an important reservoir host in Europe while the skunk, racoon and bat are important in the USA.

Rabies is a very important disease because of some unique characteristics:

- The virus has the ability to infect many different species.
- It is a zoonosis.
- The effects on the CNS often result in aggression so that animals bite each other and increase the chance of spreading the disease.
- Once clinically manifest, the disease is fatal.

Rabies can spread within wildlife and domestic dog or cat populations. **Sylvatic rabies** is the term used to describe spread of infection in wildlife; **urban rabies** describes the spread of infection in domestic dogs or cats. Domestic cats are more resistant to rabies than dogs.

Aetiology and pathogenesis

Rabies is caused by a rhabdovirus which has an affinity for cells of the nervous system. The virus is present in the saliva of infected animals and is readily transmitted by biting. Usually rabid dogs or cats will be showing clinical signs when they have bitten someone but the saliva may contain virus for up to 14 days before clinical signs develop. Being bitten by an apparently normal dog or cat in an endemic area should be viewed with suspicion.

The virus cannot penetrate intact skin but it can cross the oral or nasal mucous membrane, so that infection following ingestion and inhalation (via aerosol) is possible although a very large dose of virus is required. The virus is very labile and survives poorly off the host.

The incubation period can vary from 2 weeks to 4 months, with a mean incubation period of 3 weeks. The speed at which clinical signs develop depends on:

- The site of infection (virus reaches the CNS more rapidly if the bite is to the head or neck).
- The severity of the bite.
- The dose of virus.

Once a dog or cat is bitten, the virus remains at the site of inoculation during the incubation period. Viral replication takes place in the muscle tissue and eventually virus penetrates the neuromuscular tissue and so gains entry into the nervous system.

Infection now spreads rapidly to the central nervous system by axonal flow along nerve fibres. There is no lymphatic or blood-borne dissemination of infection. Once in the CNS, the virus replicates within the neurones and infection then spreads centrifugally to the peripheral nervous system. Eventually peripheral nervous tissue and the organs it supplies will become infected. This is how the salivary glands become infected and contain large amounts of virus.

Normally there is inadequate virus production in the muscle tissue to provoke an immune response and subsequent antibody production. However, if the patient is vaccinated an immune response will be produced and protection given *before* the virus enters the nervous system. Once the virus is in the nervous system, antibody is unable to provide protection.

The rabies virus is *only* vulnerable while in the muscle tissue and *before* it enters the nervous system.

Clinical signs

There are two recognised forms of clinical rabies:

- Furious rabies.
- Dumb rabies.

Initial clinical signs include pyrexia and a change in temperament. Dogs may become more placid and seek affection or they may hide away in corners or under beds. The site of infection may become intensely pruritic. As virus may be present in saliva before these signs develop, it is very important to isolate dogs that have been bitten and observe them for these changes in temperament.

In **furious rabies** the animal will now become progressively hyperexcitable. These episodes may last for only a short period or for many hours. During the episodes the animal may become aggressive; it may snap and bite at even imaginary objects; it may develop a depraved appetite and chew and eat anything. If free to do so, dogs will walk or run many miles before trying to return home. In between these periods the animal may be friendly, placid and calm.

As the disease progresses, there are signs of paresis of the legs and tail. There may be difficulty in swallowing and asymmetry and distortion of the face. In dogs and cats there is *no* evidence of the hydrophobia that is a feature of human rabies. Eventually the animal will die during a violent seizure.

Dumb rabies is much more common, with little or no evidence of the signs described above. There is a progressive paralysis involving the limbs and distortion of the face with drooping of the jaw and eyelids, squinting of the eyes, drooling of saliva and difficulty in swallowing. Great care should be exercised when examining such dogs, which may initially appear to have some oral or pharyngeal foreign body. If the examiner has any cuts or abrasions, this will allow easy access by the virus. In dumb rabies the animal will eventually become comatose and die.

Although these descriptions indicate that there are two clear-cut forms of rabies, it is important to emphasise that such clear-cut divisions do not always occur in reality. There may be cases with features of both forms of the disease. In all cases, death usually occurs within 7 days following the onset of clinical signs.

Where rabies is suspected, the dog should not be killed but should be kept in isolation and prevented from escaping or injuring someone. The Ministry of Agriculture Fisheries and Food (MAFF) should be contacted immediately. If the dog cannot be caught safely other appropriate action will be required, and in such circumstances great care is required to ensure the brain is not damaged.

Diagnosis

After the animal has died or been destroyed, its head is removed by an MAFF veterinary officer and transported to a Ministry laboratory. The diagnosis of rabies is achieved by examining the brain for negri bodies, which represent accumulations of virus protein in the neurones. A fluorescent antibody test is also available which can detect disease in neurones at a much earlier stage. Virus isolation can also be carried out by inoculating mice with brain suspension.

Treatment

Although there are reports of dogs and cats recovering from rabies, such situations are very rare. Generally there is no treatment for rabies and, because of the serious risk of human infection, all dogs and cats should be destroyed if rabies is suspected.

Control

Control is achieved by vaccination. Inactivated and live vaccines are available but in the UK only the former is used. There are reports of live rabies vaccination causing disease in cats which have concurrent FeLV or FIV infection (due to immuno-suppression). Initial vaccination involves a single injection. Puppies of 3–4 months of age can be vaccinated and boosted regularly.

Foxes are the most important reservoir host in Europe. In order to control the spread of rabies in Europe, oral vaccines have been produced which allow foxes to be vaccinated by means of baits. This form of vaccination appears to have been effective in controlling the spread of rabies.

Safe human inactivated vaccines are also available for persons considered to be at risk of infection. Personnel should receive an initial vaccination course followed by regular booster vaccination to maintain protection.

Diseases of the Alimentary Tract

Changes in eating behaviour are common reasons for owners to seek veterinary advice. These changes may include an increase or decrease in appetite, a depraved appetite or inability to eat. This subject is covered in greater detail in Chapter 17 (Nutrition).

DEFINITIONS

Dysphagia is the physical inability to eat food, usually as a consequence of mechanical or neurological disorders. The animal is often hungry but is simply unable to eat or swallow food. Dysphagias are usually classified into problems within the oral cavity, pharynx or oesophagus. Owners often refer to this as **inappetence**.

Anorexia is the loss of the desire to eat, while retaining the physical ablity to do so. This is also sometimes described as inappetence by the owner. Cases are associated with systemic diseases and nausea.

Polyphagia is an increased appetite beyond the amount the animal would normally consume. In some cases animals not only consume all their food but may steal food or become scavengers. Disorders such as exocrine pancreatic insufficiency, Cushing's disease and diabetes mellitus may exhibit polyphagia.

Pica describes a depraved appetite. Examples include animals eating their own faeces (**coprophagia**), eating soil or licking concrete. This often distresses owners, who may be reluctant to discuss the problem. The behaviour is often associated with some form of nutritional deficiency.

Anorexia

There are specific instances where anorexic animals should not be fed (such as acute pancreatitis) but most animals should be encouraged to eat, although the final decision rests with the veterinary surgeon. Prolonged anorexia will result in the utilisation of body fat and protein stores for energy. This will lead to not only a loss of adipose tissue and lean body mass but also:

- poor immune response to infection;
- poor wound healing;
- slower recovery;
- increased metabolic load on the kidneys and liver.

Treating the underlying cause of the anorexia will have the greatest impact on appetite but owners should also be encouraged to improve the nutritional intake of their pet by using a highly palatable and digestible diet. This can be achieved by:

- warming the food;
- using strong smelling foods;
- providing a moist food rather than a dry food;
- using high-fat diets;
- liquidising the food;
- hand-feeding while talking to the animal;
- offering several types of fresh food to determine preference.

Where these methods fail, the veterinary surgeon may use drugs to stimulate the appetite or insert a feeding tube into the alimentary tract and initiate further feeding.

Conditions of the Oesophagus and Stomach

Although owners may present their pets with a history of 'vomiting', sometimes this does not truly reflect what the animal is actually doing. Careful collection of the history may reveal the animal is actually regurgitating its food rather than vomiting. Such a differentiation can provide important information regarding the location of the problem.

Regurgitation is a passive process in which food and fluid are passed back up the oesophagus and out through the mouth. It is always associated with undigested food or liquids and often occurs shortly after feeding. No abdominal contractions are involved in this process.

Regurgitation may be associated with oesophageal disease (Fig. 23.11) such as **megaoesophagus**. In this condition there is a failure of peristaltic contractions to move a food bolus from the pharynx to the stomach. The food remains in the oesophagus, which rapidly becomes a large flaccid sac. Eventually the volume of food and fluid in the oesophagus stimulates regurgitation through the mouth.

Vomiting is an active process involving cessation of breathing, closure of the epiglottis, fixation of the diaphragm and contraction of the abdominal muscles. This squeezes the stomach and ejects food along the oesophagus and out of the mouth. Frequent retching precedes actual vomition. The vomitus may contain food, bile-stained fluid, water, blood or intestinal contents. Vomiting may be the result of primary gastric disease or may be secondary to a systemic disease (Fig. 23.11).

SOME OF THE CONDITIONS WHICH MAY BE ASSOCIATED WITH REGURGITATION OR VOMITING IN DOGS AND CATS		
	Vomiting	
Regurgitation	**Primary disease**	**Secondary vomiting**
Oesophageal FB	Acute gastritis	Azotaemia
Megaoesophagus	Chronic gastritis	Pyometra
Vascular ring	Gastric ulceration	Drug toxicity
Oesophageal stricture	Gastric neoplasia	Motion sickness
Reflux oesophagitis	Gastric foreign body	Colitis
		Pancreatitis
		Hepatitis

Primary vomiting is associated with gastric disease; in secondary vomiting there is no gastric pathology.

Fig. 23.11. Regurgitation and vomiting: associated clinical conditions.

Persistant regurgitation or vomiting can lead to serious complications:

- Loss of water and electrolytes—dehydration.
- Inhalation of food—aspiration pneumonia.

Persistent vomiting leads to excess loss of water and electrolytes. As the animal cannot drink to replace this loss, it becomes **dehydrated**. The degree of dehydration can be determined in the laboratory by measuring the packed cell volume (PCV) and total plasma protein levels. Clinically, the degree of dehydration can be detected by testing skin elasticity:

- 5%: slight loss of skin elasticity.
- 10%: skin inelastic, stays 'tented' for a few seconds and slowly returns to normal. Oral mucous membrane dry; eyes lacks lustre.
- +12%: skin stays tented permanently. Eyes become sunken; oral mucous membrane very dry; animal collapses.

Aspiration pneumonia occurs when some food is inhaled during regurgitation or vomiting. As food is not sterile, this can result in a serious infection of the lungs. It is common in animals with persistent regurgitation and can occasionally be fatal.

Treatment

The treatment prescribed for the vomiting patient depends on the underlying cause. In general, vomiting will cease once the underlying cause has been identified and treated. Symptomatic therapy for primary gastric disease includes:

- Complete dietary rest.
- Provision of fluids by intravenous route. Avoid oral fluids while still vomiting.
- Treat the underlying cause.
- If required, feed intravenously.
- Anti-emetics may be of value in specific cases.
- Antacids (cimetidine) to prevent gastric acid production.
- Surgery (foreign bodies, neoplasia).
- Protectants such as bismuth preparations.

Conditions of the Small Intestine

Diarrhoea may defined as the passage of unformed faeces of increased bulk or fluid content. Diarrhoea may be life-threatening, acute, secondary to systemic disease or chronic (Fig. 23.12). When diarrhoea is associated with intestinal disease, the character of the diarrhoea can often indicate whether it originates from the small or large intestine (Fig. 23.13).

Blood is occasionally observed in the faeces. When this is due to large intestinal disease it is usually fresh blood that is passed. **Melaena** describes the passage of changed blood in the faeces, which may be black or tarry-looking. This blood has usually originated from the stomach or small intestine.

In **life-threatening diarrhoea** the animal is usually systemically ill and will exhibit clinical signs which include persistant vomiting, marked dehydration, anorexia, abdominal pain and the passage of faeces which may contain blood. Any animal exhibiting these signs should be examined as soon as possible. Aggressive therapy is required if the animal is to be saved. Intensive intravenous fluid therapy together with antibiotics and nil-by-mouth may be followed by the use of oral anti-diarrhoeal drugs once vomition ceases. Oral fluids followed by a low-fat veterinary diet can be introduced slowly once vomiting and diarrhoea cease.

In **acute diarrhoea** the animal may remain bright and continue to eat. Vomiting and dehydration are unlikely and although treatment is required it is less urgent. It should include dietary rest for at least 24 hours together with the use of anti-diarrhoeal drugs. Systemic antibiotics should *not* be used, as primary bacterial infections are very rarely present. When faecal output has been reduced, the animal may be given a low-fat veterinary diet and a slow return to normal feeding can be permitted as long as the diarrhoea does not recur.

Chronic diarrhoea may be associated with maldigestion or malabsorption of nutrients:

- **Maldigestion** is usually associated with failure of the exocrine pancreas to produce adequate levels of digestive enzymes.
- **Malabsorption** is associated with damage to the small intestinal villi, preventing adequate absorption of nutrients.

In either case the clinical signs are very similar, so that the conditions cannot be differentiated on clinical signs alone. They include:

SOME OF THE CAUSES OF ENTERITIS OR DIARRHOEA IN THE DOG AND CAT. IN SOME CASES DIARRHOEA IS SECONDARY TO DISEASE OF OTHER ORGANS			
Enteritis			
Life-threatening	Acute	Chronic	Secondary
HGE Parvovirus Distemper	Dietary Worms Colitis Giardiasis	Malabsorption Neoplasia Colitis Dietary hypersensitivity	Addison's disease Liver disease Pancreatic disease Kidney disease

Fig. 23.12. Causes of enteritis and diarrhoea.

- Chronic diarrhoea, often containing undigested/absorbed food.
- Marked weight loss.
- Polyphagia.

Animals with maldigestion or malabsorption require low-fat veterinary diets fed at least twice daily. In the case of exocrine pancreatic insufficiency the diet must be supplemented with proprietary enzyme replacer. In malabsorptive states, anti-inflammatory drugs and occasionally antibiotics are required.

Colitis is another common cause of chronic diarrhoea, especially in dogs. Weight loss is not a feature of colitis but tenesmus, urgency and the passing of faeces containing blood and/or mucus are common. Treatment involves the use of a non-steroidal anti-inflammatory drug and dietary correction. Both high fibre diets and hypoallergenic diets have been recommended in the treatment of colitis.

Nursing care in vomiting and diarrhoea

- If an infective disease is suspected, provide isolation facilities and maintain high levels of hygiene to prevent the spread of infection.
- Ensure that the prescribed treatment is carried out.
- Monitor and maintain intravenous fluid therapy.
- Ensure that the patient is not allowed to lie in its vomit or diarrhoea and that any such clinical waste is disposed of properly.
- Record all incidents of vomiting or diarrhoea on a kennel sheet.

- Ensure that the animal receives nil by mouth initially.
- Be responsible for the careful introduction of oral intake once this has been approved by the veterinary surgeon.
- Advise owners regarding the animal's progress and treatment.
- Report any deterioration to the veterinary surgeon.

Foreign Body Obstruction

Foreign bodies are relatively common in the dog and cat, although the type of foreign body and its location vary according to the species involved. They may be found in the oral cavity, pharynx, oesophagus, stomach and small intestine. The large intestine is the least likely site for such obstructions although rectal foreign bodies involving bone fragments do occur.

Examples of possible foreign bodies in cats include:

- Fish bones stuck at tooth/gum margins of the oral cavity.
- String looped round the tongue and passing down the oesophagus.
- Needles and fish hooks in the pharynx, oesophagus or stomach.
- Chicken bones lodged in the oesophagus.
- Fur balls in the stomach.
- Needles lodged in the stomach with string attached and trailing along the intestine, creating the classical linear foreign body.

SOME CLINICAL FEATURES WHICH MAY PERMIT DIFFERENTATION BETWEEN DIARRHOEA ORIGINATING FROM THE SMALL OR LARGE INTESTINE		
Clinical sign	Small intestine	Large intestine
Faecal volume	Increased	Normal/reduced
Faecal frequency	increased	increased
Faecal fat	present	absent
Tenesmus	absent	may be present
Blood	black/tarry	fresh
Mucus	absent	present
Weight loss	present	absent

Fig. 23.13. Differentiation of diarrhoea from small and large intestines.

Examples of possible foreign bodies in dogs include:

- Stick wedged across the hard palate.
- Balls, bone or hard food lodged in the pharynx.
- Chop bones, potatoes, chicken bones lodged in the oesophagus.
- Balls, bones, and almost anything within the stomach.
- Stones and balls in the intestine.
- Bone fragment lodged in the rectum.

The clinical signs (Fig. 23.14) depend on the site and degree of the obstruction. Complete obstructions will lead to the most severe signs; partial obstruction may be better tolerated. The diagnosis is based on a thorough examination of the patient and radiographic examination. Treatment depends on the type and location of the foreign body (Fig. 23.14).

Constipation

Constipation is a associated with impaction of the colon and rectum with faecal material. Many animals with constipation will strain in an attempt to pass faeces and this is often referred to as **tenesmus**. The causes of constipation and tenesmus are similar (Fig. 23.15).

Treatment for constipation depends on the underlying cause. Many cases require surgical correction, including castration for prostatic hyperplasia, rectal strictures, perineal hernias or rectal neoplasia. In cases of simple impaction, the animal may be sedated or given a general anaesthetic so that the colon can be emptied manually.

It is important to ensure that further access to agents causing impaction is prevented, i.e. the feeding of bones should be discontinued. Prevention of impaction can also be achieved by providing bulking agents or softening agents in the diet, including methylcellulose, psyllium and dietary fibre.

> **THE FEEDING OF BONES**
> Veterinary nurses are quite often asked for advice about giving bones to pets. Although some dogs (and cats) tolerate eating bones, others do have problems. Chicken and chop bones have sharp edges which can tear the alimentary tissue or cause obstruction. Marrow bones can be beneficial but the consumption of too much bone can lead to an accumulation in the large intestine and constipation. Marrow bones many also irritate the large intestine, leading to tenesmus and haemorrhagic diarrhoea.

Administration of enemata

An **enema** is a liquid preparation which is passed into the rectum and colon and is most commonly used for the purpose of treating constipation. Details of administration are given in Chapter 20 (General Nursing).

Conditions of the Liver

Hepatitis may be defined as inflammation of the liver. It is usually associated with micro-organisms such as adenovirus or leptospiral infection but may also follow toxic damage to the liver.

FOREIGN BODIES OBSTRUCTING THE ALIMENTARY TRACT		
	Clinical signs	Treatment
Oral foreign bodies	Sudden onset of excess salivation, Pawing the mouth, Champing the jaw, Possibly bleeding from the mouth.	Remove with care under sedation or general anaesthetic.
Pharyngeal foreign bodies	Sudden onset of choking, retching, gagging, Pawing at mouth, Salivation, Possible difficulty in breathing.	Must be removed under general anaesthetic but great care needed to ensure that patent airway maintained at all times.
Oesophageal foreign bodies	Regurgitation of food associated with recent feeding, Possible aspiration pneumonia.	Remove by mouth under general anaesthetic using fibre optic endoscope or rigid endoscope. Gently pushing foreign body into stomach, or by thoracotomy.
Gastric foreign bodies	May remain asymptomatic if pylorus not obstructed, Persistent vomiting where the pylorus is involved, Occasionally clinical signs will present intermittently when foreign body moves in and out of pylorus.	Remove by fibre optic endoscopy or gastrotomy.
Small intestinal foreign bodies	Persistent vomiting, Dehydration and electrolyte loss, Abdominal pain.	Remove by enterotomy.
Rectal foreign bodies	Pain on defecation, Tenesmus, Blood may be present in the faeces.	Remove foreign body from rectum after sedation or general anaesthesia.

Fig. 23.14. Foreign bodies obstructing the alimentary tract.

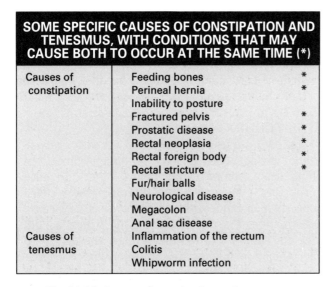

SOME SPECIFIC CAUSES OF CONSTIPATION AND TENESMUS, WITH CONDITIONS THAT MAY CAUSE BOTH TO OCCUR AT THE SAME TIME (*)		
Causes of constipation	Feeding bones	*
	Perineal hernia	*
	Inability to posture	
	Fractured pelvis	*
	Prostatic disease	*
	Rectal neoplasia	*
	Rectal foreign body	*
	Rectal stricture	*
	Fur/hair balls	
	Neurological disease	
	Megacolon	
	Anal sac disease	
Causes of tenesmus	Inflammation of the rectum	
	Colitis	
	Whipworm infection	

Fig. 23.15. Causes of constipation and tenesmus.

Jaundice and **icterus** are terms used to describe elevated levels of bilirubin in the circulation, which leads to a yellow coloration of the mucous membranes and skin. There are three possible causes of jaundice:

- Prehepatic—following excessive breakdown of red blood cells.
- Hepatic—primary liver disease leading to stasis of bile flow.
- Post-hepatic—associated with obstruction of the bile duct.

Cirrhosis of the liver develops when healing occurs by fibrous tissue formation rather than by production of new liver cells. The result is a loss of functional liver, interference with bile flow (causing jaundice) and portal hypertension, leading to ascites. The liver is reduced in size and ultimately there is liver failure.

Ascites refers to a fluid accumulation within the abdominal cavity. Several different types of fluid may accumulate, including blood, transudates, exudates, urine and gut contents. It is usual to determine the type of fluid present by inserting a sterile needle attached to a syringe through the abdominal wall and withdrawing some of the fluid for analysis. This procedure is called **paracentesis**.

Signs of Liver Disease

The liver has a massive functional reserve and considerable powers of regeneration, even following major damage. Over 70% of the liver must be lost before signs of liver failure develop.

Many of the clinical signs associated with liver disease are non-specific—vomiting, diarrhoea, anterior abdominal pain, weight loss—but more specific signs may include jaundice, ascites and pale faeces.

The final diagnosis of liver disease relies heavily on blood biochemistry, radiographs, ultrasound and ultimately biopsy of the liver.

Signs of Acute Pancreatitis

The exocrine pancreas produces and stores large amounts of digestive enzymes. They are normally stored in an inactive form within small granules called zymogens so that they cannot become active in the gland and digest the pancreatic tissue. Occasionally the protective mechanisms fail and pancreatic enzymes become activated within the gland, leading to the condition called acute pancreatitis.

The clinical signs associated with acute pancreatitis include:

- Persistent vomiting.
- Anterior abdominal pain.
- Dehydration and shock.
- Anorexia.
- Occasionally diarrhoea.
- Varying degrees of ascites and peritonitis.

A diagnosis of acute pancreatitis is usually made by detecting the following changes:

- Localised peritonitis in the anterior abdomen, often revealed by abdominal radiographs.
- Serum amylase and lipase levels are usually elevated, although in some cases only one of these enzymes may be increased in value at any given stage of the condition.
- A leucocytosis, often revealed by routine haematology.

Diseases of the Respiratory Tract

Nasal Discharge

Rhinitis is inflammation of the nasal mucous membrane. **Sinusitis** is inflammation of the sinuses, in particular the maxillary and frontal sinuses of the skull.

Nasal discharge is a common manifestation of rhinitis and sinusitis. It is often described as being **serous**, **mucoid** or **mucopurulent** in character. Occasionally the discharge involves the passage of blood and this is referred to as **epistaxis**:

- Serous nasal discharges are a feature of early infections involving viruses. Secondary bacterial infection is a common complication, when the discharge frequently becomes mucopurulent.
- Fungal infection (particularly *Aspergillus* spp.) usually start as a mucoid discharge which rapidly becomes mucopurulent due to secondary bacterial infection and haemorrhagic due to ulceration of the mucosa.
- Epistaxis may be associated with trauma, neoplasia, clotting disorders or ulceration of the mucosa following infection.

Nasal discharges are usually **bilateral** when associated with viral and bacterial infection but may be **unilateral** when associated with fungal infection, neoplasia and trauma. Occasionally discharges are initially unilateral but become bilateral with the passage of time.

Inflammation

Inflammation of other parts of the respiratory tract are described according to the region involved:

- **Tonsillitis**: inflammation of the local lymphoid tissue at the entrance to the pharynx.
- **Pharyngitis**: inflammation of the pharynx.
- **Laryngitis**: inflammation of the larynx.
- **Tracheitis**: inflammation of the trachea.
- **Bronchitis**: inflammation of the bronchi.
- **Pneumonia**: by strict definition, inflammation of the lungs, but often used to describe invasion of the lung by micro- organisms.
- **Pleurisy**: inflammation of the pleural lining between the lungs and the thoracic wall; may be 'dry' or 'wet' according to absence or presence of effusions.

Coughing

Coughing is a classical clinical sign associated with inflammation of the respiratory tract, Conditions which may be associated with coughing include:

- Cardiac failure.
- Neoplasia.
- Foreign bodies.
- Tonsillitis.
- Tracheal collapse.
- Pulmonary oedema.
- Pulmonary haemorrhage.
- Lungworm infection.
- Infections leading to pharyngitis, bronchitis, tracheitis, pneumonia.

Treatment of the coughing patient relies on determining and treating the underlying cause. The types of treatment which may be employed depend on the diagnosis but include:

- Anthelmintics for lungworm.
- Antibiotics for primary and secondary bacterial infections.
- Bronchodilators.
- Anti-tussants to suppress the cough.
- Corticosteroids to reduce inflammation.
- Environmental adjustments such as even air temperature, reduction of exercise, avoidance of airborne irritants.

Respiration

Various terms are used to describe the character and rate of breathing:

- **Dyspnoea**: difficulty in or laboured breathing.
- **Tachypnoea**: an increased rate of breathing.
- **Apnoea**: cessation of breathing, usually due to depression of the respiratory centre.
- **Orthopnoea**: breathing through an open mouth (the animal assumes sternal recumbancy with the neck extended and elbows abducted).

Acute Respiratory Failure

Acute respiratory failure represents a true emergency requiring urgent medical treatment. It implies that the lungs are no longer able to oxygenate the blood or allow exchange of carbon dioxide in order to sustain life. There are many causes of acute respiratory failure, including those shown in Fig. 23.16.

Clinical signs associated with respiratory failure vary according to the specific condition involved but may include:

- cyanosis;
- tachypnoea, dyspnoea, orthopnoea;
- tachycardia, weak pulse;
- assuming a 'dog sitting' position with abducted elbows;
- eventual collapse and unconsciousness.

Rapid and effective treatment (Fig. 23.17) is essential if the patient's respiratory function is to be improved and in some cases to save life.

SOME CAUSES OF ACUTE RESPIRATORY FAILURE	
Trauma	Ruptured diaphragm. Pneumothorax. Haemothorax.
Airway obstruction	Foreign body, Pulmonary oedema, Laryngeal paralysis.
Pulmonary embolism	
Neoplasia	Primary or secondary metastasis.
Overdose of anaesthetics	Depressing the respiratory centre.
Pneumonia	Viral or bacterial.
Pleural effusions	Hydrothorax.
Paralysis of respiratory muscles	Tetanus. Botulism.
Laryngeal paralysis	
Poisoning	Paraquat.
Pressure on diaphragm	Gastric torsion.

Fig. 23.16. Some causes of acute respiratory failure.

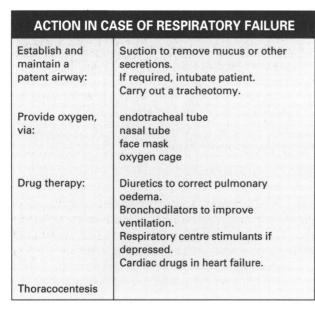

ACTION IN CASE OF RESPIRATORY FAILURE

Establish and maintain a patent airway:	Suction to remove mucus or other secretions. If required, intubate patient. Carry out a tracheotomy.
Provide oxygen, via:	endotracheal tube nasal tube face mask oxygen cage
Drug therapy:	Diuretics to correct pulmonary oedema. Bronchodilators to improve ventilation. Respiratory centre stimulants if depressed. Cardiac drugs in heart failure.
Thoracocentesis	

Fig. 23.17. Action in case of respiratory failure.

Nursing role

- Ensure that therapy is carried out.
- Monitor patient's vital signs.
- Keep careful records of patient's condition.
- Advise owner regarding patient's condition.

Pneumothorax and Hydrothorax

Pneumothorax describes the accumulation of air within the pleural cavity. In **open pneumothorax** air moves freely in and out of the pleural cavity through an opening in the thoracic wall. A **closed pneumothorax** occurs when there is physical damage to the lung leading to the escape of air into the pleural spaces as the animal breathes. In this case the air cannot escape from the pleural cavity during respiration (tension pneumo-thorax) and accumulates, causing increased breathing difficulties and eventual lung collapse.

Hydrothorax is the accumulation of fluid within the pleural cavity. The various types of fluid which may so accumulate are indicated by specific names:

- **Haemothorax**: accumulation of whole blood in the thorax, usually associated with trauma, bleeding disorders or neoplastic states.
- **Chylothorax**: accumulation of lymphatic fluid or chyle in the thorax, resulting from rupture of the thoracic duct.
- **Pyothorax**: accumulation of purulent material in the thorax, associated with bacterial infection.
- **Exudates** may also be associated with pleurisy rather than pyothorax, depending on the type of organism involved.
- **Transudates** are serum-like fluids often associated with congestive heart failure or hypoproteinaemia.

The clinical signs associated with pneumothorax and hydrothorax, which depend on the amount of air or fluid accumulating in the pleural cavity, are shown in Fig. 23.18 along with diagnosis and treatment.

Thoracocentesis involves placing a thoracic drain into the chest or using a needle and syringe on a three-way tap to aspirate the pleural space. This procedure yields valuable diagnostic information regarding the type of fluid accumulation (Fig. 23.19). It also assists in relieving the clinical signs by removing the air or fluid which is interfering with breathing.

Diseases of the Circulatory System

Congenital Heart Disease

Although not common causes of heart disease, specific inherited or congenital cardiac conditions that are most likely to be encountered include:

- Patent ductus arteriosus
- Pulmonary stenosis
- Aortic stenosis

PNEUMOTHORAX AND HYDROTHORAX

Clinical signs (varying degrees)	Diagnosis	Treatment
Dyspnoea and tachypnoea. Hypoxia and cyanosis. Tachycardia and weak pulse. Orthopnoea. Sucking sounds on inspiration. Collapse and unconsciousness. Pallor of the mucous membranes.	Careful examination of thoracic wall for injuries. Percussion of chest. Radiographs. Thoracocentesis.	Provision of therapy as for acute respiratory failure. Closure of any thoracic injury. Aspiration of fluid and or gas from pleural space. Monitoring of vital signs. Keep owners informed of current situation. Surgical correction of any lesions. Provide oxygen therapy. Inform VS if occurs unexpectedly.

Fig. 23.18. Pneumothorax and hydrothorax.

FLUID SAMPLES COLLECTED BY THORACOCENTESIS CLASSIFIED BY CERTAIN PARAMETERS TO AID IN DIAGNOSIS				
Parameter	True Transudate	Modified Transudate	Exudate	Chyle
SG	≤1.015	≤1.015	>1.015	<1.015
Colour	Clear/pink	Pink	Red	Milky
Protein	<30g/l	30g/l	>30g/l	<30g/l
Bacteria	–	–	yes	–
Clotting	–	–	may clot	–
Cells	–	some	many	some

Fig. 23.19. Thoracocentesis: fluid samples and diagnosis.

- Ventricular septal defects
- Mitral and tricuspid dysplasia
- Tetralogy of Fallot
- Persistent right aortic arch.

Patent ductus arteriosus

In this condition the fetal blood vessel that connects the aorta with the pulmonary artery fails to close after the animal is born. Normally all that remains is a ligament called the ligamentum arteriosus. Where the vessel remains open, blood shunts from the aorta to the pulmonary artery. Whether the animal exhibits clinical signs depends on the degree of blood shunting from the left to the right side of the heart. Some puppies die suddenly after birth; others show signs of heart failure at some time between birth and adulthood. Clinical signs include weakness, exercise intolerance, coughing and dyspnoea because of left heart failure, and cyanosis only if there is a right–left shunting of blood. On auscultation a classical machinery or continuous murmur is heard throughout systole and diastole.

Pulmonary stenosis

Blood leaves the right side of the heart via the pulmonary artery and its semi-lunar valve. Narrowing or stenosis of this valve leads to high pressure in the right heart and thickening or hypertrophy of the right ventricle wall. Lung perfusion may be adequate but the right ventricle has to work much harder than normal in order for this to be maintained. Where this compensatory mechanism fails, right-sided congestive heart failure develops.

Aortic stenosis

Blood leaves the left side of the heart via the aorta for the general circulation. Narrowing at the aortic valve causes high pressure in the left ventricle and poor cardiac output. Rarely this may lead to left-sided congestive heart failure. More commonly there will be episodes of fainting (syncope) on exercise and occasionally animals may die suddenly without developing signs of cardiac failure.

Ventricular septal defects

This describes an interventricular defect between the left and right ventricles. The size of the hole varies and will determine the degree of heart dysfunction that may occur. Generally blood shunts from left to right, leading to mixing of venous and arterial blood in the right ventricle. Congestive heart failure is again a likely outcome.

Mitral and tricuspid dysplasia

This is a relatively common cause of heart disease in young dogs and especially in the retriever. Deformity and incompetence of these valves leads to regurgitation of blood and a systolic murmur. The result of these changes is a progressive development of cardiac failure.

Tetralogy of Fallot

In this condition several heart defects are present at the same time. Usually there is a combination of pulmonary stenosis, interventricular septal defect, dextraposed aorta and thickening or hypertrophy of the right ventricular wall due to outflow resistance. The clinical signs depend on the severity of the lesions but are likely to include cyanosis, weight loss, exercise intolerance, harsh systolic murmur and heart failure.

Persistent right aortic arch

Occasionally, during the development of the major blood vessels supplying the heart, the right aortic arch persists instead of the left aortic arch. This leads to the ligamentum arteriosus lying across the dorsal part of the oesophagus while the remainder of the vascular ring around the oesophagus is formed by the pulmonary vein lying to the left, the aorta to the right and the heart base ventrally (Fig. 23.20). The stricture thus formed interferes with swallowing and food becomes trapped in front of the vascular ring. This leads to the development of megaoesophagus and regurgitation of food. Aspiration pneumonia is a likely complication.

Acquired Heart Disease

Acquired heart diseases include:

- Pericarditis: inflammation of the serous membrane covering the heart.
- Cardiomyopathy: disease of the cardiac muscle.

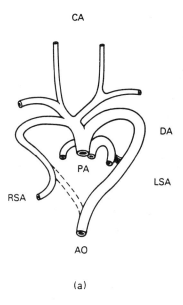

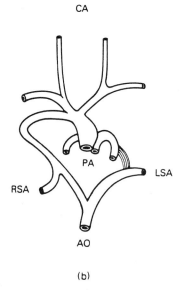

Fig. 23.20. (a) Normal aortic position and (b) persistent right arch. (Reproduced with permission of Blackwell Scientific Publications.)

- Myocarditis: inflammation of the heart muscle, usually associated with infection (e.g. parvovirus); now very rare.
- Endocarditis: inflammation of the inner lining of the heart, particularly the heart valves.
- Endocardiosis: progressive nodular thickening of the heart valves.

Pericarditis

Pericarditis is usually accompanied by pericardial effusion, which may result from tumours such as haemangiosarcomas but many are described as idiopathic in origin. The effusion itself is often sero-sanguineous in nature. The clinical signs exhibited depend on the amount of effusion, which compresses the heart and impedes its function. The heart sounds are muffled on auscultation and some degree of right-sided congestive heart failure develops in the majority of cases.

Myocardial disease

Cardiomyopathy may be primary, or secondary to some systemic disorder. The cause of primary cardiomyopathy is rarely determined but secondary cardiomyopathy can be associated with malnutrition (taurine deficiency in cats), hyperthyroidism, hypertension and viral infections.

The two forms of cardiomyopathy are:

- **Dilated** (more common in dogs), in which the heart muscle becomes thinned, with a loss of contractibility.
- **Hypertrophic** (more common in cats) in which the heart muscle becomes excessively thickened, reducing the size of the ventricular lumen and so reducing cardiac output.

Clinical signs are those of congestive heart failure.

Endocarditis

This condition is associated with bacterial infection which has spread to the heart valves from some other septic focus. Septic emboli dislodge from the damaged valves and migrate to other sites, including the myocardium, resulting in myocarditis. Clinical signs exhibited by animals with endocarditis include pyrexia, heart murmur, coughing, dyspnoea and signs associated with the original septic focus. These animals are systemically unwell and may show other signs, such as lameness.

Endocardiosis

There is often confusion between endocarditis and endocardiosis. In the latter condition, the progressive nodular thickening of the heart valves in due course renders them physically unable to function correctly and they leak severely when they should be closed. Congestive heart failure often follows. It appears to be more common in males, especially in middle to old age, and there may be a genetic predisposition in Cavalier King Charles spaniels, poodles, Pekingese and schnauzers. Clinical signs are those of congestive heart failure.

NORMAL HEART RATES

Many factors may influence the heart rate in normal dogs and cats, including the breed, age, fitness and general health, as well as excitement, stress of being examined and environmental conditions. The following figures are a guide to the range of normal heart rates for adult dogs and cats:

- Dogs: 70–140 beats/minute.
- Cats: 140–220 beats/minute.

Bradycardia, a very slow heart rate (usually less than 60 beats/minute) may be associated with conditions such as Addison's disease and excessive vagal tone.

Tachycardia, an excessively rapid heart rate, is a frequent finding in congestive heart failure, feline hyperthyroidism and some forms of adrenal tumour.

Cardiac Output Failure

This occurs as a consequence of:

- Some congenital defects
- Myocardial disease
- Electrical disturbance (**arrythmia**) including:
    Ventricular fibrillation
    Heart block
    Excessive vagal tone.

Cardiac arrest, which is rare in dogs and cats, is associated with severe arrythmias that develop when there is severe myocardial disease, excessive sympathetic stimulation or toxaemic state. Hypoxia is the most common cause and may be associated with anaesthetics or airway obstruction.

Clinical signs of cardiac failure are usually of sudden onset and occur when the animal is excited or exercising. It is unusual to have had warning signs prior to the acute episode. The animal is likely to collapse into unconsciousness, often described as **fainting** or **syncope**. This is often flaccid (unlike a fit) and is due to cerebral anoxia associated with reduced cardiac output. Animals usually recover spontaneously from these episodes and return to normal very rapidly after the event, with no lethargy or drowsiness. The clinical signs associated with cardiac arrest include lack of detectable pulse, collapse and either pallor or cyanosis of mucous membranes.

Treatment of cardiac output failure and cardiac arrest is described in Fig. 23.21.

Nursing care

In cardiac output failure, the nurse may have a vital role to play if the veterinary surgeon is unavailable when a case is presented. The nurse can:

- ensure that a patent airway is established;
- administer oxygen therapy as required;

TREATMENT OF CARDIAC OUTPUT FAILURE AND CARDIAC ARREST

1. Establish and maintain patent airway;
   – Insert endotracheal tube.
   OR – Carry out tracheotomy.
   OR – Owners should stretch out head/neck, and pull the tongue forward and remove any obvious obstructions, (warn them of being bitten).
2. Initiate ventilation at 12 ventilations/minute.
   – Use oxygen with carbon dioxide – stimulates breathing.
   OR – Blow down the ET tube.
3. Cardiac massage at 60 compressions/minute.
   – Apply pressure from lateral sides of the thorax, against table or floor.
4. Administration of drugs by veterinary surgeon.
   – Adrenaline directly into heart.
   – Possibly calcium salts intravenously.
5. Defibrillation to restart heart.
6. Fluid therapy using lactated Ringer's or saline and bicarbonate.

Fig. 23.21. Treatment of cardiac output failure and arrest.

- carry out cardiac massage to save life;
- call for veterinary assistance.

Congestive Heart Failure (CHF)

When the heart fails to function efficiently, it will compensate by changing its rate and possibly strength of contraction. If the condition progresses, clinical signs will be observed eventually and the animal will be said to have **decompensated** by developing congestive heart failure. Failure in compensation leads to pooling of blood (**congestion**) in the vascular beds. The clinical signs depend on whether the animal has left- or right-sided heart failure:

- Right-sided heart failure: poor venous return to the heart; congestion of the liver, spleen, and other viscera; ascites is likely.
- Left-sided heart failure: poor venous return from the lungs; pulmonary congestion and oedema; tachypnoea and coughing.

The reduced cardiac output also leads to reduced blood flow to the kidneys. They respond by producing **renin**, which in turn activates **angiotensin**, which stimulates **aldosterone** release from the adrenal glands. Aldosterone retains water and salt, causing further venous congestion by overloading the circulation.

Congestive heart failure may occur following cardiomyopathy, valvular stenosis, valvular incompetence, pulmonary or aortic stenosis or cardiac arrythmias.

The clinical signs observed in CHF include:

- Tachycardia.
- Weak pulse.
- Pallor of mucous membrane.
- Cyanosis if pulmonary oedema develops.
- Coughing.
- Tachypnoea.
- Ascites.
- Hepatomegaly.
- Exercise intolerance and general lethargy and weakness.
- Weight loss.

Nursing care

- Provide a quiet, stress-free environment for the patient.
- Ensure that the patient receives cage rest only.
- Restrict exercise as appropriate.
- Carry out treatments prescribed by the veterinary surgeon:
    —diuretics for pulmonary congestion/oedema;
    —glycosides for improving heart-muscle function;
    —bronchodilators to improve breathing;
    —vasodilators to reduce preload and afterload;
    —potassium supplements following use of diuretics.

- Ensure that the animal receives an appropriate veterinary diet, low in salt and containing a high biological value protein.

Diagnosis of Heart Disease

The four main aids in the diagnosis of heart disease are auscultation (listening), radiography, electrocardiogram (ECG) and echocardiogram.

Auscultation

By carefully listening to the heart with a stethoscope, the veterinary surgeon will detect heart murmurs due to valvular defects, persistent ductus arteriosus or ventricular septal defects. The heart rate may be counted and compared with the pulse rate. Any abnormal rhythms may also be detected.

Radiography

This is a valuable method of assessing the shape and size of the heart. In CHF the heart is often enlarged and this may be indicated by elevation of the trachea, and by the heart occupying more than $3\frac{1}{2}$ rib spaces. Radiographs are also useful for detecting pulmonary oedema and pericardial effusions (which cause the heart to appear globular). Ascites and hepatomegaly may also be confirmed by abdominal radiographs.

Electrocardiogram (ECG)

The ECG records the electrical activity of the heart and is therefore only useful where an arrythmia is suspected. Where CHF is due to electrical disturbances such as tachy or brady arrythmias. The ECG will record the type of disturbance and allow a diagnosis to be made. It also allows an accurate assessment of the heart rate to be calculated.

Care and use of the ECG.

- Before using the ECG, ensure that it contains adequate recording paper.
- Check the setting, including the chart speed (which should be 2.5cm/second but may be increased to 5cm/second). Centre the pen(s) on the chart paper.
- Record a 1mV trace on the recording paper, for calculation of ECG voltages following recording.
- Initially select leads 1, 2 and 3, followed by AVR, AVL and AVF.
- Apply electrode gel to the skin and then clips to hold the recording leads. The clips should be attached just below the elbow and above the hocks. The clips should hang directly downwards to stop excessive movement during recording.
- Lead positions:
  Red—right foreleg
  Yellow—left foreleg
  Green—left hindleg
  Black—right hindleg.

- Carry out the ECG recording in a quiet, stress-free room to avoid the animal moving about or shaking, as this would affect the quality of the trace produced.
- Do not sedate the animal, as this might affect the ECG trace.
- Once the recording has been completed, the leads and clips should be thoroughly cleaned and the gel should be removed from the animal.
- Always label the ECG recording with the owner's name, the case number, the breed, age and sex of animal, together with the date.

Echocardiogram

The echocardiogram allows the activity of the heart muscle or myocardium to be assessed,which is useful in cardiomyopathy. It will detect pericardial effusions and enlargement of the heart. The function of the heart valves may also be visualised using ultrasound.

Care and use of ultrasound equipment.

- Sedatives or general anaesthetics should not be used when examining cardiac patients. However, such restraint may be useful where ultrasound is used for collecting biopsy samples. (Ultrasound is now used to guide needle biopsy of organs such as the liver and kidney. This helps to prevent damage to any vital tissue and ensures that abnormal tissue is collected.)
- Shave the coat next to the area to be examined so that the probe can make good contact with the skin.
- Apply ultrasound gel to the probe and carry out the procedure.
- Always clean the gel off the patient and the probe following the examination.
- Apart from care of the probe, there is little other routine attention needed in the care of this equipment.

Anaemia

Anaemia may be defined as a decrease in the numbers of red blood cells (RBCs) below the reference range for the species concerned. Anaemia is *not* a diagnosis but a clinical sign indicating a reduction in RBCs and the oxygen-carrying capacity of the blood. It is traditional to classify anaemia into the categories shown in Fig. 23.22, which also describes clinical signs (usually sudden in onset) associated with anaemia and the basis of diagnosis and therapy. Long-term symptomatic therapy is rarely satisfactory; a definitive diagnosis is required so that specific therapy can be provided—usually specific drug therapy together with measures to alleviate the symptoms.

In general, **regenerative** anaemias are associated with haemolytic episodes or blood loos; **non-regenerative** anaemias are associated with bone

ANAEMIA			
Categories	**Clinical signs**	**Diagnosis (based on establishing category of anaemia)**	**Treatments (used singly or in combination)**
Haemorrhagic: i) Acute blood loss: – RTA trauma to major vessels. – Rupture of an internal organ; spleen, liver and kidney. – Clotting disorders; warfarin poisoning, haemophilia. – Neoplasia, haemangiosarcoma. – Haemorrhagic gastroenteritis. ii) Chronic blood loss: – Haematuria – Gastrointestinal bleeding; ulceration, hookworms. – Ectoparasites, lice. Haemolytic: – Immune mediated haemolytic anaemia. – Pyruvate kinase deficiency. – Haemobartonella infection. – Drugs; sulphonamides, anti-convulsants. Non-regenerative: – Bone marrow hypoplasia; FeLV, FIV, toxaemias, drugs such as chloramphenicol, oestrogens. – Nutritional; Iron deficiency. – Renal disease – erythropoietin deficiency. – Leukaemia, lymphosarcoma, myeloma. – Poisoning – lead.	Pallor of the mucous membranes. Jaundice. Haemorrhage either: – external, oral, nasal, body surface. – internal, into the thorax or abdomen. Lymph nodes, liver or splenic enlargement. Weakness, collapse, exercise intolerance. Tachycardia and tachypnoea.	History for knowledge of trauma, access to lead, use of drugs known to cause anaemia, detection of bleeding. Physical examination to establish evidence of haemorrhage. Routine haematology to determine number of RBCs, PCV and haemoglobin levels together with white blood cell count and platelet count. Reticulocyte count to determine if anaemia is regenerative. Coomb's test to confirm immune-mediated anaemia. Bone marrow biopsy when anaemia is non-regenerative.	Whole blood transfusions to provide immediate help in restoring oxygen carrying capacity. Ideal donors have blood groups A1 and A2 (nearly 60% of dogs). Up to 40% are ideal recipients. Single blood transfusions likely to be successful without cross-matching the blood but follow-up transfusions may be dangerous. Plasma expanders very useful where whole blood not available. They expand circulation but do not restore oxygen-carrying capacity; useful where blood transfusion unavailable and there has been major haemorrhage. Surgical correction of haemorrhage following intravenous fluid therapy to stabilise patient. Splenectomy in immune-mediated disease. Vitamin K1 for warfarin poisoning. Prednisolone therapy for immune-mediated anaemia. Erythropoietin for anaemia induced by renal disease. Stop administration of drugs known to cause anaemia. Dietary supplementation to aid red cell production – haemotinics which include high-protien diet, iron and B vitamins. Cage rest and stress-free environment. Anabolic steriods may help in non-regenerative anaemia especially associated with chronic renal disease.

Fig. 23.22. Anaemia.

marrow hypoplasia, chronic inflammatory disease, drug interations or renal disease.

Diseases of the Urinary System

Renal Diseases

DEFINITIONS

Nephritis. A general term used to describe inflammation of the kidney. It does not indicate whether the parenchyma, interstitial tissue or vascular tissue is involved. Nor does it indicate whether the inflammation is acute, chronic or progressive.

Glomerulonephritis. An inflammation associated with the capillary bed within the glomeruli with some degree of secondary tubular and/or interstitial inflammation.

Pyelonephritis. An inflammation directly associated with bacterial infection of the kidney, especially the renal pelvis. It is uncommon in dogs and cats, but when present is often associated with *E. coli*, Proteus or Pseudomonas infection.

Interstitial nephritis. An inflammatory condition of the interstitial tissues which surround the tubules. In many cases there is infiltration with inflammatory cells and healing by fibrosis.

Polyuria. The formation and excretion of increased amounts of urine. Usually associated with a compensatory increase in drinking (**polydipsia**).

Oliguria. A decreased production of urine below the values expected for the species of animal concerned.

Anuria. Cessation of urine production which is most often associated with obstruction of the urinary tract or in acute renal failure.

Dysuria. Difficulty in passing urine or pain on urination.

Haematuria. Passage of red blood cells in urine. Usually indicating bleeding into the urinary tract without specifying the location of the bleeding.

Isosthenuria. When the kidney cannot form urine with a higher or lower specific gravity than that of a protein- free plasma. The urine will remain at 1.010 irrespective of fluid intake.

Azotaemia. An increase in the waste nitrogen level in the circulation, usually measured as blood urea (BU) and creatinine. Elevations in values occur when more than 75% of the nephrons are damaged. The actual values do *not* correlate with the degree of kidney damage.

Acute Renal Failure

Acute renal failure is a condition which results in complete or almost complete cessation of renal function. The clinical signs, which occur suddenly and dramatically and vary depending on the underlying cause, are given in Fig. 23.23, which also classifies the causes of acute renal failure into groups and describes diagnosis and treatment. The latter requires a major commitment by the veterinary surgeon and nurse in order to save life.

There are generally three phases. Initially an oliguria phase occurs and occasionally anuria. This leads to retention of water, the development of acidosis and retention of potassium (**hyperkalaemia**). These changes occur because more than 75% of the nephrons are not functioning, and can be fatal.

Assuming that the animal receives prompt therapy, the oliguria phase is followed by a polyuric phase during which renal function has not been restored but fluid retention declines, together with a loss of sodium, which can lead to dehydration.

The final phase may be described as recovery when there is a gradual restoration of renal function. This may take several weeks and does not always result in the total restoration of normal renal function.

PERITONEAL DIALYSIS

Where osmotic diuresis fails to stimulate the kidneys to produce urine, peritoneal dialysis can be used to filter waste products from the blood and so reduce azotaemia. The procedure should be carried out under strict asepsic technique as there is a real risk of inducing peritonitis and shock.

The technique involves infusion of a sterile fluid into the abdomen, which will permit nitrogenous waste to leave the rich vascular bed of the peritoneum and enter the fluid. After a specified time the fluid is withdrawn (usually less than was infused) along with the nitrogenous waste, so improving the animal's condition. This may be repeated until the BU and creatinine levels fall.

Equipment required for peritoneal dialysis includes:

- Small surgical pack with drapes.
- Local anaesthetic.

ACUTE RENAL FAILURE			
Classifications	**Clinical signs**	**Diagnosis**	**Treatment**
Acute interstitial nephritis: *Leptospira canicola* infection. Acute tubular necrosis, Nephrotoxins: – mercury poisoning. – ethylene glycol poison. – gentamycin. – sulphonamides. – phenylbutazone. Ischaemic: – (results whenever renal perfusion is reduced) – prolonged anaesthetics. – acute haemorrhage. – congestive heart failure. – Addisons disease. – dehydration and shock.	Lethargy. Anorexia. Vomiting and diarrhoea. Dehydration. Halitosis. Oral ulceration. Enlarged or swollen kidneys, which are usually painful. Oliguria or anuria.	History of access to poisons, drugs or failure to vaccinate against Leptospirosis. Clinical signs. Serum biochemistry (usually reveals elevation in BU, creatinine, phosphorus, and potassium in the presence of isosthenuria).	Monitor and record vital signs regularly. Monitor urine production. Initiate intravenous fluid therapy but watch for signs of overhydration. Treat any identifiable underlying cause. Antibiotics for Leptospirosis. Stimulate kidneys to produce urine once animal is adequately hydrated by veterinary surgeon using frusemide or manitol solution (**osmotic diuresis**). Provision of comfortable stress-free accommodation. Provision of veterinary diet low in protein (14-16%DM) and in phosphorus. Protein must be of high biological value. Peritoneal dialysis.

Fig. 23.23. Acute renal failure.

- Peritoneal catheter and giving set.
- Special dialysis fluid which *must* be warmed to body temperature. The procedure is as follows:
- The hair is clipped from the ventral abdomen.
- The site is then surgically prepared.
- Local anaesthetic infiltrated into the mid line behind the umbilicus.
- The site is draped and a small incision made through the skin.
- The catheter is then inserted with the aid of a trocar into the abdomen.
- Once in place the giving set with dialysing fluid prepared to body temperature is introduced.
- The fluid is removed under gravity after 30 minutes. Occasionally this may prove difficult and the animal may have to be moved around to permit the fluid to flow.
- The procedure should be repeated as required to lower the blood urea level.

Chronic Renal Failure

Chronic renal failure may be described as a condition where there is a progressive loss of functional tissue over an undefined period. It is characterised by a slow insidious onset of clinical signs. Occasionally the owner may suggest there was a sudden onset, in which case the animal has probably had subclinical disease for some time, with the sudden development of clinical signs when the number of damaged tubules is in excess of 75%.

The numerous causes of chronic renal failure are given in Fig. 23.24, which also describes the clinical signs—these vary according to the underlying cause and many are non-specific, while others are more suggestive of renal failure. The diagnosis may be suspected from the clinical signs, history and may be confirmed from blood tests and urine analysis (Fig. 23.24). Techniques for urine analysis are given in detail in Chapter 22 (Diagnostic Samples and Tests).

Wherever possible the underlying cause of chronic renal failure should be determined and specifically treated. In the majority of cases this is not possible and treatment remains symptomatic. *Renal failure only occurs when more than 75% of nephrons are damaged.* Restoration of these nephrons is not possible and so recovery depends on the remaining healthy nephrons' ability to increase their work load. When this occurs, the animal is said to have **compensated** with restoration of renal function. If the condition progresses, eventually the animal will **decompensate** or develop renal failure again. Ultimately the kidneys will have so few healthy nephrons left that compensation cannot occur and the animal will have to be euthanased.

Symptomatic treatment which may help the kidneys to compensate is given in Fig. 23.24.

Nephrotic Syndrome

Nephrotic syndrome may be considered as an end-stage disease and is often associated with progression of glomerulonephritis. It is characterised by a severe proteinuria which leads to hypoalbuminaemia and subcutaneous oedema and ascites. The latter are due to retention of fluid which, because of the low plasma albumin, leaves the circulation for the tissue spaces. When this occurs, circulating volume falls which

CHRONIC RENAL FAILURE			
Causes	**Clinical signs**	**Diagnosis**	**Treatment**
Nephrotoxins. Ischaemia. Pyelonephritis. Congenital and hereditary disease. Idiopathic. Dietary? SLE (systematic lupus erythematosus). Glomerulonephritis.	Anorexia. Weight loss. Lethargy. Anaemia (non-regenerative). Vomiting. Halitosis. Oral ulceration and occasionally necrosis of the tip of the tongue. Polydipsia and polyuria.	Blood urea (BU), serum creatinine and phosphorus all elevated to some degree. Calcium: phosphorus ratio often changes from 1.5:1 to 1:4. Urine analysis may reveal proteinuria, granular casts, low specific gravity and sometimes haematuria.	Anti-emetics such as metoclopramide. Intravenous fluid therapy to correct dehydration and electrolyte loss. Antibiotics for primary or secondary infection. B vitamin therapy to compensate for loss in polyuria. Dietary management – by providing veterinary diet low in protein and phosphorous may be possible to halt the progression of renal failure (protein offered must be of high biological value to allow its efficient use in repair). Anabolic steroids and erythropoietin may help stimulate the bone marrow and correct anaemia.

Fig. 23.24. Chronic renal failure.

NEPHROTIC SYNDROME		
Clinical signs	**Diagnosis**	**Treatment**
Lethargy, marked weight loss, ascites, subcutaneous oedema of limbs and ventral abdomen and prepuce, polydipsia and polyuria.	Detection of a severe proteinuria on urine analysis and hypoalbuminaemia.	Dietary management involves feeding veterinary diet with very high biological value protein in reduced amounts, and low in salt and phosphorous. Aim to give as much high quality protein as possible to restore the albumin levels, without causing elevation in BU levels. Plasma expanders have been used to help correct oedema but difficult to achieve when protein loss from kidneys is so great. Anabolic steroids and corticosteroids to correct protein loss and reduce glomerular inflammation. Diuretics occasionally needed to reduce oedema if this interferes with other organ function.

Fig. 23.25. Nephrotic syndrome.

stimulates aldosterone release and further water and salt retention.

Clinical signs, diagnosis and treatment are described in Fig. 23.25. Treatment is aimed at trying to reduce the loss of protein in the urine by means of drugs and dietary management. Progress is assessed by monitoring the levels of BU, creatinine, serum proteins, sodium and potassium.

Cystitis

Cystitis may be defined as inflammation of the urinary bladder, usually associated with a bacterial infection. It is common in dogs and cats and particularly in bitches (due to the shorter urethra). Underlying causes, clinical signs (varying with the cause), diagnosis and treatment are shown in Fig. 23.26.

Incontinence

Incontinence is the inability to control the passage of urine. Animals which are incontinent may pass urine whilst walking around or whilst resting. They are

CYSTITIS			
Underlying causes	**Clinical signs**	**Diagnosis**	**Treatment**
Trauma. Calculi. Diabetes mellitus. Cushing's Disease. Obstruction. Neoplasia.	Increased frequency of urination. Urinary tenesmus (straining and difficulty in urination, often accompanied by pain on urination). 'Wetting' in the house. Apparent incontinence. Haematuria.	By urine analysis – urine collection under strict aseptic technique so that sample can be submitted for culture and sensitivity testing. Collection by either cystocentesis or catheterisation. Bacteria most often associated with cystitis include *E.coli*, *Pseudomonas* spp., *Proteus* spp. and *Klebsiella* spp.	Selection of antibiotic from the sensitivity testing. Where this is not available sulphonamides, trimethoprim, cephalosporins and synthetic penicillins are excreted in urine and may prove useful. Additional symptomatic therapy: * Increase water intake and thus urine production. * Acidify urine. * Prevention of urine scalding by application of barrier creams. * Frequent walks to encourage urination.

Fig. 23.26. Cystitis.

THE TYPES OF URINARY TRACT CALCULI ARE SHOWN TOGETHER WITH THE LIKELY URINARY pH AND DEGREE OF RADIODENSITY OBSERVED IN EACH CASE			
Type of calculi	**Likely urinary pH**	**Radiodensity**	**Species**
Struvite	alkaline	Radiodense	Dogs/cats
Oxalates	acid/alkaline	Radiodense variable	Dogs/cats
Urates	acid/alkaline	Radiolucent	Dogs
Cystine	acid	Radiolucent	Dogs

Fig. 23.27. Urinary tract calculi.

particularly likely to develop **urine scalding** (inflammation of the skin of the perineum or around the prepuce). Nursing care should include:

- Use of barrier creams to prevent urine scalding.
- Use of incontinence pads on bedding to reduce soiling.
- Frequent opportunities to attempt normal urination.
- If catheterisation is routinely required, great care must be taken to avoid introduction of infection (cystitis). For this reason an indwelling catheter may be useful.

Calculi

The most common types of urinary tract calculi are shown in Fig. 23.27. Common sites for obstruction of the urinary tract by calculi include:

- The renal pelvis.
- Ureters.

- Urethra
  —ischial arch
  —at the os penis.

Feline Lower Urinary Tract Disease (FLUTD)

This disease was previously known as feline urolithiasis syndrome (FUS). It may be caused by the formation of **uroliths** within the urinary tract, though the aetiology of urolith formation is determined in fewer than 50% of cases. Urethral plugs (22%) and uroliths (21%) account for many cases but urinary tract infection only accounts for 1–2%. Uroliths develop in the presence of an alkaline urine and in the presence of adequate magnesium and phosphates. Many cases therefore remain idiopathic.

The clinical signs of FLUTD are given in Fig. 23.28, which also describes treatment. Many cases are presented as medical emergencies, with total obstruction to urine passage, and it is essential to establish normal urine excretion in the first instance.

FELINE LOWER URINARY TRACT DISEASE (FLUTD)		
Clinical signs	**Immediate treatment (emergency cases)**	**Long-term control**
Cystitis. Urethritis. Urethral obstruction. Urinary tenesmus. Anuria. Haematuria. Enlargement of the abdomen. Azotaemia with total obstruction.	Cystocentesis to relieve urinary bladder tension. Catheterisation of urethra with Jackson cat catheter. Leave catheter indwelling until other therapy has been established. Antibiotic therapy if infection is suspected.	Urinary acidification using DL-Methionine or ammonium chloride (both drugs can be toxic and must be used with care by veterinary surgeon). Dietary management – provide a diet with low magnesium and low phosphate to reduce mineral availability, high sodium to increase urinary production and thirst, and a urinary acidifier to change pH to <6.5.

Fig. 23.28. Feline lower urinary tract disease (FLUTD).

Diseases of the Nervous System

Fits

Several terms are used to describe the fitting animal. **Convulsions** are violent or uncoordinated contractions of the muscles due to abnormal cerebral stimulation. The muscle activity is described as **clonic** when the contractions are interspersed with periods of relaxation, or **tonic** when the muscle contraction is sustained without periods of relaxation.

Epilepsy is a central nervous disorder in which an irritable focus within the brain causes disorganised electrical activity which results in convulsions. **Status epilepticus** occurs when the convulsions are continuous or where one fit follows directly upon another.

There are many causes of fits. Those described as primary are directly associated with disorders of the brain. Secondary disorders include conditions of other body organs which influence the brain in some way. Some of the most likely causes of fits include:

- Viral or bacterial infections.
- Intracranial trauma.
- Brain tumours.
- Hydrocephalus.
- Cerebral anoxia.
- Idiopathic epilepsy.
- Portosystemic shunts.
- Hypocalcaemia.
- Hypoglycaemia.
- Chronic liver disease.
- Hypokalaemia.
- Poisons (cyanide, metaldehyde, lead).
- Renal disease.

Phases

The clinical signs exhibited by animals having a fit are divided into three phases:

- An initial phase before the fit actually occurs: pre-ictal phase.
- The actual fit: ictal phase.
- The behaviour immediately after the fit: post-ictal phase.

In the **preictal phase**, animals may be asleep or resting just prior to a fit and may wake suddenly and appear restless or anxious, or seek attention.

In the **ictal phase (collapse)**, the animal collapses onto its side, champing its jaws, salivating, vocalising, urinating and defecating. The eyes usually remain open and staring. In addition the limbs often start to 'paddle' or may exhibit tonic or clonic contractions. The animal is unaware of its environment and is unable to prevent injury to itself during the fit.

In the **post-ictal phase** immediately after the fit, the animal may appear dazed, exhausted and anxious again before returning to normal over a variable period.

IMMEDIATE ACTION AND ADVICE

If an owner telephones the practice for help whilst their pet is fitting, it is important for the nurse to be able to offer the following sound advice:

- The owner will be distressed. The nurse must take control and remain calm.
- The owner should *not* touch the animal but should:
  —move items away from the animal to prevent injury;
  —clear the room of people;
  —reduce the noise and draw the curtains to provide a quiet environment;
  —stay with the animal until the fit is over and then offer comfort and reassurance.
- The owner should never:
  —try to move or handle the animal, as there is considerable risk of personal injury;
  —attempt to drive to the surgery with a fitting animal in the car, as there is a serious risk of causing an accident.
- When the animal has recovered, it should be brought to the surgery for examination by the veterinary surgeon.
- If the animal has status epilepticus, the veterinary surgeon and nurse may have to attend the owner's home to provide treatment.

The same routine should be used if a patient starts fitting in the surgery, until a veterinary surgeon can be called to administer intravenous anticonvulsant therapy.

Anticonvulsants

Long-term therapy for fits depends on finding and correcting the underlying cause. For example, there is little point in providing anticonvulsant therapy for a patient with renal disease when control of renal function will prevent the fits from continuing.

If the fit is due to idiopathic epilepsy, anticonvulsant drugs can be of considerable value. The majority of these drugs are available in tablet form and are therefore of little use during a fit. In these circumstances intravenous anticonvulsants are required. Ideally diazepam should be given by the veterinary surgeon directly into a vein with the assistance of the nurse. If this drug is unavailable, pentobarbitone sodium may be used instead. Both these drugs will normally control the fit and calm the animal.

Long-term therapy requires the use of oral anticonvulsants such as primidone phenobarbitone. Anticonvulsants are generally not provided if fits occur less frequently than every 3–6 months. This is because the interval between fits is so long that more problems exist from daily drug administration than from the fits. The dose required by any individual is variable and trial doses must be used in order to find the level of drug which just prevents fits from occurring. This approach will prevent unnecessary overdosing and allow early detection of progression as the threshold for fits tends to increase with time.

Although anticonvulsants are safe and may be used over a long period, they can have an initial sedative effect and a long-term effect on the liver. In addition owners must be particularly careful about keeping these powerful drugs away from children, as improper use can have fatal consequences.

Owners should be asked to watch for signs of the fits recurring which might change in character following drug therapy and include:

- Sudden episodes of seeking affection, restlessness or anxiety.
- Short-duration fits which may only be manifest as muscle tremors ('petit mal' fits).
- Sudden recurrence of typical fits, indicating loss of control.

UNCONSCIOUSNESS
Common Causes

Cerebral anoxia.	Barbiturate poisoning.
Trauma to the brain.	Heat stroke.
Circulatory collapse – heart disease.	Airway obstruction. Hypocalcaemia. Narcolepsy.
Hypoglycaemia. Hypokalaemia.	

Additional clinical signs
Association with exercise. Very sudden onset with no pre- or post-ictal phases (as occurs with fits). Flaccid, no muscle activity. Unaware of surroundings. Cyanosis of mucous membranes possible. Stridor – increased inspiratory noise, with airway obstruction. Spontaneous, rapid and complete recovery.

Fig. 23.29. Unconsciousness: causes and signs.

Loss of Consciousness

Syncope, or fainting, is a transient loss of consciousness due to generalised cerebral ischaemia, secondary to a major reduction in cerebral perfusion.

Unconsciousness may be defined as a state of insensibility or a loss of awareness. Animals are usually unresponsive to external stimulation during these episodes.

> **The clinical signs associated with unconsciousness must** *not* **be confused with convulsions. With unconsciousness there is** *no* **clonic or tonic muscle contractions. The animal usually collapses and lies still without signs of abnormal motor activity.**

Additional clinical signs, which depend on the underlying cause of unconsciousness, are shown in Fig. 23.29 along with the most common causes.

When confronted with an unconscious patient, take the following action:

- Try to obtain help from a veterinary surgeon as quickly as possible.
- Monitor vital signs.
- Ensure that the animal has a patent airway:
  —Remove harness or collar and extend the head and neck.
  —Clear any obstructions observed in upper airway.
  —If the obstruction cannot be removed, carry out emergency tracheotomy.
- Supply oxygen once airway is patent. This may be carried out by face mask, endotracheal tube or oxygen cage.
- Artificial respiration should be provided if the animal fails to breathe for itself. Inflate lungs 12 times per minute, either via an anaesthetic machine or by compression of the chest.

- If the heart has stopped, apply cardiac massage at 60 lateral compressions of the lower third of the thorax per minute.

Chapter 3 (First Aid) gives more detail of these procedures.

Paresis or Paralysis

Injury to the spinal cord or brain may result in limb weakness (**paresis**) or inability to move (**paralysis**). **Paraplegia** usually describes paralysis of the hind limbs. **Tetraplegia** (or quadriplegia) describes paralysis of all four limbs. Paralysis that involves a forelimb and a hindlimb on the same side is called **hemiplegia**.

Clinical signs such as these occur most commonly following trauma to the brain or spinal cord. In the latter case this is most often because of an intravertebral disc protrusion. The problem can be recognised by observing:

- The animal's inability to walk, support its weight or move its limbs.
- A loss of sensation in the affected limb(s).
- In tetraplegia or paraplegia, there may also be a loss of control over urination and defecation. In other cases there may be retention of urine or faeces.

Neurological tests, carried out by the veterinary surgeon to gauge the extent of nerve damage and also to act as a baseline from which to monitor progress, might include those shown in Fig. 23.30.

Emergency transport

If owners telephone for emergency help regarding an animal with a possible spinal injury, they should be warned not to lift the animal directly into a vehicle

NEUROLOGICAL TESTS IN CASES OF PARESIS OR PARALYSIS	
Withdrawal reflex	Lay animal on its side and prick foot with needle. Limb should be withdrawn immediately and animal consciously aware of your action.
Anal reflex	Gently insert thermometer into rectum. Normal animals will respond with pronounced contraction of anal sphincter.
Tail sensation	Prick the skin of tail and observe for signs of recognition.
Patella reflex	Hold the hind limb partially extended with animal lying on its side. Tap patellar ligament with patella hammer. Limb should extend and return to normal position.
Panniculus reflex	Sensory reception along flanks manifests as twitch of skin to pin prick.

Fig. 23.30. Neurological tests in cases of paresis and paralysis.

but to slide it gently on to a board or similar structure to keep its spine straight and prevent further injury (see Chapter 3, First Aid). Then the animal can be loaded into the vehicle on the board and brought to the surgery for examination.

Nursing care of a paraplegic patient

- Help the veterinary surgeon to carry out a baseline neurological examination, repeated at regular intervals to monitor progress.
- Regularly monitor the temperature, pulse and respiratory rates. These animals are prone to secondary infections.
- Place the animal in a comfortable, clean and dry cage.
- Keep the spine straight and prevent unnecessary movement.
- Assist in the provision of any specific treatment required (usually surgical intervention).
- Ensure that the animal receives adequate nutrition.
- Assist in the passage of urine and faeces, manually if required or by assisting the animal to posture by supporting with a blanket under its abdomen. It may be necessary to catheterise the patient regularly to prevent urine retention, infections and development of an atonic bladder.
- If the animal is incontinent, steps must be taken to prevent urine scalding by applying barrier creams and regularly changing the bedding. Incontinence pads are useful in this situation.
- Turn the animal regularly to prevent development of pressure sores or hypostatic congestion. Ideally place patient in sternal recumbency.
- Physiotherapy of limbs may be beneficial in some cases.

Muscle Disorders

Muscle conditions observed in dogs and cats include:

- **Myositis**—inflammation of muscle tissue.
- **Polymyositis**—a diffuse inflammatory disorder of skeletal muscle often associated with autoimmune diseases. Results in weakness, lameness and pain on movement and palpation.
- **Metabolic myopathy**—muscular disorders associated with such conditions as Cushing's disease, hypothyroidism, glucocorticoid use, hypokalaemia, leading to weakness and muscular atrophy.
- **Muscular dystrophy**—a rare condition that may be inherited and is characterised by progressive degeneration of skeletal muscles in dogs. Clinical signs include weakness, dysphagia and muscle atrophy.

Electromyography (EMG) may be used to identify disease of muscle fibres, neuromuscular junctions, spinal nerves and peripheral nerves:

- Normal muscle is electrically silent. Normally the introduction of a needle into muscle tissue evokes electrical activity which stops when the needle stops moving.
- Where there is damage to a peripheral nerve supply to a muscle, the electrical activity on introducing the needle is prolonged.
- Similar changes occur in primary muscular disease such as myositis.

Diseases of the Endocrine System

Diabetes Mellitus (DM)

Diabetes mellitus is a condition most commonly seen in middle-aged entire bitches, especially of the terrier breeds. Animals with diabetes mellitus have problems with carbohydrate metabolism. The blood sugar level increases (**hyperglycaemia**) because the cells are unable to take up **glucose** from the circulation due to a deficiency in **insulin** (Fig. 23.31). When hyperglycaemia reaches the renal threshold, glucose appears in the urine.

The most common cause of DM is degeneration of the beta cells of the endocrine pancreas, leading to insulin deficiency. There are other causes:

- DM often occurs shortly after the bitch has been in season. This is due to the effect of **progesterone**, which stimulates growth hormone which is diabetogenic and causes insulin resistance and hyperglycaemia.
- In **Cushing's disease**, cortisol also causes hyperglycaemia and signs of DM.
- **Obesity** causes insulin resistance and may lead to DM.

COMMON DISORDERS OF THE ENDOCRINE GLANDS		
Condition	**Gland**	**Hormone deficiency**
Diabetes mellitus	Pancreas	Insulin deficiency
Diabetes insipidus	Pituitary	ADH deficiency
	Kidney	Fail to respond to ADH
Cushing's disease	Pituitary	Excess ACTH → cortisol
	Adrenal tumour	Excess cortisol
Addison's disease	Adrenal	Deficiency of aldosterone
		Cortisol deficiency?
Hyperthyroidism	Thyroid	Excess thyroxine
Hypothyroidism	Thyroid	Deficiency of thyroxine
Hyperparathyroidism	Parathyroid	Excess parathormone

Fig. 23.31. Common disorders of endocrine glands.

- The use of **progestagens** to control oestrus may act in a similar way to natural progesterone and induce DM. This is especially important in cats.
- Excess **glucagon** activity which is also produced by the pancreas to antagonise insulin.
- Administration of **glucocorticoids** causes hyperglycaemia, which can be confused with DM although the blood sugar level is usually lower than the renal threshold.

The clinical signs exhibited by animals with diabetes mellitus depend on the duration of the condition. Initially animals will be presented with polydipsia, polyuria and polyphagia but remain bright and active. The clinical signs change as the condition advances, with the development of anorexia, vomiting, diarrhoea, dehydration, weakness and lethargy. These symptoms develop because the animal needs an energy source but cannot utilise glucose. Therefore it starts to break down protein and fat as alternative energy sources. This results in a metabolic acidosis and a toxic build-up of ketones, called **ketoacidosis**.

The initial treatment of diabetes mellitus depends on the clinical signs exhibited. Therapy can be divided into:

- Emergency treatment for ketoacidosis.
- Standard treatment for diabetes mellitus.

Emergency treatment of ketoacidosis

These animals require urgent treatment with intravenous fluids (see Chapter 21), initially using Hartman's solution to correct the metabolic acidosis and 0.9% saline for maintenance. In addition they should receive a short-acting soluble insulin administered intravenously to provide good control. The veterinary surgeon will be responsible for this therapy, which must be given with care to avoid the development of hypoglycaemia. Once the clinical signs of ketoacidosis improve and the animal starts eating, the standard therapy for diabetes mellitus can be instigated.

Standard treatment for diabetes mellitus

This requires the establishment of a strict daily routine:

- Collection of a urine sample first thing each morning and measurement of the glucose level.
- A *strict* dietary regime. Feed a high-fibre veterinary diet in exact amounts and at the same time each day.
- Subcutaneous injections of insulin each day.
- Female diabetics should be spayed before their next oestrus, to prevent instability of their condition.

Urine samples. The daily routine should start with collection of a free-flow urine sample each morning using a clean container (free from any chemical contamination). The glucose level is measured with ketodiastix, which also have a strip to measure ketones. Once the animal is stabilised, owners should be advised to observe the ketone strip: it will not change colour unless the animal has become unstable. If this occurs, owners should seek veterinary assistance immediately.

Calculation of insulin dose. The amount of insulin should be calculated from the level of glucose in the urine sample each day. The calculations are based on an initial dose of 0.5IU per kg body weight.

- Glucose > 1%: give previous day's dose plus 2IU.
- Glucose 0%: give previous day's dose less 2IU.
- Glucose 1/10% (one tenth per cent): give previous day's dose.

Injection of insulin. Before injection, the animal should be fed one quarter of its daily ration. *Only if this is consumed should the animal be injected with insulin.*

- Insulin is supplied in bottles containing 100 IU/ml as a suspension. (Some veterinary insulins contain 40 IU/ml.)
- The insulin must be kept at +4°C and gently mixed but not shaken before use.

- Insulin syringes for human use are graduated in 50 divisions from zero to 1.0ml, so that each division is equivalent to 2/IU of insulin.
- The correct dose of insulin is injected under the skin anywhere along the animal's back. A new site is selected each day to reduce localised pain.

Diet. The remaining three-quarters of the daily ration should be given 8 hours after the insulin injection, so that the timing of the meal coincides with the peak effect of the insulin on the blood sugar level.

Diabetics should receive a high-fibre diet for the following reasons:

- Many animals with diabetes mellitus are obese and need to lose weight. The diet assists in a weight-control programme.
- High-fibre diets slow the rate of gastric emptying, reduce the speed of glucose absorption from the small intestine and prolong the time during which glucose is absorbed. This reduces the surges in blood glucose which can follow a meal and therefore assists insulin in controlling blood glucose levels and tissue uptake of glucose.
- It is very important that the diet is not changed from day to day and that no additional food is offered. Either situation may result in instability.

Hypoglycaemia

The most likely complication associated with the standard routine for diabetics is the occurrence of hypoglycaemia. This may be as a result of:

- injecting too much insulin;
- injecting the right amount of insulin but the animal fails to eat (this is why it is important to feed the animal before giving the insulin);
- the peak effect of insulin occurs before the animal receives the main part of the daily ration.

The most likely time for hypoglycaemia to occur is when the peak insulin effect is expected, some 8 hours after feeding. Owners should be advised to watch for the signs of hypoglycaemia—including muscle tremors, anxiety, weakness, ataxia, collapse and coma.

Therapy for hypoglycaemia depends on whether the animal is still conscious:

- If the animal is conscious, it should immediately be given sugar, chocolate, honey or similar food to counteract the low blood sugar level.
- If the animal is unconscious, the owner should take it to a veterinary surgeon urgently for an intravenous infusion of glucose.

Over-exertion of an animal with diabetes mellitus may lead to hypoglycaemic crisis and instability. The animal should be permitted to enjoy a moderate amount of exercise but this should be regular and of the same type and duration each day.

Diabetes Insipidus (DI)

Diabetes insipidus occurs when there is a failure in the production of ADH (antidiuretic hormone) from the pituitary gland or failure of the kidneys to respond to ADH—hence the terms **central diabetes insipidus** and **nephrogenic diabetes insipidus**, which describe the location of the problem.

Normally ADH is produced by the pituitary gland in order to concentrate the urine when the body needs to conserve water. If the animal consumes excessive amounts of water, ADH production falls and a more dilute urine is produced. In this way water balance within the body can be controlled.

The clinical signs associated with diabetes insipidus are marked polydipsia and polyuria. They occur because the animal can no longer conserve water due to a defects in the ADH system. Consequently the animal produces very dilute urine all the time, and requires a compensatory increase in water intake to correct the loss. The amounts of water ingested can be dramatic: for example, a dachshund may drink up to 7 litres of water a day.

Urine analysis in animals with DI will be negative except for a very low specific gravity (in the order of 1.000 to 1.007). Repeated measurements of urine specific gravity will confirm that the animal is unable to concentrate its urine. The diagnosis is based on confirming that the animal is unable to concentrate its urine, by carrying out a water deprivation test.

WATER DEPRIVATION TEST
This must always be carried out by a veterinary surgeon and with *great care*. Animals with suspect DI will be deprived of water and can become seriously dehydrated. Constant monitoring is required and the test *must* be stopped if the animal becomes distressed. The procedure is as follows:

- Ensure that the animal is well hydrated and has a normal blood urea level.
- Empty the animal's bladder of urine and measure its specific gravity.
- Weigh the animal and calculate 5% of its body weight.
- Place the animal in a kennel without food or water.
- Every 60 minutes: empty the bladder, measure the specific gravity of the urine and weigh the animal again. Repeat until 5% of the body weight has been lost.
- After 5% of the body weight is lost, the normal animal will have concentrated its urine to > 1.020. Animals with DI will continue to produce dilute urine (< 1.007).
- Once the test is completed the animal should be allowed free access to water.

Treatment of diabetes insipidus depends on which form is present:

- In central DI, the administration of ADH by nasal drops will result in a restoration of normal water balance.
- In nephrogenic DI, there is adequate ADH but the kidneys will not respond to the hormone and so replacement hormone therapy will not work. Paradoxically, thiazide diuretics may reduce urine output by 50% in some cases. However, the prognosis for this form remains guarded.

Cushing's Disease

Cushing's disease, or **hyperadrenocorticalism**, is associated with the production of excessive levels of cortisol from the adrenal glands. This may occur because there is:

- a tumour of the adrenal gland, with excess production of cortisol; or
- a pituitary tumour, resulting in too much ACTH, which stimulates the adrenal glands to produce excess cortisol (this form of Cushings disease is more common).

Clinical signs and treatment are given in Fig. 23.32. The diagnosis is based on hormone tests such as the ACTH test and the dexamethasone screening and suppression tests, which determine whether Cushing's disease is present and, if so, in which form so that the appropriate treatment can be given.

CUSHING'S DISEASE	
Clinical signs	
Polyphagia Polydipsia and polyuria. Pot-bellied because of enlarged liver, loss of abdominal muscle tone and fat deposition in abdomen. Bilateral alopecia of flanks. Change in coat colour in some cases. Muscle wasting and weakness in some cases. Calcium deposit in the skin (*calcinosis cutis*).	
Treatment	
Adrenal tumour	Usually only one adrenal gland involved, which should be removed surgically; other gland will slowly start to function again in most cases.
Pituitary form	Oral mitotane given daily to suppress adrenal function – must be given with food for adequate absorption, and gloves must be worn when handling tablets. Animal must also be carefully monitored to determine when adequate amount of drug has been given: Measuring water intake and use ACTH test. Drug therapy to reduce water intake to 50ml/kg/day; When target is reached, once-weekly mitotane therapy to maintain control.

Fig. 23.32. Cushing's disease.

Hypothyroidism and Hyperthyroidism

Over 80% of naturally occurring cases of **hypothyroidism** are associated with autoimmune disease or atrophy of the thyroid glands. Hypothyroidism is the most common endocrine disorder of dogs (usually 6–10 years of age, either sex) but is rare in cats.

Hyperthyroidism, on the other hand, is extremely rare in dogs but is now quite commonly diagnosed in cats (usually over 6 years of age, either sex). Benign thyroid tumours account for over 95% of clinical cases and lead to excess thyroid hormone production.

Thyroid hormone is important for the function of many body organs and deficiencies or excesses result in numerous possible clinical signs, as set out in Fig. 23.33, which also describes diagnosis and treatment of both diseases.

Skeletal System

Calcium, Phosphorus and Vitamin D

The majority of calcium and phosphorus in the body is found in the bones and teeth (> 90%). Apart from their importance in forming the skeleton, calcium and phosphorus have other important functions:

- Calcium: blood clotting; nerve and muscle function.
- Phosphorus: involvement in enzyme systems throughout the body.

Although there are individual dietary requirements for calcium and phosphorus, the relationship between the two minerals is also very important—as explained in Chapter 17 (Nutrition).

Vitamin D is synthesised in the skin by action of ultraviolet light. There may also be a dietary requirement which is to some extent dependent on the dietary content of Ca:P. Following formation in the skin, vitamin D is modified by the liver and kidney to produce the physiologically active form which plays an important part in calcium:phosphorus metabolism by:

- increasing the absorption of both calcium and phosphorus from the intestine;
- decreasing excretion of calcium and phosphorus from the kidney;
- Increasing mineralisation of bone or bone resorption.

Hyperparathyroidism

An imbalance in the Ca:P ratio will result in the stimulation of the parathyroid glands and a marked increase in circulating parathormone (which is secreted by the parathyroid and controls the metabolism of calcium and phosphorus). This

HYPOTHYROIDISM AND HYPERTHYROIDISM			
	Clinical signs	Diagnosis	Treatment
Hypo-thyroidism	Cool feel to the skin Poor appetite in spite of increasing weight gain. Lethargy and increased sleeping time. Muscle weakness. Loss of temporal muscle mass. 'Tragic' facial expression. Bilateral alopecia especially of the flanks of hind limbs.	Suggested by low thyroxine (T4) levels and confirmed by carrying out a **TSH test**. TSH normally stimulates thyroid gland to produce more thyroid hormone. This fails to occur in hypothyroidism, with little or no increase in T4 levels after administration of TSH.	Hormone replacement therapy: Ideally thyroxine (T4), rather than T3, given daily and treatment continued for minimum of 12 weeks before assessing effectiveness. Response in most cases good but treatment required for life. Thyroid extract may also be used but varies from batch to batch and so tends to give poor results.
Hyper-thyroidism	Restlessness, overactivity, aggressive behaviour. Polyphagia, Tachycardia. Weight loss. Diarrhoea. Poor coat and skin condition. Palpable mass in neck (goitre).	Measure basal T3 or T4 levels (elevated). Unilateral or bilateral disease assessed by scanning thyroids after giving Technetium 99M intravenously. Over-active glands take up radioactive isotope, which can be photographed with gamma camera.	Surgical removal of over-active thyroid glands gives best results. Radio therapy using iodine 131 destroys thyroid tissue. Long-term drug management using carbimazole (CBZ) tends to result in problems with maintaining control long term.

Fig. 23.33. Hypothyroidism and hyperthyroidism.

response may be induced secondary to nutritional deficiency or renal disease.

Secondary nutritional hyperparathyroidism is also known as **juvenile or nutritional osteodystrophy**. A dietary deficiency in calcium or an excess in phosphorus, most commonly associated with feeding all-meat diets, results in hyperphosphataemia and hypocalcaemia and leads to hyperparathyroidism. A similar response may occur when other un-balanced diets are fed or following inappropriate use of dietary supplements. The animal responds by increasing renal excretion of phosphorus and retaining calcium, together with resorption of calcium from the bones.

Secondary renal hyperparathyroidism is also known as **renal osteodystrophy**, **rubber jaw** and **renal rickets**. Animals in renal failure retain phosphorus, which accumulates in the circulation resulting in a change in the Ca:P ratio from 1.5:1 to values as high as 1:4, effectively causing hypocalcaemia. This stimulates the parathyroid glands to produce para-thormone. In addition the renal disease may result in failure to activate vitamin D, which in turn compromises Ca:P metabolism. Parathormone attempts to correct the imbalance by improving absorption from the intestine and liberating calcium from the bones. Although all bones are affected, demineralisation most severely affects the mandible and maxilla.

Clinical signs associated with hyperparathyroidism (which depend on whether nutritional or renal hyperparathyroidism is present and on the age of the animal) are given in Fig. 23.34.

Hypervitaminosis A

This condition is clinically more important in cats than dogs and is associated with feeding diets rich in vitamin A. This may result from feeding cats a diet rich in liver. Excessive quantities of vitamin A are absorbed and accumulate until toxic changes are observed.

Vitamin A is required for normal endochondrial ossification but excessive amounts provoke periosteal new bone formation. Changes associated with vitamin A toxicity are characterised by the develop-ment of multiple exostoses, especially involving the cervical and thoracic vertebra and the fore limbs in young growing animals. They are particularly common around articular surfaces, leading to ankylosis at the attachments of ligaments and tendons.

Typical clinical signs (Fig. 23.34) are observed in adult cats after ingesting vitamin A rich foods for several months.

Chronic Pulmonary Osteoarthropathy

Chronic pulmonary osteoarthropathy is also known as hypertrophic pulmonary osteoarthropathy or **Marie's disease**. In this condition limb swelling due to periosteal new bone formation along the distal bones of the forelimbs occurs secondary to a mass within the thorax and more rarely the abdomen (especially bladder tumours). The reason for the association between a space-occupying lesion in the thorax and bony changes in the limbs is not fully

SKELETAL DISEASES: CLINICAL SIGNS	
1. Hyperpara-thyroidism	(a) *Nutritional forms* most common in growing puppies fed diets with incorrect balance of calcium and phosphorous: usually depressed, lame and exhibit pain on moving; Incomplete and compression fractures lead to additional clinical signs. (b) *Chronic renal failure*: tend to be middle-aged or older. In addition to signs associated with renal failure, may develop rubber jaw due to demineralisation of mandible, which becomes pliable. Teeth may become loose and in some cases fall out; spontaneous fractures due to osteoporosis (demineralisation).
2. Hypervitamin-osis A	Signs include, lethargy, poor coat condition (due to inability to groom), reluctance to move, lameness and pain on moving especially neck and head.
3. Chronic pulmonary osteoarthro-pathy	Classically bilateral, painful soft tissue swelling occurs in the distal forelimbs leading to varying degrees of lameness. These clinical signs may occur BEFORE those associated with changes in the thorax.
4. Metaphyseal osteopathy	Mild to severe lameness together with limb pain, in some cases leading to collapse and inability to walk. Joints of distal fore and hindlimbs usually involved: painful, hot and swollen. Puppies usually depressed, anorexic and often pyrexic (106°F). Clinical signs may wax and wane, with periods of complete remission. Risk of limb deformity requiring surgical correction. Clinical signs often disappear as dog matures but many are euthanased due to the severity of the condition.
5. Rickets	Obvious enlargement of growth plates, bowing of the limbs and enlargement of the costochondral junctions ('rickety rosary'), often lead to varying degrees of lameness, fractures, lordosis and loss of teeth.

Fig. 23.34. Musculoskeletal disorders.

understood. There is no joint involvement and it is rare to observe bony changes in the hindlimbs. Clinical signs are given in Fig. 23.34.

Metaphyseal Osteopathy

This is also known as **Möller–Barlows disease**, **juvenile scurvy** and hypertrophic osteodystrophy. In all cases clinical signs are associated with the metaphysis of long bones in rapidly growing dogs of large breeds. Although the true cause is not known,

vitamin C deficiency, overnutrition and excessive dietary supplementation have been implicated. In particular there appears to be an association between high levels of dietary protein, energy, calcium and vitamin D and metaphyseal osteopathy. Great care is needed in feeding puppies and it is undesirable to feed for maximum rate of growth in large breeds of dog.

A necrotic band of tissue develops adjacent to the growth plate followed by the deposition of a band of osseous material in the soft tissue along the metaphysis. There is periosteal new bone formation and infiltration with many inflammatory cells. Eventually the necrotic tissue is replaced by healthy bone.

Clinical signs, which are most frequently observed in rapidly growing puppies between 3 and 7 months of age, are described in Fig. 23.34.

Osteochondrosis

This general term is used to describe disturbances in endochondrial ossification. It is sometimes further defined as degeneration of bone and cartilage but this is misleading as only cartilage is primarily involved. Various conditions are considered to be manifestations of osteochondrosis, including osteo-chondritis dissecans involving the shoulder joint, medial humeral condyle, lateral femoral condyle, cervical intravertebral joints and un-united anconeal process.

Normal epiphyseal growth takes place by pro-liferation of chondrocytes near the surface of the joint. This is followed in time by degeneration and calcification of the chondrocytes, a condition called **endochondrial ossification**. In osteochondrosis this differentiation of chondrocytes is disturbed and the cartilage becomes thicker than normal. At points of high pressure in the joint, poor vascularisation occurs and the basal layer of the thickened cartilage becomes necrotic. This leads to cracks and fissures in the cartilage. Once these fissures reach the surface of the joint, **osteochondritis dissecans** is said to be present. This is confirmed by joint pain due to a marked inflammatory reaction. A flap of cartilage often forms or breaks off, forming a 'joint mouse' which floats around in the joint space.

Rapid growth appears to be very important in the aetiology of osteochondrosis—hence the increased number of cases seen in males. Overnutrition and dietary supplementation leading to imbalances in calcium, phosphorus and vitamin D have also been implicated. Genetic predisposition may also be important.

Rickets

This term usually describes the disease in young animals—in adult animals the term **osteomalacia** is used. In this condition, mineralisation of newly formed osteoid tissue (and of cartilage matrix in young animals) does not occur around the growth plate.

The cause of these changes remains controversial. Some studies suggest that there is a deficiency in dietary vitamin D while others suggest that there may be deficiencies in dietary calcium and phosphorus. In any case it appears that the relationship between calcium, phosphorus and vitamin D is upset.

Clinical signs of rickets are given in Fig. 23.34.

Osteomyelitis

This condition may be defined as an inflammatory condition of bone which involves both the cortex and the medulla. Osteomyelitis can be classified as follows:

- Infectious:
  —Bacterial infections (Staphylococci, Streptococci, *E. coli*, *Pseudomonas* spp., *Proteus* spp.)
  —Fungal infections (especially *Aspergillus* spp.).
- Non infectious:
  —Sequestria (bone fragments with poor blood supply).
  —Trauma to bone.
  —Foreign bodies, implants.

Treatment involves culture of infected material together with sensitivity testing in order to determine the most effective antibiotic, which should be administered for at least a month.

In addition to antibiotic therapy, surgical intervention may be required in order to remove sequestria, implants or foreign bodies associated with the osteomyelitis.

Bone Tumours

There are many tumours which can affect bone. As with other tissues, tumours may be primary (arising from the tissue itself) or secondary (metastatic spread of tumours from another tissue). The most important primary bone tumours are osteoma and osteosarcoma.

Osteoma is a slow-growing, hard but benign tumour which only causes problems due to mechanical interference with function, i.e. interference with joint movement or adjacent tissues such as muscle or nerves. These tumours may occur anywhere in the axial or appendicular skeleton.

Osteosarcoma is a primary, highly malignant and usually solitary tumour with very aggressive growth characteristics. The tumour most frequently spreads to local lymph nodes and the lungs. There appears to be a greater incidence in St Bernards, Dobermanns, Irish wolfhounds and Great Danes. Dogs over 7 years old are more often affected. The most common sites involved are the proximal humerus, distal radius and ulna, and the distal femur and proximal or distal tibia.

Other primary bone tumours include:

- **Chondrosarcoma**—often involves flat bones and is slow to spread.
- **Fibrosarcoma**—rare, affects growth plates and periosteum.
- **Chondroma**—affects the skull, with local invasion to brain.
- **Osteochondroma**—affects the limbs and vertebra and occurs most frequently during active bone growth.

Arthritis

Arthritis may be defined as inflammation of a joint. There are several different types of arthritis and consequently several different aetiologies. The classification of arthritis includes degenerative and inflammatory conditions described in Fig. 23.35, which also gives treatment for different types.

Exercise

It is very important that exercise in dogs or cats with osteoarthritis should not be totally restricted, as this will result in reduced joint mobility. However, it is equally important not to provide excessive exercise, as this will exacerbate the condition. Short frequent walks are more beneficial than single long walks. In other forms of arthritis a restriction on exercise may be important especially in the early stages of therapy.

Diet

The dietary management of every case should be carefully examined. Those on an unsatisfactory diet should be placed on one that is suitable for the animal's life stage. Animals which are obese must be placed on a reducing diet, as obesity exacerbates arthritis and reduces the long-term prognosis.

Mucocutaneous System

Various descriptive terms are used when discussing disease of the mucocutaneous system. **Alopecia** is a general term that describes a loss of hair from any site and for any reason. **Pruritus** is a sensation within the skin that produces the desire to scratch in order to relieve the irritation. **Seborrhoea** describes an abnormally copious excretion of sebum which may make the skin appear oily. **Pyoderma** describes any pyogenic (pus-forming) skin infection, usually secondary to some other skin condition.

Parasitic Skin Disease

There are several ectoparasitic conditions which are of importance in dogs and cats (Fig. 23.36). Each ectoparasite has a different life cycle and host specificity which influence the clinical signs exhibited by the host and the methods of treatment employed.

ARTHRITIS: CLASSIFICATION AND DESCRIPTION OF TYPES		
Classification	**Description**	**Treatment**
Degenerative Osteoarthritis – Primary: Aetiology not known. – Secondary: Hip dysplasia. Cruciate rupture. Inflammatory: Infective – Bacterial, viral, fungal, Mycoplasma. Crystals – Gout. Immune: Erosive – Non-erosive – Rheumatoid arthritis. – Polyarthritis. Non-erosive – SLE – Polymyositis – Polyarteritis nodosa.	(a) *Osteoarthritis* Chronic condition, insidious in onset, leading to lameness, pain, crepitation and joint instability. Progressive; leads to thickening of joint and eventually limited joint movement. (b) *Infective or septic arthritis* Usually occurs in single joint; results in pyrexia, joint swelling, heat and pain in joint. Severe cases may become anorexic and depressed. (c) *Immune-mediated arthritis* Part of a systemic disease with signs involving other tissues. With regard to joints, lamensss (single or multiple) may shift (involve different joints on different occasions). Pyrexia, stiffness, depression and associated muscle atrophy; muscle pain, pyrexia, clotting defects, renal disease, splenomegaly, anaemia, skin changes.	Depends on underlying cause: definitive diagnosis important. *Osteoarthritis*: non-steroidal anti-inflammatory drugs such as phenylbutazone and piroxicam. *Infective arthritis*: important to determine the type of micro-organism and its antibiotic sensitivity; give for minimum of 3-4 weeks. *Immune-mediated arthritis*: high doses of corticosteroids such as prednisolone depress the immune response and improve overall condition.

Fig. 23.35. Arthritis.

These signs are given in Fig. 23.37, along with general descriptions of each species and the appropriate treatment after diagnosis.

The diagnosis of ectoparasites usually depends on the collection and examination of **skin scrapings**. This is a relatively simply procedure but can produce inaccurate results if it is carried out incorrectly. The procedure is detailed in Chapter 22, which also describes microscopic examination of the samples for different ectoparasites.

Hormonal Alopecia

There is a specific group of hormonal diseases which tend to cause bilaterally symmetrical alopecia. Hormonal alopecia is usually associated with the

A LIST OF THE MOST COMMON ECTOPARASITES FOUND ON DOGS AND CATS TOGETHER WITH SOME DETAILS OF THEIR EPIDEMIOLOGY				
Clinical signs	**Live off Host**	**Host Specificity**	**Life Cycle**	**Surface of deep dwelling**
Cheyletiella spp.	Possible	Dog, cat, rabbit	5weeks	surface
Sarcoptic mange	Possible	Primary dogs	3-4weeks	deep
Neotrombicula spp.	Yes	Not specific	50-70days	surface
Otodectes spp.	Yes	Dog/cat only	3weeks	surface
Demodex spp.	No	Dog/cat only	–	hair follicle
Fleas	Yes	Not specific	3weeks/2years	surface
Lice	No	Specific	14-21days	surface
Ticks	Yes	Not specific	2months/2years	surface
Notoedres spp.	No	Primary cats	–	surface

Fig. 23.36. Common ectoparasites and epidemiology.

flanks and/or ventral abdomen and inner aspect of the hindlimbs. In advanced cases it may involve the whole body but usually spares the head and forelimbs.

It is rarely associated with pruritus, self-trauma or inflammation. Conditions which may be included in this category are:

ECTOPARASITE SPECIES			
Species	**Clinical signs**	**Diagnosis**	**Treatment**
Cheyletiella spp. Mites that live on skin and cause 'walking dandruff' on dogs, cats, rabbits and (transiently) humans.	Generalised pruritus and excessive scaling. Lesions in cats can appear like miliary dermatitis. Some remain asymptomatic.	Sellotape preparations or superficial skin scrapings.	Cases respond well to most insecticidal shampoos (pyrethrin, carbamate and organophosphorus) given weekly for 6 weeks.
Sarcoptes scabiei Primarily a burrowing mite found on dogs (human cases also occur). Extremely contagious, spread by direct or indirect contact.	Alopecia, papules and crust formation which often starts on ears, elbows, brisket and legs; sites often severely pruritic. Generalised lymphadenopathy may develop in severe cases.	Mites difficult to find; may require examination of 12-20 skin scrapings.	Clipping out coat to ensure insecticidal shampoo (used weekly for 4 weeks) makes good contact with skin. Treat all in-contact animals. Antiseborrhoeic shampoos also useful to remove scale and crusts (sulphur/salicylic acid).
Neotrombicula autumnalis Also called harvest mite or chigger; natural host small rodents but may cause clinical signs in dogs, cats and humans.	Seasonal, normally summer and early autumn. Pruritus generalised, or lesions restricted to feet with excessive biting and licking causing acute moist dermatitis. In cats, non-pruritic papular disease can occur.	Close examination of the animal, especially between the toes where clusters of red-orange mites will be found.	Insecticidal shampoos or sprays.
Otodectes cynotis Mite is found in dog and cat; usually lives in ear but occasionally causes lesions on neck, gluteal region and tail.	Typically associated with outer ear infection (otitis externa), resulting in alopecia next to ear canal, head shaking, pawing the ears, head tilt, and presence of thick waxy discharge. Lesions on body include crusts and papules.	Careful visual examination for white pinhead-sized mites.	Proprietary insecticidal ear preparations such as gamma BHC or Monosulfiram preparations, and whole-body shampoos in some cases.
Demodex canis Obligate canine ectoparasite found in hair follicles; life cycle is poorly understood, but mite can *only* be passed from bitch to puppies during the first 3 days of life. Thereafter not contagious.	Localised form typically in puppies between 3 and 6 months of age: lesions on head, forelimbs and neck as areas of alopecia with scaling, erythema, and pigmentation. Generalised disease at any age: in young animals localised lesions may coalesce and become generalised or adult onset disease may occur. Secondary deep pyoderma and generalised lymphadenopathy common. Demodecosis does occur rarely in cats.	Deep skin scrapings, or expressing pus onto a microscope slide (usually heavily contaminated with mites).	Not required for localised lesions. Generalised cases: clip out completely, then repeated application of Amitraz shampoo. Pyoderma: culture and sensitivity of purulent material; administer suitable antiboitic, often for months, until negative scrapings obtained on three occasions. Up to 70% of adult onset disease related to an underlying disorder.
Ctenocephalides felis Most common ectoparasite of dog and cat, one of several species of flea. Causes irritation, and flea saliva may cause hypersensitivity reaction.	Seasonal in the UK. Include erythema and papule formation at location of each bite, anywhere on the animal and in particular along back, tail, head, hindlegs and ventral abdomen. Self trauma common, may lead to alopecia and bleeding. Cats: miliary dermatitis, granulomata (eosinophilic granuloma complex) or symmetrical alopecia.	Physical examination for presence of fleas or flea dirt; positive reaction to intradermal flea antigen if hypersensitivity is suspected.	Sustained and simultaneous assault on patient and environment: *Animal*: suitable insecticideal preparation; shampoos, sprays, powders, flea collars or systemic insecticide. Pyrethrin products safest to use in young and debilitated animals. Other parasiticides include organophosphorus and carbamate preparations. Regularly worm for *Dipylidium caninum*. *Bedding material*: destroy or thoroughly wash in a hot wash at the same time.

Fig. 23.37.—continued ◆

ECTOPARASITE SPECIES			
	Clinical signs	Diagnosis	Treatment
Trichodectes spp. and *Linognathus* spp. Lice found on dogs and cats include sucking (*Linognathus*) and biting (*Trichodectes*) spp.; life cycle 21 days, entirely on host.	Asymptomatic, or varying degrees of pruritus, alopecia (secondary to self trauma), and in cats miliary dermatitis. In severe infestations, may become anaemic.	Close examination for evidence of adult lice or eggs (nits) attached to hairs.	*House*: thoroughly vacuumed; apply insecticidal spray to carpets, paying particular attention to corners and under furniture. Discard vacuum bag to prevent reinfestation. *Owner also has lesions*: advise to seek medical attention. It is often necessary to repeat this protocol at 14 days intervals until the problem is brought under control. Lice susceptible to almost all parasiticidal agents. Suitable insecticidal shampoo, spray or powder; repeated 14 days later to destroy hatched larvae.
Ixodes ricinus Most common tick on dogs in the UK; presence depends on geographical location and climate. Much of life cycle off host: tick only seeks host during spring or autumn, for a meal.	Factors include: Number of ticks present. Animal's individual reaction to ticks. Whether ticks are carrying any viral, bacterial, protozoal or rickettsial diseases. Owners often seek veterinary advice because suddenly observed 'cyst like' structure on skin. Individual hypersensitivity may cause local pruritus so that animal removes tick by pawing the site; mouth parts may remain in place and subsequently cause granulomatous reaction and secondary infection.	Easily made from visual examination of animal.	If required, tick can be removed after initially soaking it in alcohol: grasp firmly with forceps and remove in a twisting action. Ensure mouth parts also removed to avoid secondary infection. Insecticidal sprays prevent future problems when entering tick area.
Notoedres cati Rare mite in UK, primarily infects cats, dogs or rabbits; life cycle very similar to *Sarcoptes scabiei*.	First appear on pinna and may extend to include face, neck and forelimbs. Skin becomes crusted and thickened with areas of alopecia; intense pruritus.	Skin scrapings.	Insecticidal shampoo (Selenium sulphide) or sulphur-based alternative.

Fig. 23.37. Ectoparasite species.

- Hypothyroidism.
- Hyperadrenocorticalism.
- Sertoli cell tumour.
- Canine ovarian imbalances.
- Feline symmetrical alopecia.

Hypothyroidism and hyperadrenocorticalism have already been described under diseases of the endocrine system.

Sertoli cell tumour

This is the most common testicular tumour to induce alopecia in middle-aged to old male dogs. Cryptorchid animals are 13 times more likely to develop this tumour. Oestrogen levels may or may not be elevated.

Clinical signs, when present, are associated with hyperoestrogenism and include bilateral non-pruritic alopecia involving the perineal region, inner aspect of the hindlimbs, ventral abdomen and flanks. Gynaecomastia, pendulous prepuce and attractiveness to other male dogs are other hallmarks of this condition. The neoplastic testicle is often enlarged while the other testicle is atrophied. In advanced cases a non-regenerative anaemia develops due to the effect of oestrogen on the bone marrow.

Diagnosis is based on clinical history and physical examination and plasma oestrogen assay. Treatment involves castration, which is usually beneficial.

Canine ovarian imbalance

The aetiology of this condition is not known but may involve either an oestrogen responsive dermatosis or dermatosis induced by hyperoestrogenism.

Hyperoestrogenism (classified as type I) is usually associated with cystic ovarian disease or ovarian tumour. Clinical signs include generalised bilaterally symmetrical alopecia which starts in the perineal region. There is usually vulval enlargement, abnormal oestrus cycles and secondary seborrhoea. The treatment of choice is ovariohysterectomy although clinical signs may take up to six months to decline.

Oestrogen responsive dermatosis (classified as type II) is a rare condition of the bitch occurring after ovariohysterectomy. Clinical signs include perineal alopecia which spreads to the inner aspect of the hindlimbs and ventral abdomen and also juvenile vulva and nipples. The remainder of the coat becomes soft and 'puppy like' in character. Treatment involves oestrogen or testosterone replacement therapy.

Feline symmetrical alopecia

This was also called **feline hormonal alopecia** and is a condition of complex aetiology which is not clearly understood and is very rare. It is seen more commonly in neutered cats. Alopecia initially involves the perineal region but rapidly extends to the inner aspects of the hind limbs and ventral abdomen. In some cases generalised alopecia develops. Diagnosis is based on clinical examination and is generally one of exclusion (hair regrowth will not occur when an Elizabethan collar is worn). Various treatments have been suggested including:

- Thyroid hormone replacement.
- Megoestral acetate therapy.
- Testosterone therapy in males and females.

Pyoderma

Pyoderma is rare in the cat. In the dog it is usually associated with an underlying predisposing disease. The most common pathogen isolated in canine pyoderma is *Staphylococcus intermedius.* Secondary opportunist bacteria such as Proteus, Pseudomonas and Corynebacterium may also be isolated, usually in association with Staphylococcus. Resident bacteria, including coagulase negative Staphylococci, are thought to be important to normal skin defence mechanisms. The severity of the infection depends on how deep the infection penetrates the skin and this is used to classify pyodermas (Fig. 23.38).

PYODERMAS	
1. Surface pyodermas:	(a) Acute moist dermatitis Usually occurs following self trauma when skin becomes physically damaged, wet due to serum exudation, painful, with areas of hair loss and hair matting on skin. Most common sites include face, feet, hindquarters, tail. *Treatment*: remove underlying cause such as ear infection, impacted anal glands or harvest mites; clip hair from site and start topical cleansing with antibacterial agents such as chlorhexidine. Prevent further self trauma by using Elizabethan collar. (b) Skin fold dermatitis Conformational problem where folds in skin occur at various sites including lip fold, vulval fold, tail fold dermatitis, most commonly in breeds such as the Pekingese and Sharpei but may affect others. Acute moist dermatitis develops within fold of skin which rapidly becomes infected. Only when fold is opened can full extent of dermatitis be seen. *Treatment*: surgical correction of skin fold and use of chlorhexidine washes or benzoyl peroxide gel (if not ulcerated).
2. Superficial pyodermas:	(a) Impetigo Also known as juvenile pustular dermatitis or puppy pyoderma. Most often observed in young growing puppies, especially on their ventral abdomen. Multiple pustules and yellow scabs. Treatment: antibacterial shampoos i.e. Benzoyl peroxide or ethyl lactate and, where extensive, systemic antibiotics such as erythromycin. (b) Folliculitis Infection of hair follicle. Formation of pustules with a hair protruding. Sometimes lesions assume ring formation, especially on the ventral abdomen. Coat may have 'moth eaten' appearance. Many underlying causes. Treatment: detect and remove the underlying cause; antibiotic therapy.
3. Deep pyodermas:	(a) Interdigital pyoderma Also known as pododermatitis; seen in short-haired breeds of dog. Paws become swollen, painful; exude pus. Areas of alopecia and in severe cases ulceration and fistulas. *Treatment*: long-term antibiotic therapy; surgical drainage of purulent material; correction of any detectable underlying cause, such as removal of foreign bodies. (b) Furunculosis Most serious form of pyoderma, often associated with Demodecosis, ringworm, hypothyroidism or general debility. Pustules, discharging pus, fistulas, alopecia and pain. Lesions most often found on nose, muzzle and flanks but can extend to any area. *Treatment*: correct any underlying cause; long-term systemic antibiotic therapy; whirlpool baths beneficial as part of the treatment regime.
4. Feline Pyoderma	Bacteria such as *Pasteurella*, *Staphylococcus* and *Fusiformis* spp. commonly found in oral cavity of cats: when cat bites, its long sharp canines inoculate infection deep within skin, commonly resulting in cellulitis (diffuse infection of subcutaneous tissue). Cats exhibit signs of pyrexia, anorexia, depression, pain and swelling at site of bite wound. Treatment: systemic antibiotics; drainage usually successful.

Fig. 23.38. Pyodermas.

Ringworm

Ringworm, also known as **dermatophytosis**, may infect the skin, nails and/or hair. It is a fungal disease caused by only two organisms of major significance in the dog and cat: *Microsporum* spp. and *Trichophyton* spp. (Fig. 23.39). More details of these species are given in Chapter 16 (Parasitology and Fungi).

Ringworm is not common in the dog but it is a common cause of skin disease in the cat. Infection is acquired by direct contact or through fomites. It is important to remember that ringworm is a *zoonosis*— owners might become infected and should be advised accordingly.

THE PREVALENCE OF *MICROSPORUM* AND *TRICHOPHYTON* SPECIES IN THE DOG AND CAT WITHIN THE UK (% CASES)		
	Microsporum canis	*Trichophyton* spp.
	Clinical signs	
Cats	94.5–98.5%	1.5–5.0%
Dogs	37.8–88.0%	12.0–62.0%

Fig. 23.39. Prevalence of *Microsporum* and *Trichophyton* spp.

Clinical signs. In dogs, clinical signs include circular areas of alopecia which may appear grey or erythematous with scaling and crusting. Lesions may be confined to specific areas such as the head or forelimbs or may be generalised. In cats, lesions may appear as circular areas of grey scaling or as miliary dermatitis, or the animal may remain asymptomatic. Details of diagnosis for ringworm are given in Chapter 22 (Diagnostic Tests).

Treatment. Many cases of ringworm are self-limiting and will ultimately settle without treatment. However, because this is a zoonosis and because cases can become severe, it is usual to treat clinical cases. As ringworm can survive off the host it is necessary to carry out a detailed programme as follows:

(1) Treat the animal with oral griseofulvin, given with a fatty meal to improve absorption of the drug. Maintain treatment until all the lesions have regressed. Griseofulvin should not be used in pregnant animals.
(2) Clip away the hair from lesions, especially in long-haired animals, to allow access for topical treatments.
(3) In dogs, apply enilconazole directly to the lesions. This is particularly useful where there are only a few lesions present. In cats, apply chlorhexidine washes.
(4) All in-contact animals should be checked for ringworm and treated at the same time. Burn all contaminated material such as bedding. Thoroughly disinfect the premises using sodium hypochlorite, formalin or imaverol solutions. Paint all woodwork. Advise the owner to seek medical advice if they develop skin lesions.

Allergic Dermatitis

Allergic skin conditions include:

- Urticaria (uncommon).
- Atopic dermatitis (common, inherited).
- Food hypersensitivity (true incidence not known).
- Contact dermatitis (uncommon condition due to delayed hypersensitivity reaction).

Figure 23.40 describes typical allergens, clinical signs, diagnosis and treatment for each group.

Intradermal skin testing

(1) Only xylazine and atropine sulphate should be used as sedatives—other drugs may interfere with the test.
(2) Lay the animal on its side.
(3) Clip the flank completely.
(4) Use a felt tip pen to label the flank for each allergen to be tested.
(5) Inject 0.05ml of allergen intradermally together with a positive control (histamine) and negative control (sterile diluent).
(6) After 30 minutes read the test by examining each site for a wheal formation. A positive result is where the wheal is greater than half the difference of the diameter of the positive and negative control.

ALLERGIES			
Allergic reactions	**Clinical signs**	**Diagnosis**	**Treatment**
Urticaria Wide variety including drugs, vaccines, insect bites/stings.	Appear suddenly as multiple swellings or wheals on the skin where the hair becomes erect and stands out. May be pruritic.	Based on clinical signs.	Remove cause and administer corticosteroids.
Atopic dermatitis Wide variety in the environment – most common include house dust, house dust mites, fungi, danders and pollens.	In dogs: 1-3 years of age, often initially seasonal but in some cases rapidly become permanent. Pruritus, especially face, feet, axilla and ventral abdomen. Self trauma may lead to secondary infection, alopecia and pigmentation of the skin. Some dogs develop ocular discharge and otitis externa. In cats: similar clinical picture, or atopy associated with miliary dermatitis, symmetrical alopecia, eosinophilic granuloma complex or facial pruritus.	Intradermal skin tests with multiple allergens.	Usually life-long. May involve corticosteroids, antihistamines, hyposensitisation, essential fatty acid supplements or topical shampoos such as colloidal oatmeal every 3 days.
Food hypersensitivity Individual cases reported following sensitisation to specific foods such as beef, horse meat, milk, eggs and fish.	May be associated with pruritic skin disease and occasionally gastroenteritis.	Difficult; may be achieved by feeding 'elimination diet' composed of single protein and carbohydrate source to which animal has no previous exposure. No other food (including titbits) should be permitted. Clinical signs should regress within 6 weeks but may be as long as 8 weeks, at which point single food items can be reintroduced to the diet in order to determine allergens involved. (	Long-term therapy: avoid specific allergens identified by the dietary trials.
Contact dermatitis Soaps, detergents, shampoos, topical drugs, plastic, rubber, nylon and other synthetic agents.	May develop after only 4-6 weeks exposure to allergen but usually follow a period of over 2 years. Lesions (most frequently on feet, ventral abdomen, neck and chin) are pruritic, erythematous, and often secondarily infected following self trauma.	a) Patch testing: suspect allergen is applied to clipped area of skin and held in place with bandage; patch is removed after 48 hours and skin examined for erythema. (b) Hospitalising animal in kennel without access to any bedding or other items from own environment: if clinical signs resolve, circumstantial evidence of contact dermatitis. Animal should now be introduced to single items from home environment until allergen(s) identified.	Avoid contact with identified allergens.

Fig. 23.40. Allergies.

24
Surgical Nursing

C. MAY

Inflammation

Inflammation may be defined in two ways:

(1) Inflammation is the reaction of normal tissues to an irritant.
(2) Inflammation is a process which begins following injury to a tissue and ends with healing or the eventual death of the tissue.

The second definition, though more cumbersome, is useful because it emphasises the dynamic nature of inflammation by referring to it as a process.

There are many different causes of inflammation, but they can all be divided into a few basic categories (Fig. 24.1).

The signs that characterise inflammation are known as the **cardinal signs**. They are:

- Redness.
- Swelling.
- Heat.
- Pain.
- Loss of normal function.

The cardinal signs of inflammation have been recognised for almost 2000 years. The redness, heat and swelling are all associated with an increase in blood flow to the inflamed tissues. Swelling occurs because fluid, rich in protein and white blood cells, leaves the blood vessels and enters the tissue spaces. Sometimes inflammation is classified by the nature of this exudate (Fig. 24.2).

The inflammatory exudate serves a number of important functions:

- It dilutes irritating substances in the tissues.
- It delivers cells of the immune system to the tissues.
- It delivers immunoglobulins and other immune substances to the tissues.

THE CAUSES OF INFLAMMATION	
Cause	Examples
Pathogenic organisms	Viruses, bacteria, fungi, external and internal parasites.
Mechanical trauma	Blunt (direct) trauma, indirect trauma, lacerations, chemical injury.
Thermal injuries	Heat (burns), cold (frostbite), electrical burns, radiant energy (X-rays, sunburn).
Immune reactions	Serum sickness, delayed hypersensitivity, autoimmune diseases (e.g. rheumatoid arthritis, systemic lupus erythematosus).
Foreign material	Foreign bodies, tumours.

Fig. 24.1. Causes of inflammation.

CLASSIFICATION OF INFLAMMATION BY THE NATURE OF THE INFLAMMATORY EXUDATE	
Type	Notes
Serous	Serum is exuded from blood vessels into the interstitial space.
Fibrinous	The exudate has a high fibrinogen content and clots spontaneously. Especially seen at mucous and serous membranes (e.g. pericardium; pleura; peritoneum).
Purulent	The exudate consists of pus. Also called suppurative.
Haemorrhagic	Large numbers of erythrocytes are present together with some, or all, of the other constituents of exudates.
Mucus	Also called catarrhal. Characterised by the presence of mucus secreted from epithelial mucosa. Therefore restricted to mucous membranes. There may also be cell debris.

Fig. 24.2. Classification of inflammation by the nature of the inflammatory exudate.

- It delivers fibrinogen to the area to commence 'walling off' the inflamed site.

The pain associated with inflammation is due to increased pressure on nerve endings because of the swelling and to a direct irritating effect of toxic products. The toxins may arise from the cause of the inflammation (e.g. a bacterium) but they are more commonly a by-product of the inflammatory process itself.

The loss of function with inflammation results from pain-induced inhibition of muscle activity ('guarding'), the mechanical effects of swelling and tissue destruction.

Inflammation may also be classified by its duration as either acute or chronic.

Acute Inflammation

Acute inflammation is a process of short duration in which the cardinal signs of inflammation are usually obvious. There may also be systemic signs of illness including:

- Fever
- Increased pulse rate
- Increased circulating white blood cells, especially polymorphonuclear leucocytes (PMNL).

In most cases acute inflammation is a beneficial process leading to the elimination of the initiating factor and to eventual healing. However, there are several other possible outcomes and these are summarised in Fig. 24.3.

POSSIBLE SEQUELS TO ACUTE INFLAMMATION	
Sequel	**Notes**
Resolution	The acute inflammation subsides without significant tissue injury.
Healing	There is regeneration and repair of tissues damaged by the inflammatory process.
Abscessation	There is accumulation of pus which persists.
Degeneration	Damaged cells degenerate. This is most commonly seen in the liver and may be associated with fatty deposition in the cells.
Mineralisation	Mineral deposits in soft tissues are especially seen in chronic inflammation and in inflamed connective tissues.
Necrosis	Cell death occurs and the affected tissue is sloughed. Examples are seen in inflammation of the skin or intestinal lining.
Gangrene	Gangrene is cell death associated with the loss of local blood supply and putrefaction of the tissues by bacteria.
Chronic Inflammation	(See main text).

Fig. 24.3. Possible sequels to acute inflammation

Treatment of acute inflammation

There are two aims in the treatment of acute inflammation:

- Removal of the inciting cause.
- Limitation of the body's inflammatory response.

The method of removing the inciting cause depends on the particular initiating factor. For example, antibiotics may be prescribed when the initiating factor is a bacterium, or injurious chemicals may be washed away by lavage.

It is not always desirable to reduce the inflammatory response of the body, but when this is appropriate it is achieved by administering inhibitory drugs. The most commonly used drugs in the treatment of acute inflammation are corticosteroids and the non-steroidal anti-inflammatory drugs such as aspirin, carprofen, flunixin, ketoprofen, meloxicam and phenylbutazone. These drugs have potential toxic side effects and should only be used under the direction of a veterinary surgeon.

In superficial acute inflammation caused by trauma, damage can sometimes be limited in the early stages by the application of cold compresses to the inflamed area.

Chronic Inflammation

In some cases, the acute inflammatory phase fails to eliminate the inciting cause of the inflammation. Chronic inflammation is an ongoing response to persistent irritants. It is characterised by a marked mononuclear cell reaction and by proliferation of fibroblasts. The fibroblasts are a manifestation of repair. In chronic inflammation the processes of repair and inflammation occur together.

Chronic inflammation is a notable feature of certain diseases in which the inciting agent is of low toxicity and fails to elicit a sufficiently vigorous acute response in the host. Three major categories of this type of disease can be identified:

- **Persistent infections**, for example by intercellular organisms and by fungi.
- **Prolonged exposure to non-degradable material**, for example non-absorbable suture materials or inorganic foreign bodies.
- **Autoimmune disease**, for example rheumatoid arthritis and systemic lupus erythematosus. In these diseases, some of the inciting factors of inflammation are the animal's own body tissues. These can obviously not be eliminated and thus give rise to a chronic inflammatory response.

It is sometimes difficult to classify a particular inflammatory response as either 'acute' or 'chronic' because there is no clear dividing line between the two and both processes may occur simultaneously.

Tissue Type and Inflammation

The type of tissue in which an inflammatory response occurs can affect the structural changes and the course of events that ensue. **Abscesses** and **ulcers** are good examples.

Abscessation

Tissues such as the dermis, liver and kidney may be regarded as 'solids'. The presence of a pyogenic organism within these tissues can lead to the formation of pus which can be either localised (abscess) or diffusely distributed throughout the tissue (cellulitis).

DEFINITIONS

Abscess: A localised inflammatory reaction with a necrotic pus-filled centre.

Cellulitis: A diffuse inflammatory reaction with pus distributed through cleavage planes and tissue spaces.

Pus: An inflammatory exudate containing partially or completely liquified dead tissue mixed with large numbers of dead or dying PMNL.

Within an abscess, several different stages of inflammation and repair can be recognised at a single moment. Adjacent to the pus-filled centre is a layer of fibrin within which there are more PMNL. Peripheral to this zone is a layer of capillary and fibroblast formation. This outermost layer represents repair and serves to 'wall off' the inflammatory process to prevent it spreading to neighbouring tissue.

Toxins may sometimes be released from the abscess causing toxaemia which is potentially life-threatening. It is therefore helpful to encourage healing of abscesses as soon as possible. Healing of an abscess only occurs once there is discharge of its content. This sometimes occurs naturally by rupture of the abscess at a point.

Treatment of abscesses. Abscesses are treated by encouraging them to discharge their contents in one of two ways:

- By the application of hot compresses.
- By perforating (lancing) the abscess to drain it.

Hot compresses are only applicable to abscesses of the skin. They encourage eruption of the abscess at the skin surface, beneath the compress. More commonly, abscesses are treated by **lancing**. The abscess cavity is then drained and can be flushed with either sterile saline or with antiseptic solutions. Following the initial incision, **drainage** is encouraged by the continued application of hot compresses, or by leaving in place a surgical drain. The drained abscess collapses and heals by the deposition of scar tissue in the abscess cavity. Once drainage has been established, antibiotics may be administered to help eliminate causative bacteria.

In deep tissues, for example in the abdomen, it may not be possible to treat an abscess by drainage. In these circumstances the abscess may be completely excised along with a margin of normal tissue.

Chronic abscesses. A chronic abscess forms when an abscess fails to heal after it has drained. Chronic abscesses may result from incomplete drainage of the abscess at the time of discharge, or from the persistence of a foreign body in the abscess.

Chronic abscesses are characterised by a thick, fibrous wall enclosing granulation tissue. A sinus tract, lined by granulation tissue, may communicate from the abscess to the skin or a mucosal surface.

Treatment of chronic abscesses relies on removing the inciting cause (for example, by surgically removing a foreign body) and by providing adequate drainage.

Ulceration

An **ulcer** is a local excavation of the surface of an organ or tissue resulting from the sloughing of inflammatory necrotic tissue.

Ulcers particularly occur in the skin and mucous membranes, but they are also seen in other structures (e.g. the cornea of the eye). Ulcers usually result from mechanical injury, infections or damage by chemical irritants. Poor local blood supply may also contribute to their formation and they often become secondarily infected by bacteria regardless of the initial cause.

Ulcers contain inflammatory exudate within the crater and the edges are ragged after sloughing of the surface layers. In the healing phase, the base of an ulcer becomes covered with granulation tissue and there is re-epithelialisation from the edges.

Treatment of ulcers. There are three main aims during treatment of ulcers:

(1) To remove the inciting cause.
(2) To treat any secondary bacterial infections.
(3) To provide temporary protection for the healing surfaces.

Protection may be provided by dressings or by using the animal's own tissues. A good example of the latter technique is the suturing of the third eyelid over the eye in the treatment of corneal ulcers. It is not always possible to provide temporary protection of the healing surfaces. In situations (such as the mouth) where it is impractical to cover an ulcer, the surface may be kept clean with a suitable antiseptic solution until healing occurs.

Wound Healing

In most cases, acute inflammation is followed by healing. The precise outcome of healing varies depending on the nature and severity of the initial injury and the tissue involved. However, a number of basic processes can be recognised:

- Removal of dead and foreign material.
- Clearance of the inflammatory response.
- Regeneration of lost tissue components if possible.
- Replacement of lost tissue components by connective tissue.

The different outcomes can be summarised in three categories:

- **Resolution**—the return of tissue to its state prior to the onset of inflammation.
- **Regeneration**—the replacement of tissue destroyed by the inflammatory process with similar functional tissue.
- **Organisation**—the replacement of tissue destroyed by the inflammatory process with connective (scar) tissue.

For **resolution** to occur, there must be no tissue destruction by the inflammatory process and this is only likely to occur in mild injuries.

Regeneration of tissues is dependent on two factors:

- The lost cells must be capable of being replaced.
- The connective tissue framework and the vascular supply on which the tissue depends must both be intact.

Cells may be classified into three basic groups, based on their ability to regenerate:

- **Labile cells** normally divide and proliferate throughout life. They are highly capable of regeneration and include all epithelial cells, blood cells and lymphoid tissue.
- **Stable cells** are normally quiescent, but are capable of increased mitosis in response to certain stimuli and may therefore regenerate in some circumstances. They include cells of the liver, kidney, endocrine glands, bone and fibrous tissue.
- **Permanent cells** normally only proliferate in foetal life and are incapable of regeneration. They include neurones and cardiac muscle cells. Skeletal muscle has limited powers of regeneration.

When tissues are unable to repair by regeneration, they will undergo **organisation**. The initial step in organisation is invasion by macrophages, fibroblasts and new capillaries. This new tissue is the **granulation tissue**. Gradually, the granulation tissue is replaced by **collagen fibres**. The blood vessels regress and there is shortening of the collagen fibres which causes the scar to contract.

This type of repair by connective tissue can be further classified into two subgroups:

- First intention healing (healing by primary union).
- Second intention healing (healing by secondary union).

First Intention Healing

First intention healing of tissues is seen in clean, surgical wounds when the wound edges are **coapted** (brought together) by sutures. The events in first intention healing are conveniently illustrated by considering such a wound in the skin:

- **Day 1**: The incision fills with blood clot which dries to seal the wound. There is an acute inflammatory reaction at the wound margins.
- **Day 2**: The surface of the epithelium begins to heal by regeneration. Damaged hair follicles, sebaceous glands and sweat glands may also begin to regenerate. The underlying connective tissue cells cannot regenerate, but there is hypertrophy of fibroblasts.
- **Day 3**: The inflammatory response begins to subside. Macrophages begin removal of dead tissue debris.
- **Day 5**: The tissue space below the regenerating epithelium is filled by highly vascular granulation tissue.
- **Day 7** Epithelial regeneration is almost complete. Collagen fibrils are deposited in the underlying tissue space.
- **Week 2** Fibroblast proliferation and collagen deposition continue. Contraction of the collagen and regression of the blood vessels begins.

Second Intention Healing

Second intention healing occurs when there is significant loss of the tissue, thus preventing coaptation of the wound edges. Second intention healing is a prolonged process involving the removal of dead material and the filling of a large tissue defect.

In the early stages, the base and margins of the wound are filled with granulation tissue. This process often starts whilst there is still active inflammation in the wound. As debris is gradually removed, the granulation tissue migrates in from the wound margins to fill the defect. Re-epithelialisation, by regeneration, starts at the wound margins on the bed of granulation tissue that is laid down. Fibroblasts in the granulation tissue undergo contraction and this serves to shrink the size of the wound considerably (**wound contraction**). Granulation and epithelial proliferation continue in the wound until repair is complete.

The Management of Wounds

Wounds are generally classified into four categories based on the degree of contamination of the wound:

- **Clean wound**. A relatively non-traumatic surgical wound, made under aseptic conditions and not entering the oropharynx or the respiratory, alimentary and urinogenital tracts. Clean wounds may be closed by suturing without drains.
- **Clean-contaminated wound**. An operative wound, made under aseptic conditions, penetrating the oropharynx, respiratory, alimentary or urinogenital tracts but without undue contamination.
- **Contaminated wound**. A fresh traumatic wound or a surgical wound with a major break in aseptic technique. Also surgical wounds which encounter acute non-purulent inflammation, such as cystitis.
- **Dirty (infected) wound**. Includes old traumatic wounds (more than 6 hours) or surgery for perforated viscera in the abdomen. The organisms which cause wound infection are already present in the field of surgery before operation.

Post-operative Management of Surgical Wounds

Wound dehiscence and infection are prevented partly by attention to pre-operative preparation of the patient and by good surgical technique, but also by good post-operative care of surgical wounds. The main principles of managing a clean surgical wound are:

- Dressing the wound.
- Observation of the wound and patient.
- Prevention of self-mutilation.
- Suture removal.

Dressing of surgical wounds

The purposes of wound dressings are:

- To absorb exudate from the wound.
- To protect the wound from contamination.

Some surgical wounds require no post-operative dressings. In many other cases, a simple dressing of an absorbent pad and non-adhesive surface in contact with the wound can be held in place with adhesive tape. Alternatively a spray-on film dressing is preferred by some surgeons. In some cases additional padding is required by providing a thick cover of absorbent material such as cotton wool or cast padding. Particular indications for additional padding in wound dressings include:

- Over wounds at sites exposed to trauma, such as the limbs.
- Over wounds which have a heavy exudate.
- Beneath pressure bandages.

Once in place, most dressings can be left until the time of suture removal.

Observation of the wound and patient

Nurses are very well placed to detect early signs of wound complications by careful observation of the surgical wound. If a dressing is placed on the wound it may not be possible to observe the wound directly, but the skin surrounding the wound and the dressing itself can be observed. The factors to pay particular attention to are:

- **Exudate**: Note the amount, colour and type (e.g. serous, purulent). If exudate continues to leak through a dressing, the dressing should be removed to observe the wound.
- **Erythema**: Note whether limited to the vicinity of the sutures or whether it extends further. Has the erythematous area increased or decreased in size since the surgery?
- **Oedema**: Note how severe the oedema is and whether it is increasing or reducing.
- **Haematoma**: Note how severe the haematoma is and whether it is increasing or reducing.
- **Pain**: Note the severity of the pain (a subjective 1–10 scale is sometimes helpful) and whether the pain is continuous, intermittent, only present when the wound is handled or if there is no pain.
- **Odour**: Note if there is a foul odour from the wound.

In addition to monitoring the wound, good post-surgical wound care involves monitoring the patient for any signs of systemic illness which may be associated with wound complications. Both subjective and objective assessments should be performed:

- **Subjective assessments**: Note whether the animal is bright, alert and responsive or whether there has been a change in demeanour since before the surgery. Also note progressive changes in demeanour throughout the post-operative recovery phase.
- **Objective assessments**: Daily monitoring of temperature, pulse and respiration, a note of appetite, defecation and urination should constitute the minimum daily assessment of hospitalised patients in the postoperative phase. In some cases a more detailed clinical examination including other factors such as water intake or blood parameters may be indicated.

Prevention of self-mutilation

Self-mutilation at the surgical incision may lead to wound dehiscence. Some tendency to lick the wound is common in many animals post-operatively and need not necessarily give cause for concern. Persistent licking or chewing at the wound is an indicator of wound complications developing in some animals. In other cases an individual animal will continuously lick or chew at the surgical site for no obvious reason.

Prevention of self-mutilation begins in the operating theatre with good surgical technique. Wounds closed under tension, or with sutures placed too tightly, are more likely to irritate the animal and lead to excessive chewing at the wound. A good post-operative dressing will help in some measure to protect a wound from self-mutilation, but a determined animal will soon destroy most bandages

Many devices exist for the prevention of self-mutilation and all rely on preventing the animal traumatising the wound by either chewing or scratching. The Elizabethan collar (Fig. 2.12) is one of the most useful and commonly employed devices to prevent chewing or alternatively the use of bitter tasting substances painted on the dressing. Damage by scratching can often be prevented by covering the feet with well-padded foot bandages.

Removal of sutures

The purpose of sutures is to approximate the wound edges to allow rapid first intention healing with minimal scarring. Alternatives to sutures which may be used in some cases include metal clips, or staples and wound tapes.

Skin sutures should be removed as soon as there is adequate healing of the wound. In most cases this will be between the 7th and 10th post-operative day. However, in some young animals wound healing may be quicker and in old or otherwise debilitated animals it may be necessary to leave skin sutures in for longer. Some surgeons may use subcuticular sutures (placed in the dermis rather than through the epidermis and dermis) to close certain wounds. Absorbable sutures are often used for subcuticular sutures and these do not require removal. However, the wound should still be inspected at 7–10 days post-operatively to ensure that adequate healing has occurred.

Complications of Surgical Wounds

The main complication of surgical wound closure is **dehiscence** (the breakdown of a wound along all or part of its length). Several factors increase the chances of dehiscence:

- Infection of the wound.
- Seroma formation.
- Decreased blood supply to the wound.
- General health of the patient.
- Poor pre-operative preparation of the patient.
- Poor surgical technique.
- Poor suture technique or inappropriate suture materials.
- Poor post-operative care of the wound.

Of these, infection is by far the most common cause of wound dehiscence.

Other complications of wound healing include:

- **Sinus**, a late infective complication of surgery. A sinus is a blind-ending tract, lined by granulation tissue and usually ending in an abscess cavity. Sinuses in surgical wounds are often focused on suture material or other foreign material left in the wound at the time of surgery.
- **Fistula**, an abnormal tract connecting two epithelial surfaces, or connecting an epithelial surface to the skin. This may be a complication of wound healing or, rarely, a congenital abnormality. An example of a congenital fistula is the rectovaginal fistula in which a tract connects the lumen of the rectum to that of the vagina.
- **Incisional hernia**, a late complication of abdominal surgery in which there is dehiscence of the incision in the muscle layers whilst the overlying skin remains intact. Abdominal contents will often occupy the space between the dehisced muscles.

Some specific factors which influence wound healing include:

- The site of the wound.
- Local wound factors.
- Systemic factors.
- Duration of pre-operative stay.
- Pre-operative bathing of the patient.
- Hair removal at the operation site.
- Bowel preparation.
- Operative factors.
- Wound closure techniques.

The site of the wound

Surgical incisions should normally be made along lines of natural cleavage in the skin. Incisions along these lines fall naturally together and tend to heal more rapidly than incisions across the lines of natural cleavage. Another good example of how the site of incision can affect wound healing is found in limb surgery. Approaches to joints usually avoid crossing the flexor surface of the joint where there is increased risk of post-operative contracture leading to deformity and loss of function.

Local wound factors

Poor blood supply (as occurs in some areas of the body), dehydration of the wound, excessive exudation, foreign bodies, necrotic tissue, recurrent trauma and prolonged exposure to low temperatures can all delay wound healing and increase the risk of wound breakdown.

A **seroma** is a collection of serum or, more frequently, blood and serum in tissue spaces. The formation of a seroma at the wound site increases the risk of wound complications for several reasons:

- It is an excellent medium for the growth of micro-organisms.
- It increases tension on the wound.

- It can interfere with re-vascularisation, particularly in certain skin grafting techniques when it is important that the grafted skin acquires a new blood supply.

Seromas tend to develop in surgical wounds when large gaps (known as **dead spaces**) are left between the tissue layers. They are prevented by either scrupulous attention to wound closure and elimination of dead space or, where this is not possible, by the use of a drainage tube placed at the time of surgery.

When they do occur, seromas are treated by drainage under strict aseptic precautions. The seroma may be drained surgically, or by aspiration with a needle and syringe.

Systemic factors

Generalised systemic disorders (such as malnutrition, haematological, cardiovascular or respiratory disease causing reduced oxygen supply to the tissues, renal disease, liver disease, chronic infection) and certain therapies (including steroids, cytotoxic drugs and radiotherapy) may all result in delayed or impoverished wound healing.

Duration of pre-operative stay

Longer stays in hospital before operations increase the risk of wound infection and breakdown. The reasons for this are not fully understood, but it may be that hospitalisation reduces general fitness and causes endogenous release of steroids through stress. Alternatively, the patient's skin may become colonised with micro-organisms other than its normal skin commensals.

Pre-operative bathing of the patient

Pre-operative bathing with non-medicated soap does not reduce the incidence of wound infection and breakdown. However, pre-operative bathing with an antiseptic solution, such as 4% w/v chlorhexidine may be of benefit in reducing the incidence of wound infection.

Hair removal at the operation site

Shaving the operative site actually increases the risk of infection in clean surgical wounds. Hair should be clipped with electric clippers in the preparation room prior to surgery.

Bowel preparation

The normal colon contains large numbers of micro-organisms and some of these are potential pathogens. Some form of cleansing of the bowel may be indicated before elective colonic surgery, but the requirements vary with different surgical conditions and, to some extent, with the personal preference of the surgeon. The surgeon should be consulted about the precise requirements in each case.

Operative factors

Longer operation times, greater degrees of trauma inflicted by the surgery and increased amounts of foreign material (such as sutures) left in the wound all increase the probability of subsequent wound breakdown. Preparation of the operative site by cleansing with an antiseptic solution such as chlorhexidine or povidone iodine and the use of sterile drapes, gowns, gloves, theatre hats and masks all restrict the contamination of wounds by bacteria from the skin of the patient and the surgical team, thereby decreasing the chances of wound breakdown.

Wound closure technique

Most surgical wounds are closed by suturing. The aim is to restore functional integrity to the sutured tissues and encourage first intention wound healing with minimal scarring. Poor suture technique can lead to a wound which is more likely to break down. Examples of poor technique include:

- Overtight sutures leading to tissue necrosis below the suture material.
- Small 'bite' of tissue; larger bites generally result in stronger wounds than small bites.
- Inappropriate distance between sutures. Different wounds require different spacing of the sutures. Placing too few sutures, or placing too many sutures, can both lead to an increased risk of wound breakdown.
- Continuous sutures lead to a weaker wound than interrupted sutures.

Treatment of Wound Breakdown

First aid for wound dehiscence requires covering the wound with a clean, preferably sterile, dressing until definitive therapy can be instigated. In the case of abdominal wounds, dehiscence may lead to expulsion of viscera from the abdominal cavity through the wound. This clearly constitutes an emergency and the animal may require intensive therapy for shock. The exposed abdominal contents should be enclosed and supported in a clean, preferably sterile sheet until definitive treatment is available. The management of the infected or dehisced wound will be decided by the veterinary surgeon. However, the general principles of treatment are similar to those for all contaminated wounds.

The Management of Contaminated Wounds

The basic principles of managing contaminated wounds are:

(1) Cleanse the wound of all organic debris and necrotic, devascularised tissue. Surgical debridement may be needed to achieve this.

(2) Facilitate wound drainage, either by placing drainage tubes, or by treating the wound as an 'open wound' to allow second intention healing.
(3) Administer systemic antibiotics.
(4) If large areas of skin are missing, skin grafts may be used once the wound is clean and has filled with healthy granulation tissue.

Dressing Contaminated Wounds

Specific dressings may be of help in managing contaminated wounds. For the purposes of dressings, contaminated wound management can be considered in three stages:

(1) Cleansing and removal of necrotic debris.
(2) Granulation.
(3) Re-epithelialisation.

Cleansing and removal of necrotic debris

The dressings of use in this stage are:

- Occlusive dressings (hydrocolloids).
- Hydrogels.
- Wet packs.
- Alginate dressings.

Occlusive dressings are dressings which retain moisture in the wound, which rehydrates necrotic tissue and encourages it to slough. These dressings are usually **hydrocolloids**, which are left in place for a few days before removing. In superficial injuries, repeated hydrocolloid dressings will successfully debride the wound, leaving a healthy bed of granulation tissue. If the areas of necrosis are extensive, the hydrocolloid dressings may be combined with periodic debridement with a scalpel.

Hydrogel dressings are an alternative to hydrocolloid dressings. They contain significant amounts of water, which contributes to rehydration of necrotic tissue. Hydrogels dry if left exposed to the air and so they should always be covered with a secondary dressing that prevents moisture loss.

Hydrogels and hydrocolloids are also available in bead or paste forms which are sometimes convenient for large or particularly deep wounds. In some cases they are combined with iodine which is released into the wound and has an antibacterial effect.

A cheap but less satisfactory way of rehydrating black necrotic tissue and encouraging it to slough is by repeated application of **wet packs** made of gauze soaked in sterile saline.

Alginate dressings are especially useful for wounds with significant tissue loss which have a heavy discharge of exudate.

Granulation

The requirements for a dressing to encourage granulation are:

- To provide a moist environment.
- To provide a warm environment.
- To have reasonable absorptive capacity.

Several dressings fulfil these requirements, many of which are also used in the cleansing stage of wound healing. Alginate dressings may be used if excessive exudation persists. If there is only slight or moderate exudation, hydrocolloid or hydrogel dressings may be continued even after all dry necrotic tissue has sloughed. When granulation is to be encouraged in a clean, low exudate wound, such as that created surgically, then a cavity foam dressing may be used as an alternative to hydrocolloids or hydrogels.

Re-epithelialisation

The requirements of a dressing to encourage re-epithelialisation are:

- To provide a moist environment.
- To be non-adherent.

There are many products available which satisfy these needs. The older types are paraffin-impregnated tulle, perforated film absorbent dressings, and semi-permeable film dressings. These are still very useful general purpose non-adherent dressings. More modern alternatives include polyurethane foams, hydrophilic materials and some other products specifically indicated for use on high exudate wounds such as burns.

Skin Grafts

Superficial wounds in which there is considerable loss of skin may not heal completely, or may heal unsatis-factorily, if left to reepithelialise from the wound edges. These animals are candidates for skin graft surgery, in which a portion of skin is taken from one body area to fill the deficit in another body area on the same animal. There are many different ways of forming a skin graft, but they can all be divided into two broad categories: skin flaps (pedicle grafts) and free skin grafts.

Pedicle grafts involve moving an entire portion of skin and subcutaneous tissue complete with an intact blood supply from one body area to another. The flaps survive because of their intact circulation. They are created from areas with a well-defined blood supply which can be preserved and which have sufficiently loose skin to enable the donor site to be closed by first intention. Common donor sites for pedicle grafts include the skin over the shoulder blade and skin over the rump.

Free skin grafts lack a blood supply of their own and must initially survive by absorbing fluid from the recipient site. They will only do this successfully if the site is clean and revascularised. Free skin grafts must therefore be made on to a fresh, clean surgical wound, or on to a well-established bed of granulation tissue. Free grafts can be classified in a number of ways:

- By the source of the graft.
- By the thickness of the graft.
- By the 'design' of the graft.

The graft may come from one of three sources:

- **Autogenous graft** from skin elsewhere on the same animal.
- **Allografts** from another animal of the same species.
- **Xenografts** from an animal of a different species.

Allografts and xenografts are rarely used in veterinary medicine. They may be used as a temporary cover, but permanent grafts are invariably of autogenous tissue.

Free grafts may be of either full thickness or split thickness. **Split thickness grafts** include only the epidermis and parts of the dermis, whereas **full thickness grafts** include the whole of the epidermis and dermis. Split thickness grafts are usually harvested with a special instrument designed for the purpose, called a **dermatome**, but they can be collected with a graft knife or a scalpel. The thickness can be varied so that different amounts of dermis are included in the graft. Split thickness grafts 'take' more readily than full thickness grafts, but they are not as strong and the hair growth on them is poor. They are also more likely to undergo contraction after they are placed at the recipient site.

Free grafts may be applied as one complete piece, or they may be divided into various shapes before being placed in the recipient bed. Commonly used designs include:

- **Pinch grafts**—composed of small plugs of dermis and epidermis which are implanted in matching holes cut in the granulation bed.
- **Mesh grafts**—the donor sheet of skin is 'meshed' using a scalpel or a purpose-designed machine. The end result resembles a string vest and can cover quite large areas.
- **Strip grafts** – the donor graft is cut into strips which are laid on the recipient bed of granulation tissue with small gaps in between each strip.
- **Stamp grafts** – like strip grafts, but each piece approximates to the size and shape of a postage stamp.

The aim of these different graft patterns is to create open spaces between the donor tissue to allow drainage until the whole area is covered by re-epithelialisation which progresses from the margins of the donor tissue.

Drainage Systems

Drainage is indicated for:

- Prophylaxis, to abolish dead-space in wounds.
- Therapeutic drainage of contaminated wounds.
- To remove fluid or air from the body cavities (e.g. the chest, or bladder).

Some drains are only needed for a few hours. Most wound drains are left in place for a period of 3–5 days. All drainage systems can be categorised as open or closed.

Closed drains

Closed drains can be further classified as either active or passive. **Active** drainage systems employ some form of suction device. This may be a high pressure system driven by a pump or a low pressure system. A simple low pressure, closed, active drain can be created from a plastic catheter and syringe (Fig. 24.4). Closed, **passive** systems of drainage employ a simple collection bag which usually relies on gravity, rather than suction, to encourage drainage. A simple closed drainage system for the urinary bladder can be created by connecting an indwelling urinary catheter to the end of a giving set with an empty intravenous fluid bag attached.

Open drains

Open drains are most commonly used for prophylactic drainage of wounds or for therapeutic drainage of contaminated wounds. All open drains are passive. There are many different types but all are made of soft plastic materials, such as latex, which will not irritate the tissues. The Penrose drain is probably in most common usage in veterinary practice. Open drains rely on capillary action to remove fluid from a potential space in the tissues. Their ability to drain fluid is therefore directly proportional to the surface area of drain exposed to the tissues. Open, passive drains have the advantage of being cheap and simple.

Disadvantages of drains

The main disadvantages of drains are:

- They can act as retrograde conduits for secondary infections to gain access to a body cavity or wound space. This risk is greater with open drains than it is with closed drains.
- They are foreign bodies. The mere presence of a drain reduces the local resistance of local tissues to infection.
- They can cause damage to the tissues if they are made of hard materials or are incorrectly placed. Tissue damage may lead to fistulae or secondary haemorrhage because of blood vessel injury.

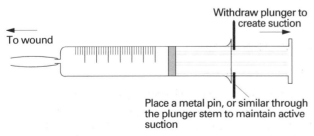

Fig. 24.4. Syringe and catheter drain.

The management of drains

Many drains, particularly the more complex active drains, are supplied with manufacturers' instructions and these should always be read and adhered to. However, some general principles of drain management can be outlined:

- Document the volume and the nature of the fluid exuding from the drain.
- Ensure that drainage tubes are not obstructed.
- When changing bottles or bags on closed drainage systems, it is important to avoid reflux of fluid which may introduce infection to the drainage site.
- Dressings should be changed before they become soaked in exudate. Great care must be taken to maintain cleanliness around the drain and the associated wound at all times.
- Wound drain sites should be observed for leakage and signs of local wound infection. The patient should be observed for signs of systemic illness.
- Passive, open drains in wounds may be shortened to minimise the risk of accumulating infected material. The end of the drain should be anchored to the skin to prevent it being retracted into the wound.
- An Elizabethan collar, or similar device, is usually essential to prevent the animal removing the drain prematurely.
- Drains are removed using aseptic technique. The procedure is well tolerated and no sedation or anaesthesia is required.

Hypothermia

Hypothermia is an abnormally low body temperature. It occurs in warm-blooded animals whenever there is a reduction in heat production by the animal or when there is excessive loss of heat. Normal heat production occurs as a result of metabolic activity and through normal muscle activity. Animals with an abnormally low metabolic rate, such as those with malnutrition or with hypothyroidism, are more likely to be hypothermic. Similarly animals which are inactive are more likely to be hypothermic. Heat losses are increased when there is a low ambient temperature, when the skin is damp and when there is a draught. Considerable heat losses can also occur through evaporation of moisture from the respiratory tract.

Many of the conditions which lead to hypothermia are present when an animal is anaesthetised for surgery. The metabolic rate is lowered, the animal may be inactive for a prolonged period, hair is clipped from a large area of skin and the skin is soaked during routine pre-operative scrub procedures. During the surgery, much heat is lost through evaporation resulting from the externalisation of tissues and internal organs. Heat losses from the respiratory tract are greater when a non-rebreathing anaesthetic circuit is used and the animal constantly breathes cold gases.

Small animals are more prone to such heat losses than large animals because they have a relatively large ratio of body surface area to weight, giving proportionately greater heat losses. Unfortunately, it is often impossible to use rebreathing anaesthetic circuits for such animals because of the excessive resistance to breathing inherent in such devices. In very small animals, such as hamsters and budgerigars, heat loss under hypothermia is a significant risk even under the shortest anaesthetic.

The clinical signs of a hypothermic animal include:

- Shivering.
- Cold extremities.
- Pallor of the mucous membranes.
- Reduced pulse rate.
- Subnormal core temperature (rectal or oesophageal).

Prolonged or severe hypothermia leads to the death of the animal, but in many more cases hypothermia is responsible for a poor or delayed recovery from anaesthesia.

Treatment of Hypothermia

Treatment centres on reducing further heat losses and *slowly* restoring the animal's body temperature to normal. It is very difficult to influence heat production by the animal. The following steps are useful:

- Wrap the animal in an insulating material such as a blanket, bubble packing or a 'space blanket' (reflective foil)
- Warm all intravenous fluids to 37°C by running a coil of tubing from the giving set through a basin of warm water placed close to the animal, or by using a purpose-made electric fluid warmer if this is possible.
- Ensure that the animal is kept in a warm room.
- *Gently* warm the animal using hot water-bottles or a hair dryer. Care must be taken in such procedures. Hypothermic animals have a reduced peripheral circulation and are very prone to being burned by the direct application of heat. Water-bottles should be insulated in blankets and constantly checked to ensure that they are not overheating the animal's skin. Hair dryers should be used on a low setting and the direction of air flow should be constantly moved so that it does not centre on one portion of skin.
- Many hypothermic animals shiver violently during the recovery period. This markedly increases oxygen consumption and it may be necessary to provide oxygen at this time.

Prevention of Hypothermia

Prevention is preferable to treatment. Many of the steps outlined above can be used as preventive measures and a few extra precautions can be taken during prolonged anaesthesia or anaesthesia of very small animals:

- Purpose-made heating pads can be used on the operating theatre table.
- A rebreathing circuit can be used if this is practical. Alternatively a suitable humidifier can be incorporated into nonrebreathing circuits to minimise heat losses by evaporation from the airway.
- The ambient temperature of the operating room should be kept as high as possible, whilst remaining suitable for working conditions.
- During skin preparation wet the skin as little as possible and cover the animal completely with drapes. The drapes should be kept dry throughout the surgery.

It is usually necessary to continue these precautions until the animal is completely recovered from anaesthesia.

Fractures

A fracture is a complete or incomplete break of bone continuity, with or without displacement of the resulting fragments.

Fracture Classification

An extensive classification system exists to describe different fracture types. Some of the more common and important terms are listed below:

- **Simple**: An uncomplicated fracture in which there is only one fracture line. Further terms are used to describe the direction of the fracture line relative to the bone. These include **transverse**, **oblique** and **spiral**.
- **Comminuted**: A complex fracture creating three or more fragments.
- **Open**: A fracture with an overlying open wound allowing potential contamination of the fracture with bacteria. Even pinpoint wounds are enough to justify classifying a fracture as open.
- **Closed**: A fracture which is not open.
- **Greenstick**: A fracture which is incomplete. The bone is fissured, but the fragments are not completely separated by the fracture line. Greenstick fractures are most common in immature animals.
- **Pathological**: A fracture resulting from normal use of a bone weakened by a disease process. The disease process may be generalised (for example a nutritional deficiency of calcium and phosphate causing weak bones), or localised (for example a tumour affecting the bone).
- **Avulsion**: A fracture in which a bone prominence is torn away from the rest of the bone, usually by the pull of a muscle.

Fracture Sites

In dogs and cats, most fractures affect the long bones of the limbs. Various terms exist to define the site of fractures in long bones and some of the more common terms are listed below:

- **Diaphyseal**: A fracture in the diaphysis, or midshaft, of the bone.
- **Physeal**: A fracture through the growth plate of an immature animal. Sometimes called a **Salter–Harris** fracture because a system of classification of this type of fracture was described by Salter and Harris.
- **Epiphyseal**: A fracture of the epiphysis.
- **Condylar**: A fracture of the epiphysis when condyles are involved (for example the distal humerus or distal femur).
- **Supracondylar**: A fracture through the shaft of the humerus or femur, just above the condyles.

Other common sites of fractures include the pelvis, the mandibles and the ribs.

Causes of Fractures

Except for pathological fractures, all fractures are caused by excessive trauma of the bone. Different types of trauma can cause different types of injury, so it is always important to know the cause of the injury. The type of trauma that causes a fracture is most commonly classified as either direct or indirect:

- **Direct trauma**: A physical blow to the bone causes it to break. Examples include the bumper of a car in an RTA (road traffic accident), kicks and gunshot injuries.
- **Indirect trauma**: The bone is broken by excessive leverage exerted upon it. Examples include avulsion fractures, limb bones broken if an animal puts its leg in a hole whilst running, or fractures sustained as a result of twisting of the leg after a fall from a height.

In general, direct trauma is more likely to cause a complex fracture which is comminuted or open and indirect trauma is more likely to cause a simple fracture.

Clinical Signs of Fractures

In most fracture cases there is a history of trauma. In the initial phases a fracture is an inflammatory lesion and many of the clinical signs can be attributed to acute inflammation. The major clinical signs seen in fractures are:

- Localised heat.
- Pain localised to the affected bone.
- Local swelling.
- Bruising at the fracture site leading to discoloration of the overlying soft tissues.
- Marked loss of function.
- Visible or palpable deformity of the affected bone.
- Abnormal mobility at the fracture site.
- Crepitus when the injured part is moved.

Radiographs should always be taken to confirm the presence of a fracture before definitive treatment is given.

Fracture First Aid

As described in Chapter 3, the pain suffered by animals with fractures may cause them to bite those who offer well-meaning efforts to help them. It is essential that the animal is adequately restrained before attempting any first aid. A muzzle is often needed (Chapter 1).

In many cases, animals with fractures have co-existing soft tissue injuries which may be more life-threatening but less obvious than the broken limb. Often, it is these soft tissue injuries which take priority in first aid. The first steps are always to ensure that there is an adequate airway, that the animal is breathing and that there is a good circulation. Shock is a major problem for fracture patients and fluid therapy may be an early requirement (Chapter 21).

The following specific first aid steps may be taken for the fracture itself.

(1) Cover any open wounds with a clean, preferably sterile, dressing.
(2) Provide some form of immobilisation for the fracture before attempting to move the animal.
(3) Special care is needed when a spinal fracture is suspected. The entire spine should be immobilised by strapping the animal to any straight and rigid structure of suitable length.
(4) In most cases, haemorrhage is adequately controlled by firmly bandaging a sterile pad over the wound. A tourniquet is only needed if there is pulsatile arterial bleeding which cannot be controlled by pressure pads.
(5) If a tourniquet is used, the time of its application should be noted so that it is not left in place too long (maximum 20 minutes).
(6) If possible, all drug therapies should be avoided until the patient has received a full clinical evaluation. Opiate analgesics may be given at the discretion of a veterinary surgeon. The time of administration and the dose of all drugs given in a first aid situation should be noted for later reference.

Splints in fracture first aid

This subject is covered in more detail in Chapter 3. In an emergency, almost any rigid structure of suitable dimensions can be used to immobilise a fracture. Some splints are used for definitive treatment of fractures (external co-aptation is described later). Two types of commercially available splints are useful in fracture first aid:

- **Zimmer splints** are made of malleable aluminium, backed by a foam composite. They can be shaped to conform with the limb and incorporated into a bandage to increase its rigidity. The foam backing is always placed towards the limb.

- **Gutter splints** are straight, non-malleable splints of rigid plastic, backed by a thin foam cushion. Like the Zimmer splint, they can be incorporated into a bandage to increase rigidity. They are stiffer than the Zimmer splint, but their use is limited because they are not malleable.

An alternative to splinting is the **Robert Jones** dressing described in Chapter 3. This is a bulky bandage applied firmly to the limb as a means of temporary stabilisation. The dressing both immobilises the injured limb and provides comfort because of its snug fit.

Fracture Repair

Following successful first aid and stabilisation of any life-threatening soft tissue injuries, definitive fracture fixation is required. An understanding of fracture fixation techniques requires a knowledge of both normal anatomy and the processes involved in fracture healing.

Fracture healing

The bone, its periosteum and the surrounding soft tissues are all damaged at the time of fracture. There is often considerable haemorrhage which, after 6–8 hours, coagulates to form a **haematoma** (Fig. 24.5). Some fragments of bone and connective tissues die as a result of the blood vessel damage and the dead tissues elicit an inflammatory response.

The haematoma is gradually replaced by granulation tissue and by the invasion of **stem cells** which will effect repair of the fracture. The stem cells migrate into the fracture gap, especially from the periosteum and the endosteum. Along with the stem cells there is a migration of new blood vessels derived from periosteal blood vessels and from blood vessels within the medullary canal of the bone.

The cells migrating into the area synthesise a tissue known as **callus**. Callus is composed of fibrous tissue, cartilage and immature bone. The callus envelops the bone ends, leading to an increase in stability at the fracture site. With time, the callus contains less fibrous tissue and more cartilage and bone. The stiffness of the callus thus increases and this further improves stability at the fracture site. Eventually the bone fragments are rigidly united by the callus. This is the point of **clinical union**.

Clinical union is followed by a prolonged period of bone remodelling. **Remodelling** is a process by which the initial callus is gradually removed and new bone is deposited. If the fracture fragments are accurately aligned, remodelling will restore the original shape of the bone. However, if the fragments are not kept in alignment during healing, the direction of the forces acting on the bone will change. The remodelling process will re-shape the bone to maximise its resistance to the new forces.

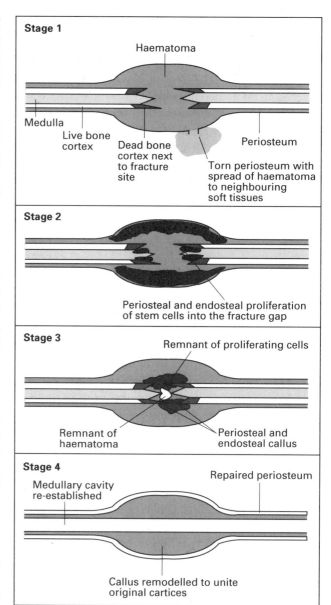

Fig. 24.5. Fracture healing stages.

The principles of fracture fixation

The primary aim of fracture fixation is to restore the functional anatomy of the fractured bone. This is achieved by:

- Restoring continuity of the bone.
- Restoring the length of the bone.
- Restoring the functional shape of the bone.
- Maintaining essential soft tissue functions.

Essential soft tissues include the blood vessels supplying the bone, muscles acting on the bone and nerves supplying the muscles. Any techniques for fracture repair must be sympathetic to these soft tissues because without them there is no chance of restoring function to the injured limb.

Many techniques exist for successfully restoring bone continuity, length and shape. However, the same basic principles apply to all the techniques:

- **Reduction**: The fracture fragments should be brought together in correct anatomical alignment. This may be done 'closed', by traction and manipulation of the limb, or 'open' by performing surgery at which the fracture is visualised and the individual fragments manipulated back into position.
- **Fixation**: The fragments should be immobilised in correct alignment until clinical union occurs.
- **Blood supply**: The blood supply to the bone fragments must be preserved. Fractures will only heal if there is an adequate blood supply.

The rate of fracture healing

Provided that there are no complications, clinical union is usually achieved in 12–16 weeks in adult dogs and cats. Remodelling may persist for many months, or even years, after clinical union has occurred. The rate of fracture healing is assessed by clinical examination to detect the increase in stiffness and the firm swelling associated with union by callus formation. Radiographs are taken to assess the degree of callus formation and the extent of mineralisation within the callus.

Many factors influence the rate at which fractures heal and it is important to be aware of these when contemplating fracture repair:

- Fractures of immature animals heal more quickly than adult animals.
- Geriatric animals heal fractures more slowly.
- Osteomyelitis interferes with healing and is one of the most common causes of poor fracture healing after surgical fracture repair. Healing can progress once the infection is overcome.
- Debilitated animals heal fractures more slowly. Debilitation may be due to poor nutrition or systemic illness such as hormonal disorder or kidney failure.
- Fractures in cancellous bone (epiphyses of long bones) heal more quickly than fractures in cortical bone (diaphyses of long bones).
- Fractures with access to a good blood supply heal more quickly than those in areas with a poor blood supply. For example, the pelvis and scapula are covered by large muscle masses which have a good blood supply. Fractures in these bones heal well. The distal one-third of the radius and ulna has little muscle cover and a poor blood supply. Fractures at this site heal poorly, especially in very small breeds of dog.
- Oblique fractures heal more quickly than transverse fractures because there is a larger area to promote tissue re-growth.
- Poor reduction or fixation of a fracture will result in a slow rate of healing.

Complications of fracture healing

In some cases, fracture healing does not progress normally. The complications that can occur in fracture healing include:

- **Non-union**: Complete failure of the fractured ends of the bone to unite. This is usually caused by one or more of the factors which slow down the rate of fracture healing.
- **Delayed union**: Fracture healing progresses slowly. Clinical union is not achieved within the expected time.
- **Mal-union**: Fracture heals in poor alignment. This is caused by inadequate reduction or fixation.
- **Osteomyelitis**: Infection of bone. Bacterial osteomyelitis is commonly caused by inadequate asepsis during fracture repair surgery. It is more likely to occur if there is also damage to the local blood supply.
- **Short limb**: Limb shortening occurs if there is healing with inadequate reduction of overriding fracture fragments. Limb function may be severely compromised.
- **Fracture disease**: Fracture disease describes an inability to flex the joints in a limb after fracture repair. One or more joints in the affected limb may be held rigid due to scar formation within the joints or within muscles surrounding the fracture site. Fracture disease is more common after fixation by external coaptation or when there is inadequate reduction.

Fracture Fixation Techniques

After reduction of a fracture, the bones must be held in position until healing occurs. In some cases, such as greenstick fractures and some fractures of the pelvis, immobilisation may be unnecessary and simple restriction of activity will suffice. The indications for immobilisation at a fracture site are:

- To relieve pain.
- To prevent displacement of the fragments (loss of reduction).
- To prevent movement that might cause delayed union or non-union.

Fracture fixation techniques are broadly classified into three groups:

- External coaptation, using casts or splints.
- Internal fixation, using pins, plates, screws and other devices
- External–internal fixation, using 'external fixators'.

External coaptation

Methods of external coaptation fall into three main groups: splints, casts and extension splints.

THE MAIN ADVANTAGES OF EXTERNAL COAPTATION TECHNIQUES

- They are technically simpler than some internal fixation techniques.
- They are economical.
- They are non-invasive compared with internal fixation.

DISADVANTAGES

- They have limited applications. For example, casts are most useful below the stifle in the hindlimb or below the elbow in the forelimb.
- They do not provide sufficient stability for some fractures, particularly comminuted or severely oblique fractures.
- They are prone to cause pressure sores.
- They restrict activity of joints and muscles in the limb and are therefore prone to cause fracture disease.

Splints. The splints described for use in fracture first aid may be used as definitive fixation in some fractures, particularly those occurring below the carpus or hock in cats and small dogs.

Casts. An ideal casting material should be:

- Strong and relatively light in weight.
- Easy to mould to the desired shape.
- Simple to handle.
- Waterproof, but sufficiently porous to prevent maceration of the skin.
- Rigid but not so brittle that it will splinter in normal use.
- Radiolucent (and, perhaps, amenable to imaging by other techniques such as ultrasound).
- Cost-effective.

Plaster of Paris bandages are still the most common casting material used, though recently many alternatives have been introduced. These are mainly polyurethane-based materials or thermoplastic polymers. They have the advantage of being light, waterproof and durable and have rapid drying times so that they reach full strength quickly (usually 10–30 minutes). They are also more radiolucent than plaster of Paris and less messy. However, the modern casting materials have the disadvantages of being more expensive and more difficult to apply than plaster of Paris.

Plaster of Paris

THE ADVANTAGES OF PLASTER OF PARIS

- Safe and non-allergenic.
- Easily moulded.
- Easy to use and does not need gloves in handling.
- Cheap.

DISADVANTAGES

- Slow to dry and to reach its full strength.
- Weakened if it becomes wet again.
- Heavy when wet (but does become lighter when dry).
- Not completely radiolucent.

Plaster of Paris setting times vary with the temperature and with the type of solution used for immersion. Low temperatures and sugar solutions slow the setting time, whilst warm temperatures and salt or borax solutions accelerate the setting time. In most cases plaster of Paris sets in a few minutes, but drying takes much longer. Often more than 24 hours is needed for complete drying of a limb cast. The cast does not reach full strength until it is completely dry.

APPLICATION OF A PLASTER OF PARIS CAST

A cast should normally stabilise at least one joint proximal to the fracture and one joint distal to the fracture.

Usually a cast extends from the foot to cover one joint proximal to the fracture.

(1) After reduction of the fracture, the injured limb is first covered with a tubular gauze.
(2) The tubular gauze is covered by a layer of cast padding material placed with 50% overlap at each successive turn. A provision should be made to allow 2 cm of cast padding and tubular gauze to protrude from either end of the plaster bandage.
(3) The plaster bandage is unwound by about 10 cm and the roll and the free end are immersed in water for a few seconds until air bubbles cease to rise. Cold water is used for longer setting times and hot water for shorter times.
(4) The plaster bandage is removed from the water, then squeezed *gently* to expel excessive water.
(5) The plaster bandage is applied from the distal limb working proximally. This encourages smoother application and reduces venous congestion resulting from application of the cast. At either end of the plaster bandage, 2 cm of cast padding and tubular gauze are left protruding.
(6) The overlap of plaster bandage is kept at a constant 50% or 60%. Gussets or tucks are created to keep this overlap constant at areas where the circumference of the limb changes.
(7) Once the layers of plaster bandage are in place, the cast is smoothed and moulded to fit the limb accurately. The cast padding and tubular gauze are turned back at each end of the plaster bandage to create a smooth edge. It is normal to leave the middle two toes just protruding from the cast distally.
(8) The limb is checked at regular intervals to ensure that circulation is adequate. The animal is not allowed to weight-bear until the cast has reached full strength.

When the animal is discharged, the owner should be given written instructions about care of the cast, potential problems with the cast and how to seek advice if problems arise. Figure 24.6 is an example which may be adapted for use in many practice situations.

INSTRUCTIONS FOR OWNERS TAKING A PET HOME WITH A BANDAGE OR CAST

1. The success of the surgery performed on your pet may depend on good care of the dressing. Much of this care is given by you at home, but your veterinary surgeon will need to check the bandage from time to time and the bandage may need to be changed. Bandage materials are expensive and bandaging is a skilled and time consuming job. A charge will be made for bandage changes.
2. If the animal goes outside in wet weather, cover the end of the dressing with a plastic bag held in place by string or a loose elastic band. **Remove the bag and elastic band as soon as the animal returns to the house.**
3. Check the dressing daily for evidence of swelling of the limb or chafing at the edges of the bandage. A small amount of talcum powder may help to stop chafing. If you are worried, consult your veterinary surgeon.
4. You should seek prompt attention from your veterinary surgeon if there is any evidence of problems with the wound or with the general well being of your animal. This might include, staining of the bandage with discharge from the wound, a foul smell from the bandage, slipping of the bandage from its original position, excessive chewing at the bandage or other signs of discomfort, general illness in the animal such as depression, lethargy or lack of appetite.
REMEMBER – IF YOU ARE WORRIED AT ANY STAGE, CONTACT YOUR VETERINARY SURGEON.

Fig. 24.6. Instructions for owners taking a pet home with a bandage or cast.

Application of plaster slabs (plaster splints). The indications for plaster slabs are:

- Slabs can be used on their own as initial splinting of an injury. They are more easily applied and allow more swelling than a normal cast. However, a plastic splint incorporated into a bandage is more frequently used in this situation.
- Slabs are more often used to reinforce a normal cast, especially at weak points such as joints.

To create slabs:

(1) Unroll plaster of Paris bandage on a dry surface.
(2) Double the plaster bandage backwards and forwards to provide a stack of suitable length.
(3) Hold the splint at both ends and immerse in water until bubbles cease to rise.
(4) Hold it vertically above the water to allow it to drain.
(5) Squeeze it dry, keeping hold of each end at all times.
(6) Stretch slab to its original shape.

The limb is prepared as for a normal cast and a single layer of circular cast applied first. Slabs are laid on the limb lengthways and may be held in place by a layer of wet cotton bandage. The cast is completed as before.

Application of modern casting materials. The basic principles of application of thermoplastic and polyurethane based casts are similar to those for plaster of Paris casts but the immersion and application requirements of these materials may be different. The manufacturer's instructions should always be consulted. It is usually necessary to wear gloves when applying resin-based casts. Conformation of the cast can often be helped by wrapping it in a wet cotton bandage during the hardening period. Often, the polyurethane materials are stronger, less bulky and lighter than a Plaster of Paris.

Some of the modern cast materials are amenable to the formation of a **split cast**. The cast is applied normally and allowed to set. It is then immediately removed by a single straight cut along its length which allows it to be eased off the limb if desired. When replaced it is encircled by strong adhesive bandage which holds it in place. This technique is useful when frequent inspection of the limb is needed during the healing phase. The split cast will also 'give' a little if required and so the method is useful for growing animals. The adhesive bandage is removed and replaced every 1 to 2 weeks, allowing the cast to expand as necessary in order to incorporate growth of the limb.

Cast removal

> WARNING
> Care must be taken not to damage the skin and other soft tissues during cast removal.

It is advantageous to have the animal sedated, and sometimes anaesthetised, when removing a cast. An assistant is often useful to hold the cast steady whilst it is being cut.

The most commonly used tools for removing casts are plaster shears and electric oscillating saws. The line of cut is chosen carefully to avoid any bony prominences. **Plaster shears** are inserted at the distal end of the cast and the cut is advanced proximally in small regular steps. As the shears approach the more fleshy proximal limb, the skin can be stretched by the assistant to minimise the risk of damage. Final cutting of the tubular gauze and cast padding can be made with scissors.

The **oscillating saw** is held so that there is no danger of coming into contact with either the skin or the electrical cable supplying the saw. Only the *plaster* is cut—the plaster padding will catch in the oscillating blade and not be cut. The circular blade gets quite hot as a result of its rapid oscillation in contact with the cast and so the saw should be gradually rotated to use a cooler part of the blade. It is often helpful to combine initial oscillating saw cuts with the use of plaster shears to remove a cast quickly and safely.

Extension splints. Extension splints (**Schroeder–Thomas splints**) have largely been superseded by internal fixation techniques and external fixators, but they are still used occasionally. Extension splints are most commonly applied to the hindlimb, but similar structures exist for use in forelimbs.

Extension splints are traction devices designed so that soft bandages act as slings to position the limb on a metal frame and counteract the pull of muscles. In this way the skeleton is immobilised. Indications for extension splints:

- Immobilisation of fractures distal to the middle of the femur in the hindlimb or the middle of the humerus in the forelimb.
- Immobilisation of joints at, or below, the level of the stifle in the hindlimb and the elbow in the forelimb.

Successful use of extension splints is completely dependent on accurate construction, tailored to the size of each individual animal and on accurate positioning of the completed splint on the limb. Failure to use the device properly may increase the risk of non-union. They are difficult to manage and require frequent adjustment to ensure that their position on the limb is maintained.

Internal fixation

Internal fixation, using pins, plates, screws and other devices, has both advantages and disadvantages compared with external coaptation.

ADVANTAGES

- They are suitable for fractures in any bone;
- They are more versatile than external coaptation for handling the full range of fracture types;
- They allow accurate reduction and relatively rigid fixation when compared to casting;
- Internal fixation often allows an early return to full functional limb use—this encourages fracture healing and minimises the risk of fracture disease.

DISADVANTAGES

- It is relatively expensive and time-consuming;
- Some internal fixation techniques are technically demanding;
- There is capital expenditure in the equipment;
- The risks of surgery (wound healing problems, infection) is inherently greater in an open reduction and fixation than in closed reduction and fixation.

In some cases. internal fixation methods may be supplemented with external coaptation or by an external fixator.

Implants used in internal fixation. The commonly used implants for internal fixation of fractures in dogs and cats are:

- Intramedullary pins (Steinman pins, Kirschner wires, arthrodesis wires and Rush pins).
- Cerclage wire.
- Bone plates (Venables plates, Sherman plates, Compression plates).
- Screws (tapped or self-tapping).

All of these implants can be sterilised and stored in a routine manner used for any surgical steel instruments.

Other internal fixation devices exist but are less commonly used in veterinary practice. These include intramedullary nails, locking nails and absorbable implants.

Intramedullary pins. The **Steinman pin** is perhaps the most commonly used internal fixation device for dogs and cats. Steinman pins are straight pins with sharpened, trocar-point ends. They are driven down the medulla of a fractured bone and across the fracture gap to hold the fragments together. A range of sizes are available to suit different sizes of animal and to fit into the many different sizes of medullary cavity. Selection of the right length and diameter of pin is important for successful fracture repair.

Kirschner wires and **arthrodesis wires** are really thin versions of the Steinman pin. Like Steinman pins, arthrodesis wires have a trocar point, but Kirschner wires have a flattened point instead. They may be used as intramedullary pins in small bones, but they also have many other applications in fracture repair.

Rush pins are highly specialised curved pins often used in pairs to anchor small epiphyseal fragments back on to the shaft of a bone. The point of the Rush pin is flattened to form a 'sledge', which is important to the way the pin functions when used in fracture repair.

Cerclage wire. Cerclage wire is malleable monofilament wire which comes in several different sizes suitable for use in different sized animals. It is most often supplied on a reel. Cerclage wire is usually used in combination with pins or plates to increase the stability of a fracture. Suitable lengths of wire are cut from the reel as required and they are anchored in place by twisting them with a pair of surgical pliers.

Bone plates and screws. Bone plates are rectangular plates of surgical steel which are fastened to bone using screws. They come in a range of sizes to suit different sizes of dog and cat. Plates are used to 'bridge' fracture gaps and therefore hold fracture fragments together. Screws may also be used to fasten fracture fragments together.

Two common patterns of bone plate are the **Venables plate** and the **Sherman plate**. These plates are held in place using 'self-tapping' screws. A hole is drilled in the bone and the screws are inserted into the holes. The screws cut their own way into the bone as they are tightened with the screwdriver in the same way that wood screws cut their own way into wood.

A more sophisticated type of plate is the **compression plate**. These plates are more rigid than the others and are specially designed in a way which allows fracture fragments to be compressed together. This helps to improve rigidity at the fracture site. Compression plates are used in conjunction with tapped screws. Unlike self-tapping screws, the tapped screws are not designed to cut their own way into the bone as they are driven with the screwdriver. Once a hole has been drilled, a special device (the 'tap') is used to cut a thread in the bone to the same shape as that of the screw. The screw is then placed into the 'tapped' hole. The tapped screws have greater holding power in the bone than self-tapping screws. Compression plate systems are more versatile than other plate systems and are capable of handling most fracture situations. However, the equipment for compression plating is very expensive, and the method for using the system is technically demanding.

Aftercare of patients following internal fixation

Immediate post-operative management of animals with internal fixation of fractures includes:

- Post-operative radiographs to check that the fracture repair is adequate.
- Monitoring carefully to ensure that the animal is maintaining airway, breathing and circulation and to ensure that it is normothermic.
- Analgesia may be required using either non-steroidal anti-inflammatory drugs or opiate analgesics at the discretion of the veterinary surgeon in charge of the case.
- The use of antibiotics post-operatively is controversial, but most veterinary surgeons will prescribe some antibiosis either pre-operatively or post-operatively.

When the animal returns home, its owner, plays a critical role in its aftercare. They have a natural tendency to be more cautious with animals that are in a cast or splint, which they can see, than with an animal after internal fixation, which they cannot see. The following advice should be given to all owners of animals after internal fixation:

- Although repaired, the fracture is a long way from healed. The animal must be restricted to the house or to a cage. Exercise periods should be on the leash and only for long enough to allow the animal to urinate and defecate (often less than 1 minute).
- Instructions for administration of any medication must be made clear.
- Regular post-operative check-ups will be necessary in the interests of the well-being of the animal and further radiographs will usually be needed. The importance of attending clinics for such check-ups must be emphasised.
- The owners should be instructed about possible complications (see below), how to recognise them and how to seek veterinary advice if these occur.
- In most cases active rehabilitation is not necessary. Some cases may benefit from passive flexion/extension exercises or from non-weightbearing exercise such as swimming once healing is under-way. These exercises should only be performed under advice from the veterinary surgeon in charge of the case.
- During the recovery phase, the animal should be fed adequate amounts of a well-balanced diet. Except for certain pathological fractures, the addition of mineral or vitamin supplements is of doubtful benefit.
- Suture removal will be necessary 7–10 days after the surgery.

Complications of internal fixation

The complications of internal fixation are those associated with wound healing and with fracture healing. The two most common complications are osteomyelitis and implant failure.

Osteomyelitis. Osteomyelitis may present shortly after internal fixation as an acute inflammation in the region of the fracture. The limb will be hot, swollen and painful. The animal may become systemically ill, inappetent and feverish. In the event of suspected osteomyelitis, veterinary attention is needed to decide the best course of treatment.

Implant failure. The metal implants used for internal fixation may fail either by breaking or by coming adrift from the bones. This will result in a sudden deterioration, with instability and pain returning at the fracture site. Some implant failures are associated with osteomyelitis. Further investigations will be needed to find the cause of the failure and to plan a suitable course of treatment.

Luxations and Subluxations

A **luxation** (also called **dislocation**) is a persistent and complete displacement of the opposing articular surfaces of the bones forming a joint.

A **subluxation** is an incomplete displacement of the opposing articular surfaces of the bones forming a joint.

Luxations and subluxations may be classified according to their aetiology into two types: congenital and acquired.

Congenital luxations or subluxations arise as anatomical abnormalities present at birth. The abnormality may or may not be inherited. The most common congenital luxation is that of the patella. This is usually amenable to surgery to replace the patella in its normal position. However, some congenital luxations are so severe that they cannot be corrected. Some small dogs and cats are able to cope with the permanently luxated joint, but in larger animals severe congenital luxation may be a cause of great disability.

Acquired luxations and subluxations result from some form of trauma, such as a road traffic accident. The ligaments restraining the joint in its normal position are damaged and the joint is forced out of alignment. Acquired luxations most commonly occur in the hip and elbow joints. Less commonly affected are phalangeal joints and the hock and acquired luxations of the shoulder are rare. The stifle is a common site for acquired subluxation as a result of rupture of the cranial cruciate ligament.

Treatment of luxations requires restoration of the normal anatomical relationship of the bones of the joint and stabilisation of any ligamentous injuries. Like fracture reduction, reduction of luxations may be achieved in one of two ways:

- **Closed reduction** is reduction of the joint by manipulation of the limb. Specific manipulations, depending on the joint involved and the direction of displacement of the bones, are essential for successful closed reduction. Simple brute force is unlikely to succeed and may cause further injury.
- **Open reduction** is a surgical approach to the joint: the luxated bones are visualised and manipulated back into the joint.

Closed reduction is preferable to open reduction whenever possible. Reduction is more successful if performed early—a delay of several days results in contraction of the surrounding soft tissues which renders closed reduction difficult, or impossible.

Radiographs should always be taken before any attempt is made at reduction. This allows the diagnosis to be confirmed and also determines whether there is any other damage, such as a fracture. Fractures affecting the joint surface will complicate any attempts to reduce the luxated joint.

For many luxations, *general anaesthesia* is required before reduction can be attempted. Some luxations, such as the patella, phalangeal joints and shoulder, may be reduced in conscious animals.

Post-operative care is similar after both open and closed reductions except that open luxations require the added precautions taken following all surgery. The main postoperative aim is to avoid forces that could cause a recurrence of the luxation. Support bandages, or non-weightbearing slings are useful for 5–7 days to prevent overuse of the joint. Exercise should be restricted, as for fracture healing, for a period of 3–4 weeks; thereafter, the animal's exercise can be slowly increased again.

Complications that may arise following treatment of luxations include:

- Re-luxation is the most common complication, especially if activity is not sufficiently restricted, or if there is other pathology in the joint, such as a fracture.
- Joint infection is a risk, especially if an open reduction has been performed.
- There may be injury to surrounding soft tissues, associated either with the original trauma or with the reduction of the joint. These injuries may not be obvious at first. They include damage to nerves in the region of the joint.

Orthopaedic Instrumentation

Orthopaedic surgery is technically complex and involves a wide range of instruments in addition to the standard surgical instrumentation (Chapter 26). It is beyond the scope of this text to provide a fully comprehensive review of orthopaedic instruments, but a brief discussion of the more common instruments is relevant. Care of most of the instruments is routine: they can be cleaned, sterilised and stored like any other surgical instrument (Chapter 25). Some require special attention.

The pin introducer

This consists of a drill chuck on a handle. It is primarily used for driving intramedullary pins into bone, but may be used as a drill on some occasions. The pin introducer is sometimes (incorrectly) referred to as a **Jacob's chuck**, which is actually the part of the introducer that grips the pin. Jacob's chucks may also be found on drills.

Orthopaedic drills

Three basic types of orthopaedic drill are available:

- Hand drills.
- Air drills (driven by compressed air).
- Electric drills (with rechargeable batteries).

Hand drills and air drills can be autoclaved. The moving parts require periodic oiling and specific instructions are provided by the manufacturers for individual drills. Electric drills cannot be immersed in solutions or autoclaved; they are supplied with a cloth 'sock' (shroud) which is autoclaved and encloses the drill when it is in use.

Depth gauge

This is a calibrated instrument used to measure the depth of a drill hole so that the appropriate length of screw can be selected.

Screwdrivers, mallets, chisels and saws

These instruments are surgical steel equivalents of normal carpentry tools. Chisels have one edge of the instrument blade bevelled. This differentiates chisels from osteotomes which have both edges bevelled.

Retractors

Retractors are useful in all sorts of surgery for restraining tissues in the surgical field. Many different types are available and they can broadly be divided into two groups:

- **Hand-held** retractors are held by the surgeon or an assistant to restrain tissues.
- **Self-retaining** retractors have a scissor-like action and some form of ratchet which locks them in place. Once inserted and locked they will remain in place and restrain tissues without being held. Self-retaining retractors are especially useful for surgeons working alone.

Patterns of retractor particularly useful in orthopaedic surgery include **Langenbeck** retractors, **Hohman** retractors (both hand-held) and **Gelpi** retractors (self-retaining).

Bone-holding forceps

Bone-holding forceps are designed to grasp bones during open reduction of fractures and to hold them in a reduced position whilst definitive fixation is applied. They all have a scissorlike action and some have a ratchet or similar device to enable them to be locked in place. There are many different patterns. The choice of instrument depends partly on the needs of the particular fracture and partly on the personal preference of the surgeon.

Bone-cutting forceps and rongeurs

Bone-cutting forceps are shearing tools designed specifically for cutting through bone. Rongeurs are scissor-action tools designed for nibbling away at bone and removing small bits.

Common Surgical Conditions

In addition to anatomical terminology and the pathological terms outlined above, surgery has its own extensive terminology (Fig. 24.7). Surgical terms with similar meanings often share a common suffix such as -otomy, -ostomy, -ectomy, -centesis, -oscopy (which each indicate a different type of surgical procedure) or -itis (which indicates inflammation).

Some of the more common surgical conditions of the dog and cat will now be considered.

Surgery of the Eye

Common conditions of the eye amenable to surgery include conjunctivitis, keratitis, entropion, ectropion, distichiasis, tumours and cataracts. There are also several emergency conditions.

Conjunctivitis. Conjunctivitis is inflammation of the conjunctival membrane characterised by reddening of the conjunctiva. It is a frequent sequel to many other ocular diseases, including ocular infections, foreign bodies in the eye, entropion, ectropion and inflammatory diseases of the eyeball.

Keratitis. Keratitis is inflammation of the cornea, which may be accompanied by ulceration. The inflamed cornea is cloudy. The addition of fluorescein to the eye allows better visualisation of corneal ulcers. In severe cases, corneal ulcers may perforate causing the cornea to rupture. Ulcers are treated medically, or by creating a protective flap from the conjunctiva or third eyelid. Keratitis and ulceration is often secondary to some other disease of the eye which may also require treatment.

Entropion. Entropion is inversion of the eyelid margin such that the eyelashes rub on the cornea. There is often secondary conjunctivitis and keratitis. Entropion is treated by surgery to return the eyelid margin to its normal position.

Ectropion. Ectropion is eversion of the eyelid margin. In most cases, ectropion does not require surgical attention, but in some dogs it gives rise to chronic conjunctivitis or keratitis, thus requiring surgical correction. Certain breeds of dog exhibit both ectropion and entropion at different points along the margins of one or both eyelids.

Distichiasis. Distichiasis is the most common of a group of disorders characterised by abnormal growth of hairs at the eyelid margin so that the hairs rub against the cornea. In many cases, the hairs do not cause a clinical problem, but in some cases they cause chronic keratitis requiring treatment. Several surgical techniques exist for treating distichiasis, but all centre on removal of the offending hairs.

Tumours. Tumours on the margin of the eyelid are common in dogs. They are treated by excising a small wedge of the eyelid margin containing the tumour.

Cataracts. A cataract is the opacification of the fibres or capsule of the lens of the eye. This can occur for many different reasons. Cataracts may be left untreated or they may be treated by surgical removal of the cataract.

OCULAR EMERGENCIES

- **Eyeball prolapse.** Complete prolapse of the eye out of its socket (proptosis of the globe) can occur, especially in brachycephalic dogs. *First aid treatment is important if there is to be any chance of saving the eye.* The eye should be kept moist with KY jelly or something similar and gently supported in saline soaked swabs. Definitive surgery to replace the eye in its socket should be performed as soon as possible.
- **Glaucoma**, an acute elevation in the pressure within the eye which *can lead to permanent blindness within 24 hours if not treated.* There are several causes of glaucoma, but two of the most common are anterior uveitis and dislocation of the lens of the eye from its normal position. This is especially seen in the terrier breeds. In glaucoma, the eye is painful, the sclera is engorged and the pupil is usually dilated.
- **Ocular trauma.** Foreign bodies (including grass seeds, glass and gunshot pellets) may lodge behind the eyelids or they may penetrate the orbit itself. The eyeball may also be lacerated, for example by claws or teeth during fights with other animals. All these conditions are potential emergencies and require prompt veterinary attention.
- **Chemical irritation** of the eye by contact with noxious substances may also require emergency treatment. As a first aid measure, the eye should be irrigated with copious amounts of water or saline to remove as much of the offending chemical as possible.

SURGICAL TERMINOLOGY	
Terminology	**Meaning**
TEMPORARY OPENINGS	The suffix **-otomy** denotes a procedure for temporarily opening or dividing a tissue during surgery. The tissue is closed by allowing it to heal naturally, by suturing it or, in the case of bone, by reuniting it with pins, wires, screws or plates. Many of these terms describe common surgical approaches.
Laparotomy	A temporary opening into the abdomen.
Thoracotomy	A temporary opening into the thorax.
Cystotomy	A temporary opening into the urinary bladder.
Urethrotomy	A temporary opening into the urethra.
Enterotomy	A temporary opening into the intestines.
Gastrotomy	A temporary opening into the stomach.
Arthrotomy	A temporary opening into a joint.
Rhinotomy	A temporary opening into the nasal chambers.
Osteotomy	A temporary division of a bone.
Myotomy	A temporary division of a muscle.
Tenotomy	A temporary division of a tendon.
	Some surgical approaches can be further classified by the precise way in which the procedure is performed. For example, a laparotomy may be made in a number of ways:
Midline laparotomy	By an incision through the linea alba.
Paramedian laparotomy	By an incision slightly to one side of the ventral midline.
Parapreputial laparotomy	By an incision to one side of the prepuce in male dogs.
Pararectal laparotomy	By an incision just lateral to the rectus abdominis muscle.
Paracostal laparotomy	By an incision just caudal to, and parallel with, the last rib.
PERMANENT OPENINGS	The suffix **-ostomy** denotes the surgical creation of an opening, or **stoma**, which has the potential to be permanent.
Urethrostomy	A permanent opening in the urethra.
Tracheostomy	A permanent opening in the trachea.
Gastrostomy	A permanent opening in the stomach.
Pharyngostomy	A permanent opening in the pharynx.
	In some cases, the stoma is left permanently open, but in others further surgery is performed at a later date to close the stoma once again. Stomata are almost always into the airway, gastrointestinal tract or urinary tract. They allow access to these structures for special reasons. For example, animals unable to chew or swallow may be fed through a pharyngostomy or gastrostomy; animals with blocked urethra will be able to pass urine through a urethrostomy and animals with a blocked upper airway will get air into their lungs through a tracheostomy.
REMOVAL OF STRUCTURES	The suffix **-ectomy** denotes the surgical removal of all or part of a structure. This is commonly performed when neutering animals.
Enterectomy	Removal of a length of bowel.
Gastrectomy	Removal of a portion of stomach.
Lum lobectomy	Removal of a lung lobe.
Ovariohysterectomy	Removal of the ovaries and uterus (spay).
Orchidectomy	Removal of the testis (castration).
Ostectomy	Removal of a portion of bone.
	Enterectomies and gastrectomies are performed to remove irreparably damaged parts of the gastrointestinal tract. When this is done, the remaining ends of the gastrointestinal tract must be sutured back together, a procedure known as **anastomosis**. Although most commonly used in the gastrointestinal tract, anastomosis can be performed in any tissue where free ends can be rejoined; for example, blood vessels, nerves, ureters, urethra, etcetera.
INFLAMMATION OF TISSUES	The suffix **-itis** denotes inflammation in a given tissue.
Oesophagitis	Inflammation of the oesophagus.
Gastritis	Inflammation of the stomach.
Enteritis	Inflammation of the small intestine.
Colitis	Inflammation of the colon.
Cystitis	Inflammation of the urinary bladder.
Hepatitis	Inflammation of the liver.
Pancreatitis	Inflammation of the pancreas.
Rhinitis	Inflammation of the nose.
Tracheitis	Inflammation of the trachea.
Dermatitis	Inflammation of the skin.
Arthritis	Inflammation of a joint or joints.
Conjunctivitis	Inflammation of the conjunctiva.

Fig. 24.7.—Continued

SURGICAL TERMINOLOGY	
Terminology	**Meaning**
ASPIRATION OF FLUID	The suffix **-centesis** denotes the aspiration of fluid from a body cavity.
Cystocentesis	Aspiration of urine from the bladder.
Arthrocentesis	Aspiration of synovial fluid from a joint.
Pericardiocentesis	Aspiration of fluid from within the pericardium.
Thoracocentesis	Aspiration of fluid from the thoracic cavity.
	Fluid may be aspirated so that it can be analysed for diagnostic reasons or it may be aspirated for therapeutic reasons. For example, fluid is not normally present in either the pericardium of the thoracic cavity. The presence of fluid at these sites can be life-threatening and in such cases pericardiocentesis or thoracocentesis are life-saving procedures.
ENDOSCOPIC PROCEDURES	The suffix **-oscopy** denotes examination by various devices.
Endoscopy	An endoscopic examination.
Gastroscopy	Endoscopic examination of the stomach.
Cytoscopy	Endoscopic examination of the urinary bladder.
Arthroscopy	Endoscopic examination of a joint.
	Endoscopy is examination by the use of a fibre-optic device, the endoscope. Endoscopes are available in many different sizes, some small enough to fit into a joint or up the urethra, others long enough to reach down the oesophagus, through the stomach and into the small intestine. Other examination devices include:
Bronchoscope	A device for examining the trachea and bronchi via the mouth.
Laryngoscope	A device for examining the larynx via the mouth.
Proctoscope	A device for examining the rectum and distal colon via the anus.
Auroscope	A device for examining the ear canal.
Ophthalmoscope	A device for examining the eyes.

Fig. 24.7. Surgical terminology.

The retina

Although not amenable to surgery in most cases, the retina is an important site of disease in the eye. Of particular importance are a group of inherited diseases of the retina collectively known as **progressive retinal atrophy (PRA)**. These diseases occur in certain breeds. The British Veterinary Association and the Kennel Club check for PRA by running eye examination schemes, performed by specialist ophthalmologists.

Surgery of the Ear

DEFINITIONS

- **Aural haematoma**: A discrete collection of blood in the pinna (ear flap).

- **Otitis**: Inflammation of the ear.

  Three subgroups of otitis are recognised:

- **Otitis externa**: Inflammation of the external auditory meatus (ear canal).

- **Otitis media**: Inflammation of the middle ear cavity.

- **Otitis interna**: Inflammation of the inner ear, affecting the organs of balance and, less commonly, hearing.

Aural haematoma. Aural haematoma is the most common injury of the dog's pinna. It is generally believed to be self-inflicted as a result of scratching or head shaking which damages a blood vessel in the pinna. It is most commonly seen on the concave surface of the pinna, but may occur on either or both sides. The injury is usually secondary to otitis and treatment of aural haematoma must also concentrate on treating the primary cause of the otitis.

Haematomas resolve spontaneously if left alone, but the blood is a good medium for potential infection and the scar tissue that forms during resolution may lead to deformity of the pinna. For these reasons, most aural haematomas are treated by surgical drainage either by needle aspiration, or by surgical incision.

After incision, sutures are often placed in the pinna to close the dead space and prevent recurrence. Buttons, quills (lengths of rubber tubing) or some similar devices may be incorporated into the sutures to increase the compression of the dead space and to prevent the sutures pulling through. Post-operative care includes treatment of the primary ear disease and, in some cases, the ears are immobilised in a figure of eight head bandage to prevent further damage as a result of head shaking and scratching.

Otitis externa. Otitis externa is very common in dogs and cats. Inflammation of the ear canal may occur for many reasons, including:

- Foreign bodies in the ear canal.

- Ear mites (*Otodectes*).

- Bacterial or fungal infection of the ears.

- As an extension of generalised skin disease.

- Poor ear conformation, especially in the floppy-eared breeds.

Veterinary investigation is necessary so that specific treatment can be prescribed for the problem. Animals with otitis externa show irritation, and sometimes pain, centred on the ear.

EAR DROPS

Drugs for the treatment of otitis externa are often administered by ear drops. It is important that the drug carries well down into the ear canal and the veterinary nurse must be familiar with the anatomy of the ear canal so that suitable advice can be given to owners. The drops are first placed into the canal, which is then massaged to encourage distribution of the drugs. Excessive discharge can be cleared with cotton wool or tissue, but owners must be warned against probing down the ear canal with cotton buds or anything similar. If it is necessary to probe down the ear canal, either to retrieve a foreign body or to cleanse the canal thoroughly, this should be done under the direction of a veterinary surgeon as it requires a general anaesthetic.

Cases of otitis externa that do not respond to medical therapy may undergo surgery. Several different surgeries are used for the treatment of otitis externa, including:

- **Lateral wall resection** involves removing the lateral portion of the ear canal to improve drainage from the ear and to improve air circulation in the ear canal.
- **Vertical canal ablation (VCA)** involves the total removal of the vertical part of the ear canal, thus resecting the diseased tissue.
- **Total ear canal ablation (TECA)** involves resection of both the vertical and the horizontal parts of the ear canal. This procedure is more radical and technically demanding than the VCA, but it is finding favour with many surgeons because it removes all the diseased tissue.

Post-operative care following ear surgery is similar for all surgical procedures. The ear must be protected from self-inflicted head shaking and scratching injuries by using an Elizabethan collar, figure-of-eight head bandages or by bandaging the pinnae together as necessary. There is often discharge of blood and exudate from the ear and this needs gentle cleaning. Ear surgery can be very painful and thought should be given to analgesia in the immediate post-operative period.

Otitis media. Otitis media is frequently an extension of otitis externa when infection penetrates the ear drum. In some cases it may arise because of ascending infection via the eustachian tube, from the pharynx. Otitis media is much more difficult to treat success-fully than otitis externa, and so prompt therapy of otitis externa is indicated to reduce the risk of otitis media.

Otitis interna. Otitis interna causes a loss of balance and the head tilts to one side. There are other causes of similar findings in old cats and dogs and a careful examination is necessary to tell these apart. Examination may include taking radiographs of the skull. Treatment of otitis interna may include both medical and surgical therapies.

Surgery of the Gastrointestinal Tract (GIT)

The GIT includes mouth, pharynx, oesophagus, stomach, small intestine, rectum and anus.

The mouth and pharynx

Common conditions of the mouth include:

- Dental disease
- Congenital deformities
- Labial (skin fold) dermatitis
- Foreign bodies
- Tumours
- Ulcers
- Rodent ulcers
- Stings.

Dental disease

DEFINITIONS

- **Periodontal disease**: Disease of the tissues and structures which surround the teeth.
- **Dental plaque**: A film like deposit on the surface of the tooth consisting of a mixture including salivary deposits, bacteria and food particles.
- **Dental calculus**: A stonelike concretion of minerals on the teeth.
- **Gingivitis**: Inflammation of the gums.

Periodontal disease, associated with the build-up of dental plaque, is perhaps the most common dental condition encountered in small animal practice. Periodontal disease presents with gingivitis, gingival bleeding, halitosis and, in advanced cases, inappetence because of pain on mastication. The problem is exacerbated by the formation of dental calculus. Although gingivitis is commonly associated with dental disease, it may have a much more complex aetiology, especially in cats.

Veterinary dentistry has now developed into a speciality in its own right and many complex dental procedures are performed. However, the most common dental procedures are still measures of basic dental hygiene aimed at controlling periodontal disease, particularly by dental scaling.

DENTAL SCALING

- General anaesthesia is required. This allows a full examination of the mouth, together with radiographic examination if necessary, before scaling begins.
- Scaling should *never* be performed at the same time as other major surgery. Scaling releases bacteria from the mouth into the blood stream and leads to a high risk of infection in surgical wounds.
- The operator should wear a face mask and protective glasses as defence against aerosol bacteria and calculus liberated from the animal's mouth, particularly when ultrasonic scalers are used.
- The animal's head can be placed on a grill to keep it dry.
- Precautions should be taken to ensure that the animal does not inhale particles of calculus or any other debris released during the procedure. These precautions include:
  —the use of a close-fitting, cuffed endotracheal tube for maintenance of anaesthesia;
  —packing the pharynx with 2.5 cm gauze bandage to occlude the part of the pharynx not occupied by the endotracheal tube (the end of the gauze is trailed out of the mouth as a reminder that it must be removed at the end of the procedure);
  —recovery of the animal from anaesthesia in a 'head down' position.
- Large deposits of calculus are initially removed with dental forceps. Smaller deposits are removed with a dental scraper or, preferably, with an ultrasonic scaler. The ultrasonic scaler loosens plaque by liberation of high frequency sound waves which cause the tooth to vibrate. A spray wash helps to cool the tooth and remove the loosened debris. The tip of the scaler is moved lightly and rapidly over the tooth surface. It should not be used to scrape the tooth surface, nor should it be centred in one place for prolonged periods as the build-up in heat can damage the tooth. The gingival sulcus should also be gently cleaned.
- The spray on the ultrasonic scaler may include an antiseptic (0.2% chlorhexidine is commonly used).

Owners can help to prevent the build-up of dental plaque by regularly brushing their pet's teeth, providing the animal is amenable. A 0.2% chlorhexidine solution or a proprietary pet toothpaste may be used for this procedure.

Dental extractions. Dental extractions are performed for severe periodontal disease and for tooth fractures. Recent advances in veterinary dentistry have lead to the preservation of teeth which would previously have been extracted. However, dental extraction is still a common procedure in small animal practice.

GUIDELINES APPLIED TO DENTAL EXTRACTIONS

- The general precautions of anaesthesia and pharyngeal packing are similar to those for dental scaling.
- The tooth is thoroughly loosened using a root elevator. A number eleven scalpel blade may be used as an alternative in cats.
- Every effort is made to remove the roots intact and attempts should be made to remove fragments of root should they fracture during the extraction process.
- The canines, upper fourth premolar teeth and first molars of dogs have deep roots which may require reflection of the gum and alveolar bone before they can be adequately loosened.
- Teeth with multiple roots may be sectioned with a dental saw before loosening the fragments and associated roots individually.
- Only when the tooth is thoroughly loosened by root elevation should it be grasped with dental forceps for removal. Excessive force, or rocking of the tooth from side to side with the forceps should not be necessary and may lead to complications.
- Haemorrhage from the alveolar socket is usually self limiting, or it can be controlled by packing the socket for a few minutes.

Complications of dental extractions include:

- Incomplete removal of a tooth root.
- Persistent haemorrhage, which may be indicative of a bleeding disorder.
- Iatrogenic fracture of the mandible or maxilla.
- Creation of an oronasal fistula. This is seen especially in extraction of the canine from small dogs or cats.

Congenital deformities. One of the most common congenital deformities affecting the mouth is **cleft palate** and harelip. Suckling is difficult with this deformity and there may be problems with persistent nasal discharge, Affected animals may not thrive and they are often destroyed at an early age. However, if the puppy or kitten survives to 3 months of age, anaesthesia and corrective surgery may be practical.

Labial dermatitis. Labial dermatitis associated with bacterial infection of the skin folds around the lips is particularly common in breeds with prominent jowels, such as the spaniels. The infection may be a source of irritation for the dog and also gives off a foul smell which some owners mistake for halitosis. Medical treatment may give temporary relief, but many affected animals require surgery to remove the fold of skin, so that there is adequate air circulation to the area.

Similar skin fold dermatitis problems may occur in any area of skin liable to the formation of deep folds. These include facial folds in brachycephalic dogs, inguinal folds in overweight dogs and folds at the base of the tail in screw-tail dogs.

Foreign bodies. Foreign bodies such as sticks, bones and fish-hooks can lodge in the soft tissues of the mouth or between the teeth, or even penetrate the wall of the buccal cavity or the pharynx. All will cause pain associated with the mouth, difficulty in swallowing and excessive salivation. In some cases, radiographic or ultrasonographic examination is helpful in reaching a diagnosis.

The mouth can be safely examined by inserting ropes or leashes behind the canine teeth of the upper and lower jaws. The ropes are used to pull the jaws apart. Some sticks and bones can be grasped with forceps in the conscious animal and then removed. In other cases a general anaesthetic will be required.

It is important to note that the early clinical signs of **rabies** are similar to those seen with oropharyngeal foreign bodies. Although rabies is unlikely to occur in the UK, it is such a potentially dangerous zoonosis that it must be ruled out before progressing to examine an animal closely for a possible foreign body. If the animal is unknown to the practice, the owner should be questioned carefully about its past history.

Tumours. Tumours in the region of the mouth (including the tonsils) are often locally malignant. Some are amenable to resection using radical procedures which involve removing the tumour *en bloc* with a piece of mandible (**mandibulectomy**) or maxilla (**maxillectomy**). Although these procedures may seem excessive at first, they are often the only way of effecting a cure. Furthermore, the cosmetic results are often good and the quality of life following recovery from surgery is usually excellent.

Some tumours, such as the **epulis**, are benign. Epulides are primarily found on the gum. They may be left alone or, if they present a problem, they can be surgically removed.

Ulcers. Ulcers in the oral cavity have many different causes, including:

- Viruses, such as the 'cat 'flu' infections.
- Systemic illness, such as kidney failure causing uraemia.
- Dental disease.
- Some oral tumours may ulcerate.

Treatment of the ulcer depends on recognising the underlying cause. Some ulcerative gingivitis in cats has no clear cause and can be very difficult to treat. The use of pharyngostomy or gastrostomy tubes is sometimes useful for managing animals with severe oral ulceration which refuse to eat.

Rodent ulcers are chronic, flat, ulcerated granulomatous lesions occurring on the lips of cats. The cause of rodent ulcers is unknown. They usually respond to corticosteroid therapy.

Stings. The oral cavity is a frequent site for bee and wasp stings. Although usually of little significance, stings in this area can become an emergency because the associated swelling may cause obstruction of the airway, especially in brachycephalic breeds. Treatment with corticosteroids and/or antihistamines is usually sufficient to resolve the problem, but some cases may require an emergency tracheotomy to relieve their dyspnoea.

The oesophagus

The two most common conditions encountered in the oesophagus are oesophageal foreign bodies and megaoesophagus.

Oesophageal foreign bodies. Oesophageal foreign bodies are seen far more commonly in dogs than in cats. They are usually bones and most frequently lodge in the thoracic oesophagus, at the level of the base of the heart. In most cases, they can be retrieved, or pushed into the stomach, using either long forceps under fluoroscopic guidance or oesophagoscopy. In a few cases, oesophagotomy via a thoracotomy may be needed for removal. Inevitably, oesophageal foreign bodies produce an oesophagitis and, in severe cases, there may be complete penetration of the oeosphageal wall. Post-operative nursing for the oesophagitis may include feeding liquidised food, or the placement of a gastrostomy tube.

Megaoesophagus. Megaoesophagus, a flaccid dilatation of the oesophagus, is seen as an idiopathic condition, but also in some disease states, most commonly myasthenia gravis. The flaccidity impairs passage of food from the pharynx to the stomach. This may be eased by feeding affected animals from a height, so that they stand on their hindlegs whilst eating, or by lifting the front end of the animal into the upright position after feeding.

The stomach

Common conditions of the stomach include acute gastritis, gastric foreign bodies, gastric dilation/volvulus (GDV) syndrome and pyloric stenosis.

Acute gastritis. Acute gastritis is common in dogs because their scavenging habits lead them to dietary indiscretions. The main sign is acute vomiting in an otherwise well dog. There may also be diarrhoea. These findings are not characteristic for dietary induced upsets and so persistent vomiting and/or diarrhoea should always be investigated by a veterinary surgeon. Most uncomplicated cases of dietary induced gastritis respond to complete withdrawal of food for 24 hours followed by a gradual return to normal feeding over a period of a few days. Initially, meals should be small and consist of bland foods. The animal's normal diet is reintroduced as the bland food is withdrawn. All dietary changes are made gradually to prevent recurrence. Some individuals are very prone to dietary induced gastritis; they should be kept on a very constant diet and may require special diets to control the problem.

Foreign bodies. Foreign bodies which are swallowed and reach the stomach may cause vomiting. A gastrotomy, via a laparotomy, is usually required for their removal. Post-operatively, food is withheld for 24 hours before introducing small, bland meals which may be liquidised. The normal diet is gradually reintroduced.

Gastric dilation/volvulus syndrome. GDV *is important because it constitutes an emergency.* It occurs mainly in large, deep-chested dogs but is also seen in some small breeds. It frequently presents shortly after feeding, especially if the meal was large and followed by a period of exercise. Affected dogs become rapidly depressed. They make repeated but unsuccessful attempts to vomit and they salivate profusely. The abdomen swells because of food and gas (from swallowed air) in the stomach. The abdominal swelling is usually severe enough to be noticed by the owners. The swollen stomach presses on the diaphragm and compromises breathing. Once distended, the stomach tends to rotate about its own axis forming a twist (**volvulus**). The volvulus interferes with normal blood supply to the stomach wall and, sometimes, with the blood supply to the spleen. The devitalised tissues become necrotic if the condition is not treated promptly.

WARNING

GDV has a high mortality rate and swift emergency action is essential to maximise the chances of survival. The first priorities are:

- **Decompression of the stomach**: This may be achieved by passing a stomach tube down the oesophagus, by percutaneous catheterisation of the stomach or by a keyhole laparotomy. In severe emergencies, when the animal may be dying because of respiratory distress, a wide gauge hypodermic needle can be used to penetrate the most prominent and palpable part of the gas distended stomach to provide relief until veterinary assistance arrives.
- **Vigorous fluid therapy**: Dogs with GDV develop shock rapidly. Fluid therapy to counter the shock is an important priority.

Once the animal is sufficiently stabilised, surgery is needed to decompress the stomach fully, to resect any devitalised tissues and to return the stomach to its normal position. Further procedures may be performed to anchor the stomach in place. Post-operative, fluid therapy is maintained for at least 24 hours whilst all oral food and fluids are withheld. If all progresses well, small volumes of water may be given by mouth after 24 hours and the first small amounts of food may be given 24–48 hours later.

Cardiac arrythmias are an important complication of GDV, often occurring 12–48 hours post-operatively. Frequent routine monitoring by auscultation and by ECG should be performed over this period.

Recurrence of GDV in susceptible animals is common. Precautions to minimise this risk include:

- Feed several small meals daily rather than one large meal.
- Enforce rest for 1–2 hours after feeding.
- Feed only small amounts of cereal in the diet.
- Ensure biscuit meals are thoroughly pre-soaked.
- Raise food bowl to prevent aerophagia.

Pyloric stenosis. Pyloric stenosis is a congenital deficiency in the anatomy or function of the pylorus which prevents normal emptying of the stomach. Affected puppies or kittens vomit in association with feeding. Surgical correction of the condition is possible.

The small intestine

Common conditions of the small intestine include intestinal foreign bodies and intussusception.

Foreign bodies. Swallowed foreign bodies that reach the small intestine can cause either partial or complete obstruction of the bowel, which leads to vomiting. Complete obstruction rapidly leads the animal into a state of shock requiring fluid therapy before surgery. Most intestinal foreign bodies are removed by enterotomy via a laparotomy. In cases where damage to the bowel is severe, enterectomy may be indicated. Post-operative care is as for gastrotomy (see Gastric foreign bodies).

Intussusception. Intussusception is the telescoping of one section of the bowel into an adjoining portion. The length of an intussusception may vary from less than a centimetre to several centimetres. It is associated with abnormal intestinal motility for any reason and is especially seen in young animals. It may occur as a complication in animals with diarrhoea. In some cases, the bowel can be reduced to its normal position by gentle traction. Often, however, the affected portion is badly damaged, requiring removal by enterectomy. Recurrences are not uncommon, particularly after reduction of an intussusception. Post-operative care is as for gastrotomy.

The rectum

Common conditions of the rectum include rectal foreign bodies, rectal tumours, chronic constipation and rectal prolapse.

NOTE

Most routine surgical or imaging procedures of the rectum require thorough cleansing of the rectum first by withholding food for 24 hours and administering **enemas** prior to the procedure. An enema may be a proprietary brand; or it can be warm soap-and-water which is introduced using a soft enema pump inserted gently and with plenty of lubricant, such as KY jelly. Great care must be taken not to injure or perforate the rectal wall, especially in small dogs and in cats. In very small animals, a soft catheter attached to a syringe can substitute for the enema pump. The pump should not be forced if the animal strains against it during insertion. Once in place, the soap and warm water is *gently* flushed into the rectum: it is both dangerous and unnecessary to pump vigorously.

Rectal foreign bodies. Rectal foreign bodies are most often either sharp or impacted bones. They cause constipation and pain which is exacerbated by attempts to defecate. The diagnosis is confirmed by digital palpation. In most cases, the foreign body can be manipulated through the anus with the animal under general anaesthesia.

Tumours. Tumours can arise in all sections of the gastrointestinal tract, including the rectum. In the rectum, they can be visualised by proctoscopy or by contrast radiography. Cleansing of the rectum is essential for the successful application of both these techniques.

Chronic constipation. Chronic constipation is a not uncommon disorder in dogs and cats. Many cases respond adequately to the administration of an enema, but manual evacuation is needed in some. Often the constipation is secondary to some other disease problem, such as an enlarged prostate, a tumour of the rectum, perineal rupture or narrow pelvic canal associated with an old fracture of the pelvis. If possible, the inciting disease should be treated as well as giving symptomatic relief of the constipation. The addition of liquid paraffin, or a bulk laxative, to the diet help to prevent recurrence of constipation.

Rectal prolapse. Rectal prolapse is eversion of the wall of the rectum through the anus. It is usually secondary to chronic straining and often associated with a rectal tumour. Successful management of rectal prolapse requires treatment of the primary disease as well as reduction of the prolapse itself.

FIRST AID MEASURES FOR A PROLAPSED RECTUM
- Protect everted mucosa using a lubricant (e.g. KY jelly or obstetrical lubricant) cover with saline-soaked swabs. Simple saline- or water-soaked swabs may be used if lubricants are not available.
- Protect the area from self-mutilation, e.g. by application of an Elizabethan collar.

The prolapse is normally reduced under general anaesthesia by manipulation, or by a surgical method. A temporary purse-string suture may be placed in the anus to help retain the inflamed rectum in place, but this must be removed as soon as possible to allow normal defecation.

The anus

Common conditions of the anal area include imperforate anus, anal sac disease, anal furunculosis and anal or perianal tumours.

Imperforate anus. Imperforate anus is a congenital problem in which there is failure of the anus to unite with the rectum, thus leaving a complete obstruction to the normal passage of faeces from the moment of birth. The problem can sometimes be corrected surgically.

Anal sac disease. Anal sac disease is very common in dogs. It causes irritation focused on the anal area and affected animals chew at the region or typically drag their backside along the floor. In most cases, there is simple impaction of the anal sacs, often associated with infection. Some cases may develop abscessation of the anal sac. Digital evacuation of the anal sac gives relief in simple cases and this may be combined with systemic or topical antibiotic therapy. Recurrence is common and persistent cases require surgical removal of the anal sacs. Pre-operative preparation for anal sac removal (under general anaesthesia) includes:

(1) Manual evacuation of the anal sacs.
(2) Irrigation of the sacs with saline via a fine catheter, such as a tomcat catheter,
(3) Some surgeons prefer to pack the anal sacs with wax or dental mould prior to surgery.
(4) Routine pre-operative clipping and skin preparation of the perineum.

In rare cases, the surgery is complicated by faecal incontinence. This results from damage to the nerves to the external anal sphincter during surgery and is usually only a temporary problem.

Anal furunculosis. This is a deep, chronic infection of the skin surrounding the anus. Animals with anal furunculosis may show anal irritation and often have a foul odour. Most cases occur in German shepherd dogs. Sinuses and fistulae are found in the perianal area. Treatment requires thorough surgical debridement of the area and may include cryosurgery. Recurrences are common.

Tumours. The most common perianal tumour is the **anal adenoma**. This is a benign tumour, primarily of old male dogs. It can become quite large and ulcerate, but responds well to surgical resection. Growth of the tumour is dependent on the male sex hormones and so affected dogs are castrated at the time of tumour removal to prevent recurrence.

The **perianal adenocarcinoma** is a malignant tumour. It is much rarer than the anal adenoma and occurs in both male and female dogs.

Surgery of the Respiratory Tract

The respiratory tract includes the nose, larynx, trachea and lungs.

The nose

Causes of nasal discharge include:

- Intranasal foreign bodies (especially in dogs).
- Infections:
  —viral (e.g. cat 'flu; canine distemper)
  —bacterial
  —fungal (aspergillosis in dogs)
- Tumours.

In some cases, the discharge is associated with intense sneezing and nose bleeds (**epistaxis**). Epistaxis may also be seen following trauma, such as a road traffic accident. Investigation of these problems usually requires radiography under general anaesthesia and surgical exploration by a rhinotomy may be necessary.

The larynx and trachea

Laryngeal paralysis. Laryngeal paralysis is a disease of unknown cause, affecting old dogs. The paralysed larynx impairs breathing. The condition is irreversible, but surgery can be performed to assist air flow through the larynx and thereby help the animals breathing.

Collapsing trachea. Collapsing trachea affects certain toy breeds of dog. The cervical part of the trachea, the thoracic part of the trachea, or the entire trachea may be affected. The collapsed trachea impairs breathing. Treatment may be medical, or surgery can be performed to help prevent collapse of the trachea.

Tracheostomy and tracheotomy. **Tracheostomy** is a technique for creating a permanent opening into the trachea, usually halfway down the neck, to bypass an obstruction to breathing in the upper part of the airway. Tracheostomy is rarely indicated in dogs and cats.

Tracheotomy is a potentially life-saving procedure in the event of acute upper airway obstruction: In an emergency, the veterinary nurse should be prepared to perform a tracheotomy, using only local anaesthetic (or even no anaesthetic) if necessary. If a risk of upper airway obstruction is anticipated (for example following surgery on the airway) the site on the ventral midline of the neck can be clipped in readiness for a tracheotomy if it proves necessary. In a peracute emergency, time should not be wasted in clipping and surgically preparing the skin. In most cases the airway is not completely blocked and oxygen, delivered by a face mask, provides some relief whilst the tracheotomy is being performed.

EMERGENCY

If an animal is close to death because of acute upper airway obstruction, a wide-gauge hypodermic needle pushed quickly through the ventral midline of the neck into the trachea can be life-saving until a proper tracheotomy is established.

In cats and very small dogs, a needle tracheotomy may suffice in place of an open tracheotomy if relief is only required for a short period of time.

PROCEDURE FOR TRACHEOTOMY

- The skin incision is made in the ventral midline, over the trachea, immediately behind the larynx.
- The underlying muscles are gently separated in the midline. This exposes the ventral surface of the trachea so that the cartilaginous rings can be identified,
- A scalpel (usually a number 15 blade) is used to incise the trachea between the second or third pair of tracheal cartilages.
- The incision is kept open by insertion of a tracheotomy tube which is held in place by ties around the neck, or by sutures. Tracheotomy tubes are available in a range of sizes to suit different animals.
- In the absence of a suitable tracheotomy tube, an endotracheal tube or any other suitably sized soft tubing, such as the end of a urinary catheter, can be used.
- The end of the tracheotomy tube obstructs with mucus if left without further attention. It must be cleaned at regular intervals, usually every 2 to 3 hours with saline. Some tracheotomy tubes have an inner sleeve and an outer sleeve, allowing the inner sleeve to be removed

---

for cleaning before replacing it in the outer sleeve. If this type of tube is not available, the tracheotomy can sometimes be cleared by aspirating mucus with an intravenous catheter, or a short length of fine male urinary catheter attached to a 10 ml or 20 ml syringe.

Brachycephalic airway obstruction syndrome (BAOS). BAOS is a condition of the short-nosed (brachycephalic) dogs in which the anatomical deformities which are 'normal' for these animals cause respiratory embarrassment because of obstruction of normal airway. The deformities which make up BAOS include:

- Narrow nares.
- Narrow nasal cavity and pharynx.
- An overlong soft palate.
- An overlong tongue.
- A narrow (hypoplastic) trachea.

The number and severity of the abnormalities vary between individuals. Some dogs are so severely affected that they may have acute, life-threatening respiratory distress, particularly in very hot and humid conditions. In this situation, emergency first aid may be required:

FIRST AID MEASURES FOR BAOS
(1) Extend the neck and pull the tongue forwards gently to exteriorise it, deflecting it to the side.
(2) Administer oxygen by a face mask.
(3) Perform an emergency tracheotomy if necessary.
(4) If the animal is overheated, it can be gently cooled by showering with cold water.

Some of the abnormalities that make up BAOS are amenable to corrective surgery. Care is needed with anaesthesia and recovery of these animals. They must be monitored closely until they are fully recovered from surgery and advance preparations should be made in case a tracheotomy is needed. In a small number of cases, corrective surgery is impractical because the deformities may be too extreme or they may be complicated by collapse of the larynx. Tracheostomy is the only option for such animals.

The thorax

A **thoracotomy** is a temporary opening into the thorax to allow surgery on intrathoracic organs such as the oesophagus, lungs, blood vessels and pericardium. There are several different approaches to thoracotomy:

- An incision through the intercostal muscles.
- Rib resection and incision of the underlying periosteum and pleura.
- By sternotomy (splitting of the sternum).

Of these, the intercostal approach is probably the most commonly used in dogs and cats. Following thoracotomy great care is taken to ensure a leak-proof closure, and the excessive free air in the pleural cavity must be removed to allow the lungs to re-inflate. A **chest drain** is used to remove the pleural air. This consists of a length of sterile tubing with one end placed in the thoracic cavity and the other end exiting the chest. The outer end may be linked to a water seal which allows continual aspiration of air or it may be occluded with a clamp and excessive air removed by periodic aspiration using a three-way tap and syringe. The tube is normally enclosed inside a chest bandage to keep it clean and prevent excessive movement. Most chest drains can be removed after only a few hours.

Surgery of the Urinary Tract

The urinary tract includes kidneys, ureters, bladder and urethra.

The kidneys

The kidney is not a common site for surgery. It is sometimes necessary to biopsy a kidney to help make a diagnosis. Occasionally, severe disease such as neoplasia, chronic infection or hydronephrosis requires complete removal of one kidney (**nephrectomy**). The ureter may be removed along with the kidney (**ureteronephrectomy**). The success of nephrectomy is absolutely dependent on the health of the remaining kidney, which is able to compensate for the lost function.

The ureters

One of the most common surgical conditions of the ureters is **ureteric ectopia**. An ectopic ureter is one which inserts further down the lower urinary tract than its normal insertion in the bladder. They usually insert at the proximal urethra, but may insert as far down as the vagina in females. Ureteric ectopia is a congenital condition seen especially in golden retrievers, labrador retrievers and Skye terriers. One or both ureters may be involved. The condition causes urinary incontinence which is evident from an early age. It presents as a clinical problem in females more commonly than in males. Ureteric ectopia is usually amenable to surgery to replace the ureter at its correct anatomical site in the bladder. Postoperatively it is important for the animals to be monitored to ensure that they can urinate normally. Temporary urinary obstruction sometimes occurs because of swelling of the bladder and may require careful catheterisation. In some cases of ureteric ectopia, ureteronephrectomy is necessary because of secondary damage to the ureter and its kidney.

The bladder

The most common surgery of the bladder is a **cystotomy** to remove **urinary calculi** which can cause an obstruction and/or act as a focus for repeated bladder infections (**cystitis**). As with correction of ureteric ectopia, animals should be monitored closely post-operatively to ensure that they urinate.

The urethra

The urethra of the male is very prone to blockage with **urinary calculi** in both dogs and cats. If not relieved, the obstruction will lead to rupture of the bladder, spillage of urine into the abdominal cavity, uraemia and a rapid death.

Bladder or urethral rupture is also a common complication of pelvic fractures. Animals with pelvic fractures should be monitored extremely carefully for normal urination.

Another common reason for urethral obstruction which may lead to bladder rupture is retroflexion of the bladder into a perineal rupture. An animal with urethral obstruction strains unsuccessfully to pass urine. There may be associated pain and depression. First aid is aimed at providing temporary relief for the overdistended bladder by **cystocentesis.**

CYSTOCENTESIS
- Anaesthesia is unnecessary and sedation is only required in the most fractious of animals. Sedation is contraindicated in very uraemic patients.
- Identify the palpably distended bladder and prepare a small overlying area on the ventro-lateral abdomen by clipping and surgical scrubbing.
- Use a 20 gauge (or similar) needle of suitable length for the size of animal, a large syringe and a threeway tap.
- Puncture the bladder through the prepared skin site. Aspirate urine, turn the three way tap and expel the urine into a bowl.
- Repeat until the bladder is drained.

Surgical removal of urethral calculi can often be achieved by urethral catheterisation and the forcible injection of sterile saline (**retropulsion**). If retropulsion is not successful, the calculi may be removed via a **urethrotomy**. A **urethrostomy** may be created if the calculi cannot be removed, or to minimise the risk of recurrence. The urethrostomy can be created at one of two levels, depending on the site of the obstruction:

- Low urethrostomy: in the pre-scrotal penile urethra. This is adequate for obstruction at the level of the os penis, a common site for lodgement of urinary calculi.
- High urethrostomy: in the perineal urethra. This procedure is commonly used in cats.

Post-operative care for urethrostomy patients includes:
- Prevention of self-mutilation. The sutures at the urethral stoma are frequently irritant and an Elizabethan collar or similar device is essential.
- Prevention of chafing around the urethral stoma by application of vaseline or a similar oil based cream.

Surgery of the Genital Tract

The genital tract includes testes, prostate, ovaries, uterus, vagina and vulva.

The testes

Orchidectomy is removal of one or both testes. Bilateral orchidectomy (**castration**) is most commonly performed for socialising reasons in dogs and tomcats. The greatest effects are often seen when animals are castrated at a relatively early age. Beneficial effects that may result from castration include:

- Prevention of unwanted breeding.
- Prevention of roaming.
- Prevention of territorial spraying by tomcats.
- Reduction of excessive libido.
- Reduction of aggression.

Orchidectomy may also be performed in the treatment of testicular tumours or otherwise unmanageable infections and to control testosterone dependent diseases such as anal adenoma and prostatic disease.

The prostate

The prostate is a common site of disease in older male dogs. A range of conditions affect the prostate, including:

- Benign hyperplasia.
- Infections (prostatitis).
- Cyst formation.
- Neoplasia.

These diseases may present with constipation or pain on defecation because of prostatic enlargement, or with an abnormal discharge from the prepuce. The discharge is commonly blood or pus and may be associated with urination, or independent of it. Some of these conditions are amenable to medical therapy and others require surgery. Castration is frequently indicated as part of the management of prostatic disorders.

The ovaries and uterus

Ovariectomy (surgical removal of the ovaries) and **hysterectomy** (surgical removal of the uterus) are not common procedures in dogs. Most often complete removal of both organs is performed simultaneously (**ovariohysterectomy** or spaying). Ovariohysterectomy is most commonly performed purely for neutering in females.

The advantages of ovariohysterectomy include:

- Guaranteed absence of unwanted pregnancy.
- Cessation of all oestrus activity.
- Prevention of pyometra (see below).
- Prevention of mammary carcinoma if performed at an early age.

Elective ovariohysterectomy should be avoided during oestrus, pregnancy or false pregnancy. Most surgeons prefer to perform elective ovariohysterectomy approximately 8 weeks after the end of oestrus.

Pyometra. Pyometra, the accumulation of pus in the uterus, may be an infected or a sterile condition and it is life-threatening. It occurs most commonly in middle-aged to old animals which have never had a litter. It often presents shortly after a season. Affected animals are usually depressed and polydipsic. They may have a fever and they often vomit. If the cervix is open (**open pyometra**) there is a vaginal discharge. No discharge occurs if the cervix is closed (**closed pyometra**).

Animals with pyometra frequently need intensive fluid therapy before they are fit for anaesthesia. Ovariohysterectomy is needed as a life-saving procedure as soon as the animal is stable enough for surgery. Intensive nursing is also required in the post-operative phase.

Hysterotomy. Caesarian section (hysterotomy) is performed for the relief of dystocia because of uterine inactivity or foetal obstruction. Much of the nursing associated with the procedure centres on the well-being of the young:

(1) Check that the neonate's air way is clear, and remove any remaining amniotic fluid by aspirating or by *carefully* swinging the animal by its back legs.
(2) Wrap the animal in a warmed towel and rub vigorously to dry it and to encourage respiration.
(3) Oxygen may be useful for resuscitation in some cases as are respiratory stimulants such as doxapram hydrochloride.
(4) The umbilical remnant should be ligated with a suitable material and may be treated with an antiseptic solution.
(5) Check for any obvious congenital defects such as cleft palate or imperforate anus.
(6) Keep the animal warm and encourage suckling at the earliest possible opportunity.

The vagina and vulva

Rectovaginal fistula. Rectovaginal fistula is a congenital condition which is associated with imperforate anus. Surgery can be performed to close the fistula and restore the normal anatomy of both the rectum and vagina.

Vaginal hyperplasia. Vaginal hyperplasia, seen most commonly in brachycephalic breeds, is an exaggerated hyperplastic response of the vaginal mucosa to oestrogen. During the follicular phase of the oestrous cycle, affected bitches have excessive folds of vaginal mucosa which protrude through the vulva. Many owners are concerned that this is a tumour, but the appearance of the tissue in association with the first oestrous makes this unlikely. The exposed tissue is likely to become traumatised.

Treatment of vaginal hyperplasia includes:

- Temporary relief by lubricating the exposed mucosa with KY jelly.
- Surgical resection is possible, but there is a risk of recurrence.
- Recurrences can be prevented by ovariohysterectomy or by treatment with progestagens in early proestrus.

Vaginal prolapse. Vaginal prolapse is far less common in dogs than vaginal hyperplasia, but the same breed predispositions exist. Mild prolapses may need no treatment other than protection of the exposed mucosa. Spontaneous regression occurs during the dioestrus period. Attempts may be made to replace the everted tissue under general anaesthesia. Further procedures may be needed in recurrent cases.

Inflamed vulva. In bitches with incontinence or cystitis, the vulva frequently becomes inflamed. Nursing of these cases requires:

- Regular washing and rinsing of the vulva.
- Application of a soothing antiseptic ointment.
- Covering the area with vaseline or other oily barrier cream.
- Prevention of excessive licking by use of an Elizabethan collar.

Veterinary attention is necessary to diagnose and treat the underlying condition.

Hernias and Ruptures

As defined in Chapter 3 (First Aid), a **hernia** is an abnormal protrusion of an organ or organs through a physiological opening in the lining of the cavity within which it is normally enclosed. A **rupture** is a pathological tear in the lining of the cavity, through which enclosed organs may protrude.

Most herniations and ruptures affect the abdominal cavity, but some occur elsewhere. Examples outside the abdomen include herniation of the occipital or temporal lobes of the brain under the bony tentorium cerebelli as a complication of space-occupying lesions in the CNS and rupture of the tympanic membrane in severe otitis externa.

Two groups of physiological openings are recognised through which hernias occur: normal openings which may become enlarged, such as the inguinal canals, and openings which should have closed before birth, such as the umbilicus.

Hernias and ruptures share many characteristics. However, most abdominal hernias are lined by an out-pouching of the peritoneum, whereas the peritoneum is often torn along with other structures in abdominal ruptures.

Terms used to describe hernias and ruptures include:

- **Reducible**: The contents of the hernia or rupture can be replaced in their original anatomical location via the defect itself.

- **Irreducible** or **incarcerated**: The contents of the hernia or rupture cannot be replaced, usually because of the formation of adhesions in chronic cases.

- **Strangulated**: Devitalisation of the contents of a hernia or rupture because of entrapment of the blood vessels passing through the defect. Strangulation is obviously an emergency.

Hernias and ruptures are primarily described by their location. Common examples include umbilical and inguinal hernias, and diaphragmatic and perineal ruptures.

Umbilical hernias are especially seen in puppies. Small umbilical hernias are of no consequence; hernias tend not to grow with the puppy and therefore becomes less significant with time. However, large umbilical hernias should be surgically corrected to prevent the risk of incarceration of small intestine or other abdominal organs.

Inguinal hernias are more common in bitches than in dogs. In bitches the contents of the hernia may include fat in the broad ligament, the uterus, intestines or bladder. They present as a swelling in the groin extending towards the vulva. In dogs, inguinal hernias can be an emergency because of incarceration and strangulation of a loop of small intestine through the inguinal canal and into the scrotal sac.

Diaphragmatic rupture is commonly associated with violent trauma such as a road traffic accident. The loss of a functional diaphragm hinders breathing and this may be exacerbated by incarceration of abdominal organs in the thoracic cavity. Affected animals are obviously anaesthetic risks when surgery is performed for repair of the rupture or other injuries acquired in the accident.

Perineal rupture occurs almost exclusively in older male dogs. It is associated with degeneration of the muscles of the pelvic diaphragm (primarily the coccygeus and the retractor ani muscles). Affected dogs have difficulty defaecating and an obvious swelling of the perineum on one or both sides of the anus. Surgical correction is usually necessary and castration helps to prevent recurrence. An important complication of perineal rupture is retroflexion and incarceration of the bladder causing acute urethral obstruction. This constitutes an emergency.

Pre-operative preparation for perineal rupture surgery includes thorough emptying of the rectum by enemas, starting the day before surgery. Post-operatively, bulking agents should be added to the diet to make defecation easier and minimise straining.

Principles of treatment of hernias and ruptures

Correction of both hernias and ruptures is by reduction of the organs followed by closure of the defect. Elongation of the defect and/or breaking down of adhesions may be needed to achieve reduction. Many hernias are thought to have an inherited component and neutering is routinely recommended after hernia repairs to prevent problems in future generations.

Tumours

A tumour is an abnormal swelling of tissue with no physiological use, in which cell growth and replication is uncoordinated and exceeds that of the normal tissue cells. All unexplained lumps or bumps on an animal should be considered as potential tumours until proven otherwise. Many owners are frightened by the implications of a diagnosis of tumour, but they should be reassured that many tumours are benign and, if removed completely, they will not grow again.

Tumours may occur at any site in the body and from any tissue with the potential for growth. However some sites are more common than others and these include:

- Skin.
- The alimentary canal (mouth to anus).
- Mammary glands.
- Lymphatic system (including solid tumours of lymph nodes and, less commonly, leukaemias).
- Bones.

Tumours are broadly classified as benign or malignant.

Benign tumours usually grow quite slowly. They are discrete and encapsulated, and are often movable relative to neighbouring tissues. The suffix '-oma' is often used to describe benign tumours (although there are exceptions) and examples include:

- **Lipoma**: a benign tumour of adipose cells, very common in the subcutaneous tissues in older, overweight animals.
- **Papilloma**: a benign wart-like tumour of epithelial cells, most often seen on the skin of cats and dogs (for example, at the lip margins, eyelid and ear); they also occur on the bladder epithelium.
- **Melanoma**: a benign skin tumour of melanocytes, but some melanomas (especially in the mucous membrane of the mouth) behave in a highly malignant manner (**malignant melanoma**).
- **Fibroma**: a benign tumour of fibrous tissue, present as firm, superficial tumours of the skin and may be difficult to differentiate from other, more malignant, types of tumour.

- **Adenoma**: a benign tumour of glandular tissue, may be quite common in older dogs (e.g. anal adenoma).

Malignant tumours. Malignant tumours may grow quickly or slowly. They have an indefinite capsule and are usually locally invasive so that they cannot be clearly delineated from neighbouring tissues and are not freely mobile.

Some malignant tumours spread (**metastasise**) very readily to affect other organs. Metastasis may occur in one, or all, of three ways:

- In the circulation.
- In the lymphatic system.
- By direct contact of tumour cells with neighbouring organs by direct invasion (**extension**) or by exfoliation of tumour cells into a cavity such as the abdomen (**transplantation**).

The most common site for metastases is the lungs, via the circulation.

Malignant tumours are further classified on the basis of the type of tissue from which they arise:

- **Carcinoma**: a malignant tumour arising from epithelial tissues.
- **Sarcoma**: a malignant tumour arising from mesenchymal tissues (mainly connective tissues).

Common carcinomas include:

- **Squamous cell carcinoma**: commonly found in the oral cavity.
- **Transitional cell carcinoma**: in the urinary tract.
- **Adenocarcinoma**: malignant tumour of glandular tissue.

Common sarcomas include:

- **Lymphosarcoma**: commonly seen in association with feline leukaemia virus infection in cats. Also common in dogs.
- **Fibrosarcoma**: malignant tumour of fibrous tissue.
- **Osteosarcoma**: malignant tumour of osteoblasts.

In some cases histopathological examination of sarcomas and carcinomas allows the tumour to be further 'graded' in its degree of malignancy.

Mammary tumours. Mammary tumours deserve special consideration because they are the most common site of neoplasia in female dogs. They are especially seen in older entire bitches (neutering early in life significantly reduces the risk of mammary neoplasia). Mammary tumours can appear in any of the five pairs of mammary glands in bitches, but the two caudal pairs are most frequently affected. In queens, all four pairs of mammary glands are at equal risk of developing mammary tumours.

In bitches, benign tumours (**mixed mammary tumours**) are most common, comprising almost 50% of cases. Benign mixed mammary tumours are curable by complete resection. Malignant mammary tumours include adenocarcinomas and sarcomas. Metastasis via the lymphatics or blood stream is common with all malignant mammary tumours, but survival times after surgery vary dramatically with the exact type and histopathological grade of tumour.

Most mammary tumours of queens are highly malignant mammary carcinomas or adenocarcinomas which metastasise very readily.

Biopsies and prognoses

A **biopsy** is a sample of tissue or other material obtained for diagnosis, prognosis and to aid in planning therapy. A **prognosis** is a prediction of the course or outcome of a disease.

In all cases, it is important to define the type of tumour clearly. The prognosis and treatment is very different for different tumour types. Benign tumours can often be completely cured and significant steps have now been made in the treatment of many malignant tumours. Although much can be implied from the history and examination of a tumour, the only way to type the tumour exactly is to obtain a biopsy for cytological and/or histopathological examination. Several different techniques exist for obtaining biopsies including:

- Needle aspiration.
- Needle core biopsy.
- Punch biopsy (skin and superficial lesions)
- Trephine biopsy (bone).
- Incisional biopsy.
- Excisional biopsy.

Needle aspiration. Needle aspiration involves the insertion of a fine needle into the tumour and the application of suction with a syringe to aspirate small numbers of cells for cytological examination. It is a useful preliminary examination technique for many lumps, but is especially used for collecting bone marrow for examination. There is a special bone marrow biopsy needle, consisting of a stiff outer core and an inner stylet. Bone marrow is usually obtained from the wing of the ilium, but may be collected from other sites. Sedation and local anaesthesia or general anaesthesia is necessary. The overlying skin is prepared as for surgery and a small stab incision made. The bone marrow biopsy needle, complete with stylet, is inserted through the incision and driven through the bone cortex. The stylet is removed, the syringe is attached and bone marrow is aspirated. Needle aspiration of superficial soft tissue tumours or lymph nodes may be performed with a 19 gauge needle and 10 ml syringe without recourse to sedation or anaesthesia.

Needle core biopsy. Needle core biopsies are small cylinders of tissue obtained with a purpose-designed instrument. Several patterns of core biopsy needle exist, but the 'true-cut' type is one of the most popular: it has a central obturator, which is notched and an outer sleeve or cannula with an attached handle. Local or general anaesthesia and aseptic preparation of the overlying skin is required. A stab incision is made and the obturator is inserted into the tumour tissue. The cannula is then advanced over the obturator so that a core of tissue is trapped in the notch in the obturator. The needle, and biopsy, are then withdrawn.

Punch biopsy. Punch biopsies are obtained from superficial tissues using a punch which is a small, sharp circular blade a few millimetres in diameter.

Trephine biopsy. Trephine biopsies of bone are obtained with a circular cutting tool (**trephine**) a few millimetres in diameter which removes a core from the bone in much the same way that an apple corer removes the centre section of an apple.

Incisional biopsy. Incisional biopsies involve removal of a small part of the tumour, often a wedge, by a surgical incision. They have the advantage over needle biopsy techniques of obtaining a significantly larger piece of tissue, thus improving the chances of successful diagnosis from the biopsy. However, they have the disadvantage of requiring a full surgical procedure in order to obtain them.

Excisional biopsy. Excisional biopsies involve the complete removal of all identifiable tumour tissue. They are especially useful for suspected benign lesions because, if complete, they negate the need for a second surgery to treat the tumour.

PRESERVATION OF BIOPSY SPECIMENS FOR HISTOPATHOLOGY

- Specimens should be fixed in a large volume of fixative for 24–48 hours. They may then be transferred to a smaller volume of fixative for postage to a pathologist.
- For most routine histopathology, 10% formal saline is the fixative of choice.
- Thin sections of tissue (< 5mm) are preferred to large masses because they fix more rapidly. If possible, margins of normal tissue should be included with the suspected tumour tissue.
- For large excisional biopsies, it is helpful to send the whole specimen to a pathologist so that it can be examined to determine if all tumour tissue has been removed. Rapid fixation can be facilitated by incomplete thin sectioning of the tissue. Alternatively, a single thin slice of the tissue can be fixed separately for identification and the remainder can be fixed whole.

- Care must be taken to satisfy posting regulations for pathological specimens, as described in Chapter 22 (Diagnostic Samples and Tests).
- The pathologist should be sent a detailed history of the case under separate cover (Chapter 22).
- The owner should be warned to expect a delay, usually of 1–2 weeks, before a result is obtained. Longer may be needed for bone biopsies, which must be decalcified before they are sectioned for histological examination.

Treatment of tumours

Especially when treating a tumour that is ultimately incurable, it is important to bear in mind the goal of therapy. If there is no hope for cure, the only remaining goal is preservation of an acceptable quality of life for as long as possible.

Most tumours are likely to be treated by surgical excision. **Debulking** is a procedure to remove as much tumour tissue as possible when complete excision is impractical. Other tumour therapies include:

- **Chemotherapy**: The use of drugs to kill tumour cells selectively. Chemotherapy is a successful way of treating some tumour types.
- **Radiotherapy**: The use of radiation to selectively kill tumour cells. Although a useful mode of treatment for some tumour types, radiotherapy is limited to use in a few specialised centres.
- **Hyperthermia**: The local application of heat to tumours can aid selective killing of tumour cells, particularly in conjunction with radiotherapy.
- **Cryosurgery**: Tumour tissue can be destroyed by the local application of extreme cold.
- **Combined modality**, or **multi-modality** therapy is when more than one method of treatment is used on a single tumour. An example is the combination of hyperthermia and radiation given above, but many other combined modality therapies exist.
- **Adjunctive therapy** is important in tumour therapy as it is in many other diseases. Adjuncts to the treatment of tumours are dictated by the problems of individual patients, but may include analgesia, nursing management of open wounds and antibiotics, amongst others.

Finally, **counselling** is a crucial part of successful cancer therapy. Full, frank and sympathetic discussions with the owner are necessary at each and every stage. This is usually the responsibility of the veterinary surgeon in charge of the case, but many owners gain great comfort from a compassionate, reassuring nurse.

Further reading

References prefixed by * are texts based on human nursing. Nevertheless, the general principles apply and these books remain useful because of a dearth of similar texts on veterinary nursing.

*Crawford Adams, J. and Hamblen D. L. (1992) *Outline of Fractures*. 10th edn. Churchill Livingstone, Edinburgh.

*Morison, M. J. (1992) *A Colour Guide to the Nursing Management of Wounds*. Wolfe Publishing, London.

*Westaby, S. (ed.) (1986) *Wound Care*. William Heinemann, London.

Slatter, D. H. (ed.) (1993) *Textbook of Small Animal Surgery*. 2nd edn. W. B. Saunders, Philadelphia.

Stead, C. (1988). External support for small animals. *In Practice*, July.

Taussig, M. J. (1981) Inflammation. Chapter 1, In: *Processes in Pathology. An Introduction for Medical Students*. Blackwell Scientific, Oxford.

25
Care and Maintenance of Surgical Equipment

K. A. WIGGINS

Care and maintenance of surgical equipment is generally the responsibility of the veterinary nurse. To assist with the day-to-day running of a veterinary establishment surgical equipment should be well maintained and frequently checked. Manufacturers' instructions for cleaning and general care should be carefully followed, not only to maintain a consistently low level of contamination and to keep items in efficient working order but also to extend the working life of each item.

An efficient method of maintaining surgical equipment is to compile a file of maintenance manuals and to establish a checklist of the equipment, with details of the maintenance procedures required and the intervals at which maintenance should be performed.

The following information could be collated in a maintenance file for each piece of equipment:

- Name of equipment.
- Location.
- Model number and serial number.
- Name of manufacturer.
- Name and telephone number of company from which it was purchased.
- Name and telephone number of salesperson.
- Name and telephone number of person to call for servicing.
- Date of purchase.
- Period of warranty.
- Dates of routine maintenance.

This system of recording information will save time in the future should the equipment require some form of repair.

Items that should be listed for maintenance of this type include the following:

- Anaesthetic equipment.
- Monitoring devices.
- Suction equipment.
- Ventilator.
- Diathermy equipment.
- Surgical lights.
- Surgical table.
- Air-conditioning/heating system.
- Dental scaler.
- Clippers.
- Laundry equipment (washer and dryer).
- Refrigerator.
- Ultrasound machine.

- ECG machine.
- Cryosurgery equipment.
- Endoscopes.

Care and Maintenance of Surgical Instruments

The basic rules for the care and maintenance of surgical instruments apply whether a veterinary nurse works in general practice or in a specialised institution.

Many varieties of surgical instruments feature in a wide range of instrumentation catalogues that are readily obtainable from manufacturers and wholesalers. These catalogues provide excellent descriptions of surgical equipment and are very useful for revision and training purposes.

The cost of surgical instruments may appear to be extraordinarily high but in most cases high quality is worthy of investment. Instruments of lesser quality may be cheaper to purchase but may prove to be more expensive in the long term: their performance may not meet certain needs and rapid wear or corrosion may necessitate early replacement. Good quality stainless steel surgical instruments that are handled and cared for properly will last for years before replacement becomes necessary.

Instrument Metals

Chromium-plated carbon steel surgical instruments are commonly found in veterinary hospitals. They are popular because of their low price, ease of maintenance and highly polished finished. The plated surface, however, is susceptible to attack by low pH solutions, saline and other chemicals. Early deterioration by pitting, rusting and blistering of the plated surface is a very common problem, resulting in early repair or replacement.

Better quality surgical instruments are made from **stainless steel**. Stainless steel is not a single specific material but consists primarily of iron, chromium and carbon, with other elements such as nickel combined in different proportions to achieve the desired properties.

Two major types of stainless steel are used for surgical equipment. The first is **martensitic**, a higher carbon stainless steel that provides greater hardness through heat treatment. This imparts wear resistance, which is especially important for sharp bladed surgical instruments (e.g. scissors and ophthalmic equipment) where fine edges must be maintained and strength and durability must be exhibited. The hard martensitic steels are most commonly used in the manufacture of surgical instruments.

The second type of stainless steel is **austenitic**. This is hardened, not by heat treatment but by work: as machine-forming takes place, the material gets harder. Its use is limited to the fabrication of bowls, sinks and some types of retractor blades and speculae.

The lack of hardness exhibited by these alloys is offset somewhat by their higher resistance to corrosion. Austenitic steels are often used for screws and rivets in surgical instruments.

Tungsten carbide inserts add an extra dimension to gripping and cutting surfaces. These substances are very hard and very resistant to wear. The inserts are attached to stainless steel instruments by various means and can be removed and replaced by the manufacturer. Some manufacturers identify these better quality instruments by gold-coloured handles.

Resistance to Corrosion

A stainless steel instrument attains its resistance to corrosion by passing through a series of manufacturing processes. This begins with selection of the correct material, which is then forged, descaled, machined and fitted. The new instrument is hardened by heat-treatment and then buffed and polished to a smooth surface. A highly polished finish is more resistant to spotting and discolouration but it reflects light easily and can cause mild eye irritation. More recently a dull satin finish has become popular, one advantage of which is reduced eye strain.

The final process of corrosion resistance is passivation. This involves bathing the finished instrument in a nitric acid solution, which burns out foreign particles that may have become embedded on its surface during the manufacturing process. Additionally a thin layer of chromium oxide forms on the stainless steel, providing more corrosion resistance.

Instrument Cleaning

Careful consideration should be given to the cleaning of instruments. To comply with COSHH regulations, a veterinary nurse dealing with used surgical instruments must wear protective clothing, i.e. rubber gloves and plastic apron.

- The first task should be the safe removal and disposal of **sharps** such as scalpel blades and suture needles. The safest way to attach and remove scalpel blades is with a **haemostat**. After

use, blades should be placed in a rigid clinical waste container. Bear in mind that old and worn blades can inflict serious lacerations.
- Instruments should be *separated* so that heavy pieces, especially orthopaedic equipment, are kept apart from smaller, more delicate instruments.
- All *blood and tissue debris* should be cleaned off immediately, before it dries on the instruments. Initial soaking in cold water is very effective. Hot water will cause coagulation of proteins and should not be used.
- *Saline solutions* used during surgery should be rinsed from the instruments as soon as possible. Instruments should never be soaked in saline, as this can cause pitting of the instrument surface and will lead to corrosion.
- The *washing* of instruments is carried out effectively under cool or warm running water using a hand brush with stiff plastic bristles. Particular attention should be paid to serrations, ratchets, box joints and other areas not easily exposed. A range of hand brushes for cleaning instruments is very useful. Those with long handles and round ends, used for cleaning endotracheal tubes, are very effective for instruments with tubular cavities.
- *Abrasive cleaners* should be avoided as repeated cleaning can damage the instrument surface. Ideally, a moderately alkaline low-lather *detergent* should be used, or alternatively a chemical cleaner specifically manufactured for instrument cleaning. The manufacturers' recommendations for use must be followed carefully.
- Ordinary *soap* should not be used, especially with hard water, as insoluble alkali films can form on the surface of the instrument trapping bacteria and thus protecting them from sterilisation.
- *Water* plays a major role: water alone accounts for much of the solvent action that occurs during instrument cleaning. As the quality of tap water in many areas is poor, careful consideration should be given to matching water quality with the appropriate detergent. Softened demineralised or distilled water should be considered to eliminate the deposition of hard-water salts on instruments, especially during the final rinsing.

Ultrasonic Cleaners

Ultrasonic cleaners (Fig. 25.1) are convenient, and can be used in any veterinary establishment. These small electrical units hold a wiremesh basket or perforated tray and are used with an ultrasonic detergent cleaner, especially formulated for its cleaning abilities and its chemical effects on the instruments being cleaned. The instruments are placed in the wire basket or tray and then submerged into the cleaner. The majority of these cleaners have timers, and the cleaning cycle is generally 15 minutes.

Ultrasonic cleaners are very effective for the removal of debris from areas that are inaccessible to

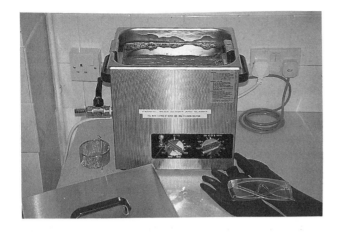

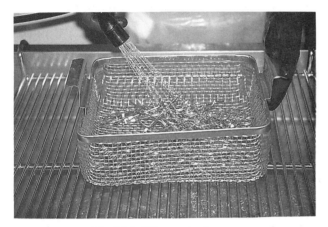

Fig. 25.1. Ultrasonic cleaner.

manual brushing, such as box joints and deep grooves. They work by the production of sinusoidal energy waves, with the frequency of vibrations in excess of 20,000 per second. The effectiveness of ultrasonic cleaning is based on a process called **cavitation**. Ultrasonic energy produces minute bubbles of gas within the cleaning solution. These bubbles form on the surface of the instruments and expand until their surface becomes unstable and then collapse by **implosion** (bursting inwards). The bubbles implode as fast as they form, creating small vacuum areas. This process releases energy and breaks the bonds that hold debris to instrument surfaces. The debris is then dislodged or dissolved into the solution.

The use of an ultrasonic cleaner is as an adjunct to the initial washing procedure rather than a replacement for it. Points to bear in mind when using the cleaner are:

- Rubber gloves should be worn, as the detergent may be harmful to the skin.
- Ensure that the manufacturer's instructions for detergent dilutions are carried out correctly.
- All instruments with joints should be opened when in the basket or tray.

- Different types of metal should not be mixed. Electrolysis may occur and the instrument surfaces may be damaged.
- Instruments removed from an ultrasonic cleaner must be rinsed thoroughly to remove residual detergent.
- The use of an ultrasonic cleaner is as an adjunct to, and not a replacement for, the initial washing procedure.

Instrument Lubrication

Surgical instruments with movable parts, particularly box joints, become stiff with repeated use. Instrument lubrication is commonly practised but can present problems if not properly performed. Mineral oil, machine oils and grease must be avoided: they leave an oily film on the instrument surface and can trap bacterial spores, preventing adequate penetration during steam sterilisation.

Instrument manufacturers recommend routine lubrication of instruments with an antimicrobial water-soluble lubricant (**instrument milk**). This is a water–oil emulsion that does not interfere with sterilisation. It is particularly important to lubricate instruments after cleaning with an ultrasonic cleaner, as the effective cleaning will remove all previous lubricants.

The lubricant bath should be prepared according to the manufacturer's recommendations. The instruments are submerged in the lubricant for at least 30 seconds (wearing rubber gloves is advisable). After removal from the bath the lubricant should be allowed to drain away without rinsing or manual drying, this gives added protection against corrosion. Follow the manufacturer's instructions for the disposal of used instrument milk to comply with COSHH regulations.

Instrument Checking before Packaging

Instruments should be checked regularly for distortion, misalignment and incorrect assembly. *Forceps* in particular should be checked:

- for tip alignment;
- that daylight cannot be seen through the serrations;
- that the ratchet grips are sound.

Needle-holders can be tested by lifting threads of suture material to test their grip. *Scissors* must be sharp: test them prior to packaging by checking that the tips will cut through four thicknesses of gauze swab or equivalent. It is advisable to have spare pairs of sharpened scissors sterilised separately for inclusion in the surgical pack should the veterinary surgeon discover the scissors in use are inadequately sharp for the surgical procedure.

Instrument Packaging for Sterilisation

Once the instruments have been cleaned and lubricated, they can be prepared for sterilisation. It is recommended that instruments that are not required on a day-to-day basis (e.g. specialised orthopaedic equipment used in elected surgical procedures) should be stored unsterilised in a clean dry environment.

There are various methods of packaging instruments prior to sterilisation. Packaging materials frequently used are textile wraps (usually cotton), paper, plastic and paper and plastic combinations.

- **Textile wraps** are commonly used for packaging instruments sets. They are easy to use, washable, flexible and long-lasting. However, they are easily contaminated by contact with moisture.
- **Double-wrapping** instrument kits with a textile wrap and a surgical paper wrap increases safe storage. The paper has a water repellency but still allows steam penetration during sterilisation.
- Double wrapping of **sterile packages** provides a

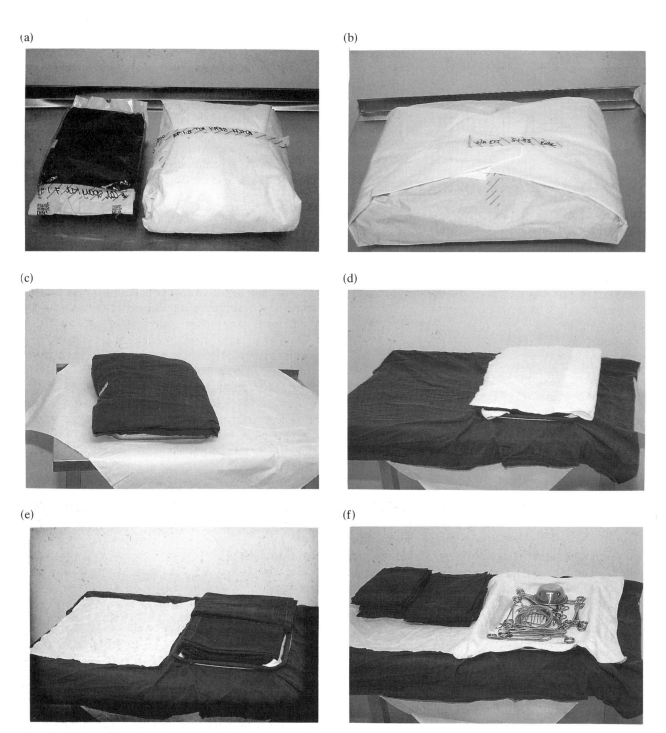

Fig. 25.2. Unpacking a small animal surgical kit. The kit has been double-wrapped to reduce contamination. Surgical drapes are sterilised with the instruments.

margin of safety during package opening. Dust contamination that has settled on a package is thrown into the surrounding air during opening, making the contamination of contents very likely, but a second wrap greatly reduces this risk.

- **Plastic and paper wraps and paper-and-plastic combinations are used extensively, especially for individual instrument packing. Packaging with peel-back openings for presentation of sterile instruments lessens the possibility of contamination.**
- **Plastic and cardboard boxes**, available in various shapes and sizes, are also used. Again, an outer wrap increases sterility.
- **Sharp and pointed instruments** should be protected to prevent accidental penetration of the surgical packaging. Various sizes of protective covers are commercially available. As an additional measure, instruments packaged in bags should always be positioned so that the instrument handle emerges from the bag first when opened (Fig. 25.3).

Instrument Identification

Date, label and initial all packages with a felt-tip marker, writing on the plastic side only or on the indicator tape to avoid puncturing or the bleeding through of ink.

Colour-coded plastic autoclavable tape is often used for the identification of instruments, especially where different surgical kits are employed.

Engraving should be avoided, as this can damage the instrument surface and predispose to staining and corrosion.

Instrument Kits

Surgical instruments should be selected to suit the purpose for which they are to be used, rather than because they were convenient to use at the time. For example, artery forceps used to extract intra-medullary pins may have the desired effect but will almost certainly be damaged.

The basic surgical kit generally consists of instruments for cutting, dissection, tissue-holding, retraction, haemostasis, ligation and suturing. Surgical kits can be assembled on this basis but also bear in mind the size of animal. For example, instruments used for a cat spay will vary in size to those used for a bitch spay. Most veterinary establishments develop surgical kits for various procedures. A basic kit is often employed, and then specific instruments for special procedures are packed and prepared either individually or in special procedure packs.

Chapter 26 (Theatre Practice) sets out suggestions for different instrument kits.

The laying out of instruments in a kit should be given careful thought. They should be placed in positions which relate to their actual requirement (Fig. 25.4). Every veterinary surgeon has personal preferences and through good communication, observation and anticipation, the veterinary nurse will help to ensure efficient and consistent surgical procedures.

Special Equipment

Ultrasound

Ultrasound is sound of frequencies higher than those audible to the human ear. Diagnostic ultrasound is a non-invasive procedure that allows the internal structures of the abdominal and thoracic cavities to be examined visually. It usually employs sound waves of frequencies between 1 and 10 MHz.

These sound waves are produced by electrical vibration of a 'piezo-electric' crystal stored in the ultrasound transducer, or probe, and they have sufficient energy to penetrate living tissue. Different structures within the body and interfaces between

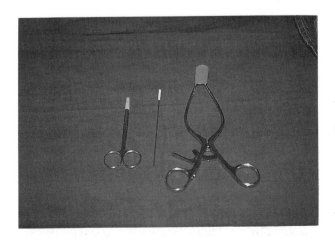

Fig. 25.3. Protecting sharp and pointed instruments to prevent accidental penetration of the surgical packaging.

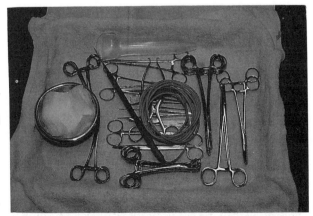

Fig. 25.4. Example of layout for a small animal surgical kit. The large empty syringe case holds the diathermy handle when not being used during the surgery.

structures and organs impede the passage of sound to varying extents. Those sound waves that are not transmitted are reflected back towards their source of origin, where their strength can be detected and thus the degree of attenuation can be recorded electronically on an oscilloscope screen.

The ultrasound scan is recorded in images of black and white with varying shades of grey:

- Fluid is recorded as black, because the sound waves pass through it unimpeded.
- Bone, other mineral densities and also gases, reflect the sound waves totally and are recorded as white.
- Soft tissues appear as various shades of grey, depending on their proportions of fat, fibrous tissue and fluid.

There are two main types of transducer: linear and sector. **Linear transducers** have the crystals arranged in a line, each producing sound waves that form a rectangular sound beam. Superficial structures can be seen well but the transducer itself is bulky and cumbersome, which limits its use with small animals.

Sector transducers contain a single crystal which oscillates or rotates to produce a fan-shaped beam. The size and manoeuvrability of these transducers allow ready access to most of the thoracic and abdominal viscera even in small dogs and cats. Superficial structures, however, are not seen so clearly because of the shape of the beam.

Transducers are also available in a selection of frequencies. A higher frequency will penetrate far less but will provide better resolution than a lower frequency. A 5MHz transducer provides an adequate depth of penetration for cats and small to medium-sized dogs. A 3.5MHz transducer is required for large dogs.

Procedure

It is very important to achieve good skin contact with the transducer when scanning an animal. Hair is better clipped, although it is possible in the longer-haired dogs and cats to part the hair (this is preferable in a show animal). The skin should be clean and free from dirt and grease—surgical spirit helps to degrease it. A proprietary aqueous gel is then applied to the skin and to the transducer, to enable efficient contact. Poor contact will result in a distorted image, often with arc-shaped or horizontal white lines.

Ultrasound is generally carried out on the conscious patient and the position of the animal depends on the area to be examined. If the animal is restrained in any type of recumbency, it will usually be more relaxed and calmer on a padded table-top. For cardiac investigations, a better image of the heart is achieved by scanning from underneath an animal in lateral recumbency, because the lungs will be slightly more compressed on the recumbent side. To achieve this position efficiently, use a table-top with side cut-outs.

Applications

The clinical applications for ultrasound are extensive. The areas in which it offers the greatest imaging advances are in:

- pregnancy diagnosis;
- evaluation of the female reproductive tract;
- investigation of cardiac function (echocardiography);
- evaluation of the architecture of parenchymatous organs, such as the liver, kidneys and spleen.

Ultrasound machines work in two-dimensional 'real time': the image appears with spatial relationships that allow direct recognition of anatomical structures and it is constantly up-dated so that movement in the patient can be recorded. 'Hard copy' can be stored on videotape, heat-sensitive paper or medical imaging film. Cytology or histology samples can be obtained in some cases with the assistance of ultrasound; the 'real time' continual monitoring enables visual precision of the placement of a needle into the area or organ of interest. Some transducers have a biopsy guide attached.

The effects of diagnostic ultrasound on living tissue have been investigated intensively and it appears to be biologically safe and without adverse clinical effects.

Diathermy

Diathermy is a method of cutting or coagulation of tissues by means of high-frequency alternating electrical currents producing local heat within the tissues at the site of application. (This technique must not be confused with electrocautery, in which the electric current creates a red-hot probe which is then applied to the tissues.)

The conventional method for achieving haemostasis during a surgical procedure is to clamp the bleeding vessel with a haemostat and then ligate with suture material. Diathermy can be applied to:

- control haemorrhage, allowing better visualisation of the surgical field;
- decrease surgical time;
- reduce the number of ligatures necessary, so that less suture material is left within the surgical site.

The nature of the waveform of the applied current used in diathermy can vary the effect from cutting to coagulating:

- Continuous waveforms are employed for cutting tissues.
- Interrupted waveforms are used for pure coagulation.
- A mixed waveform combines cutting with coagulation.

Types of coagulation

Coagulation achieved by diathermy may be described as either black or white.

Black coagulation results in the charring of the tissue surface and coagulation of the deeper tissue by the formation of an electrical arc. A crackling is often heard, with miniature explosions. Although this technique is quicker and more impressive than white coagulation, it results in greater tissue necrosis and longer wound healing.

White coagulation is the application of an electrode directly to the underlying tissues without significant arc formation. The electrical current is applied at a lower density and must be applied for longer. Heating occurs over the entire area where the electrode is in contact with the tissue and therefore the effect is more controllable and predictable than with the black method.

Applications

Diathermy currents can be applied by monopolar or bipolar electrodes.

Monopolar diathermy is the only technique that can be used for cutting and for black coagulation. The electrode for **cutting diathermy** can be a flat blade, wire or conventional scalpel blade. For **coagulation diathermy** a flat blade, ball electrode or dissection forceps electrode can be used to grasp a vessel or area of tissue and the current can be applied by touching the instrument with the electrode.

Bipolar diathermy requires two separate electrodes which are applied across the tissue. This can be achieved using either two fixed electrodes on one handle or the two points of dissecting forceps which can be used to elevate the tissue from the surrounding area. The advantage of bipolar application is that the current allows more control over the location and depth of coagulation, but it cannot be used for cutting.

Precautions

There are several designs available for surgical use and it is important that the veterinary nurse is familiar with the specifications for the particular unit being used. Most units require the patient to be 'grounded' or 'earthed' so that the electrical current is conducted to ground. This is usually achieved by placing a special diathermy plate under and in contact with the patient. The plate is connected by a wire to the diathermy unit to enable the transfer of the current to ground. An alternative is a metal rectal probe, in the shape of a thermometer, which is grounded in the same manner as the plate.

If the patient is not properly earthed, the electrical current used for diathermy will travel along the path of least resistance, which may be through the animal or through the surgeon. Serious electrical burning of the animal can be caused by improper grounding.

Alcohol, ether or other highly flammable materials should not be present when diathermy is used. A particular problem could arise with pooling of flammable skin preparations such as surgical spirit.

Care of the diathermy unit

Portions of the diathermy unit may be sterilised (usually the handles and attachments). The manufacturer's instructions concerning sterilisation techniques, maintenance and the operation of the unit must be followed carefully.

Cryosurgery

Cryosurgery destroys living tissue by the controlled application of extreme cold. The aim of cryosurgery is to kill cells in a diseased target area whilst simultaneously producing minimal damage to normal surrounding tissue. As a surgical agent, cryosurgery has the advantage of coagulant and destructive properties.

The fundamental principle is that living cells are at first injured and later die from the effects of freezing:

(1) The refrigerant or probe of the cryosurgical unit is placed in the target area, and heat is extracted from the surrounding tissues.
(2) Water is a major component of all living cells and is the first to be affected; therefore tissues that are relatively fluid-free are the least susceptible to freezing (e.g. bone).
(3) As the temperature of the tissue is reduced, the water in both the intracellular and extracellular spaces begins to freeze, with the formation of ice crystals.
(4) This affects the osmoregulation of the cells, leading eventually to cell dehydration, denaturation, anoxia and ultimately cell death.

A rapid freeze followed by a slow thaw is the best combination in destroying tissue, and repeat freeze–thaw cycles are recommended in order to achieve optimal lethal effects. The temperatures must fall to $-20°C$ or lower, and can be monitored with thermocouples (probes that can be placed into the deeper regions of the affected tissue).

Refrigerants

Cryosurgery begins with the selection of a refrigerant (freezing medium) and a method of its application. Many gases can be converted into their liquid state to serve as a refrigerant and carbon dioxide, nitrous oxide and liquid nitrogen are readily available.

Liquid nitrogen is generally the refrigerant of choice for cryosurgery: with its lower boiling point of $-195.6°C$, it is a more effective and efficient refrigerant for destroying larger areas of tissue than the other gases. It is relatively inexpensive, readily available and non-explosive (provided that it is stored correctly). It can be stored reasonably easily in narrow-necked, large-bodied metal containers with loose-fitting stoppers (dewars) which are usually provided by the main suppliers of liquid nitrogen.

If cryosurgery is only employed occasionally by a practice, it may be sensible to approach a larger institute (veterinary, medical or research) as a local source of supply of the refrigerant. Liquid nitrogen may be collected in a domestic thermos flask but to prevent explosion this must not be screwed shut. Some institutes may offer handling expertise.

Precautions

Liquid nitrogen is a powerful refrigerant and great care should be taken when handling it. The inexperienced should not take a casual approach to its use.

- Avoid splashing exposed areas of clothing in close contact with the body.
- Wear protective eye goggles, an apron or overall, and thick, well-insulated gloves (the type used for handling birds are usually suitable).
- Take even greater care to avoid skin contact with metal surfaces that have been pre-cooled by liquid nitrogen. A severe cold burn will result.

The filling of vessels with liquid nitrogen can be a problem. The situation is similar to that of filling a container with hot water: steam will be produced until the container is at the same temperature as the liquid. A considerable amount of liquid nitrogen will evaporate in this way (and this should be taken into consideration when assessing the amount that is required). Once the inner surface is at liquid nitrogen temperature, evaporation losses when topping up are minimised.

Unfortunately liquid nitrogen continues to evaporate over a period of days or weeks. The evaporation rate is influenced by the size of the storage container: the losses increase as the size of the container decreases. Dipstick indicating gauges are used to estimate levels of liquid nitrogen because a constant cloud of condensate above the surface makes viewing of the level almost impossible.

Refrigerant application

There are several methods of applying the liquid nitrogen to the area to be treated. One of the simplest is to use a probe, or even a cotton bud dipped into the liquid nitrogen and then applied directly to the treatment area. Only small lesions such as warts are suitable for this type of application.

Another method is to pour liquid nitrogen on to a mass or into a cavity however there is not much control. Efficient application requires the use of a cryosurgical unit, which provides a direct application under pressure by spray to provide a very effective form of rapid freezing. Various sizes of orifice and hollow probe are available for use with the sprays.

Preparation

Preparation of the surgical site for cryosurgery depends on the location. Oral lesions require little or no preparation. Asepsis is not necessary for surface lesions but areas covered with hair will require clipping and cleaning to allow efficient contact and application of the liquid nitrogen. Skin antiseptics can be used for cleaning. Normal aseptic precautions must be followed when deep lesions are treated.

It is important to protect adjacent tissues, as they will be vulnerable, especially if a spray application is used. Protection can be provided by petroleum jelly or vaseline; polystyrene from packaging material or disposable cups is also a suitable insulator.

Disadvantages of cryosurgery

Owners should be warned beforehand that postoperatively an area that has been treated cryosurgically is not an attractive sight, especially if a large region is involved.

- A slough occurs initially and this may become moist and discharge. This is not only unsightly but also in some cases smelly.
- Hair-covered areas may heal with unpigmented hair and this could be a problem in a show animal.
- Daily cleaning of the surgical area post-operatively is usually necessary.
- Immediately post-operatively there is likely to be a degree of erythema and oedema which could lead to problems, especially in the oral cavity.
- The procedure of cryosurgery is time-consuming. Small warts etc. are probably removed more easily and quickly with a pair of scissors.

Care of the equipment

Cleaning of the cryoprobes is essential, as a build-up of debris on the tips can lead to a build-up of corrosive deposits which may eventually weaken the tips and create a positive hazard. Washing in mild detergent, coupled with gentle polishing of discoloured areas, is normally adequate. Care should be taken not to use corrosive or abrasive polishes which, over a period, will result in thinning of metal components.

Sterilisation of some cryoprobes can be by autoclaving but as there are many different cryo-units and attachments it is advisable to check with the manufacturers for the cleaning and care of all equipment.

Endoscopes

Endoscopes are delicate and expensive instruments. They are used for visual examination of the interior of a body cavity or hollow organ. The word endoscopy is derived from the Greek prefix *endo*, meaning 'within', and *skopien*, meaning 'to view or observe with intent, to monitor'. Thus endoscopy is an apt term for the procedure of peering into the recesses of the living body. This is made possible by combining a light source with simple optical systems of lenses and mirrors, which have been available for centuries and which are present in every veterinary establishment in forms which range in complexity, e.g. auroscopes, proctoscopes and ophthalmoscopes.

Endoscopy was first introduced to veterinary medicine in the early 1970s. Its use has increased dramatically as veterinary surgeons have become aware of the diagnostic and therapeutic indications. It provides a non-invasive means of viewing and obtaining tissue samples from a variety of body organs.

Types of endoscope

There are two types of endoscope in common use: **flexible** and **rigid**. There are two types of flexible endoscope:

- **Fibre-optic** endoscopes use glass-fibre bundles for the transmission of images.
- **Video** endoscopes use television for the transmission of images.

The glass-fibre bundles, contained within an 'umbilical cord', have two functions:

- They transmit light from a remote source, through the instrument, to illuminate the tissues under inspection.
- They carry the image back to the observer's eyepiece.

Although the glass fibres are flexible and are protected within a stout outer cover, individually they are brittle so that even under careful working conditions occasional fractures of single strands occur. Each broken fibre ceases to transmit light. As it is not practical to replace individual fractured fibres, it can be appreciated that these delicate fibre-optic endoscopes must be handled with great care.

An air pump for insufflation is usually housed in the remote light source. A water bottle attached to the air pump assembly allows water to be flushed down the air/water channel for washing the lens.

Care of endoscopes

Endoscopes should be cleaned after use. If this is not done immediately, thorough cleaning will be much more difficult and the instrument will deteriorate due to the presence of dried mucus, blood etc.

> **WARNING**
> Unless the endoscope is of an immersible type, it must never be immersed completely in liquid. Extensive damage will occur if liquid enters the control section or light connector plug. The endoscope should not be autoclaved or placed in a hot air oven.

Cleaning equipment includes:

- Large bowl.
- Rubber gloves.
- Gauze swabs.
- Tap water.
- Cotton buds.
- Endoscope cleaning brush.
- Disinfectant solution (as recommended by the manufacturer).

The endoscope should remain attached to the light source with the water bottle and suction pump also attached.

(1) Prepare approximately a litre of disinfectant solution in a bowl.
(2) Place the distal tip of the endoscope in the solution, and aspirate through by depressing the suction button.
(3) Unscrew the biopsy valve and clean the inside with a cotton bud; pass the cleaning brush through the biopsy channel. Follow with a clear-water rinse by suction.
(4) Disconnect the water bottle tube from the light guide connector, block the water inlet with a finger and then depress the water/air button to blow all the water out of the channel.
(5) With gauze swabs, wipe the insertion tube with the disinfectant solution. Follow with a clear-water rinse.
(6) The control section and light guide tube/plug may be wiped with gauze that has been lightly dampened in the disinfectant. Follow with a water-dampened swab to remove residual disinfectant.
(7) The ocular lens can be cleaned with a solution of 70% alcohol applied carefully with a cotton bud.
(8) Thorough drying is recommended. Hang the endoscope on a secure hook or drip-stand to enable residual fluid to run downwards away from the control and eye-piece section.
(9) Once dry, endoscopes can be stored in carrying cases or cabinets for protection. Check that the end tip is included before closing lids or doors.

Expensive injuries can be avoided and the life expectation of the equipment can be extended if routine precautions for use and care are observed.

26
Theatre Practice

D. McHUGH

The veterinary nurse is usually given the responsibility for running the operating theatre. This involves maintenance of hygiene in the theatre; care and maintenance of instruments and equipment, preparation of theatre, the patient and the surgical team, and assistance as both scrubbed and circulating nurse.

The most important factor in successful theatre practice is the establishment and maintenance of a good **aseptic technique**, i.e. all the steps taken to prevent contact with micro-organisms.

DEFINITIONS

Sepsis: The presence of pathogens or their toxic products in the blood or tissues of the patient. More commonly known as **infection**.

Asepsis: Freedom from infection, i.e. exclusion of micro-organisms and spores.

Antisepsis: Prevention of sepsis by destruction or inhibition of micro-organisms using an agent that may be safely applied to living tissue.

Sterilisation: The destruction of all micro-organisms and spores.

Disinfection: The removal of micro-organisms but not necessarily spores.

Disinfectant: An agent that destroys micro-organisms—generally chemical agents applied to inanimate objects.

Factors Influencing the Development of Infection

Infection of a clean surgical wound is always a matter of great concern to surgeons. Obviously it is far better to prevent infection than to try and treat it. The use of antibiotics should not be relied upon to protect patients from the consequences of poor asepsis.

It has been established that most surgical wound infections occur at the time of surgery, not during the post-operative period. Poor aseptic technique will undoubtedly affect the success of any surgery and in the long term the success and reputation of the practice. Strict theatre discipline is essential if high standards are to be maintained. There has to be a specific protocol that is adhered to rigidly and that everyone involved with surgery respects. This will include correct theatre attire, scrubbing up procedures, patient preparation, draping techniques, sterilisation, organization of surgical lists, cleaning protocol and conduct during surgery.

Sources of contamination in the operating theatre include:

- Operating room and environment.
- Equipment and instruments.
- Personnel.
- Patient.

Operating room and environment

Many micro-organisms are airborne and any movement within the operating theatre will disperse them. Good ventilation is necessary as hot, humid conditions are a great threat to asepsis. Cleaning procedures should be performed first because micro-organisms from contaminated sites will remain in the air. The operating room itself must be easily cleaned and should contain as little furniture and shelving as possible.

Equipment and instruments

All equipment and instruments used in the operative site must be sterile. There must be a new set of instruments for each operation.

Personnel

The more people present in theatre, the greater the likelihood of infection. All theatre personnel should wear theatre clothing, caps, masks, scrub suits and anti-static footwear. These are only worn in the designated theatre area. In addition those who are in the surgical team should prepare their hands aseptically and wear sterile gowns and gloves.

The patient

The patient is probably the greatest source of contamination, especially as animals are covered in hair. The source of micro-organisms may be:

- **Endogenous**—those that originate from within the body of the patient.
- **Exogenous**—those that are found on the outside, i.e. the skin and coat. This term is also used with reference to environmental sources or micro-organisms (e.g., air, equipment etc.).

It does not necessarily follow that introduction of micro- organisms will result in an infected wound. Micro-organisms can and will enter any wound that has been exposed to air but whether infection follows depends on several variable factors, including the balance between the **virulence** (disease-producing ability) of the organism and the resistance of the patient. Other factors that influence wound infection include:

- Duration of surgery—bacterial contamination increases the longer the wound is open. Infection rate doubles for every hour of operative time.
- Surgical technique—excessive trauma to tissues and damage to vascular supply may increase the likelihood of infection.
- Impaired host resistance—this may increase the risk of infection if it is due to drugs, nutrition or underlying disease.
- Contamination of the wound—surgical wounds are classified with respect to their potential for contamination and infection.

Classification of surgical wounds

   Clean—where there is no break in asepsis. The respiratory, gastrointestinal and urinary tracts are not entered and there is no break in aseptic technique.

   Clean-contaminated—where a contaminated area is entered but without spillage or spread of contamination (i.e. ingesta, urine, mucus). Minor break in asepsis.

   Contaminated—where there is spillage from a viscus or severe inflammation is encountered, but no infection present. Open fresh traumatic wounds.

   Dirty—where there is pus present or viscus perforation spilling pus. Traumatic wound containing devitalised tissue or foreign bodies.

Sterilisation

All instruments, implants and equipment which are to be used during surgery must be sterilised before use. There are several different methods of sterilisation available. Choice will depend on:

- Amount and type of equipment to be sterilised.
- Financial constraints.
- Room available.

Each method has both advantages and disadvantages. Selection is based on the requirements of the individual practice or hospital. Usually several different methods will be chosen. They must be efficient, safe and economical. Sterilisation can be divided into two types (Fig. 26.1).

Cold Sterilisation

Ethylene oxide

Ethylene oxide is a highly penetrating and effective method of sterilisation. However, concerns have been expressed about its use in veterinary practice as it is toxic, irritant to tissue and a very inflammable gas. Currently its use is permitted and the danger to

COLD AND HEAT STERILISATION	
Cold sterilisation	Heat sterilisation
Ethylene oxide	Dry heat
Formaldehyde	Hot-air oven
Chemical solutions	High vacuum oven
Gluteraldehyde	Convection oven
Chlorhexidine-based	Autoclave (steam under
Alcohol-based	pressure)
Irradiation	Vertical
	Horizontal
	Vacuum-assisted

Fig. 26.1. Cold/heat sterilisation.

operators should be negligible as long as the manufacturer's recommendations are followed. COSHH regulations may however make its use impractical in some veterinary practices. Ethylene oxide inactivates the DNA of the cells, thereby preventing cell reproduction. The technique is effective against vegetative bacteria, fungi, viruses and spores. Several factors influence the ability of ethylene oxide to destroy micro-organisms, including temperature, pressure, concentration, humidity and time of exposure. As temperature increases, the ability of ethylene oxide to penetrate increases and duration of the cycle shortens. However the only system available in the UK operates at room temperature for a period of 12 hours.

Use of the ethylene oxide steriliser. The steriliser consists of a plastic container which is fitted with a ventilation system to prevent gas entering the work area. It should be located in a clean, well-ventilated area (e.g. fume cupboard) away from working areas. The temperature of the room must be at least 20°C (68°F) during the cycle.

Individually packed items to be sterilised are placed in a polythene liner bag. A gas ampoule containing ethylene oxide liquid is placed within the liner bag which is then sealed with a metal twist tie and placed in the steriliser unit. The top of the glass vial is snapped from outside the liner bag to release the sterilant gas. The door to the steriliser unit is closed and locked, the ventilator turned on and the items left to sterilise. The sterilisation process is frequently performed overnight. At the end of the 12 hour period a pump is switched on to aerate the container. The door may be opened after 2 hours and the load removed.

The items should then be left for a further 24 hours in a well-ventilated room to allow the ethylene oxide to dissipate.

Items which may be sterilised using ethylene oxide. Ethylene oxide is effective for the sterilisation of many different types of equipment but its use is limited by the size of the container, the duration of the cycle and concerns about toxicity. Its use therefore tends to be restricted to items which are damaged by heat:

- Fibre-optic equipment
- Plastic catheters, trays etc.
- Anaesthetic tubing etc.
- Plastic syringes
- Optical instruments
- High-speed drills/burrs
- Battery-operated drills.

Some commercially available products are now sterilised by this method, e.g. syringes, synthetic absorbable suture materials and catheters. Avoid sterilising equipment made of polyvinylchloride (PVC) by this method as it may react with the gas.

Preparation of materials for sterilisation. Materials to be sterilised by ethylene oxide must be cleaned and dried. The presence of protein and grease will slow the sterilisation process. Water on instruments at the time of exposure may react with the gas and reduce its effectiveness.

Occlusive bungs, caps or stylets must be removed from instruments so that gas can penetrate freely. Syringes should be packaged disassembled.

Ethylene oxide penetrates materials more readily than steam so a wider variety of packaging materials may be used when preparing items for sterilisation and storage. However, nylon film designed for autoclaving should not be used as it has been shown that there is poor penetration by ethylene oxide.

Testing efficiency of sterilisation. **Indicator tape** with yellow stripes which turn red when exposed to ethylene oxide may be used as an indicator of exposure to the gas, but they do not guarantee sterility as they give no indication that exposure was for the correct length of time. In fact, the colour change will occur after a very short period.

Chemical indicator strips which undergo a colour change when exposed to ethylene oxide for the correct time may be placed in the centre of a pack or load to test the penetration efficiency.

Spore strips placed into a load are added to a culture medium on completion of the cycle and are incubated for 72 hours. This is a useful test of the efficiency of the system but is obviously not suitable as an immediate indicator of sterility.

Formaldehyde

In the past formaldehyde gas was used in a similar way to ethylene oxide but it has been largely superceded and COSHH regulations have limited its use.

Chemical solutions

This method should really only be considered as a means of disinfection although some manufacturers guarantee sterilisation following prolonged immersion (usually 24 hours). It remains a useful method for surgical equipment which may not be sterilised by any other means. It has gained particular popularity for the disinfection of endoscopic equipment.

Care should be taken to use the specific concentrations and time stipulated by the manufacturer. The chemical solution and the article to be disinfected should be placed in a tray or bowl, preferably with a lid to prevent evaporation and contamination by airborne micro-organisms.

Gluteraldehyde

This is the most widely used commercial product available. It is extremely irritant to tissues and so articles must be rinsed with sterile water before use. Gloves and masks should be worn when using this chemical. The product is supplied as an acid solution which is activated by the addition of a powder at the time of use. It may be reused over a 2–4 week period, depending on the preparation used.

Chlorhexidine-based solutions

These have also been widely used for disinfection of surgical equipment. They have the same drawback as many other solutions, i.e. poor activity against spores, fungi and viruses.

Alcohol-based solutions

A variety of these have been used—e.g. ethyl alcohol and isopropol alcohol. They work by denaturation and coagulation of proteins.

Irradiation

This form of sterilisation is a form of gamma irradiation and can only be carried out under controlled conditions within industry.

Many pre-packaged items are sterilised by this method.

Heat Sterilisation

Dry heat

Dry heat kills micro-organisms by causing oxidative destruction of bacterial protoplasm. Micro-organisms are much more resistant to dry heat than when heated in the presence of moisture and so higher temperatures are required (150–180°C). Dry heat below 140°C cannot destroy bacterial spores in less than 4–5 hours.

The range of equipment sterilised in this way is restricted: fabrics, rubber goods and plastic cannot withstand these high, dry temperatures and are easily damaged.

There are certain items for which dry heat sterilisation is the method of choice. These include glass syringes, cutting instruments, ophthalmic instruments, drill bits, glassware, powders and oils which cannot be sterilised using any form of moisture.

Hot-air ovens. These are heated by electrical elements (Fig. 26.2). They are usually small but are economical in terms of purchase and running costs. They have been largely superseded by the autoclave, which is more efficient and suitable for most types of material.

A long cooling period is needed before the items may be used. The door should be fitted with a safety device to prevent it being opened before the oven is cool. It is important to ensure that the oven is not overloaded and that items are placed so that air can flow freely.

Spore strip tests and Browne's tubes are available which are designed specifically for testing sterility in hot-air ovens.

Other types of dry heat steriliser include high vacuum assisted ovens and convection ovens, though neither type is commonly used in current veterinary practice. **High vacuum assisted ovens** are fully automatic and incorporate a vacuum system that reduces the time required for sterilisation to approximately 15 minutes for most articles. Mechanical **convection ovens** incorporate a motor blower to circulate the air and are designed to achieve a uniform temperature in all parts of the unit.

Steam under pressure (autoclave systems)

Steam under pressure is the most widely used and efficient method of sterilisation. It is also the most economical, although the initial outlay may be large. Items which may be sterilised in the autoclave include:

- Instruments
- Drapes
- Gowns
- Swabs
- Most rubber articles
- Glassware
- Some plastic goods.

Heat-sensitive items which may be damaged in the autoclave include fibre-optic equipment, lenses and plastics (especially those designed to be disposable, such as catheters).

The three main types of autoclave are the vertical pressure cooker, the horizontal or vertical downward displacement autoclave and the vacuum-assisted autoclave.

TEMPERATURE AND TIME RATIOS RECOMMENDED FOR HOT AIR OVENS		
Item	Temperature	Time mins
Glassware Non-cutting instruments	180°C	60
Powders, Oils	160°C	120
Sharp-cutting instruments	150°C	180

Fig. 26.2. Hot-air oven temperatures.

Vertical pressure cooker. This is a very simple machine which operates by boiling water in a closed container like a household pressure cooker. It usually has an air vent at the top which is closed once the air has been evacuated, and pressure (15lbs p.s.i) is allowed to build up. As the air vent is at the top, the main disadvantage of this type of autoclave is the danger that some air will be trapped underneath the steam. The temperature in this area will be lower and sterility cannot be guaranteed. Also, as it is manually operated there is room for human error in the sterilising cycle.

Horizontal or vertical downward displacement autoclave. This type is larger and usually fully automatic. It uses an electrically operated boiler that is incorporated in the autoclave as a source of steam. Air is driven out more efficiently by downward displacement. There is an air outlet at the bottom and a steam outlet at the top.

Most of these machines are designed for loose instrument sterilisation only, rather than packs, as they have insufficient drying cycles: packs may seem to be dry but they remain damp, allowing entry of micro-organisms during the storage period.

There is usually a choice of programmes on this type of autoclave with temperatures of 112°C, 121°C, 126°C or 134°C. Although larger than the portable autoclave this type is not really suitable for a busy surgical unit needing to sterilise large amounts of instruments, gowns and drapes.

Vacuum assisted autoclave. This type of autoclave works on the same principle as the other two but uses a high vacuum pump to evacuate air rapidly from the chamber at the beginning of the cycle. Steam penetration after evacuation is almost instantaneous and sterilisation occurs very quickly. A second vacuum cycle rapidly withdraws moisture after sterilisation and dries the load. It is suitable for all types of instruments, drapes and equipment and there is a choice of cycles using different temperatures and pressures.

Vacuum-assisted autoclaves are fully automatic, with failsafe mechanisms (usually warning lights and alarms) which indicate whether the load is non-sterile or has been sterilised effectively. They are generally much larger and more sophisticated than other types and are invariably connected to a central boiler to supply steam. The cost of purchase and maintenance are higher, but the machine's efficiency and reliability in sterilisation far outweigh those of the smaller types.

Principles of sterilisation using steam under pressure

Although autoclaves vary in size and type the basic principle of function remains the same. When water boils at 100°C it is converted to steam and the temperature remains the same however long it is heated. Many bacteria, spores and viruses are resistant to heat and remain unchanged even if exposed to such a temperature for a long time. By increasing the pressure, the temperature of the steam is raised and resistant micro-organisms and spores will be killed by coagulation of cell proteins. It is the increased temperature, not the increased pressure, that leads to this destruction of micro-organisms. The higher the temperature, the shorter the time needed to achieve sterilisation (Fig. 26.3).

The autoclaving process. The central sterilising chamber of the autoclave is surrounded by a steam jacket. The pressure in the jacket is raised (depending on the cycle). Steam then enters the chamber and as it does so air is displaced downwards, because steam is lighter. When all the air is evacuated, exhaust vents are closed and steam continues to enter until the desired pressure is reached. The more sophisticated types of autoclave have a vacuum prior to introduction of steam to displace air from materials to be sterilised. If any air remains in the chamber the temperature will be lower than steam at that pressure and sterility cannot be guaranteed.

Once the air had been evacuated, steam that has entered the chamber begins to condense on the colder surfaces in the chamber, i.e. instruments etc. The steam produces heat which penetrates to the innermost layer of the pack. The moisture increases the penetrability of the heat. After the given amount of time the steam is exhausted. As the temperature drops, the pressure returns to normal. In vacuum-assisted autoclaves the instruments are then heat dried: filtered air replaces the exhausted steam. On modern machines the door cannot be opened until the end of this stage.

Effective sterilisation also depends on correct loading of packs into the autoclave. There should be adequate space between them to allow steam to circulate freely. Care should be taken to avoid overloading and blocking of the inlet and exhaust valves. Before packing for sterilisation, instruments must be free of grease and protein material to allow effective penetration of steam.

AUTOCLAVE TEMPERATURE, PRESSURE, TIME COMBINATIONS		
Temperature	Pressure	Time (mins)
121°C	15psi [1.2kg/cm²]	15
126°C	20psi [1.4kg/cm²]	10
134°C	30psi [2kg/cm²]	3½

It should be noted that this is only the sterilising time. The length of the whole cycle will vary from 15–45 minutes.

Fig. 26.3. Autoclave times and temperatures.

Maintenance of the autoclave. All types of autoclave should be serviced by a qualified engineer to ensure that they remain in good working order and remain electrically safe. Vacuum-assisted autoclaves with a separate boiler should be serviced every 3 months to comply with health and safety regulations. Thermocouple testing is recommended at least annually to ensure effective sterilisation is taking place.

Monitoring efficacy of sterilisation in the autoclave. **Chemical indicator strips** show colour changes when the correct temperature, pressure and time have been reached. A strip is placed inside each pack. It is important that the appropriate strip is used for each different pressure/time/temperature cycle otherwise a false result may be given.

Browne's tubes work on the same principle i.e. a colour change. Small glass tubes are partly filled with an orange-brown liquid which changes to green when certain temperatures have been maintained for a required period of time. Tubes are available which change at 121°C, 126°C or 134°C. It is essential to ensure that the correct type of tube is selected for any particular temperature cycle. Browne's tubes are also available for hot-air ovens.

Bowie–Dick indicator tape is commonly used to seal instrument and drape packs. It is a beige-coloured tape which is impregnated with chemical stripes that change to dark brown when a certain temperature is reached (121°C). As with ethylene oxide indicator tape, it is not reliable as an indicator of sterility as it does not ensure that the temperature was maintained for the required time.

Spore tests are strips of paper impregnated with dried spores (usually *Bacillus stearothermophilius*). A strip is included in the load; on completion of the cycle it is placed in the culture medium provided and incubated at the appropriate temperature for up to 72 hours. If the sterilisation process has been successful, the spores will be killed and there will be no growth.

Spore systems are more accurate than chemical indicators but the delay in obtaining results is a major disadvantage. A combination of both systems is recommended: chemical indicators should be included in each pack and spore strips should be used at regular intervals.

Vacuum-assisted autoclaves will usually have visible temperature and pressure **gauges** on the front. Some systems have a paper **recording chart** which indicates the efficiency of sterilisation.

Thermocouples (electrical leads with temperature sensitive tips) are placed in various parts of the sterilising chamber with the leads passed out through an aperture to a recording device outside. The temperature within the chamber can be constantly recorded throughout a cycle to check that required temperatures are received and held for the specified time.

Moist heat (boiling)

Boiling should no longer be considered as a method of sterilisation. It cannot be guaranteed to kill all micro-organisms and spores, because the maximum temperature of 100°C is insufficient to kill resistant spores. With far superior sterilisation methods available, the old fashioned boiler has no place in modern veterinary surgery.

Packing Supplies for Sterilisation

Various materials and containers are available for packing supplies for sterilisation, each having advantages and disadvantages. Choice will depend on several factors:

- Size of autoclave/gas steriliser.
- The packaging material must be resistant to damage when handled and not damage the equipment to be sterilised.
- Steam or gas must be able to penetrate the wrapping for sterilisation to occur and must be easily exhausted from the pack once sterilisation is complete.
- Micro-organisms must not be able to penetrate from the outer surface of the wrap to the inner.
- Cost.
- Personal preference.
- Time taken to achieve sterility.

Materials and containers

Nylon film. Nylon film designed specifically for use in the autoclave is available in a variety of sizes. It has the advantages of being reusable and transparent so that items can be easily seen. Its main disadvantage is that it becomes brittle after repeated use, resulting in development of tiny unseen holes and therefore contamination of the pack. It may also be difficult to remove sterile items from packs without contaminating them on the edges of the bag. The packs are often sealed using Bowie–Dick tape.

Seal-and-peel pouches. Disposable bags, consisting of a paper back and clear plasticised front with a fold over seal, are available in a wide variety of sizes. They may be used with ethylene oxide or the autoclave. The risk of contamination during opening is small. Double wrapping decreases the risk of damage to the instrument during storage or when opening the pack. They are most suitable for individual instruments.

Paper. Paper-based sheets are commonly used for packing instruments. The most suitable type consists of a crepe-like paper which is slightly elastic, conforming and is water-repellent. It is therefore ideal as an outer layer for packs. Although it is frequently reused, it is intended to be disposable. It is available in large sheets which can be cut to the appropriate size.

Textile. Textile sheets, usually linen, are commonly used to wrap surgical equipment for sterilisation. They are conforming, strong and reusable but have the major disadvantage of being permeable to moisture. Usually a double layer of linen is covered by a waterproof paper-based wrap for surgical packs.

Drums. Metal drums with steam vents in the side which are closed after sterilisation are commonly used in veterinary practice, especially with the small portable autoclaves. They can be used for instruments, gowns and drapes. Their main disadvantage is that they are frequently multi-use, so that there is a degree of environmental contamination each time the lid is opened. There is also a risk of contamination of items touching the edge or outside of the drum when they are removed. Initial outlay is relatively high but they will last for years.

Boxes and cartons. A variety of boxes and cartons are available for use in the autoclave. They are useful for gown or drape packs and for specialised kits (e.g. orthopaedic kits). They are relatively inexpensive and may be reused.

Care and Sterilisation of Equipment

Gowns and drapes

After use surgical gowns and drapes should be washed, dried and inspected for damage. Gowns should then be folded correctly so that the outside surface of the gown is on the inside (Figs 26.4 and 26.5). This is so that the surgical team can put on gowns in a aseptic fashion (described later). Plain drapes may be folded concertina-style (Fig. 26.6) or so that two corners are on the top surface (Fig. 26.7). Fenestrated drapes are usually folded concertina style.

Sterilisation. Both gowns and drapes may be sterilised by ethylene oxide but this method is often uneconomical in a large practice owing to the small size of the steriliser, duration of the cycle (12 hours) and the airing time of 24 hours. Autoclaving is a quicker, more efficient method but it is essential that the machine has a porous load cycle to ensure complete penetration and drying of the load. A hot air oven is unsuitable as it will lead to charring of the material.

Gowns and drapes may be sterilised in drums, boxes, bags or packs. A handtowel is usually placed with the gown when packing for sterilisation. Drapes are sometimes incorporated into the instrument pack.

Swabs

Swabs may be purchased pre-sterilised however they are usually purchased non-sterile because of the cost. They may be already tied in bundles of either five or ten but it is usual for the nurse to do this. Each pack

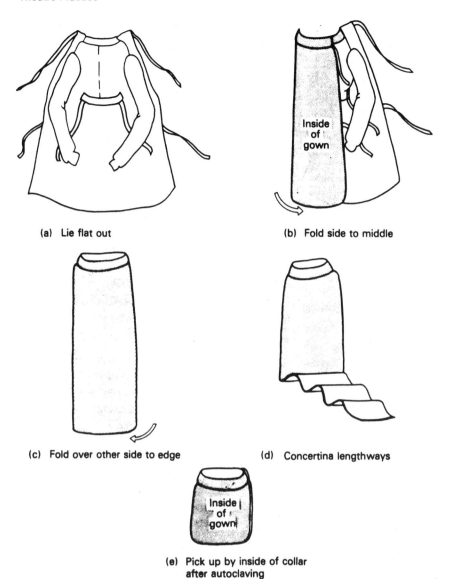

(a) Lie flat out

(b) Fold side to middle

Inside of gown

(c) Fold over other side to edge

(d) Concertina lengthways

(e) Pick up by inside of collar after autoclaving

Inside of gown

Fig. 26.4. Folding a gown.

should have a consistent number which is known to all surgery staff. Swabs may be incorporated into the instrument pack, supplied in drums or packed individually in packets.

Sterilisation. Swabs should be sterilised in the same way as gowns and drapes.

Urinary catheters

Although designed for single use, most urinary catheters may be re-sterilised once. The exception to this is the Foley catheter, which will usually be unfit for re-use. After use catheters should be washed, rinsed and then dried. They should be packed, without coiling if possible, in appropriate bags.

Sterilisation. Many brands of catheter may be sterilised by autoclaving but some will be damaged by heat. Ethylene oxide can be successfully used for all types of catheter. It is essential to ensure that they are aired for the recommended time before use.

Syringes

Plastic syringes are designed to be disposable. To ensure sterility after storage they must be packed individually. It is therefore rarely economical to re-sterilise small syringes but it may be profitable to re-sterilise 30ml and 50ml syringes. They should be disassembled, washed thoroughly and dried prior to sterilisation.

Sterilisation. Most plastic syringes can be auto-claved safely but some brands will be damaged. Ethylene oxide may be used effectively to sterilise syringes. The plungers should be removed from the barrel prior to this. Glass syringes may be sterilised using a hot air oven, autoclave or ethylene oxide.

Liquids

It is usual to purchase liquids pre-sterilised, although more sophisticated autoclaves have a cycle for the sterilisation of fluids. However, the risk of breakage

(a)   (b)

(c)   (d)

(e)   (f)

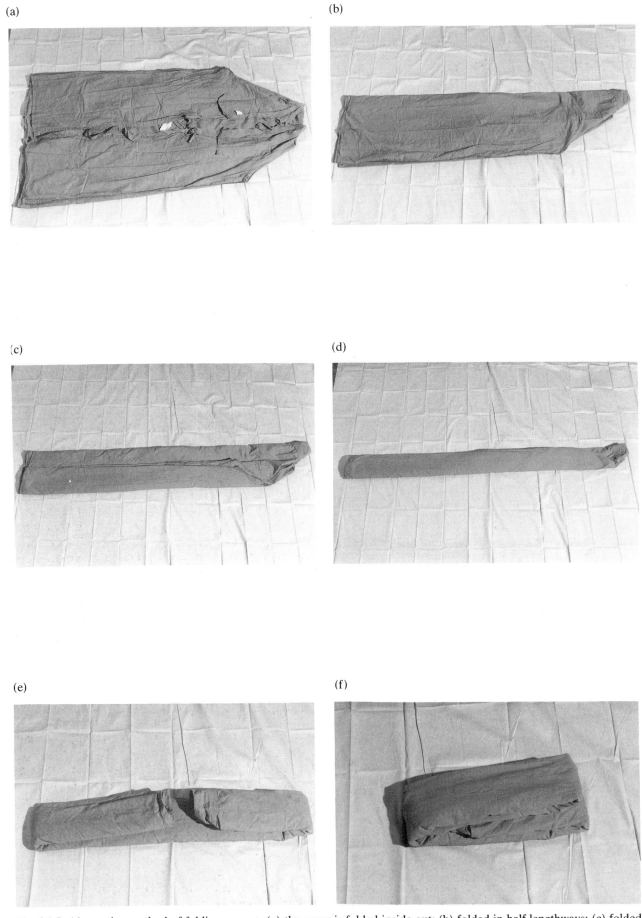

Fig. 26.5. Alternative method of folding a gown: (a) the gown is folded inside out; (b) folded in half lengthways; (c) folded in half lengthways again; (d) and again in half lengthways; (e) the top and bottom edges are folded to the middle; (f) the gown is then folded in half again.

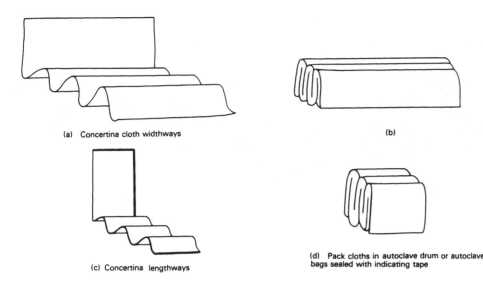

(a)   Concertina cloth widthways

(b)

(c)   Concertina lengthways

(d)   Pack cloths in autoclave drum or autoclave
bags sealed with indicating tape

Fig. 26.6. Folding surgical
drapes.

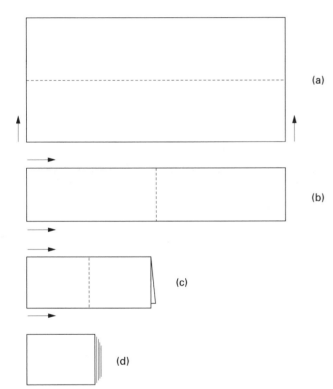

(a)

(b)

(c)

(d)

Fig. 26.7. Folding a plain drape corner to corner: (a) the
drape is folded in half widthways; (b)–(d) it is then folded
in half lengthways three times so that there are two corners
at the top.

of glass bottles is high and it is probably more
economical to purchase fluids which have been
commercially prepared.

Power tools

Air drills, saws and mechanical burrs are usually
autoclavable but individual manufacturers' instructions should always be followed. Autoclaving can in
some cases lead to jamming of the motor. Ethylene
oxide can be used for all air driven tools. Battery
drills frequently have plastic casing which would melt

in an autoclave but they can be sterilised by using
ethylene oxide. Alternatively the unsterile drill is
dropped into a sterile sleeve and a sterile chuck is
then attached.

Storage after Sterilisation

There should be a separate area for storage of sterile
packs. It should be dust free, dry and well-ventilated.
Ideally all packs should be kept in closed cupboards.
They should be handled as little as possible to
minimise risk of damage, and packed loosely on
shelves so that bags are not damaged. The length of
time for which packs may be safely stored after
sterilisation is the subject of much debate, with
recommendations varying from a few weeks to 6
months. A sealed pack should remain sterile for a
limitless period but it may become contaminated by
excessive handling, resulting in damage to the pack,
or moisture. It is therefore recommended that unused
packs should be repacked and resterilised after 6–8
weeks.

The Operating Theatre

The design and layout of the operating theatre will
rarely be within the control of the veterinary nurse. It
is important, however, to have some knowledge of
ideal requirements and desirable features in order to
appreciate differing standards or aseptic techniques
and to try and make the best of existing facilities.
The operating theatre suite should ideally consist of:

- The operating theatre
- Anaesthetic preparation area
- Area for washing and sterilising equipment
- Sterile storage area
- Scrubbing-up area
- Changing rooms
- Recovery room.

The Operating Theatre

Many practices have just one operating theatre which is used for all surgery. Larger hospitals may have theatres which are used specifically for particular types of surgery, e.g. orthopaedic work, general surgery and 'dirty' surgery such as dental work. The size of the theatre will depend on the purpose for which it is intended. If it is to be used for simple, routine surgery it can be quite compact. However, if it is to be used for orthopaedic surgery a large amount of surgical equipment may be needed. If the theatre is too small, working conditions will be compromised and it may be difficult to maintain a high standard of asepsis. It has to be large enough to accommodate the patient, anaesthetic equipment, surgical instrument trolley, other equipment and personnel.

There are several other requirements that are essential, or at least desirable:

- The operating theatre should be an end room, not a throughfare to other rooms.
- It must be easily cleaned. Walls and floors must be made of impervious, non-staining materials, floors should be non-slip and hard wearing. The use of drains should be avoided where possible but should not pose a problem if maintained properly. Walls and ceiling should be painted with a light coloured 'waterproof' paint. The corners and edges of all walls should be coved to facilitate easy cleaning.
- There should be as little shelving and furniture as possible as it will harbour dust.
- Good lighting is essential. Advantage should be taken of natural daylight. Ideally lighting should be concealed within the ceiling with additional side lights on the wall and an overhead theatre light.
- There should be a good supply of electric sockets (in waterproof casing), preferably recessed into the wall.
- Heating is an important consideration since anaesthetised animals are unable to control their own body temperature. The ambient temperature should be between 15 and 20°C. Fan heaters cause air and dust movement and should be avoided. Modern wall-mounted radiators are the most realistic method of heating. Panel heating within the walls is ideal, but expensive.
- Some system of air-conditioning and ventilation is necessary and may become mandatory under COSHH regulations.
- A scavenging system for anaesthetic waste gas will also be necessary.
- An X-ray viewer, preferably flush with the wall, is an important fixture in all operating theatres.
- An air supply for power tools may be needed. This should ideally be piped into theatre from cylinders housed outside theatre. Anaesthetic gases can be delivered in the same way.
- All equipment, including the operating table, must be easily cleaned.

- A wall clock is needed for anaesthetic monitoring and timing of surgery.
- A dry-wipe board is useful for recording details such as swab numbers, suture details, blood loss etc.
- The rooms should have double swing doors which should normally be kept closed.
- There should be no clear-glass window to the outside, as this will be distracting. Windows should not open, as this will be a threat to asepsis.
- The operating table should be adjustable to facilitate positioning of the patient and to suit the height of the surgeon. The base of the table may be static or maintained on wheels for easy moving. There is usually a hydraulically operated pump to adjust the height, and some electrically operated pumps are also available.

Anaesthetic Preparation Area

There should be a separate area where the induction of anaesthesia pre-operative procedures (e.g. clipping, catheterisation of the bladder and preparation of the surgical site) can be carried out. It should lead directly into the operating theatre.

Area for Washing and Sterilising Equipment

There needs to be a room where dirty instruments are washed, packed and sterilised. It should be situated close to the operating theatre but away from the sterile storage area. It should include a washing machine and tumble drier (specifically for theatre wear, gowns and drapes), sterilisation facilities and possibly an ultrasonic instrument cleaner.

Sterile Storage Area

Sterile supplies should be stored in closed cupboards away from the instrument washing area, but adjacent to theatre. Here instrument trolleys can be laid out prior to surgery. Entry should be directly into the theatre.

Scrubbing-up Area

There should be a separate scrub room within the theatre suite but outside the theatre itself. This should lead directly into the sterile preparation area and theatre. Swing doors which can be foot operated should separate the rooms.

Changing Rooms

Changing rooms for personnel should be situated at the entrance to theatre. It is a good idea to have a red line delineating the sterile area and appropriate notices displayed to indicate these areas. Footwear for use in theatre should be placed at the entrance to theatre beyond the red line. This barrier should be adhered to at all times. The layout of rooms within the theatre suite is important for the sake of asepsis. There should be a one-way traffic system, so that the surgical team and sterile supplies enter through one door and unscrubbed personnel enter and leave through a separate doorway.

Recovery Room

A room where the patient can recover following surgery may be situated near the operating theatre suite. It should be quiet and warm and contain essential equipment to deal with any post-operative emergencies which could occur.

Maintenance and Cleaning of the Operating Theatre

A routine cleaning programme in the operating area is essential if a high standard of asepsis is to be maintained:

* At the beginning of each day, all the surfaces and all the furniture and equipment in the theatre suite should be damp-dusted using a dilute solution of disinfectant. A dry duster would simply move dust around the room.
* In between cases, the operating table, equipment and surfaces including the floor should be wiped clean if soiled.
* At the end of the day, the floors in all rooms of the theatre suite should be vacuumed to remove debris and loose hair. They should then be either wet-vacuumed or washed using disinfectant. All waste material should be removed. Surfaces, equipment, lights and scrub sinks should all be washed down with disinfectant.
* Once a week there should be a more thorough cleaning session where all equipment is removed from the room and the floors and walls are scrubbed. A disinfectant with detergent properties which will remove organic matter and which is active against a wide range of bacteria, including *Pseudomonas* spp., should be used. After removing any excess solution, allow the disinfectant to dry on the surface rather than rinsing it off, for longer residual activity. All equipment should be meticulously wiped over.
* Cleaning utensils should be designated specifically for use in the theatre suite. They should be rinsed and allowed to dry after use. Buckets should always be emptied and rinsed out. Autoclavable mops are available and should be used whenever possible. Failing this, cloths and mop heads should be washed daily in a washing machine. All utensils should be stored away from the sterile area.

Preparation of the Surgical Team

If good surgical asepsis is to be achieved, all those involved in the surgery should change from their ordinary clothes into correct theatre attire before entering the operating theatre suite.

Theatre wear, which should be worn only within the suite, usually consists of a simple two-piece **scrub suit** or dress made of cotton or polyester. A clean suit should be worn each day, or it should be changed more frequently if it becomes soiled. Theatre **footwear** should be antistatic and traditionally has consisted of white clogs or wellingtons. These have the advantage of being easy to clean. Canvas shoes are sometimes worn but have the disadvantage of being difficult to clean on a daily basis and should be covered by waterproof over-shoes. All footwear should be wiped over with a disinfectant at the end of the day.

Various different styles of **headwear** are available to accommodate longer hairstyles and beards. These are usually disposable and paper-based.

The purpose of **masks** is to filter expired air from the nose and mouth. Masks are effective filters for relatively short periods only and so should ideally be changed between operations.

Scrubbing Up

Pre-operative scrubbing up is a systematic washing and scrubbing of the hands, arms and elbows which is performed by all members of the surgical team before each operation. As it is not possible to sterilise the skin, the aim of the scrubbing-up routine is to destroy as many micro-organisms from the surface of the arms and hands as possible, prior to donning a sterile surgical gown and gloves. Many different scrub routines have been described and no single technique is necessarily better than another. It is recommended that one of the tried and tested regimes is adopted and adhered to strictly. For example:

(1) Remove watch and jewellery.
(2) Finger nails should be cut short and any nail varnish removed.
(3) Adjust the water supply (which should be elbow or foot operated) to a suitable temperature and flow. Once the scrubbing-up routine has started, the hands should not touch the taps, sink or scrub dispenser. If they are inadvertently touched, the last stage of the procedure should be repeated.
(4) Wash the hands thoroughly using a plain soap. At this stage, clean the nails using a nail pick.
(5) Once the hands have been washed, wash the the arms up to and including the elbows. Always keep the hands higher than the elbows so that water drains down towards the unscrubbed upper arms rather than the other

way round (which would lead to recontamination). The purpose of this stage of the procedure is to remove organic matter and grease from the skin.

(6) Rinse the hands and then the arms by allowing water to wash away the soap from the hands towards the elbows.

(7) Repeat this procedure using a surgical scrub solution, e.g. povidone iodine or chlorhexidine (Fig. 26.8). Use only sufficient water to produce a lather, as bactericidal properties of the scrub solution are dependent on contact time with the skin. Excessive amounts of water will rinse away the scrub solution before it has achieved its aim.

(8) Rinse off the scrub solution as in stage 6.

(9) Take a sterile scrubbing brush and systematically scrub the hands. Scrub the palms of the hand, wrist and four surfaces of each finger and thumb (back, front and both sides) and the nails. Either rinse the brush and use it on the other hand or discard it and take a second brush. It is not recommended that the backs of the hand and arms are scrubbed as this may lead to excoriation, which predisposes to infection.

(10) The final stage is a repeat of stage 7. Wash the hands and arms in surgical scrub but this time the scrubbing process is not extended to include the elbow, so that there is no danger that a previously unscrubbed area is touched.

(11) Rinse the hands and arms as before.

(12) Take a sterile handtowel, holding it at arm's length. Use a different quarter to dry each hand and each arm. Then discard the handtowel.

The scrubbing procedure should take between 5 and 10 minutes.

Check the clock as you start and as you begin the final stage to ensure that you have not rushed the procedure.

Putting on a Surgical Gown

There are two different types of gown: back-tie and side-tie. The technique for putting on the gown is similar for both, with slight variation.

(1) The sterile gown (folded inside out) is taken from its sterile pack, held at the shoulders and allowed to fall open (Fig. 26.9a).

(2) One hand should be slipped into each sleeve (Fig. 26.9b). No attempt should be made to try and pull the sleeves over the shoulder or to readjust the gown as this will lead to contamination of the hands or outside of the gown. An unscrubbed assistant should pull the back of the gown over the shoulders (touching only the inside surface of the gown) and secure the ties at the back.

(3) With the hands retained within the sleeves, the waist ties should be picked up and held out to the sides (Fig. 26.9c).

IDEAL PROPERTIES OF SURGICAL SCRUB SOLUTIONS

Wide spectrum of antimicrobial activity.
Ability to decrease microbial count quickly.
Quick application.
Long residual lethal effect against micro-organisms.
Remain active and effective in the presence of organic matter.
Safe to use without skin irritation or sensitisation.
Economical.
Practical for veterinary use.

Commonly used agents:

Povidone iodine
Iodine combined with a detergent.
Broad spectrum anti-microbial activity – bactericidal, viricidal and fungicidal.
May cause severe skin reactions and irritation in some individuals.
Efficacy impaired by organic matter.
Chlorhexidine
Effective against many bacteria, including *E. coli* and *Pseudomonas* spp.
Viricidal, fungicidal and sporicidal properties.
Effective level of activity in the presence of organic material.
Longer residual activity than povidone iodine.
Relatively low toxicity to tissue.
Triclosan
A newer agent, claimed to be antibacterial against both Gram-positive and Gram-negative bacteria.

Fig. 26.8. Ideal properties of surgical scrub solutions.

(a)

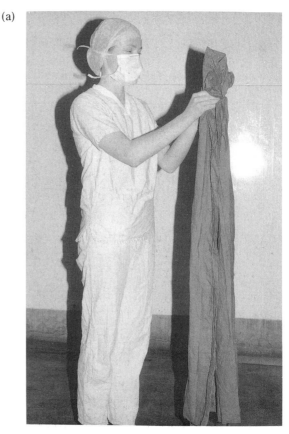

Fig. 26.9.—Continued   ▸

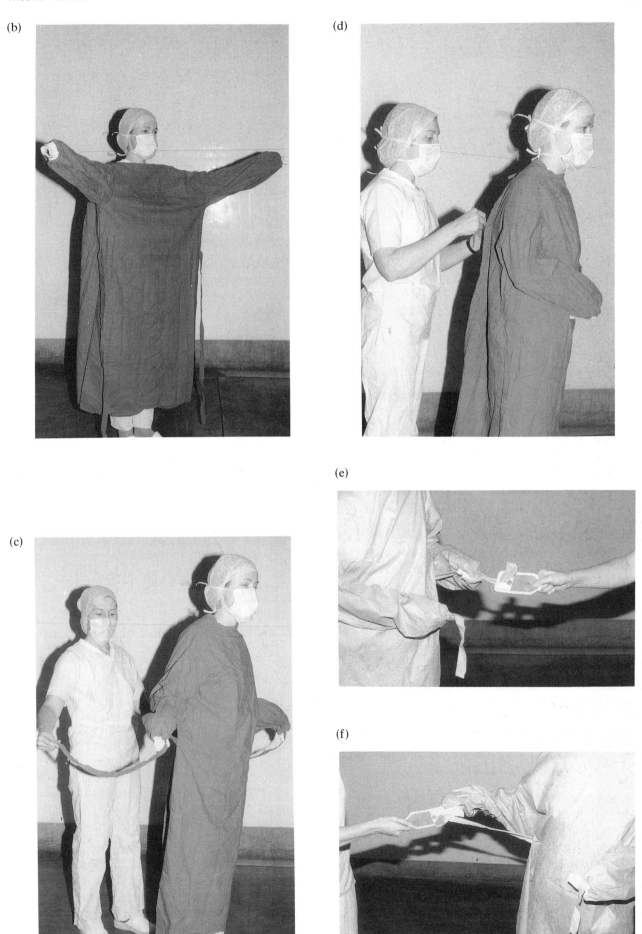

Fig. 26.9. Caption overleaf.

(g)

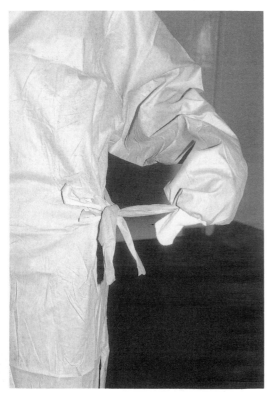

Fig. 26.9. Putting on a surgical gown.

In the case of **back-tying** gowns, the unscrubbed assistant will then take the ends of the waist ties and secure them at the back (Fig. 26.9d). The back of the gown is now unsterile and must not come into contact with sterile equipment, drapes and gowns.

In the case of the **side-tying** gown the unscrubbed assistant takes hold of the paper tape on the longer waist tape and takes the tie around the back to the opposite side (Fig. 26.9e). The scrubbed person then pulls the tape, so that the paper tape comes away (Fig. 26.9f). The gown is tied at the waist by the scrubbed person (Fig. 26.9g). This type of gown, though uncommonly used in veterinary surgery, provides an all-round sterile field.

Putting on Surgical Gloves

Three methods are available: closed gloving, open gloving and the plunge method.

Closed gloving

The hands are kept inside the sleeves while gloving takes place. This technique (Fig. 26.10) has the advantage that it minimises the chances of contaminating the gloves, since the outside of the gloves do not contact the skin.

(1) Hands remain within the sleeves of the gown. The glove packet is turned so that the fingers point towards the body. (The right glove will now be on the left and vice versa.)
(2) The glove is picked up at the rim of the cuff of the glove.

(3) The hand is turned over so that the glove lies on the palm surface with fingers of the glove still pointing towards the body.
(4) The rim is picked up with the opposite hand.
(5) It is then pulled over the fingers and over the dorsal surface of the wrist.
(6) The glove is then pulled on as the fingers are pushed forwards.

Open gloving

The hands are extended out of the sleeves while gowning. This technique (Fig. 26.11) has the disadvantage that the gloves are relatively easily contaminated by skin contact.

(1) The glove pack is opened by an assistant.
(2) With the left hand, pick up the right glove by the turned down cuff, holding only the inner surface of the glove.
(3) Pull on to the right hand. Do not unfold the cuff at this stage.
(4) Place the gloved fingers of the right hand under the cuff of the left glove and pull onto the left hand holding only the outer surface of this glove.
(5) The rim of the left glove is hooked over the thumb whilst the cuff of the gown is adjusted.
(6) Pull the cuff of the left glove over the cuff of the gown using the fingers of the right hand.
(7) Repeat for the right hand.

Plunge method

With this method (Fig. 26.12) the sterile glove is held open by a scrubbed assistant and the hand inserted. There is a risk of contaminating both personnel involved. This technique is not commonly employed in veterinary operating theatres.

Pre-operative Preparation of the Patient

Surgical cases may be categorised as follows:

- **Elective and non-urgent**: the patient is usually healthy and often young (e.g. ovariohysterectomy, castration, corrective osteotomies).
- **Necessary or urgent**: not immediately life-threatening but require prompt attention (fracture repair, airway, gastrointestinal surgery).
- **Emergency surgery**: life-threatening conditions (e.g. abdominal crisis), often traumatic (e.g. chest injury).

The time between admission and surgery will depend on various factors. In the simplest elective procedures, the patient is admitted on the morning of surgery and returns home later that day. Pre-operative preparations in these cases are minimal. In others there may be a delay before surgery is performed. Reasons for this may include:

- **Investigative procedures** e.g. blood samples, diagnostic tests, radiographic studies, e.t.c.

(a)

(d)

(b)

(e)

(c)

(f)

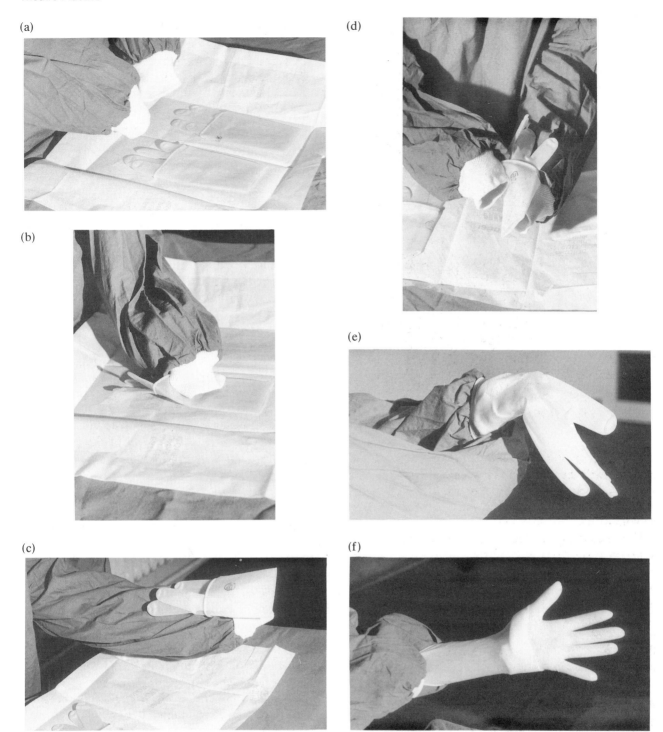

Fig. 26.10. Closed gloving technique.

- **Fluid therapy or transfusion**—to improve the patient's physiological status before surgery.
- **Presence of other injuries** which require treatment before surgery may be undertaken (e.g. thoracic trauma associated with a limb fracture).
- **To allow reduction of swelling/debridement of wounds:**— bandaging of fracture site;—application of wound dressings.
- **Stabilisation** of patient with concurrent metabolic disturbance (e.g. diabetes mellitus, renal disease, Cushing's syndrome).

Admission of the Patient

On admission of the patient:

- All relevant details must be recorded on the case records.
- Check the reason for admission.
- Where relevant, identify the site (draw a diagram if necessary).
- Ensure that the owner understands what is to be done and how the patient will look when discharged (e.g. it will have a clipped area and may

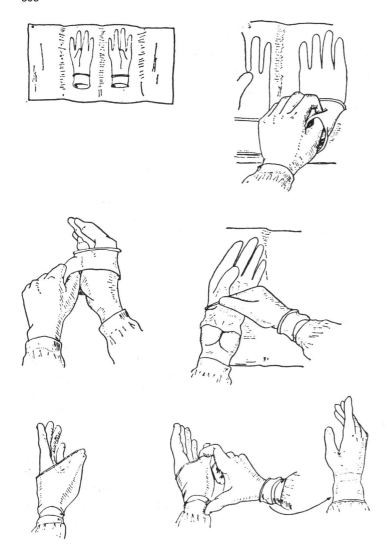

Fig. 26.11. Open gloving.

be wearing a bandage, cast, Elizabethan collar etc.).

- Ensure that the patient is in good general health or that symptoms have not changed since last seen by a veterinary surgeon.
- Always ensure that you have a contact telephone number and that an anaesthetic consent form is signed.
- The patient should then be weighed.
- It is sensible at this stage to fit a plastic identicollar containing the patient's name/number, weight, and reason for admission to minimise the risk of mistakes occurring.

Pre-operative Procedures

Starvation

Food is usually withheld for 12 hours prior to surgery. This is primarily to prevent regurgitation of food under general anaesthesia or during recovery. A full stomach could also interfere with the surgical procedure.

Clipping

Clipping the surgical site is necessary for most procedures (except intraoral). It may be carried out pre-anaesthesia or under general anaesthesia (Fig. 26.13). Certain considerations should be borne in mind when clipping:

- Clip a large area around the surgical site.
- Ensure that the clipping is neat. (This is what the owner will notice.)
- Ensure that clipper blades are in good order. Nicks in the skin will cause irritation, which may encourage post-operative licking and scratching at the site.
- When clipping around a wound, K-Y jelly placed in the wound and on the coat at the edges of the wound will help to prevent hair entering the wound.
- Clean clipper blades in between cases. It may be necessary to sterilise them after clipping contaminated sites, e.g. abscesses.
- Clipping should be performed away from the operating theatre to minimise contamination by hair.
- Some surgeons advocate shaving of the skin after clipping but this leads to severe excoriation of the skin, which may encourage post-operative licking, scratching and soreness.

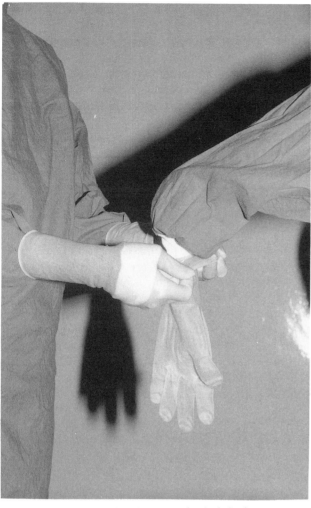

Fig. 26.12. The plunge method of gloving.

Bathing

Ideally all patients should be bathed before surgery to decrease the risk of contamination but this is not always feasible. It should be considered in elective orthopaedic procedures such as total hip replacement.

Administration of an enema

For some surgery (e.g. rectal/colonic) it is desirable to give an evacuant enema prior to surgery. A soap-and-water enema is simplest. The patient may need bathing afterwards to remove faecal contaminants from the skin.

Preparation Immediately Before Surgery

Some form of **premedicant** drug is usually given by intramuscular or subcutaneous injection, 15 minutes to 1 hour before induction of anaesthesia.

Antibiotic drugs are often given at the same time as the premedicant drugs to ensure effective antibiotic blood levels at the time of surgery. **Eye drops** are often applied immediately prior to ophthalmic surgery. **Catheterisation of the bladder**:

- monitor urine output during and after surgery;
- minimise risk of soiling during surgery;
- facilitate access to abdominal organs;
- prevent risk of bladder perforation or rupture during surgery.

Other possible preparations are described in Fig 26.14.

Preparation of the Skin

The skin and coat are two of the greatest sources of wound contamination as it is not possible to remove all bacteria from the skin. The aim is to significantly reduce the number present without damaging the skin itself. Common skin bacteria include species of *Staphylococcus*, *Bacillus* and occasionally *Streptococcus*.

As antiseptic and detergent properties are required in skin-cleansing agents, surgical scrub solutions such as chlorhexidine and povidone iodine are ideal. An antiseptic solution (which may be water- or alcohol-based) is then usually applied to give residual bactericidal activity.

Initial skin preparation should be done in the preparation room. There are several different techniques which are used commonly and one that is recommended is as follows:

(1) Surgical gloves should be worn to prevent contamination of the patient's skin from the nurse's hands. It is not necessary for the gloves to be sterile during the initial preparation.
(2) Using lint-free swabs, wash the site using a surgical scrub solution and a little warm water, beginning at the proposed incision site and working outwards. Once the edges of the clipped area are reached, discard the swab and take a new one.

CLIPPING		
	Advantages	**Disadvantages**
Under general anaesthesia	Often takes less time. Fewer people required to restrain animal. Desirable with fractious animals or painful/inaccessible sites.	Decreases asepsis: small loose hairs are extremely difficult to remove even with a vacuum cleaner. Increases anaesthetic time.
Pre-anaesthesia	Shorter anaesthetic time. Improves asepsis: loose hairs generally shed before surgery. Improves operating theatre efficiency (more operations can be performed).	Patient may be un-cooperative. Requires two or more people. Clipping more than 12 hours before surgery may increase skin bacteria.

Fig. 26.13. Clipping: advantages and disadvantages.

OTHER PREPARATIONS IMMEDIATELY BEFORE SURGERY

1) **Purse-string suture around anus**
   To prevent contamination by faecal material during surgery in the peri-anal region. The nurse should ensure that it is removed at the end of surgery.
2) **Application of Esmarch's rubber bandage and tourniquet**
   For a bloodless operating field during surgery on distal limbs.
3) **Introduction of a throat pack**
   To prevent aspiration of blood, mucus etc., during oral or nasal surgery. Usually a dampened conforming bandage is used for this purpose.
4) **Cover any additional wounds not associated with the surgery**
   To prevent risk of further contamination.
5) **Application of a foot bandage**
   To cover any unclipped areas where the surgery involves a limb.

Fig. 26.14. Other preparations immediately before surgery.

(3) Continue this procedure until the area is clean, i.e. there is no discolouration on a white swab.
(4) A small amount of a 70% alcohol solution can then be sprayed over the site to remove any remaining detergent. It should not be used on open wounds or mucous membranes.
(5) Move the patient into theatre and position for surgery. For limb surgery, a tape is applied over the foot and attached to a drip stand to allow preparation around all sides of the limb.
(6) As the site is likely to have been contaminated to some extent in the transition to the theatre, the skin is given another wash in the manner previously described. This time, however, use sterile gloves, water and swabs.
(7) The final stage of preparation is carried out by the scrubbed surgical team with an antiseptic solution using sterile swabs on sterile Rampley sponge-holding forceps, which are then discarded.

Care should be taken to avoid soaking the coat as this would increase the risk of 'strike through' from the drapes and may make the patient hypothermic.

Preparation of Eyes and Mucous Membranes

The solutions commonly used for preparation of the skin are likely to be irritant and cause damage to mucous membranes and in particular the eye. Dilute solutions of povidone iodine (0.1–0.2%) are commonly used to irrigate the eye and may also be used on oral and other mucous membranes. Chlorhexidine solutions are shown to be more irritant to the surface of the cornea. Alcohol-based solutions should not be used on this sensitive tissue.

Some surgeons do not advocate clipping around the eye for intraocular surgery but use adhesive drapes to protect the eye from the hair and skin.

Others prefer to clip a minimal amount of hair around the eye. Application of petroleum or K-Y jelly to the hair prior to clipping with a narrow fine blade will help to prevent hair being introduced into the eye. The skin around the eye is extremely thin and sensitive, and so it is important that the clippers are in good order and great care is taken when clipping. The eye should then be irrigated several times with physiological saline before irrigating with a povidone iodine solution, as described. The skin should also be prepared with the povidone iodine solution.

Positioning the Patient for Surgery

Most surgeons have individual preferences with regard to positioning of the patient for surgery, although there are some standard positions for specific operations. The veterinary nurse needs to be familiar with positioning for different surgical techniques and individual variations. When there is any doubt, the nurse should check well in advance of surgery.

Some operating tables have adjustable sides and tilting facilities which assist positioning of the patient. If not, the use of additional restraining aids such as troughs, sandbags and tapes will be necessary. Care should be taken to avoid placing heavy sandbags over limbs or tying tapes tightly, which may occlude blood supply to the area.

Draping the Patient

The reason for draping the patient is to maintain asepsis by preventing contamination of the surgical site by hair and the immediate environment. Drapes must therefore cover the entire patient and operating table, leaving only the surgical site exposed. Drapes may be disposable or reusable. The relative advantages of each type are shown in Fig. 26.15.

Disposable drapes are usually paper based. Many different types are available and cost tends to reflect the quality. Most of these are designed for the medical market but many are suitable for veterinary use.

Draping systems

Plain drapes. Four rectangular drapes are used to create a 'window' (**fenestration**) for the surgical site (Fig. 26.16). The fenestration created can be of any size. The first drape should be placed between the surgeon and the nearest side of the table. Then a drape is placed over the opposite side of the patient (i.e. furthest from the surgeon). Drapes are then placed over both ends. They are then secured in place using towel clips.

Fenestrated drapes. Fenestrated drapes achieve the same effect as the plain drapes in leaving a surgery

DRAPES		
	Advantages	**Disadvantages**
Disposable	Labour saving Less laundry Pre-sterilised Usually very water repellent Always in perfect condition	Expensive Cheaper brands can be less conforming Large stock needed
Reusable drapes	Cheaper	Porous – all fluids leak through leading to a break in asepsis Time-consuming – washing and folding Danger of threads detaching and gaining access to wounds After repeated use quality becomes poor

Fig. 26.15. Drapes: advantages and disadvantages.

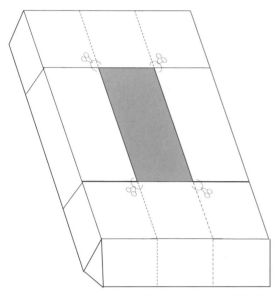

Fig. 26.16. Draping the surgical site with plain drapes, placed longitudinally on both sides of the operating table. Plain drapes are then placed over each end and secured by towel clips.

window, but the window is already formed in a single ready-made drape. Fenestrated drapes can be large enough to cover the entire animal and table top. A selection of different sized fenestrations are needed however to cater for all the different surgical sites.

Adhesive 'barrier' drapes. Sterile clear adhesive plastic sheets are sometimes placed over the surgical site. Standard drapes are then applied in the usual way. The skin incision is made through the adhesive material.

Draping limbs. There are various ways of draping limbs for surgery (Fig. 26.17). The surgeon's individual preference will govern the choice of method. Commonly, the lower limb is tied to a drip stand, using tape. A sterile drape is placed on the table top underneath the limb. Then either a sterile drape or stockinette is secured to the lower limb and the suspending tape is cut. The surgical site is then draped in a routine fashion.

Sub-draping. Additional towels are sometimes used to protect the incision site from contamination. They are applied to each side of the incision by towel clips. The towel is then folded back over the towel clips.

Surgical Assistance

The theatre nurse has two main roles: one as a circulating nurse and one as a scrubbed nurse. Duties in the respective roles are shown in Fig. 26.18.

Guidelines for the Scrubbed Nurse

The role of the scrubbed nurse is an extremely important one and requires rigid adherence to a set of rules. It is very easy to make mistakes if corners are cut or changes made. Knowledge of the procedure to be performed is important so that the needs of the surgeon can be anticipated.

(1) The instrument trolley should not be prepared until just before it is needed but it must be ready by the time the patient arrives in theatre.

(2) It is essential to know exactly what instruments and equipment are on the trolley at the start and throughout surgery.

(3) All swabs, sutures, needles etc., must be counted before surgery begins and again before the wound is closed, to prevent any items being accidentally left within a wound cavity.

(4) The nurse should watch the operation carefully in order to anticipate the surgeon's needs.

(5) Instruments should be passed to the surgeon so that they are ready to be used, i.e. not upside down.

(6) Instruments should be returned to the same place on the trolley each time so that the nurse knows exactly where they are. They should not be left around the surgical site, because they are likely to fall on the floor and because they will not be immediately to hand when needed.

(7) Instruments should be wiped over with a dry swab when they are returned to the trolley.

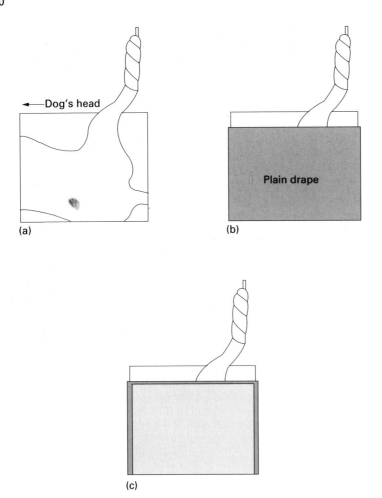

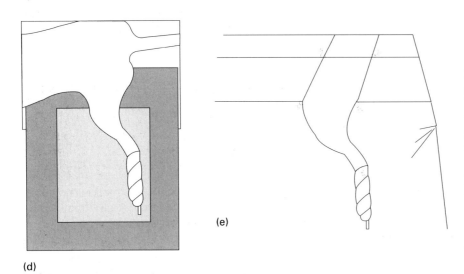

Fig. 26.17. Draping a limb for surgery: (a) the lower limb is bandaged and attached by tape to a transfusion stand; (b) a plain drape is laid over the body and the opposite limb of the patient; (c) a smaller plain drape is laid on top of this; (d) the tape is then cut and the limb lowered on to the inner drape; (e) the drape is carefully wrapped around the limb and secured with a towel clip; plain drapes or a fenestrated drape are then applied over the surgical site.

(8) Only one swab should be given to the surgeon at any time and the nurse must keep a constant check on the number of swabs.

(9) Swabs should be applied firmly to a bleeding site, without wiping across the tissue which may both damage tissue and disturb a clot.

(10) All tissues should be handled gently to avoid trauma. Viscera in particular should be handled very carefully.

(11) One of the nurse's roles may be to irrigate the tissues with warmed saline to prevent desiccation, particularly during long operations.

(12) On completion of surgery ensure that all instruments, needles and swabs are returned to the trolley and that needles, blades and glassware are safely disposed of.

Preparing an Instrument Trolley

Instrument trolleys should be prepared immediately prior to use. The longer that instruments are exposed to air, the greater the chance of contamination from the environment or personnel. If there is a delay once the trolley has been laid out, then a sterile drape should be placed over the top. Trolleys can be laid up by a scrubbed nurse or by using sterile cheatle forceps. The top of the metal instrument trolley will not be sterile and it is important to cover this with a waterproof, sterile drape first to prevent bacterial strike through from the trolley if it becomes wet.

Instrument sets may be packed in trays complete with drapes and swabs. In these cases the outer wrappings of the set can be unfolded to cover the base of the trolley.

Where instruments are taken from multi-use containers the trolley should be covered by a waterproof drape followed by two layers of linen cloth. Swabs, drapes and instruments are then added.

GENERAL RULES FOR MAINTENANCE
OF ASEPSIS
(1) Correct theatre attire to be worn at all times.
(2) There should be a minimum number of people present and movement should be kept to a minimum
(3) There should be a new set of sterile instruments for each operation, even when dealing with a contaminated site.
(4) Plan to perform 'clean' operations first, i.e. orthopaedic operations (especially when implants are used), and contaminated surgery to be carried out last (i.e. aural and oral).
(5) Wherever possible there should be a room for 'dirty' procedures.
(6) Adopt an efficient sterilisation programme.
(7) Ensure that the theatre is maintained at an ambient temperature and the ventilation is good. Hot, humid conditions will encourage the growth of pathogens, in particular *Pseudomonas* spp.
(8) Wherever possible, clip and bath the patient before taking it to theatre.
(9) The surgical team must ensure that they do not touch any non-sterile surfaces during surgery. Any break in asepsis must be reported and rectified.
(10) Ensure that any contaminated instruments or equipment are not returned to the sterile trolley.
(11) Keep a record book of all operations so that if any sepsis problems arise the cause can be detected.
(12) Maintain a strict cleaning protocol.

DUTIES OF NURSES
Duties of a circulating nurse
1. Help prepare theatre, instruments and equipment for surgery.
2. Tie the surgical team into gowns.
3. Help position the patient on the table.
4. Preparation of the surgical site.
5. Connect apparatus (diathermy, suction, airlines etc.).
6. Open packs of sutures/instruments etc.
7. Count swabs, sutures etc., with the scrubbed nurse.
8. Be in theatre at all times when surgery is in progress.
9. Assist the anaesthetist.
10. Prepare post-operative dressings.
11. Help clear theatre at the end of surgery.
Duties of the scrubbed nurse
1. Prepare the instrument trolley.
2. Assist in draping the patient.
3. Pass instruments, swabs etc., to the surgeon.
4. Assist with surgery: retract tissue, cut sutures etc.
5. Be responsible for all equipment, swabs, sutures, needles etc.

Fig. 26.18. Duties of a circulating nurse and of the scrubbed nurse.

Hazards in the Operating Theatre

The avoidance of accidents to patients and staff in the operating theatre is of the utmost importance. The Health and Safety at Work Act and the COSSH regulations are designed to ensure safety in the work place, including the operating theatre.

Equipment

With the increasing use of new and sophisticated equipment, the risk of accidents has also increased. It is very important that all nursing staff are instructed in the use and maintenance of all new equipment. It is also important that all equipment is serviced regularly and tested for electrical safety to minimise risks.

Pollution from anaesthetic gases

All staff should be aware of the dangers associated with inhaling anaesthetic gases. An anaesthetic gas scavenging system must be fitted or absorptive filters used to minimise exposure to gases.

Disposal of needles/sharp instruments

Many sharp blades, needles and stylets are used in the surgical unit. The disposal of these can create a major and serious hazard. They should be placed in commercially produced sharps containers which, when full, are sealed and disposed of as 'clinical waste'.

Clinical and pathological waste

It is a requirement of the COSSH regulations that all clinical and pathological waste is separated from ordinary refuse using colour coded bags.

- **Clinical waste** (i.e. anything contaminated by blood, body fluids or tissue) should be placed in yellow bags, sealed with Biohazard tape and incinerated.
- **Pathological material** (i.e. gross tissue) should be placed in red bags and sealed. This too should be disposed of by incineration.

Chemicals

In the operating theatre nursing staff will be exposed to various chemicals. Protective clothing, masks and gloves should be worn where appropriate.

Care of the Patient During Surgery

It is important to remember that underneath the drapes is a live patient! Care must be taken to avoid leaning on the animal's chest, which may compromise breathing in a small patient. Careful positioning of towel clips is important to avoid delicate structures such as the eye, which cannot be seen once drapes have been placed. Attention should be paid to the conservation of heat especially in the small or very young. The use of heated water beds, insulation (e.g. bubble-wrap) and warmed intravenous and irrigation fluids should be encouraged. Careful positioning of the animal on the table is also important to avoid post-operative complications.

Immediate Post-operative Care

Recovery from Anaesthesia

The patient should not be left unattended until it is conscious and sitting up. The endotracheal tube is usually removed just before the cough reflex returns. The animal should be watched closely to ensure that an adequate airway is maintained once the tube has been removed especially in brachycephalic breeds or following airway surgery. A source of oxygen and a means of ventilation should be available during this time in case any problems arise. Colour of the mucous membranes, presence or absence of respiratory noise and effort will be indicators of effective ventilation by the animal. The ability to maintain body temperature is lost under anaesthesia, so steps should be taken to prevent hypothermia.

Haemorrhage

During recovery the patient should be observed for signs of external haemorrhage (which is usually obvious) or internal haemorrhage (development of shock).

Recognition of Pain

It is important to be able to recognise when an animal is in pain (see Chapter 27). The nurse should obtain instructions from the veterinary surgeon regarding post-operative analgesia.

Application of Dressings or Casts

Many orthopaedic and some soft tissue cases will require post-operative bandages or casts. This should be done before the animal regains consciousness. Take care not to apply too tightly (especially head and ear dressings).

Comfort

Make sure that the animal has comfortable bedding, especially orthopaedic patients. Turn the animal regularly if it is disinclined or unable to do so by itself. Give opportunities for the animal to urinate, or empty the bladder manually if necessary. Do not forget to offer food and drink if this is allowed, especially in young and old patients.

Instrumentation

The cost of good quality surgical instruments is extremely high but they will last for years if handled correctly, whereas cheaper instruments of poor quality will require early replacement.

Stainless steel is the material of choice for most surgical instruments. It combines high resistance to corrosion with great strength and it has an attractive surface finish.

Tungsten carbide inserts are often added to the tips of stainless steel instruments that are used for cutting or gripping, such as scissors and needle-holders. They are very hard and resistant to wear but tend to be expensive. Instruments with tungsten carbide inserts are often identified by their gold-coloured handles.

Chromium-plated carbon steel surgical instruments are commonly used in veterinary practice because they are lower in price. However, they will rust, pit and blister when in contact with chemicals and saline and they tend to blunt quickly.

Care and Maintenance of Surgical Instruments

Surgical instruments should be handled carefully at all times, both during use and after. They should not be dropped into trays and sinks or on to trolleys. Special care should be taken of sharp edges and pointed instruments.

Care of new instruments

Most new instruments are supplied dry without lubrication. Before use, therefore, it is recommended that they should be carefully washed and dried and their moving parts should be lubricated.

Cleaning after use

To comply with the COSHH regulations, the veterinary nurse must wear protective clothing (i.e. a plastic apron and rubber gloves) when dealing with surgical instruments.

Sharp items such as needles, glass vials and scalpel blades should be safely disposed of before removing other disposable items such as suture packets, swabs etc., from the instrument trolley. Any specialised or delicate equipment should be separated from the general instruments and cleaned separately.

Instruments should be cleaned as soon as possible on completion of surgery to prevent blood, tissue debris or saline drying on them, as this will lead to pitting of the surface and subsequent corrosion. Initial soaking or rinsing in cold water is extremely effective for this. Hot water should not be used as it causes coagulation of proteins (e.g. blood). Alternatively instruments may be initially soaked in a chemical cleaning solution specifically manufactured for instrument cleaning. Where indicated instruments should be dismantled and ratchets and box joints opened before immersion.

Instruments should then be cleaned under cool or warm running water, using a hand brush with fairly stiff bristles. Particular attention should be paid to ratchets, box joints, serrations etc. Abrasive chemical agents or materials should never be used as they may damage the surface of the instrument.

Ordinary soap should also be avoided as it causes an insoluble alkali film to form on the surface, thus trapping bacteria and protecting them from sterilisation.

After washing, instruments should be rinsed thoroughly—preferably in distilled or deionised water—and then dried prior to packing.

Ultrasonic cleaners. Bench-top ultrasonic cleaners suitable for veterinary use are readily available. They are extremely effective at removing debris from areas inaccessible to brushes (e.g. box joints). They work by the production of sinusoidal energy waves with a vibration frequency in excess of 20,000/second.

Following an initial rinsing or soaking in cold water to remove excess blood and debris the instruments are placed in the wire mesh basket of the ultrasonic cleaner. The unit is filled approximately half full with water to which a specific ultrasonic cleaning detergent has been added. The basket is placed in the solution, the lid replaced and the unit switched on. Usually a period of approximately 15 minutes is sufficient. On completion of the cycle, the basket is removed and the instruments rinsed individually under running water.

All instruments should be dried after washing, as water collecting in trapped areas may lead to corrosion. After cleaning, each instrument should be inspected for distortion, misalignment and incorrect assembly. Pivot movements should be checked.

Lubrication

Lubrication of instruments on a regular basis is recommended, particularly after using an ultrasonic cleaner. It is important to use lubricants which are recommended by the manufacturer. Mineral oils and grease must be avoided as they leave a film on the surface under which bacterial spores may be trapped, preventing adequate penetration during sterilisation. Antimicrobial water-soluble lubricants (instrument milk) available: instruments are dipped into the solution for a short period and then removed and allowed to dry. They do not need to be rinsed.

Cleaning of compressed air machines

Compressed air machines should never be immersed in water or ultrasonic cleaners. The machine's detachable parts (drills etc.) can be cleaned in standard fashion. The instrument itself should be detached from the air hose and wiped over thoroughly with disinfectant, paying particular attention to triggers and couplings. Use of a handbrush may be necessary. It should then be rinsed without immersing it completely. The air hose should be cleaned in the same way and then both should be dried. The machine should be lubricated, using the manufacturer's recommended lubricant, before packing for sterilisation.

General Surgical Instruments

There is a wide variety of different surgical instruments available. It is not expected that the veterinary nurse should be familiar with them all but a broad knowledge of general instruments can be gained by reference to manuals and catalogues to learn the names and appearance of the more common ones.

Scalpel

The scalpel is the best instrument for dividing tissue with minimal trauma. Usually scalpel blades with interchangeable disposable blades are used (Fig. 26.19). A size 3 handle is commonly used for small animal surgery with blade sizes 10, 11, 12 and 15. A size 4 handle is used for large animal surgery with blade sizes 20, 21 and 22. The primary advantage of disposable blades is consistent sharpness. A scalpel with a blade and handle as a disposable package is available, as is a small, rounded (Beaver) handle with smaller disposable blades which has gained popularity with ophthalmic surgeons.

Dissecting forceps

These are commonly referred to as thumb forceps (Fig. 26.20) and are designed to hold tissue. They

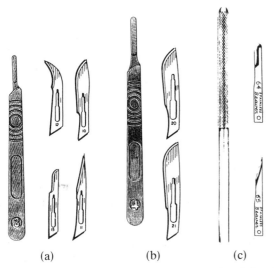

Fig. 26.19. Scalpel handles and blades: (a) size 3 handle and sizes 10, 11, 12 and 15 blades; (b) size 4 handle and sizes 21 and 20 blades; (c) Beaver handle with two different blades.

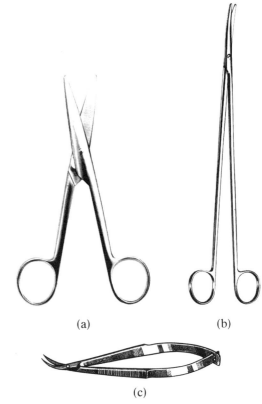

Fig. 26.21. Surgical scissors: (a) Mayo; (b) Metzenbaum; (c) corneal.

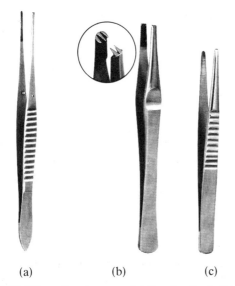

Fig. 26.20. Dissecting forceps: (a) fine-toothed; (b) heavy-duty toothed; (c) plain dressing forceps.

have a spring action and the jaws are opposed by holding the metal blades together. They may have plain or toothed ends. Generally forceps with plain ends are used for handling delicate tissues such as viscera whilst toothed forceps are used for denser tissues. Dissecting forceps should be held like a pencil.

Scissors

Operating scissors are available in various lengths and shapes (Fig. 26.21). Mayo dissecting scissors are commonly used for routine surgery; the finer, long-handled Metzenbaum scissors tend to be used for more delicate work. Special suture scissors (e.g. Carless scissors) should be used for cutting sutures to prevent unnecessary blunting of dissecting

scissors. For removal of sutures, Paynes scissors are used. These are small and curved with the cutting surface of one blade hollowed out to fit under the suture easily. Scissors should be held with the ring finger and thumb inserted in the ring of the scissor and the index finger placed on the shaft to guide the scissors.

Haemostatic or artery forceps

Artery forceps (Fig. 26.22) are designed to clamp blood vessels and thus stop bleeding. They come in several different lengths and shapes. Most have transverse striations to facilitate holding tissue. There are many different patterns of artery forceps. Some of those commonly used include the Spencer Wells, Dunhill, Crile, Cairns and Kelly. Mosquito forceps are very small artery forceps for finer blood vessels, the most common type being the Halstead forceps. Like scissors, artery forceps should be held with the ring finger and thumb using the index finger to steady the forceps.

Tissue forceps

Allis tissue forceps and Babcock's forceps are the most commonly used type of tissue forceps (Fig. 26.23). They are designed to grasp tissue with minimal trauma but neither should be used to grasp and hold viscera; more specialised forceps such as Duvall's should be used for this.

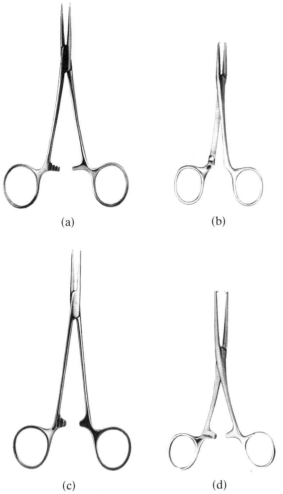

Fig. 26.22. Artery forceps: (a) Cairn's, with a fine, slightly curved blade; (b) Spencer Wells, with a short, stubby blade; (c) Crile's, similar to Mayo but longer and finer; (d) Kocher's, with a toothed end and long serrated jaw.

Towel clips

These are used to attach drapes to the patient and instruments to the operating site (Fig. 26.24). Backhaus and Mayo forceps have a ringed handle and curved, pointed, tong-like tips. Gray's cross-action forceps, commonly used in veterinary surgery, have a strong spring-clip attachment.

Needle-holders

Needle-holders are forceps that are specifically designed for holding suture needles during suturing and for knot tying (Fig. 26.25).

- Gillies needle-holders are very commonly used in veterinary surgery. They have a scissor action as well for cutting the suture ends. Their major disadvantage is that they have no ratchet, so that the needle has to be held in place by gripping the blades tightly.
- Olsen–Hegar needle-holders also have a cutting edge but have the advantage of a ratchet to hold the needle securely in place. The disadvantage of the scissor edge is that the suture material may be inadvertently cut.
- Mayo–Hegar needle-holders resemble a pair of long-handled artery forceps. They have a ratchet but no scissor action. This is one of the most popular types of needle-holder.
- McPhail's needle-holders traditionally have copper inserts in the tips, although those with tungsten carbide inserts are of superior quality. The handles have a spring ratchet so that by squeezing them together the jaws open and release the needle.

Retractors

These are used to facilitate exposure of the operating field (Fig. 26.26). They may be hand-held or self-retaining. Hand-held retractors include Langenbek, Senn and Czerny; muscle and joint retractors include Gelpi, West's and Travers; Examples of abdominal wall retractors are Gossett and Balfour; and Finichietto retractors are used for the chest.

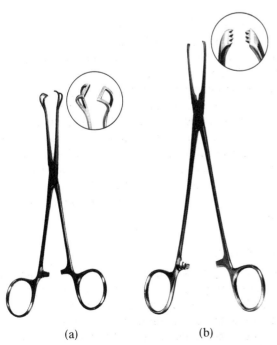

Fig. 26.23. Tissue forceps: (a) Babcock's; (b) Allis.

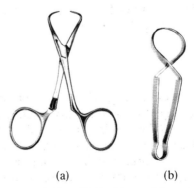

Fig. 26.24. Towel clips: (a) Backhaus; (b) cross-action.

(a)

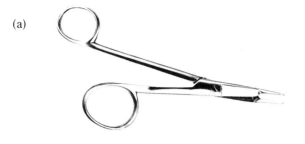

(b)

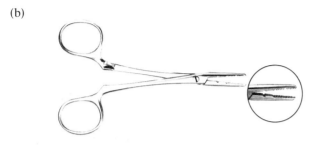

(c)

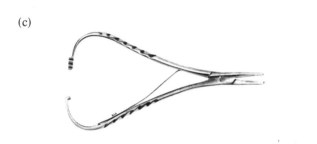

(d)

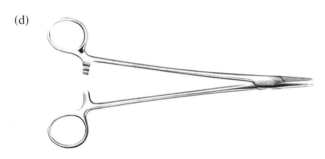

Fig. 26.25. Needle-holders: (a) Gillies; (b) Bruce Clarke's;
(c) McPhail's; (d) Mayo–Hegar.

Orthopaedic Instruments

Osteotomes, chisels and gouges

These are used to cut or shape bone or cartilage (Fig. 26.27). They are available in a wide variety of sizes. The cutting edge of the osteotome is tapered on both sides whereas the chisel is tapered on one side only. The gouge has a U-shaped edge to remove larger pieces of cartilage or soft bone.

Curettes

These have an oval-shaped cup. They scoop the surface of dense tissue to remove loose or degenerate tissue (e.g. cartilage flaps, necrotic bone). The cup has a sharp cutting edge and is available in various sizes (Fig. 26.27).

Periosteal elevators

These are used to lift periosteum and soft tissue from the surface of bone (Fig. 26.28).

Bone-holding forceps

These are designed to grip bone fragments during reduction and alignment in fracture repair (Fig. 26.29).

Bone cutters and rongeurs

Bone rongeurs (Fig. 26.30(a)) are used to cut out small pieces of dense tissue such as bone or cartilage. Bone cutters (Fig. 26.30(b)) are designed to cut larger pieces of bone.

Bone rasps

Bone rasps may be used to remove sharp edges following arthroplasty procedures.

Retractors

Standard retractors are commonly used in orthopaedic surgery but in addition hand-held Hohmann retractors are often used for retracting muscle, tendons and ligaments (Fig. 26.31).

Drills, saws and burrs

Hand, battery and air drills are commonly used in orthopaedic surgery (Fig. 26.32). Hand drills are useful around delicate structures and when only minimal drilling is required but for most major surgery a battery-operated or air drill should be a pre-requisite. These allow more speed and precision than hand drills. Battery drills tend to be slower and more cumbersome than most of the compact air drills available but they are suitable for most veterinary procedures and are less expensive. They should be recharged after each use.

Oscillating saws and mechanical burrs are either air or electrically driven. Great care should be taken when connecting attachments and during use. The power supply should not be applied until the couplings are assembled.

Wire forceps

Various wire-cutting and twisting forceps are available for applying cerclage wires and for stabilising bones with wire.

Gigli wire and handles

These are used in osteotomy techniques to saw through bone with a cheese-wire effect.

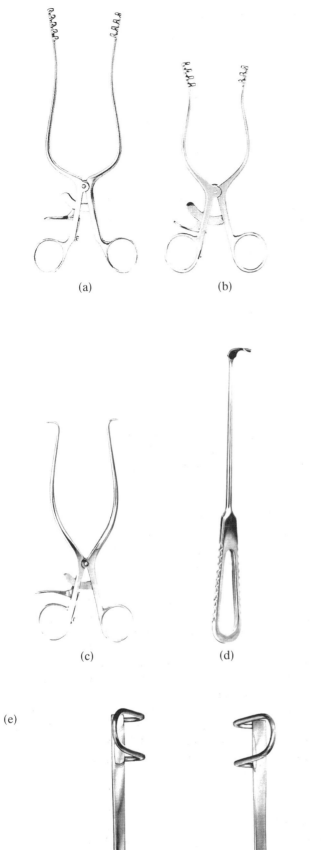

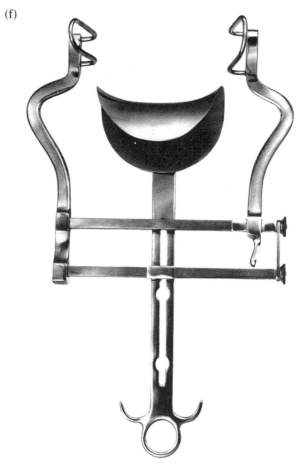

Fig. 26.26. Retractors: (a) Travers; (b) Weitlander's; (c) Gelip; (d) Lagenbek; (e) Gossett; (f) Balfour.

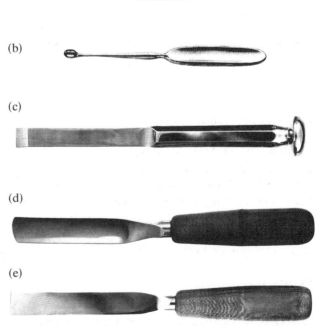

Fig. 26.27. Some basic orthopaedic instruments: (a) Volkman's scoop; (b) curette; (c) chisel; (d) gouge; (e) osteotome.

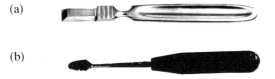

Fig. 26.28. Periosteal elevators: (a) Farabeuf's rugine; (b) straight periosteal elevator.

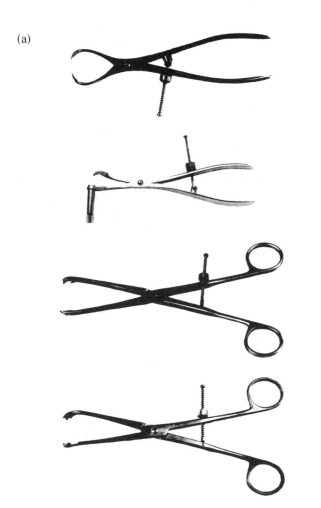

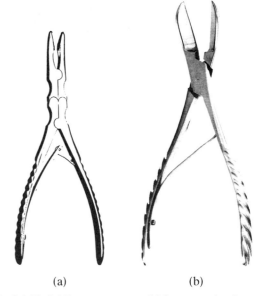

Fig. 26.30. (a) Bone rongeurs; (b) bone-cutting forceps.

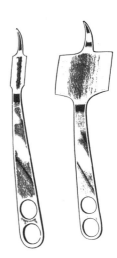

Fig. 26.31. Hohmann retractors.

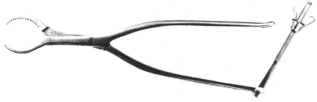

Fig. 26.29. Bone-holding forceps; (a) self-centring forceps with speedlock fastening.

Instrumentation for Fracture Repair

The instruments required for fracture repair depend on the technique which is to be used and are described in Chapter 25 (Surgical Equipment). Materials used to repair fractures internally include Steinman pins, orthopaedic wire, bone plates, screws and external fixator apparatus.

Packing a Surgical Set

Instrument sets are often packed together with swabs, drapes, suction tubing etc. They are usually wrapped so that, when unfolded, the layers of wrapping will cover the base of the instrument trolley. A metal or plastic tray is usually lined with a towel or linen sheet. The instruments should then be laid out in a specific order. This is usually the order in which they are likely to be used (Fig. 26.33). Swabs, drapes etc. are then added. A water-resistant paper wrap is then laid over the top of the trolley, followed by two layers of linen sheet. The tray is placed on this and the pack is then wrapped (Fig. 26.34). The set is secured with Bowie-Dick tape and tied with string. It should then be labelled and dated prior to sterilisation.

(a)

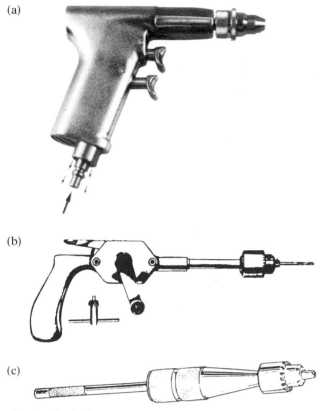

(b)

(c)

Fig. 26.32. Orthopaedic drills: (a) hand drill; (b) air drill; (c) Jacob's chuck.

Instrument Sets

Instrument sets are made up to suit individual requirements and they vary from one practice to another. Some practices have sets for specific procedures (e.g. bitch spay set). Others have a standard instrument set that is used for all operations, to which other instruments will be added depending on the procedure. Often a smaller set will be available for minor procedures such as a cat spay. It is important that each of the standard instrument sets should contain the same number and type so that the surgical team always know what instruments they will have and so that it is easy to check that all are present at the end of the procedure. Fig. 26.37 lists suggested contents for various instrument sets required for surgical procedures but these are only guidelines.

Suction Apparatus

A suction unit in the operating theatre is important for several reasons. It may be used for aspiration of the oropharynx and nasopharynx during or after surgery. It may be used for thoracocentesis following surgery or for suction of fluids and blood during the surgical procedure. Various suction machines are available and a size suitable for individual requirements should be chosen. It is sensible to choose a unit with two bottles so that there is always a spare when one bottle becomes full.

Suture Materials

The ideal suture material should:

- be suitable for use in any situation;
- be readily available and inexpensive;
- be readily sterilised by steam or ethylene oxide;
- show high initial tensile strength, combined with small diameter material;

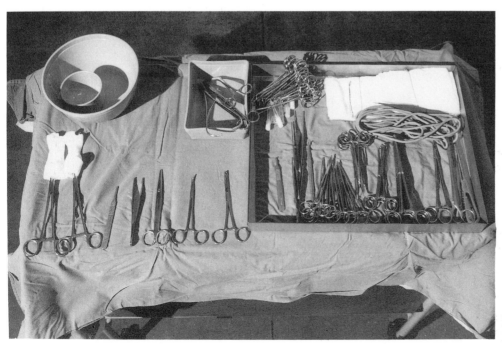

Fig. 26.33. Instruments laid out ready for use.

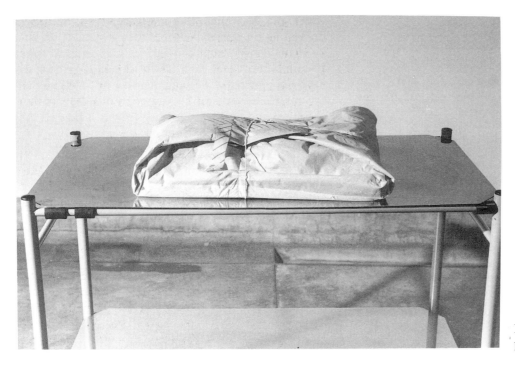

Fig. 26.34. Instrument set packed and ready for use.

- have a good knot security—it should tie easily, with no tendency to slip or loosen, and the knot should hold securely without fraying;
- produce minimal tissue reaction—it should be inert (i.e. not cause pain or swelling or delay healing), non-allergenic, non-carcinogenic and non-electrolytic;
- show good handling characteristics—it should be easy to handle when wet or dry and pass through tissue without friction or cutting;
- not create an environment for bacterial growth, i.e. not show capillarity or wicking of fluids (ideally monofilament);
- be absorbed after its function has been served.

No single suture material in the wide range available possesses all of these ideal characteristics. Selection tends to depend on the surgeon's teaching and preference. Fig. 26.38 gives the terms used to describe the characteristics of suture materials.

Classification of Sutures

Suture material are either absorbable or non-absorbable. They may be further classified as natural or synthetic, and as monofilament or multifilament. Examples of each category are shown in Fig. 26.39.

Common Suture Materials

Absorbable sutures

These materials are degraded within the tissues and lose their tensile strength by 60 days. The natural fibres (i.e. catgut) are removed by phagocytosis, which tends to produce some degree of tissue reaction. The synthetic absorbable materials are hydrolysed and tend to produce minimal tissue reaction. In general, absorbable suture materials are used when closing internal tissue layers or organs which do not require long-term support.

Catgut. Catgut is a derivation of the word 'kid-gut'. It is made from the submucosa of sheep small intestine or the serosa of cattle intestines. 'Plain catgut' is untreated; 'chromic catgut' is tanned with chromic salts to slow its absorption, increase its strength and decrease the tissue reaction (Fig. 26.40). Catgut is absorbed by phagocytosis and enzyme degradation. The rate of absorption is influenced by infection, blood supply and tissue pH.

- It loses its initial tensile strength very rapidly.
- It always causes a mild to severe inflammatory reaction.
- In contaminated sites it may act as a nidus for infection.
- It handles well, the knots are secure when dry but may loosen as it swells when it becomes wet.
- It also tends to break if pulled sharply during knot tying.

Polyglactin 910. This material is a co-polymer of lactide and glycolide and is absorbed by hydrolysis. It is available in dyed and undyed preparations the latter causing less tissue reaction; it is coated to improve its handling characteristics and it is braided.

- It has a higher initial tensile strength than catgut.
- It loses 50% of its strength in 14 days and is totally absorbed in 60–90 days.
- There is considerable tissue drag and careful placement of knots is necessary.

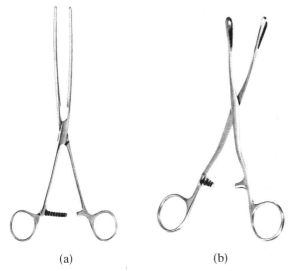

(a)   (b)

Fig. 26.35. (a) Doyen bowel clamps; (b) Rampley's sponge-
holding forceps.

Polyglycolic acid. This is an inert, non-antigenic, non-pyrogenic polyester made from hydroxyacetic acid and it is braided. It is absorbed by hydrolysis; the hydrolysed breakdown products have been found to be bacteriostatic experimentally, therefore its use has been advocated in infected sites.

- It loses approximately 30% of its strength in 7 days and 80% in 14 days.
- Tissue drag is considerable even in the coated formulation.
- It has poor knot security.

Polydioxanone. This is a monofilament absorbable suture which is absorbed by hydrolysis.

- It loses only 30% of its strength in 2 weeks and is minimally absorbed at 90 days.
- Tissue reaction is minimal.
- As it is monofilament, tissue drag is reduced.
- It is ideal in infected sites and where an absorbable material is required for a long period of time.
- Its main disadvantage is its springiness.

Polyglyconate. This is also a synthetic mono-filament absorbable suture which is very similar to polydioxanne. it is slightly less springy and therefore easier to handle than polydioxanone.

Non-absorbable sutures

These maintain their strength for longer than 60 days. The material is neither hydrolysed nor phagocytosed: it becomes encapsulated within fibrous tissue. Non-absorbable sutures are used where prolonged mechanical support is required. The main indications for use are:

- In skin closure, where sutures are generally removed after 10 days.
- Within slow healing tissues.

Silk. This is available as braided or twisted strands. It is obtained from threads spun by the silkworm larvae. It may be coated with silicone or wax to minimise the capillarity which may promote infection.

Silk has good handling characteristics, excellent knot security and good tensile strength. It is relatively inexpensive. Its main uses include cardiovascular and thoracic surgery, genital mucosa and adjacent to

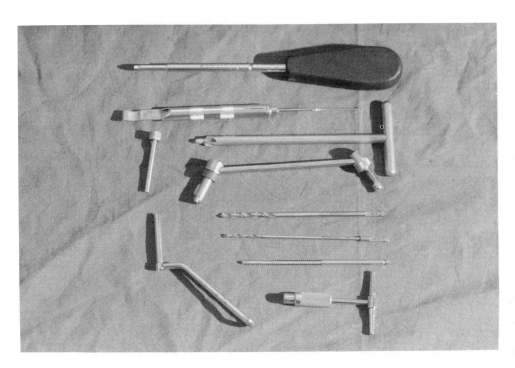

Fig. 26.36. ASIF (Association for the Study of Internal Fixation) instruments for internal fixation.

eyes. It should not be used in infected sites, oral mucosa or hollow organs where it may act as a nidus for infection.

Linen. This is twisted from long strands of flax. It is easily sterilised, handles well and has excellent knot security. It does show capillary properties however and has been shown to contribute to sinus formation. It has become less popular since the advent of the synthetic absorbable materials.

Polypropylene. This is an inert, non-absorbable, monofilament material. It has high tensile strength but tends to stretch and will snap if crushed by

---

SURGICAL INSTRUMENTS

			No. of pairs
Standard instrument set	Scalpel handle no. 3		x 1
	Dissecting forceps – rat toothed fine		x 1
	rat toothed heavy duty		x 1
	fine plain		x 1
	Mayo scissors – straight		x 1
	Metzenbaum scissors		x 1
	Artery forceps		x 10
	Mosquito forceps		x 5
	Allis tissue forceps		x 4
	Suture scissors		x 1
	Needle-holders		x 1
	Langenbeck retractors		x 2
	Gelpi retractor		x 1
	Probe		x 1
	Backhaus towel holding forceps		x 10
	Gallipot		x 1
	Receiver		x 1
	Suture tray		x 1
	Suction tubing and tip		x 1
	Electocautery and handle		x 1
	Swabs (X-ray detectable)		x 10
	Scalpel blades size 10, 15		x 2
	Different types of surgery may require the addition of other instruments:		
Abdominal surgery	Self retaining retractors (e.g. Gossett)		
	Doyens bowel clamps (Figure 26.36)		
	Long dissecting forceps		
	Long artery forceps (e.g. Roberts)		
	Towels to pack abdomen		
Thoracic surgery	Rib cutters		
	Finichietto rib retractors		
	Periosteal elevator		
	Chest drain		
	Suture wire ⎱ If sternotomy approach		
	Oscillating saw ⎰		
	Lobectomy clamps		
	Long-handled artery forceps (e.g. Roberts)		
	Rib raspatory		
Orthopaedic surgery	General:		
	Osteotome	Gigli wire and handles	
	Chisel	Periosteal elevator	
	Curette	Hand drill	
	Gouge		
	Mallet		
	Hohmann retractor		
	Putti rasp		
	Hacksaw		
	Liston's bone cutting forceps		
	Bone rongeurs		
	Power tools:		
	Battery drill		
	Air drill		
	Mechanical burr		
	Oscillating saw		
	Implants:		
	Stainless steel wire		
	Intramedullary pins		
	Kirschner wires		
	Rush pins		
	Staples		
	Screws		
	Plates		
	In addition to general orthopaedic instruments:		
	Bone Pinning:		
	Jacob's chuck and key		
	Pin cutters		

Fig. 26.37.—continued ◆

SURGICAL INSTRUMENTS

	Steinmann pin
	Wire fixation:
	Stainless steel wire
	Wire-holding forceps
	Wire-cutting forceps
	Bone staples:
	Bone staples
	Staple introducer
	Staple remover
	External fixator:
	Steinmann pins
	Kirschner Ehmer rods
	Kirschner Ehmer nuts
	Pin cutter
	Drill or Jacob's chuck
	Bone plating or screw fixation:
	Venables/Sherman bone plates
	Sherman screws
	Drill bit
	Air/hand drill
	Depth gauge
	Screw driver
	Plate bender
	A.S.I.F. technique (Figure 26.37)
	(Association for the Study of Internal Fixation)
	Dynamic compression plates and screws
	Bone drills: standard and overdrill
	Bone tap and handle
	Drill guide – neutral and loaded
	Tap sleeve
	Drill insert
	Depth gauge
	Counter sink
	Screw driver
	Plate bender or irons
Ophthalmic instruments	No. 3 scalpel handle
	Scalpel blade sizes 11, 15 or Beaver handle and blades
	Fine dissecting forceps
	Fine scissors
	Corneal scissors
	Capsular forceps
	Vectis
	Iris repositor
	Castroveijo needle-holders
	Eyelid speculum
	Irrigating cannula
	Distichiasis forceps
Dental instruments	Mouth gag
	Dental scalers
	Dental elevators
	Dental chisels
	Dental forceps
	Ultrasonic descaler

Fig. 26.37. Instrument sets for various surgical procedures: some suggested contents.

needle-holders. The knot security is varied and a bulky knot may be formed. It is very springy but shows little tissue drag. It becomes encapsulated in a thin fibrous covering.

Polyamide. This may be either monofilament or braided. The monofilament form causes little tissue reactions, has little tissue drag and is non-capillary. Its handling characteristics are not good and knot security can be poor. It loses approximately 15% of its tensile strength each year. It can be used on fascia and muscle, but the buried ends can be irritant in serous or synovial cavities. The braided form is usually sheathed in an attempt to decrease capillarity but its use as a buried suture is not recommended. It shows more tissue drag than the monofilament variety, although it handles better.

Polyesters. Various braided polyesters are available. They are easy to handle and retain their tensile strength well. Some are coated with silicone, teflon or polybutylate to reduce tissue drag. They tend to have poor knot-tying quality and some have shown signs of capillarity.

Stainless steel. This is available in monofilament or braided varieties. It is very strong, inert and non-capillary. It is relatively difficult to handle as the wire lacks elasticity and knots may be difficult to tie, but knot security is good. It is useful in slow-healing tissues such as bone, tendon and joint capsules, and in contaminated sites. It has become less popular in recent years as newer materials have become available.

CHARACTERISTICS OF SUTURE MATERIALS: TERMINOLOGY

Tensile strength	The breaking strength per unit area of tissue.
Knot security	Related to the surface frictional characteristics of the material. Every suture is weakest where it is tied. Often the strongest sutures have the poorest knot security.
Tissue reaction	The response of the tissue to the suture material involved.
Tissue drag	The degree of frictional force developed as the material is pulled through the tissue.
arity	The extent to which tissue fluid is attracted along the suture material. Materials with high capillarity act as a wick and encourage fluids to move along them. Such materials should not be used in the presence of sepsis.
Memory	The tendency of the material to return to its original shape. A material with high memory tends to unkink during knot tying i.e., knot security is poor with materials possessing high memory.
Chatter	The lack of smoothness as a throw of a knot is tightened down.
Stiffness and elongation	The less force required to stretch a suture, the more it will elongate before it ruptures.
Sterilisation characteristics	The ability of the material to undergo sterilisation without deteriorating. Autoclaving is satisfactory for the nylon materials. Repeated autoclaving will however weaken them. The natural products and synthetic absorbable materials should not be steam sterilised. Ethylene oxide sterilisation is safe for all sutures provided the packs are sufficiently aerated.

Fig. 26.38. Characteristics of suture materials: terminology.

ABSORBENCY OF SUTURES

	Natural fibres	Synthetic	
Absorbable sutures	Multifilament: Catgut: plain Chromic	**Monofilament** Polydioxanone Polyglyconate **Multifilament** Polyglactin 910 Polyglycolic Acid	[PDS II]** [Maxon] [Vicryl]** [Dexon]*
Non absorbable sutures	Multifilament Silk Linen	**Multifilament** Braided polymide Polyester Coated polyester **Monofilament** Polyamide Polypropylene Polybutester Polyethylene **Stainless steel**	[Nuralon]** [Supramid] [Mersilene]** [Ethibond]** [Ethilon]** [Prolene]** [Novafil]* [Dermalene]**

*Trademark Davis & Geck Ltd.
**Trademark Ethicon

Fig. 26.39. Examples of suture categories.

SURGICAL GUT: APPROXIMATE ABSORPTION TIMES

Plain gut	3–7 days	Severe tissue reaction
Mild treatment	14 days	
Medium treatment	21 days	Most commonly used
Prolonged treatment	40 days	

Fig. 26.40. Catgut: approximate absorption times.

Alternatives to Sutures

Staples

Metal clips or staples for use in skin and other tissues have gained popularity in the field of veterinary surgery over the last few years. Staples designed for skin closure are packed in a gun-like applicator for rapid insertion. These instruments are intended to be disposable, although they may be safely sterilised by ethylene oxide.

The main advantage of staples is speed of insertion. They are inert and well-tolerated. A special instrument is needed to remove them although this can be done efficiently using a pair of artery forceps.

Stapling machines have also been designed for gastro-intestinal anastomosis. Although designed for the human market, they are suitable for veterinary applications and are gaining popularity. They may permit resection of areas of bowel that are inaccessible to routine suturing, particularly in the equine abdomen. Their major disadvantage is cost, but their ease of use and the shortened surgery time have much to recommend them.

Metal clips are also available for use as ligatures. They come in various sizes with reuseable applicators. They are simple and quick to use.

Tissue glue

There are cyanoacrylate monomers which polymerise on contact with moisture in the wound. They have been found useful by some surgeons.

Adhesive tapes

Designed for use in humans, these have been of limited use in animals as they do not adhere well to moist skin.

Suture Selection

The veterinary surgeon will normally select the suture material but the veterinary nurse should have some idea of which materials may be used in different tissues (Fig. 26.41) and the sizes that will be required (Fig. 26.42).

When selecting suture sizes, small diameter materials should be chosen. These cause less tissue reaction, form smaller knots, knot more easily and are less likely to tie too tight (because they will break). If sutures are tied too tight, they will cut through friable tissue.

Packaging of Suture Materials

Individual packets

Most suture materials are purchased in pre-sterilised individual packets. This guarantees a sterile suture (unless the packet is damaged) and a needle in perfect condition where one is attached. The only

SIZES OF SUTURE MATERIAL		
Metric	USP – non absorbable Synthetic absorbable	Catgut
0.2	10/0	
0.3	9/0	
0.4	8/0	
0.5	7/0	8/0
0.7	6/0	7/0
1	5/0	6/0
1.5	4/0	5/0
2	3/0	4/0
3	2/0	3/0
3.5	0	2/0
4	1	0
5	2	1
6	3 & 4	2
7	5	3
8	6	4

Sutures come in either metric or USP (US Pharmacopeia) sizes

Fig. 26.42. Sizes of suture material.

disadvantage is that of cost. Synthetic absorbable suture materials are only available packaged in this way.

Cassettes

Multi-use cassettes are frequently used in veterinary practice for packaging catgut, nylon and stainless steel sutures. The disadvantage of these is the likelihood of contamination of cassettes during use—they often become damaged. It is also easy to contaminate the material as it is cut from the reel and transferred to the instrument trolley.

Suture Needles

Suture needles are designed to pass through tissue easily. They must be sharp enough to penetrate tissues with minimal resistance, rigid enough to prevent excessive bending and yet flexible enough to bend before breaking. They should be made from corrosion resistant stainless steel.

Swaged needles

Swaged or atraumatic needles are attached to the suture material, i.e. they do not require threading. The advantage of this is that a needle in perfect condition is available with each strand and tissue trauma is minimised by the passage of material and needle of a comparative size. All of the pre-packed suture materials are available with a variety of different needle shapes and sizes.

Eyed needles

This type of needle requires threading. The primary indication for its use is economy of suitable material or use of speciality needles, e.g. for large animal work. The disadvantages are increased tissue trauma

SUTURE MATERIALS SUITABLE FOR DIFFERENT TISSUES	
Skin	Monofilament nylon or Polypropylene Metal staples Avoid materials with capillary action
Subcutis	Fine synthetic absorbable material with minimal tissue reaction e.g. polydioxanone polyglactin, polyglycolic acid
Muscle	Synthetic absorbable, non absorbable e.g., nylon
Fascia	Synthetic non-absorbable if prolonged suture strength required
Hollow viscus	Synthetic absorbable or polypropylene. In bladder: monofilament synthetic absorbable
Tendon	Nylon, polypropylene, stainless steel
Blood vessels	Polypropylene: least thrombogenic is silk
Eyes	Synthetic absorbable e.g., Polyglactin, Polydioxanone
Nerves	Nylon or polypropylene: minimal tissue reaction

Fig. 26.41. Suture materials suitable for different tissues.

due to the eye size, loss of sharpness of the needle tip, bending and corrosion following repeated use. The needle shape refers to both the longitude shape of the shaft and the cross-sectional shape.

Longitudinal shape

Of the great variety of different sizes and shapes that are available, some of those used in veterinary surgery are shown in Fig. 26.43.

Cross-sectional shape

Round-bodied. These are designed to separate tissue fibres rather than cut them, and are used for soft tissue or in situations where easy splitting of tissue fibres is possible.

Modified point. The **taper-cut** needle has a cutting tip on the point of the needle and a round body. This provides increased penetration of the needle without increase tissue trauma.

The **trocar-point** needle has a strong cutting head and a robust round body. This is useful in dense tissue.

Cutting needles. These are required wherever dense or tough tissue needs to be sutured. The cross-sectional appearance of the needle is usually a triangular cutting edge which extends at least half-way along the shaft. The reverse cutting needle has the cutting edge on the outside of the needle curvature to improve strength and resistance to bending.

Micro-point needles. These are very fine needles with a sharp cutting edge. They are designed for ophthalmic and micro-surgery.

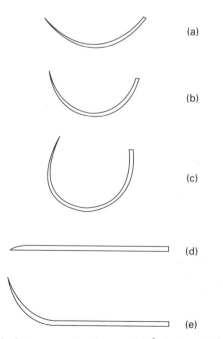

Fig. 26.43. Suture needle shapes: (a) $\frac{3}{8}$ circle; (b) $\frac{1}{2}$ circle; (c) $\frac{5}{8}$ circle; (d) straight; (e) $\frac{1}{2}$ curved.

Selection of needles

The use of swaged needles is to be encouraged—their advantages far outweigh those of eyed needles. Other needles should be as close as possible in diameter to that of the suture. A large needle tract invites bacteria and foreign substances to enter the wound, thus delaying healing. The needle should be of the appropriate shape and size to enable the veterinary surgeon to close the wound accurately and precisely.

The smaller and deeper the wound, the greater the curve should be. Straight needles are designed to be hand held and tend to be used in the skin. Half-curved cutting needles have been commonly used in veterinary surgery but have little to recommend their use. The tissue type will determine the necessary point of the needle. Generally speaking:

- Round-bodied needles are used for viscera, subcutaneous and friable tissue.
- Taper-tip needles are used for easily penetrated tissue. i.e. for denser tissue.
- Cutting needles are generally used in the skin.

Suture Patterns

Veterinary nurses maintained on the list held by the RCVS are now legally allowed to perform minor acts of surgery, including the suturing of wounds, and it is important that they should be familiar with basic suturing techniques. The veterinary surgeon should give practical instruction and reference should be made to surgical technique textbooks.

Suture patterns (Fig. 26.44) may be interrupted or closed, and may be further classified as apposing, everting or inverting:

- **Apposing** sutures bring the tissues in direct apposition.
- **Everting** sutures tend to turn the edges of the wound outwards.
- **Inverting** sutures turn the tissue inwards (e.g. towards the lumen of a viscus).

Surgical knots

A surgical knot has three main components:

- The **loop** is the part of the suture material within the opposed or ligated tissue.
- The **knot** is composed of a number of **throws**, each throw being the linking of two strands of tissue around each other.
- The **ears** are the cut ends of the suture which prevent the knot coming untied.

Knots can be tied by hand or by an instrument. Hand ties may be single- or two-handed.

The basic surgical knot is the reef knot or square knot. A surgeon's knot has an initial double throw instead of a single throw. This reduced the risk of the first throw loosening before the second throw is placed.

Hand-tying helps to prevent slippage of the first throw, since tension can be kept on both ends of the suture throughout the procedure. However, it tends to be wasteful on suture material.

The knots of skin sutures should be pulled to one side of the incision and the suture loop should be loose. Sutures which are too tight compromise the vascular supply, enhance infection and delay healing. They are also uncomfortable and encourage the patient to interfere with the wound.

Suture material should not be crushed in the jaws of needle-holders. When tying knots, only the end of the suture material should be grasped. Needle-holders should not be clamped on to the eye of swaged needles as this will cause damage or breakage of the needle.

Interrupted sutures

The main advantage of the interrupted suture is its ability to maintain strength and tissue apposition if part of the suture line fails. Each suture is individually tied and cut distal to the knot. Its main disadvantage is the amount of suture material used and left within the tissue and the time required to suture.

Continuous sutures

These are neither knotted nor cut, except at each end of the suture line. The advantages of the continuous suture line are ease of application, use of minimal amount of suture material and ease of removal. The main disadvantage is that slippage of either the beginning or end knot is likely to cause failure of the entire suture line.

Common suture patterns

Skin. Common suture patterns used in the skin (Fig. 26.44) include:

- Simple interrupted
- Simple continuous
- Ford interlocking
- Interrupted vertical mattress
- Interrupted horizontal mattress
- Cruciate mattress.

Skin sutures should be placed at least 5mm from the skin edge and be placed squarely across the wound. The skin should be handled gently with fine rat-toothed forceps. The wound edges should be apposed or slightly everted with no gaping or over-lapping.

Muscle and fascia

- Simple interrupted
- Simple continuous
- Ford interlocking
- Cruciate mattress

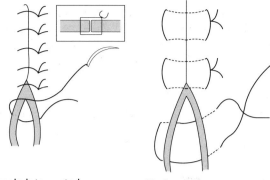

Simple interrupted   Horizontal mattress

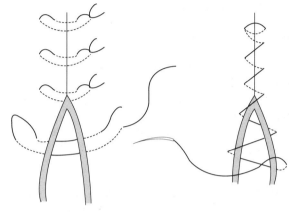

Vertical mattress   Simple continuous

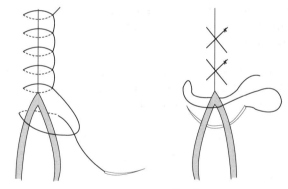

Ford interlocking suture   Cruciate mattress

Fig. 26.44. Common suture patterns used in the skin.

- Horizontal mattress
- Vertical mattress
- Mayo mattress.

Hollow organ closure

- Simple interrupted
- Parker kerr
- Purse string
- Connell
- Cushing
- Lembert
- Gambee
- Halstead

Further Reading

Knecht, C. D., Allen, A. R., Williams, D. J. and Johnson, J. H. (1987, 3rd edn) *Fundamental Techniques in Veterinary surgery*. W. B. Saunders Company, Philadelphia.

McCurnin, D. M. (1990, 2nd edn) *Clinical Textbook for Veterinary Technicians*. W. B. Saunders Company, Philadelphia.

Tracey, D. *Small Animal Surgical Nursing*. Mosby's.

27
Anaesthesia and Analgesia

R. E. CLUTTON

Anaesthesia and the Central Nervous System

Anaesthesia means the elimination of sensation by the controlled, reversible suppression of nervous function with drugs. To understand anaesthesia, it is necessary to understand the nature of sensation.

Sensations like touch, pressure, temperature and pain begin with the stimulation of peripheral nerve endings in sense organs (Fig. 27.1). From these, impulses travel through sensory, or afferent, nerves to the spinal cord and then ascend to the brain, terminating in cerebrocortical projection areas dedicated to appreciating the particular sensation. Special senses like olfaction (smell) do not enter the spine; impulses travel (almost) directly to the associated projection area.

Anaesthesia occurs when sensory pathways are blocked anywhere between the peripheral sense organ and projection area. Local anaesthetics block sensation in peripheral nerves (after conduction block) or in the spinal cord (after extradural local anaesthetic injection). In contrast, general anaesthetics affect the brain, especially the particularly sensitive projection areas and produce unconsciousness. They also reduce activity in the ascending reticular formation, a part of the neuraxis that increases cortical sensitivity to incoming stimuli.

In addition to sensation, anaesthetics depress the function of subcortical centres receiving afferent information about unconscious stimuli such as blood pressure, plasma levels of oxygen (O_2) and carbon dioxide (CO_2), and blood temperature. These 'vital centres' are relatively resistant to anaesthetics but become increasingly depressed as anaesthesia deepens; at deep levels, significant hypoventilation and hypotension occur and animals are predisposed to hypothermia.

The ways in which drugs produce anaesthesia are not fully understood but depend partly on the drug involved. Some, like α_2-agonists and ketamine, act via specific receptors; others such as volatile agents and barbiturates probably act in a non-specific way on cell membranes. Some drugs acting via receptors may be antagonised.

Drugs Affecting Central Nervous Function

These can be divided broadly into depressants, which reduce nervous activity, and stimulants, which increase it and oppose the effects of anaesthetics.

Depressants

General anaesthetics. General anaesthetics like thiopentone and halothane eliminate sensation by causing unconciousness; the animal is unaware of and largely unresponsive to events and is unable to remember the experience afterwards. Righting reflexes concerned with maintaining posture are lost and so animals become recumbent.

Anaesthetics are classified by their physical properties: volatile liquids (halothane), gases (nitrous oxide), water-soluble (thiopentone) or water-insoluble drugs ('Saffan').

Cyclohexanones like ketamine produce a unique state in which humans would feel dissociated from the environment and be unconscious but experience vivid dreams and profound analgesia. Such drugs are known as 'dissociative' anaesthetics.

Sedatives. Drugs like xylazine produce non-selective, dose-dependent central nervous depression producing drowsiness, lethargy, indifference to the environment and reduced activity. Consciousness is lost at high doses; low doses have a tranquillising effect.

Hypnotics. Drugs like thiopentone produce sleep or 'hypnosis', a term synonymous with anaesthesia as hypnosis is drug-induced sleep. The 'depth' of sleep produced is dose-dependent.

Narcotics. Narcosis is a drug-induced stupor characterised by insensibility and paralysis. Effects are non-selective and dose-dependent. Basal narcosis is complete unconsciousness induced as a preliminary to surgical anaesthesia. Narcotics are any

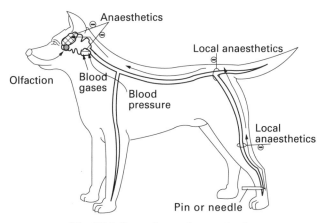

Fig. 27.1. Sensation and anaesthesia.

drugs producing these conditions and so the term includes anaesthetics, hypnotics and sedatives.

Ataractics. Ataractics, or tranquillisers, exert a quietening effect that calms aggressive animals and reduces anxiety. In high doses they cause catalepsy, a state in which the animal, though conscious, can be 'moulded'. Strong stimuli arouse tranquillised animals, whereas in sedated ones the responses, if present, are sluggish. This group is divided into 'major' or 'minor' ataractics, based on effects; major tranquillisers are also called neurolepts.

Neurolepts. These produce neurolepsy, a state of apathy and mental detachment. Neurolepts like acepromazine also relieve emotional distress and disturbed behaviour without clouding consciousness.

Neuroleptanalgesics. Neuroleptanalgesia is a state produced by the combined effects of a neurolept and an opioid analgesic, e.g. acepromazine and morphine. Neuroleptanalgesics cause dose-dependent effects and high doses produce unconsciousness (neuroleptanaesthesia).

Stimulants

Drugs that increase nervous activity oppose the effects of anaesthetics. They are classified according to their site of action. Analeptics (medullary stimulants) are the most commonly used. Others have undesirable side-effects and, with the exception of doxapram, are not licensed for animal use. Some are controlled substances.

Drug Interactions

Usually, drugs depressing central nervous function act in an additive or synergistic fashion. If a sedative drug (A) produces an effect (e), and if drug (B), which is more potent, causes an effect 2(e), then after (A) and (B) are given:

- **Additive** effects occur when the level of sedation equals 3(e).
- **Synergy** occurs when the level of sedation is greater than 3(e).
- **Antagonism** occurs if the level of sedation achieved is less than 3(e).

Inhalation anaesthetics act in an additive fashion; neurolepts and opioids act in a synergistic way.

The Blood–Brain Barrier

In order to affect brain activity, anaesthetics must first cross the blood–brain barrier, a conceptual anatomic feature formed by 'tight' junctions between endothelial cells of capillaries and envelopment of brain capillaries by glial cells.

Drugs that are non-ionised, small, fat-soluble (or lipid-soluble) and unbound from albumen cross the blood–brain barrier rapidly. In some conditions (e.g. encephalitis), the blood–brain barrier is disrupted and the patient becomes more sensitive to anaesthetics.

Analgesia

Analgesia is a state of reduced sensibility to pain. Painful (noxious) stimuli reach the brain in similar ways to other sensations but are amenable to interruption by a greater range of drugs. An animal's response to pain depends on the level of the central nervous system to which the pain message ascends (Fig. 27.2):

- Spinal responses include, for example, reflex limb withdrawal.
- Medullary responses include increased heart rate, blood pressure and respiratory rate.
- Hypothalamic responses take several forms. The hypothalamus initiates catecholamine release from the adrenal medulla and nerve endings of the sympathetic nervous system. This further increases heart rate and blood pressure and causes piloerection. Less obviously, the hypothalamus secretes releasing factors which cause the pituitary gland to release 'stress' hormones such as adrenocorticotropic hormone ACTH. Other pituitary hormones like thyroid stimulating hormone (TSH), anti-diuretic hormone (ADH) and prolactin (PRL) are also released.
- Cortical responses are the most complex; they include activity like vocalisation and voluntary acts such as attempting to escape or to bite at the noxious stimulus.

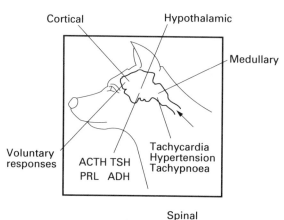

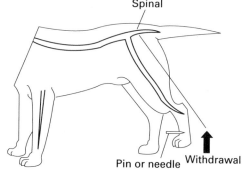

Fig. 27.2. Responses to pain.

Analgesics

Analgesics interrupt the ascending pain pathway at various levels (Fig. 27.3) and suppress the sensation of pain. After analgesics are given, pain responses are modified according to the level of interruption, which in turn depends on the sensitivity of that level to the analgesic. For example, general anaesthetics like halothane exert their greatest effect on the cortex. Therefore, in the halothane-anaesthetised animal, complex responses like vocalisation or escape will not occur. However, if anaesthesia is very 'light', limb withdrawal from noxious stimuli (e.g. toe-pinches) may still be seen. Traditionally, analgesics have been categorised as anti-pyretic analgesics (or non-steroidal anti-inflammatory drugs) and narcotic or opioid analgesics. This classification is of limited use because several drug groups suppress pain. These include:

- Non-steroidal anti-inflammatory drugs (NSAIDs)
- Glucocorticoids
- Local anaesthetics
- Benzodiazepines
- Opioids
- General anaesthetics

Each group operates at specific levels of the pain path. Some, like the opioids, act at several points along this path.

Peripheral nerve endings

Glucocorticoids and NSAIDs reduce nerve-ending sensitivity to pain-sensitizing chemicals released from damaged tissue (autocoids). Topical local anaesthetics block nerve endings.

Glucocorticoids. These drugs suppress inflammation and the generation of autocoids.

NSAIDs. These drugs inhibit mediators of inflammation and ideally should be given before surgery

begins. Drugs available include acetylsalicylate, phenylbutazone, paracetamol, flunixin, carprofen, ketoprofen and meloxicam.

Peripheral nerves

Local anaesthetics block the nerve impulse in peripheral nerves.

Spinal cord

Pain can be suppressed in the cord by the extradural injection of several drug types:

- Local anaesthetics block all nerve fibre types producing anaesthesia, analgesia and muscle relaxation.
- Opioids diminish sensitivity to pain but do not eliminate sensation, proprioception or muscle function. Animals are therefore free from pain but can walk.
- Benzodiazepines, NMDA (*N*-methyl-D-aspartate (involved in allowing calcium ion entry into the post synaptic ganglion)) receptor antagonists and α_2-agonists have analgesic effects at spinal level although they are currently experimental.
- Combinations of drugs that are compatible *in vitro* may be injected in order to capitalise on the desirable properties of each, e.g. lignocaine, bupivacaine, morphine.

Brain

Opioids, α_2-agonists and general anaesthetics cause analgesia through effects on the brain. Consciousness need not be lost for analgesia to be present.

Central Analgesia: Anaesthesia versus Analgesia

During surgery, general anaesthetics prevent the appreciation (and subsequent memory) of pain by affecting projection areas. However, subcortical centres like the medulla and hypothalamus still respond, causing heart and respiratory rate increases, hormone release and, when anaesthesia is very 'light', limb movement. Under these conditions, anaesthesia is present but analgesia is poor.

Conversely, low concentrations of some local anaesthetics (0.25% bupivacaine) only block pain fibres, leaving other sensations 'intact'. If this formulation is used extradurally, the hindquarters become analgesic but sensitive to sensations like touch and pressure. The animal remains conscious.

Surgical Anaesthesia

This is a state of insensibility which allows surgery to be performed. In addition to unconsciousness (general anaesthesia), adequate analgesia is required to suppress undesirable responses (increased blood pressure) while muscle relaxation is needed to prevent movement and to facilitate surgery.

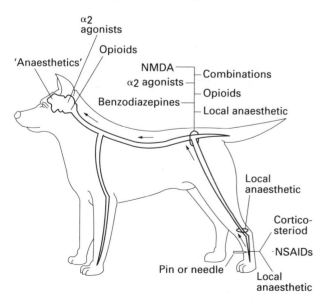

Fig. 27.3. Pain pathways and analgesia.

Balanced Anaesthesia

Surgical anaesthesia can be produced with high doses of general anaesthetic. This may be safe in healthy animals undergoing surgery but the high doses required may jeopardise vital functions in ill patients, causing critical ventilatory and cardiovascular depression. Balanced anaesthesia describes the use of several drug types to achieve the goals of surgical anaesthesia: unconsciousness (anaesthetics/hypnotics), analgesia and muscle relaxation. By relieving general anaesthetics from the task of producing analgesia and muscle relaxation, lower doses of anaesthetics are needed and so vital centre activity is preserved.

Types of Anaesthetics

The route of drug administration forms a basis for describing anaesthetics. Importantly, the route of administration affects drug activity.

Enteral

The gastrointestinal tract is seldom used to administer anaesthetics or pre-anaesthetic medication because absorption is unpredictable and onset times are slow. Aggressive animals may be given oral acepromazine before presentation. Caged, aggressive animals are subdued if medetomidine (dogs) or ketamine (cats) is squirted on to the oral mucous membranes.

Parenteral

Drugs can be injected, or inhaled into the respiratory tree.

Injection

Drugs may be given by intravenous (IV), intramuscular (IM), subcutaneous (SC) or intraperitoneal (IP) routes. Pre-anaesthetic medication is often given IM or SC while induction agents are usually given intravenously. In laboratory animals, IP injections are sometimes used. The advantages of the various routes are given in Fig. 27.4.

Intravenous. Poor intravenous technique may damage veins and preclude later use. Veins must be regarded as 'sacred'; they allow the most rapid drug responses and so are used for emergency drug administration. This route must be used for irritant drugs like thiopentone.

Intramuscular. Some drugs (e.g. diazepam) are poorly absorbed after IM injection. In general, up to 3 times the IV dose may be needed to produce the same effect. Some drugs (e.g. morphine, ketamine) cause pain on injection. In obese animals, inadvertent

COMPARISON OF DRUG ADMINISTRATION ROUTES	
Convenience	SC > IP > IM > IV
Pain on injection	IM > IP + IV > SC
Restraint needed	IV > IP > IM > SC
Animal tolerance	SC > IP > IM > IV
Onset of action	IV > IM > SC > IP
Duration of action	IP + SC > IM > IP
Predictability	IV > IM > SC > IP
Relative dose required	IP + SC > IM > IV
Risk of complications	IP > IV > IM > SC
Technical ease	SC > IM > IP > IV

Fig. 27.4. Comparison of drug administration routes.

injection into fat deposits may account for poor responses.

Subcutaneous. For animals in 'shock', the blood supply to the skin is poor so that drug absorption after subcutaneous injection will be poor. In fat animals, drugs may be injected inadvertently into fat, which is a relatively avascular tissue and so drug absorption may be severely retarded.

ADVANTAGES OF INJECTABLE ANAESTHETICS

- Convenient; simple to inject.
- Inexpensive—less equipment needed.
- Intravenous injection usually causes a rapid loss of consciousness.
- No airway irritation.
- No explosion/pollution hazard.
- Rapid recovery.
- Some drugs can be antagonised.
- Endotracheal intubation is less necessary.
- Rapid deepening of anaesthesia is possible.
- Respiratory function does not influence drug behaviour.

DISADVANTAGES

- Stressful restraint may be required.
- Myositis and pain may result from injection.
- Effects may be irreversible; for drugs without antagonists, recovery depends on cardiovascular, hepatic and renal function.
- Anaesthesia is readily deepened, but not 'lightened'.
- Wide dose-range requirements.
- Self-administration is hazardous with some drugs.
- Repeated doses may cause drug accumulation and prolonged recoveries.
- Injectable drugs have widely different side-effects.
- Airway protection is often neglected.

Inhalation

Inhalation, volatile or 'gaseous' anaesthesia refers to the inhalation of anaesthetic vapours or gases delivered into the respiratory tract. Anaesthesia is commonly maintained with inhalation agents although they can also be used to induce anaesthesia.

Some emergency drugs like adrenaline, lignocaine, atropine and methoxamine are given by the intra-tracheal route if venous access is unavailable.

ADVANTAGES OF INHALATION OF ANAESTHETICS

- Recovery depends on respiratory function and is normally rapid and predictable.
- The depth of anaesthesia is readily controlled.
- Single dose rate; MAC is similar in most species.
- Concurrent oxygen delivery; volatile agents are usually 'carried' in oxygen.
- Volatile agent activity is independent of hepatic and renal function.
- Continued administration does not necessarily cause prolonged recoveries. Surgery may be prolonged without complication.
- Inhalational drugs have broadly similar effects.
- The airway is usually protected.

DISADVANTAGES

- Recovery may be delayed by inadequate ventilation or lung pathology.
- A considerable range of equipment is required; some items are expensive.
- Intubation usually necessary.
- Knowledge of breathing systems and anaesthetic machines is required.
- Hazards associated with compressed gas.
- Fire and explosion risks with some agents.
- Possible health-risk associated with exposure to volatile agents.

Regional (Local) Anaesthesia

With regional anaesthesia, the loss of sensation is restricted to a body region, or part, rather than the whole body. It may be achieved by several techniques. Regional anaesthesia has considerable advantages.

ADVANTAGES OF REGIONAL ANAESTHESIA

- Lower equipment requirement.
- Excellent anaesthesia and muscle relaxation when technique is satisfactory.
- Consciousness is retained; there is no loss of protective reflexes.
- There is little cardiopulmonary depression; techniques are relatively safe in ill animals.
- Techniques are inexpensive.
- Some techniques allow titration: the degree, duration and anatomic 'level' of block can be increased by repeat injections.

DISADVANTAGES

- Not all procedures can be performed with local anaesthetic techniques.
- Some techniques are difficult to perform and subsequent block may be incomplete.
- Some techniques are painful to perform; animals may require sedation.
- Active animals may require physical or chemical restraint for surgery.
- Overdosage and toxicity is possible with some drugs.
- Some techniques (e.g. extradural anaesthesia) produce untoward cardiovascular effects.
- Some local anaesthetics have a short duration of action.

The Objectives of Anaesthesia

In veterinary practice, anaesthetics are used for several reasons:

- To permit surgery. In the UK, the 'carrying out of any operation with or without the use of instruments, involving interference with the sensitive tissues or the bone structure of an animal shall constitute an offence unless an anaesthetic is used in such a way as to prevent any pain to the animal during the operation.'
- To facilitate examination. Anxious, aggressive or painful animals may not allow examination.
- To control pain. Opioids, benzodiazepines, local and general anaesthetics are used to control pain.
- To facilitate handling. Controlling strong, aggressive animals with drugs reduces risk of injury to handlers and the need for physical restraint. Drugs for chemical restraint are chosen for potency, predictability, efficacy and speed of onset after intramuscular injection and not necessarily for safety. Drug combinations for restraint should be reserved for unmanageable cases and not regarded as anaesthetics in tractable subjects.
- To control seizures. Diazepam and pentobarbitone are used to control status epilepticus in animals.
- To perform euthanasia. Commercially available euthanasia solutions consist of concentrated anaesthetic (pentobarbitone) occasionally combined with a local anaesthetic (e.g. cinchocaine) and/or an anticonvulsant (e.g. phenytoin).

The Anaesthetic Period

The anaesthetic period is conveniently separated into five time divisions. Patient risk, the responsibilities of surgeon, anaesthetists and nurses, and the drugs and equipment used are different in each period.

R. E. Clutton

Pre-operative period (preparation)

Animals are examined and prepared for anaesthesia and surgery. Drugs may be given to control pre-existing medical conditions. Anaesthetic equipment is checked and prepared for use.

Pre-anaesthetic period (pre-anaesthetic medication)

Drugs (pre-anaesthetic medication, or 'premeds') are given to sedate the animal and for other reasons.

Induction

The animal is rendered unconscious with 'induction' agents.

Maintenance period

Unconsciousness is maintained with 'maintenance' agents, allowing surgery or examination to be performed.

Recovery period

Drug administration ceases and the animal is allowed to regain consciousness.

The Anaesthetic Technique

Anaesthesia can be produced in many ways because of the range of drugs and drug combinations, doses, routes of administration and techniques available. Selection of the optimum technique is based on:

- Patient species. Drugs are not equally safe in all species: ketamine and 'Saffan' are unsafe in dogs although satisfactory in cats.
- Patient individuality. Some breeds do not tolerate certain drugs (e.g. sight hounds and barbiturates). Breed-related conditions complicating the management of anaesthesia may be present (e.g. Von Willebrand's disease in Dobermann pinschers). Also individual animals may have specific diseases, or be old and fat.
- The nature and duration of surgery. Greater risk is associated with invasive, prolonged surgery and so anaesthesia will be more complicated. Anaesthesia must also produce adequate conditions in terms of duration. In all cases, the magnitude and duration of physiological perturbation must be kept to a minimum.

Anaesthesia and the Respiratory System

The respiratory and cardiovascular systems operate in concert to oxygenate blood and then deliver it to peripheral, metabolically active tissue. Here, energy-rich substrate (glucose) is oxidised (with O_2) to produce CO_2. The metabolic requirements of organs like the brain are such that diminished O_2 or glucose supplies will rapidly cause cell death.

Understanding the respiratory system during anaesthesia is important because anaesthetics depress ventilation, causing or contributing to cardiac arrest. The system also takes up and eliminates volatile anaesthetics.

Ventilation

The respiratory system must provide enough fresh gas to the alveoli per minute to ensure that blood is oxygenated, and 'purged' of CO_2. The volume of gas inspired per breath is the tidal volume (V_t), measured in millilitres or litres. The volume of gas inspired per minute—the 'minute volume' (V_m) of ventilation—is given by:

$$V_m = V_t \times R,$$

where R is the respiratory rate in breaths per minute.

Dead-space. Not all inspired gas reaches the alveoli and participates in gas exchange. At the end of inspiration, the last portion resides in the volume of the respiratory tree down to the level of conducting bronchioles. This does not participate in gas exchange and is called the **anatomic dead-space** volume (Vd_{anat}).

Anatomic dead-space is augmented by excessive equipment attached to the proximal end of the airway; overlarge masks and overlong endotracheal tubes are examples of **mechanical** (or apparatus) **dead-space** volume (Vd_{mech}).

Some inspired gas reaches alveoli that are not perfused with blood and so does not contribute to gas exchange. This is known as **alveolar dead-space** (Vd_a). Anatomic and alveolar dead-space constitute physiologic dead-space.

$$Vd = Vd_{anat} + Vd_a + Vd_{mech}.$$

The remaining volume reaching alveoli is the alveolar volume (V_A).

$$V_A = V_t - Vd,$$

and the volume of gas usefully inspired per minute is given by:

$$V_A = R(Vt - Vd).$$

The importance of dead-space is now apparent: when excessive, it reduces alveolar ventilation.

The elimination of carbon dioxide (CO_2), the normal determinant of respiration, is directly proportional to V_A:

$$PaCO_2 = k \times VCO_2/V_A,$$

where VCO_2 is the volume of CO_2 produced by the body per minute, k is a constant and $PaCO_2$ is the partial pressure or 'level' of CO_2 in arterial blood. Consequently, under normal conditions $PaCO_2$ is an indicator of the adequacy of ventilation. Normal $PaCO_2$ is 5.33 kPa (40mm Hg).

Control of Ventilation

The contraction of ventilatory muscles (most importantly the diaphragm and external intercostal muscles) causes lung inflation and the inspiration of tidal volume. The activity of these muscles, and therefore the level of ventilation, is driven by nerve fibres whose origin lies in the 'respiratory centre' of the medulla oblongata, located in the brain stem. Activity in these fibres is controlled by several factors such as body temperature and pain, but the most important are blood levels of CO_2 and O_2. These levels are monitored by two types of receptors known as **chemoreceptors**:

- Zone of Central Chemoreceptors (ZCC). This area of tissue lies in the brain stem close to the respiratory centres and is sensitive to the pH of surrounding cerebrospinal fluid (CSF). Carbon dioxide diffuses from blood into CSF, lowering its pH. The ZCC responds by increasing respiratory drive to the respiratory centres.
- Peripheral chemoreceptors. The carotid bodies are sited near the carotid bifurcation and respond to falling oxygen tensions in blood. In conscious animals their activity increases dramatically when PaO_2 falls below 8kPa (60mm Hg). (Normal O_2 levels are 13kPa (100mm Hg).)

Normally, $PaCO_2$ levels are the major determinant of minute ventilation; when CO_2 rises, alveolar ventilation rises, restoring $PaCO_2$ to normal. Blood oxygen levels only become important in driving respiration when they are critically reduced.

Hypoventilation

Hypoventilation means inadequate ventilation and causes plasma CO_2 levels to rise—a state known as **hypercapnia** (or hypercarbia). Carbon dioxide tensions in excess of 5.33 kPa (40 mm Hg) indicate hypoventilation. Hypoventilation occurs when:

- Respiratory rate (R) is too low (e.g. anaesthetic overdose).
- Tidal volume (V_t) is reduced (e.g. heavy drapes on chest wall).
- Dead-space (Vd) increases (e.g. endotracheal tube projects too far from mouth, hypovolaemia reduces alveolar perfusion).
- A combination of these.

Hypercapnia can also result from increased production of CO_2. This may occur in the pyrexic animal or during malignant hyperthermia, a rare condition in companion animals but not uncommon in certain pig breeds. Carbon dioxide dissolves in blood to produce carbonic acid:

$$CO_2 + H_2O = H_2CO_3 = H^+ + HCO_3^-.$$

This increases the acidity (and lowers the pH) of blood—a state of acidosis. Because the state is caused by hypoventilation, the ensuing condition is called **respiratory acidosis**. Hypercapnia and respiratory acidosis have important effects:

- Modest levels increase heart rate and blood pressure (and bleeding at the surgical site).
- High levels depress the heart, cause arrythmias and enhance narcosis.

Anaesthetics reduce chemoreceptor sensitivity to CO_2 and O_2 (some more than others) with the result that anaesthetised animals are usually hypercapnic.

Hyperventilation

This is an excessive level of breathing that drives off CO_2 and causes hypocapnia (or hypocarbia) and respiratory alkalosis. Pain and 'light' anaesthesia are common causes. Excessive manual or mechanical ventilation also causes hypocapnia; after periods of hyperventilation, animals usually will not breathe until $PaCO_2$ levels rise again.

Hypoxia

Hypoxia means abnormally low oxygen tensions in arterial blood (PaO_2). (Anoxia is an obsolete term meaning no oxygen.) Hypoxia is important because inadequately oxygenated haemoglobin means active tissues may become deprived of oxygen (tissue hypoxia). If the heart becomes hypoxic, cardiac arrest will occur. Lowered tissue oxygen delivery can result from several causes:

- Reduced oxygen in inspired gas (e.g. oxygen cylinder empties).
- Reduced alveolar ventilation (e.g. reduced rate, tidal volume or increased dead-space).
- Lung pathology (e.g. pneumonia).
- Insufficient haemaglobin to carry oxygen from lungs (e.g. anaemia).
- Insufficient cardiac output to deliver oxygenated blood to tissue (e.g. anaesthetic overdose).
- Increased tissue demand for oxygen (e.g. increased work—the myocardium becomes hypoxic at high heart rates).

Anaesthesia and the Cardiovascular System

The cardiovascular system consists of the heart, blood vessels, blood and elements of the autonomic nervous system that control its activity. The heart is considered in two parts: the right pumps un-oxygenated blood to the lung, the left pumps oxygenated blood to peripheral tissue.

The goal of cardiovascular activity is **perfusion**—the movement of sufficient volumes of blood containing metabolic reagents (oxygen and glucose) through tissue capillary beds per unit time.

Anaesthetics depress many facets of cardio-vascular function and, in combination with respiratory effects, may cause vital tissue to become deprived of oxygen (or glucose) and fail. Central nervous tissue hypoxia and hypoglycaemia rapidly cause irreversible damage.

Perfusion

Blood movement through capillaries depends on three factors (Fig. 27.5):

- High upstream (arterial) pressure (blood pressure).
- Low downstream (venous) pressure.
- Low resistance through tissue (relaxation of the pre-capillary sphincter).

Local tissue perfusion largely depends on local requirements. When metabolic activity is high, O_2 tensions fall and CO_2 accumulates. Both local hypoxia and hypercapnia cause pre-capillary sphincters to relax. Provided that upstream pressure is adequate, the blood flow will increase, delivering oxygen and removing CO_2.

Cardiovascular activity aims to ensure 'adequate upstream pressure' (or arterial blood pressure) so that tissues receive blood in inverse proportion to the resistance they offer, that is, according to their requirements. For non-vital tissue, 'whole-body' needs often override local requirements.

Systemic vascular resistance (SVR)

Arterial blood pressure is determined by cardiac output and systemic vascular resistance (Fig. 27.5): an increase in either raises blood pressure. Systemic vascular resistance is governed by the collective state of precapillary sphincters throughout the body. When these are closed, or in a state of vasoconstriction, SVR is increased and blood pressure rises. Precapillary sphincter diameter is controlled by:

- Local metabolic factors (PO_2, PCO_2).
- Tonic vasoconstrictor nerve discharge.
- Hormones and drugs:
  —endogenous: angiotensin, adrenaline;
  —exogenous: drugs (e.g. acepromazine, methoxamine).

Throughout the body, SVR is controlled by tonic, vasoconstrictor discharge from nerves of the sympathetic nervous system. This activity originates from the vasomotor centre of the medulla and is of fundamental importance in maintaining blood pressure by increasing SVR. It should be appreciated that perfusion downstream from constricted precapillary arterioles is reduced. Not surprisingly, vasoconstrictor fibres project principally to blood vessels of non-vital tissue, including the gastrointestinal tract and skin, the perfusion of which is reduced when 'whole-body' needs dictate. During haemorrhage, vasoconstrictor nerve activity increase in these tissues, preserving blood pressure and maintaining perfusion of vital tissue (brain and heart).

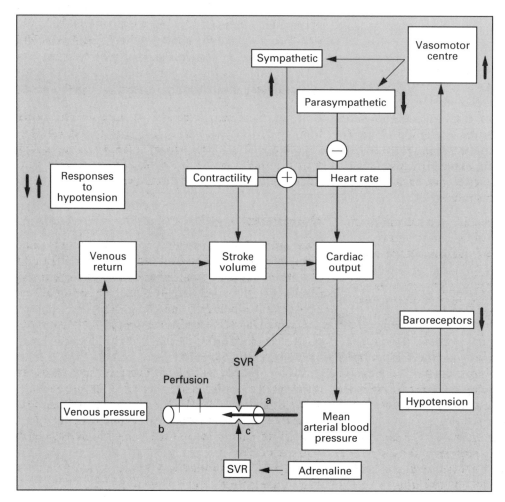

Fig. 27.5. The control of blood pressure.

Vasomotor centre function is depressed by general anaesthetics, which lower SVR and therefore blood pressure. Extradural local anaesthetics block vasoconstrictor fibres leaving the spinal cord; SVR is therefore lowered in areas affected by the block.

Cardiac output

Cardiac output, the volume of blood ejected by the heart per minute (measured in l/min) is the product of stroke volume (volume of blood ejected per beat) and heart rate. Variations in either component influence cardiac output.

Heart rate is governed by relative activity in either division of the autonomic nervous system; cardiac accelerator fibres (sympathetic) increase heart rate, while vagal (parasympathetic) activity slows heart rate. The rate also increases in response to circulating adrenaline. Stroke volume is governed by myocardial contractility and venous return—the volume of blood returning to the heart. Venous return depends on several factors including the circulating blood volume. Myocardial contractility is increased by circulating adrenaline.

Rapid heart rates reduce the time available for ventricles to fill with blood and lower stroke volume. At very high heart rates, cardiac output is reduced.

Control of blood pressure

Arterial blood pressure is sensed by baroreceptors (or mechanoreceptors), which are stretch-sensitive nerve endings lying within the elastic walls of the arterial tree. The most important group lie in a dilatation of the internal carotid artery known as the carotid sinus. These stretch when exposed to high pressure, and activity in baroreceptor nerve fibres increases. These fibres project to the medulla where their activity initiates three responses:

- Reduced activity in cardiac sympathetic nerves lowers heart rate and the force of contraction.
- Increased parasympathetic (vagal) activity causes slowing of the heart.
- Vasomotor centre activity is suppressed; reduced vasoconstrictor activity causes vasodilation in mesenteric and cutaneous vascular beds, lowering SVR and blood pressure.

During haemorrhage, blood pressure falls because venous return is reduced. Normally, this would lower baroreceptor activity, initiating an increase in heart rate and contractility, a reduction in vagal tone and increased vasoconstrictor activity and so restore blood pressure. During anaesthesia, these responses are depressed for several reasons: general anaesthetics suppress vasomotor centre sensitivity, while SVR and cardiac output are lowered by drugs.

Hypotension

Hypotension, or low blood pressure, results from:

- Reduced cardiac output. Most anaesthetics depress heart rate and contractility. Surgical haemorrhage lowers venous return.
- Reduced SVR. Volatile agents especially isoflurane, lower blood pressure by causing vasodilation as does acepromazine.
- Both of these.

Hypertension

Elevated blood pressure results predictably from increased cardiac output and, SVR. It occurs when animals are inadequately anaesthetised during surgery because of adrenaline release. On recovery, it indicates pain. Hypertension can follow excessive transfusion of colloids or blood, or overdosage with drugs increasing cardiac output (inotropes).

Tachycardia

Tachycardia (excessive heart rate) is caused by adrenaline release. This preserves blood pressure and is desirable when it occurs in response to physiological changes like hypotension, hypercapnia or hypoglycaemia. In response to pain, however, severe tachycardia is undesirable because cardiac output and coronary perfusion is reduced while myocardial work and oxygen consumption are elevated. Subsequent hypoxia causes arrythmias and eventually arrest.

Bradycardia

Bradycardia means excessive slowing of the heart. Slow heart rates are not always undesirable: ventricular filling and stroke volume are increased, while cardiac work is lowered. However, very slow rates reduce output and cause hypotension.

Oxygen Flux

The combined function of cardiovascular and pulmonary systems is to deliver oxygenated blood to peripheral tissue and can be expressed as **oxygen flux** (DO_2). This is the volume of oxygen reaching peripheral tissue per minute.

Oxygen flux (DO_2) = Cardiac output (Qt) × oxygen content of blood (CaO_2)

$CaO_2 = SaO_2 \times [Hb] \times 1.34$

Where SaO_2 is the percentage saturation of haemoglobin by oxygen (when PO_2 is normal this value is nearly 1.0); [Hb] is the haemoglobin concentration in blood (which is normally 12–15 g/dl). The figure 1.34 is the ml of O_2 combining with each gramme of Hb.

Oxygen flux is lowered by reduced cardiac output (e.g. anaesthetics) and reduced oxygen content of blood. The latter results from lowered SaO_2 (lung disease) or Hb (e.g. anaemia).

Pre-operative Period (Preparation)

Pre-operative examination may indicate that some individuals are poor candidates for anaesthesia and surgery. In these cases, adequate preparation is required to minimise the risk of untoward events. The degree of preparation depends on several factors:

- Animal health
  Healthy animals need little preparation. High-risk cases may require considerable preparation before minor surgical procedures.
- Surgery
  Prolonged and, or invasive procedures require more preparation than superficial operations.
- Elective vs emergency
  Emergency cases requiring immediate surgery may receive only cursory preparation. Elective procedures may be postponed without compromising the animal.

Pre-operative Examination

The animal's medical condition is determined by history-taking, physical examination and, when necessary, further tests.

- Physical examination
  This concentrates on the organ systems affected principally by anaesthesia: central nervous; cardiovascular; respiratory; haematologic; hepatic and renal.
- History
  Useful information is gleaned from questioning the owner.
- Further tests
  —Haematology
  A blood sample should be examined if history or physical examination raises the suspicion of anaemia, polycythaemia, hypoproteinaemia, coagulation disorders or hyperkalaemia.
  —Electrocardiography
  Abnormal pulse rhythms require further investigation.
  —Radiography
  Animals involved in road traffic accidents, those with neoplastic disease and those with signs of cardiovascular or pulmonary disease should undergo radiographic examination of the thorax.

Establishing a full medical history requires additional information

- Duration of ownership
- Previous medical history
- Previous anaesthetic history
- Vaccination status

- Current medication, including 'over-the-counter' products. The dose, dosing frequency and duration of treatment should be established. Drugs of particular concern are listed in Fig. 27.6.

Pre-operative Preparation and the High-Risk Case

High-risk cases may be defined as those with pathological changes which exacerbate the effects of anaesthetics and anaesthesia.

Central Nervous System

- Behaviour better indicates an animal's suitability for surgery than chronological age: a tail-wagging, active 15-year-old is a better risk than the depressed, small, inactive 8-month-old with a porto-systemic shunt.
- Depression increases patient sensitivity to anaesthetics and may indicate the presence of intracranial pathology (tumours, meningitis), systemic disease (pyrexia, hyperkalaemia, toxaemia) or cardiovascular problems (anaemia).
- Excitable, nervous or aggressive animals may require profound sedation.
- Epileptic animals are sensitive to anaesthetics if anti-convulsant therapy has only recently begun. In time, liver enzyme induction occurs and accelerates the metabolism of some anaesthetics.

Cardiovascular and Respiratory Disease

Signs of cardiac and respiratory disease (including exercise intolerance), are always important. When disease is present, the fundamental goal of preparation is to optimise the factors contributing to oxygen flux, i.e. cardiac output, haemoglobin and pulmonary function.

Cardiac disease is not a contraindication to anaesthesia if the effects on cardiac function and blood flow are appreciated and drugs selected accordingly. In general, 'stress', pain and volume losses are less well tolerated by animals with cardiovascular disease. Drugs used for treating cardiac disease (e.g. digoxin, β antagonists) may interract with anaesthetics.

DRUGS POTENTIALLY AFFECTING ANAESTHESIA

Antibiotics
Glucocorticoids
Non-steroidal anti-inflammatory drugs
Organophosphorus compounds, flea collars, parasiticides
Anticonvulsants
Digoxin
Frusemide and other diuretics
β-blockers or ACE-inhibitors
Endocrine supplements e.g. thyroxin
Antihistamines
Antitussives/bronchodilators
Sex hormones

Fig. 27.6. Drugs potentially affecting anaesthesia.

Cases with congestive failure may require cage-rest, sodium restricted diet and digitalisation. Pre-existing arrythmias may require treatment.

Respiratory disease predisposes the animal to hypoxia and hypercapnia. It may contribute to secondary right ventricular changes (cor pulmonale) or polycythaemia. A common form of restrictive respiratory disease is morbid obesity. Animals unable to breathe adequately during surgery must be intubated and have respiration supported.

Causes of respiratory embarrassment (e.g. pneumothorax, gastric tympany), must be relieved pre-operatively. Otherwise the airway should be rendered as dry and as dilated as possible with the aid of antibiotics and bronchodilators. Excessive alveolar transudate may be cleared with diuretics and, or drugs that improve cardiac contractility and function (inotropes).

Hypovolaemia or Dehydration

In dehydrated and hypovolaemic animals, tissue perfusion may become compromised during anaesthesia. Animals with chronic fluid loss (e.g. those with chronic vomiting and diarrhoea) may have electrolyte and, or pH disturbances.

Animals with nephritis cannot concentrate urine and become dehydrated if access to water is restricted. Dogs with chronic renal failure, or any disease characterised by polyuria and polydipsia, must not have water withheld pre-operatively; if necessary, parenteral fluids may be given.

When reduced, circulating blood volume must be restored pre-operatively with appropriate fluids. Oral, intravenous, intraperitoneal, intraosseous or subcutaneous routes may be used, depending on the fluid type.

Animals with unstable blood glucose levels

Diabetes mellitus causes hyperglycaemia with diuresis, fluid loss and keto-acidosis. Severe hypo-glycaemia resulting from insulinomata or liver disease causes considerable neuronal damage if brain glucose supply is curtailed. Glucose levels must be controlled with soluble insulin or dextrose solutions pre-operatively.

Anaemia

Low haemoglobin levels (< 8 g/dl) caused by blood loss or renal disease must be resolved before surgery; oxygen flux may become inadequate when compensatory changes (increased cardiac output and modest hyperventilation) are depressed by anaesthetics. In elective cases, low haemoglobin levels may be raised by treating the underlying cause; otherwise blood transfusion, preferably with 'packed' cells, may be required.

Polycythaemia

Haematocrit values in excess of 0.55 make blood hyperviscous, causing it to 'sludge' in capillaries. They may also indicate that the animal is dehydrated or suffering from chronic hypoxia (cardiopulmonary disease). High haematocrits are lowered by the process of normovolaemic haemodilution. This involves the withdrawal of whole blood and simultaneous replacement with plasma or fluids.

Pyrexia

Pyrexia increases metabolic rate; there are rises in the consumption of O_2 and glucose and in the production of CO_2. The cause of pyrexia should be sought because, while there is little problem anaesthetising animals with superficial abscesses, there is considerable risk when pyrexia results from endocarditis or meningitis. Pyrexia is treated with antibiotics if the cause is infective.

Hypoalbuminaemia

This indicates liver or renal disease and has two consequences. First, the albumen-bound fraction of drugs normally bound (e.g. thiopentone) is lowered and so more free drug is available. Second, plasma oncotic pressure may be lowered, promoting oedema and increased diffusion distance for gases in the lung.

Coagulation problems

Clotting failure may be genetic (von Willebrand's disease in Dobermanns) or indicate liver failure. Fresh blood transfusion may be required pre-operatively.

Electrolyte and pH abnormalities

High potassium levels resulting from Addison's disease or renal failure must be lowered pre-operatively, while low serum potassium should be raised. Normal pH should be restored by treatment of conditions causing alkalosis or acidosis.

High potassium levels are lowered with sodium bicarbonate solutions, calcium gluconate, insulin–glucose solutions or cation-exchange resins. In extreme cases, peritoneal dialysis may be required. Potassium is raised by infusing solutions at rates not greater than 0.5 mmol/kg/h. Extremes of pH are ameliorated by treating the underlying cause.

Any 'emergency' case

These are cases where surgical delay is unacceptable:

- Thoracic visceral damage
- Airway obstruction
- Uncontrollable haemorrhage
- Obstetric emergencies in which neonates are at risk

In emergencies, preparation may be limited to catheterising a vein, administering fluids and enriching inspired breath with oxygen.

Final Details

Before admitting normal animals for surgery, owners must:

- Be informed of the risks and possible outcomes;
- Have signed an anaesthetic consent form;
- Be asked to withhold food the night before (water can be given).

Food and Water Deprivation

A full stomach reduces lung volume, limits breathing and predisposes to vomiting; this may result in fatal aspiration. If an animal scheduled for surgery has received a large meal pre-operatively, the options are:

- Cage the animal in a calm environment and place it at the end of the surgical list.
- Postpone surgery.
- Induce vomiting. Morphine inclusion (0.50 mg/kg) in premedication is probably safer than α_2-agonists such as xylazine.

Premedication

Pre-anaesthetic medications ('premeds') are drugs given before surgery to smooth subsequent events. The objectives of pre- medication are:

- To reduce anxiety.
  Nervous animals may resist restraint for induction, and possess undesirable catecholamine levels. In any case, intravenous injection is easier in calm animals. For animals excited by pain, analgesics will reduce anxiety.
- To enable 'smooth' induction.
- To reduce induction agent dose.
- To reduce associated side-effects of the anaesthetic to be given.
- To reduce maintenance agent requirement.

In providing 'background' narcosis, premedication and analgesics lower the requirement for maintenance agents and consequently the incidence of associated side-effects. However, certain premedications may be more hazardous than the induction or maintenance agents themselves.

- To reduce adverse effects of surgery.
  It is alleged that some surgical procedures cause vagal activity, in which case atropine or glycopyrrolate are given beforehand.
- To smooth recovery.

Long-acting drugs like acepromazine smooth recovery after induction with methohexitone and other drugs. Similarly analgesics smooth recovery after painful procedures.

Not all animals require pre-anaesthetic medication e.g. those already depressed by toxaemia, shock or head trauma. After haemorrhage or in shocked animals, normal doses produce more profound effects.

Pre-anaesthetic Medication

Drugs maintaining the health status of the patient (Fig. 27.6) are not usually recognised as 'premedication' because most are pharmacologically unrelated to anaesthetics. Their consideration is important because they may:

(a) have adverse pre-operative effects (e.g. digoxin may cause intraoperative arrythmias);
(b) interract with anaesthesia (e.g. propranolol may block pressor responses of hypercapnia).

Despite this, it is generally true that withdrawing medication pre-operatively is likely to cause more problems than are possible through adverse drug interraction.

A range of drugs (Fig. 27.7) is used to achieve the classical goals of pre-medication:

The route by which pre-anaesthetic medication is given influences time to peak effect, duration of action (Fig. 27.4) and the incidence of side-effects.

Phenothiazines

Acepromazine. This phenothiazine neurolept is available for small animals as a 2 mg/ml solution; it remains a popular and useful drug despite important side-effects. At normal doses the drug is safe but does not usually produce profound sedation. Increasing the dose does not increase the degree of

PRE-ANAESTHETIC MEDICATIONS		
Drug class	**Type**	**Examples**
Phenothiazines	Neurolept	Acepromazine, chlorpromazine
Butyrophenomes	Neurolept	Azaperone, fluanisone
Opioids	Narcotic-analgesic	Morphine, methadone, pethidine, butorphanol, papaveretum, pentazocine, buprenorphine
α_2-Agonists	Sedative	Xylazine, medetomidine
Benzodiazepines	Tranquiliser	Diazepan, midazolam
Anti-muscarinics (also known as anti-cholinergics)		Atropine, glycopyrrolate

Fig. 27.7. Range of pre-medicant drugs.

sedation but extends the duration of action and increases the severity of adverse reactions.

ADVANTAGES
- Synergism; improves sedative effects of opioids.
- Antiarrythmic; low doses exert antiarrythmic activity.
- Antiemetic; offsets the emetic effects of some opioids.
- Safety; doses do not cause coma in overdose.
- Spasmolytic; reduces discomfort when 'colic' results from gastrointestinal spasm.
- Antihistamine; potentially useful with some histamine-releasing opioids.

DISADVANTAGES
- Hypotension
  This side-effect, which causes most concern, results from vascular smooth muscle relaxation. Problems occur when high doses (> 0.15 mg/kg) are used or when normal doses are used in hypotensive (e.g. hypovolaemic) animals. It causes acute decompensation and hypotension when blood pressure relies on increased SVR (e.g. hypovolaemia, cardiac failure).
- Unpredictability
  Failure to produce dose-dependent sedation. Terriers and aggressive dogs are resistant.
- Long-acting
  Normal long (dose-dependent) duration of action; clinical sedation lasts 4–6 hours after 0.20 mg/kg.
- Slow onset.
  Peak effect does not occur for 10–20 min.
- Syncope
  In some breeds, syncope occurs after rapid IV injection. Some breed-lines of Boxers collapse after low doses.
- No analgesia
- Hypothermia
  Cutaneous vasodilation and (hypothalamic) thermoregulatory depression cause heat loss.
- Poor muscle relaxation
  The drug has no relaxant effects but reduces hypertonicity with ketamine.

Butyrophenomes

These behave like phenothiazenes. There are no butyrophenomes licensed for sole use in animals, but fluanisone and droperidol are available combined with opioids.

Opioid analgesics

Opioids are often included in premedication:

- To relieve pre-operative pain and therefore anxiety.
- To contribute to sedation.
- To provide analgesia during maintenance.

Non-steroidal anti-inflammatory drugs do not have obvious sedative effects in pain-free animals and are not usually given as premedication. This is short-sighted, however, because high plasma levels are desirable before surgery begins.

While the properties of individual opioids differ there are common advantages and disadvantages.

ADVANTAGES
- Profound, drug and dose-dependant analgesia.
- Benign cardiovascular effects. With some exceptions, opioids slow heart rate. In high doses, bradycardia and bradyarrythmias may occur. Cardiac output is usually maintained.
- Anaesthetic-sparing effect. Opioids reduce dose requirements of induction and maintenance agents.
- Sedation. Some opioids produce sedation in non-painful animals.
- Positive ventilatory effects. By reducing chest-wall pain after thoracotomy or trauma , opioids improve ventilation. Sedative and respiratory depressant effects are useful in cases of tracheal collapse.

DISADVANTAGES
- Dysphoria. In pain-free animals, opioids may stimulate rather than sedate and cause excitation on overdosage. Central nervous effects depend on dose, species and degree of pain present. At normal analgesic doses, opioids in pain-free animals do not cause marked stimulation. Stimulation is also unlikely when neurolepts are given concurrently.
- Respiratory depression. Probably a greater problem in people than animals, pre-anaesthetic opioids prolong apnoea after induction with thiopentone. Intra-operative alfentanil and fentanyl often eliminate breathing, mandating ventilatory support.
- Antitussive effects. Opioids suppress the coughing reflex, which may be useful in animals requiring analgesia and prolonged intubation. However, accumulated bronchial secretion may impair respiration.
- Gastrointestinal effects. Morphine causes vomiting in dogs which does not appear distressing. Other opioids are less likely to cause vomiting. With the exception of pethidine, opioids increase non-propulsive segmenting intestinal contractions leading to constipation with prolonged use. Opioids cause contracture of the sphincter of Oddi, and increased pressure in the biliary tree. They should not be used in pancreatitis and obstructive jaundice.
- Urinary retention. Opioids cause urinary retention which seems to be of little clinical importance. However, the urethra should be catheterised after surgery on the bladder.

- Tolerance. The diminishing effect of constant opioid doses is unlikely to occur in animals, as prolonged administration is not practised.
- Dependence. Animals are unlikely to become 'addicted' to opioids as long-term administration is rarely required.

Individual properties. Opioids have slightly different properties (Fig. 27.8) and their use in any situation is governed by several factors.

- Potency
  Although drugs vary in anaesthetic potency, this is of little relevance as 'weaker' opioids like pethidine are given at greater doses. The quality of analgesia is more important. Pure agonists (morphine, fentanyl) should be chosen if severe pain is anticipated.
- Pharmacodynamic effect
  The central nervous, autonomic, cardiopulmonary and gastrointestinal effects of individual drugs may render them useful or hazardous under different circumstances.
- Pharmacokinetic factors
  Onset time, duration of action and elimination pathways may be important considerations in choosing specific opioids.
- Others
  Personal preference, cost and controlled drug status may also influence choice.

Drug legislation. Because of their abuse potential, most opioids are controlled drugs (CD)—that is, their use is controlled by the Misuse of Drugs Act 1971.

Controlled drugs are 'scheduled' according to the degree of control applied to their use. Schedule 1 agents (e.g. LSD) are stringently controlled but unused in veterinary practice. Schedule 2 drugs like morphine, etorphine ('Immobilon'), fentanyl, alfentanil and pethidine are regulated in terms of:

- Special prescription requirements.
- Requisition requirements.
- Record keeping: acquisition and prescription must be recorded in a controlled drugs register (CDR).
- Safe custody. Schedule 2 drugs must be kept in a locked receptacle.
- Destruction of expired stocks.

Schedule 3 drugs include pentobarbitone and phenobarbitone, pentazocine and buprenorphine. These are subject to prescription and requisition requirements but transactions do not have to be recorded in the CDR. With the exception of buprenorphine, they do not have to be kept in a locked receptacle.

Neuroleptanalgesia. Phenothiazines and butyrophenomes mixed with opioids create a neuroleptanalgesic (NLA) combination. The two components are synergistic; lower doses of each are needed, which lowers the incidence and severity of side-effects. Commercially available mixtures are convenient but effects are sub-optimal in about 40% of recipients.

- Small Animal Immobilon (etorphine 74 μg, methotrimeprazine 18 mg/ml).
- Hypnorm (fentanyl 0.315 mg, fluanisone 10 mg/ml).

Neuroleptanalgesics may be 'home-made'; doses and drugs are modified to suit the individual case.

ADVANTAGES
- Lower incidence of side-effects.
- Increased degree of sedation.
- Increased predictability.
- Stable cardiopulmonary performance.

DISADVANTAGES
- Animals remain sensitive to, and are aroused by, certain stimuli (e.g. acoustic).
- Neuroleptanalgesics provide little more sedation in non-painful cats than neurolepts alone.
- Only opioid antagonism is possible. The neurolept is not antagonised and is the longer-acting component.
- Behavioural changes are alleged to have occurred after neuroleptanalgesia in dogs.

α_2-Agonists

Xylazine (2%) and medetomidine (1 mg/ml) are α_2-agonists licensed for use in companion animals. Medetomidine is more potent and longer acting.

ADVANTAGES
- Profound, dose-dependent sedation.
- High doses produce basal narcosis. Duration of action is also dose-dependent.
- Marked drug-sparing effect.
- Doses of induction and maintenance agents are considerably reduced. Circulation time is prolonged, accelerating the uptake of volatile anaesthetics. A greater lag time elapses before effects of induction agents are seen.

COMPARISON OF SELECTED FEATURES OF OPIOID ANALGESICS

Drug	Controlled ?	Potency	Efficacy	Duration
Morphine	Yes (Sch 2)	1	+++++	2 – 4 h
Pethidine	Yes (Sch 2)	0.1	+++	30 min – 1 h
Papavertum	Yes (Sch 2)	0.5	++++	2 – 4 h
Methadone	Yes (Sch 2)	1	++++	2 – 4 h
Butorphanol	No	5	++	2 – 4 h
Buprenorphine	Yes (Sch 3)	5	++	3 – 7 h

Fig. 27.8. Comparison of selected features of opioid analgesics.

- Muscle relaxation.
- Relaxant effects offset muscle rigidity seen with ketamine, making α_2/ketamine combinations popular.
- Visceral analgesia
- The α_2-agonists are thought to provide useful visceral analgesia.

DISADVANTAGES
- Cardiovascular depression.

    There are dose-dependent and profound cardiovascular effects—hypertension then hypotension, bradycardia and hypoventilation. Antimuscarinic pre-treatment, which counteracts bradycardia (the most worrying aspect of α_2 activity), is controversial. Injected by the intramuscular route, medetomidine has only a modest hypotensive effect.

    In dogs, xylazine sensitises the myocardium to adrenaline-induced arrythmias during halothane anaesthesia.
- Respiratory depression

    While breathing is periodic with apnoeic pauses of 45 seconds and mucous membranes turn grey, PaO_2 is often satisfactory.
- Emesis

    Vomiting occurs in dogs and cats after xylazine and, to a lesser extent, after medetomidine.
- Diuresis

    This occurs because of ADH inhibition and insulin suppression, causing hyperglycaemia.
- Gut motility

    This is reduced or abolished and barium meal interpretation may be confused. Because aerophagia occurs, some say α_2-agonists should not be used in breeds predisposed to gastric dilation—volvulus complex.
- Thermoregulation

    α_2-agonists impair thermoregulation, allowing hypo- or hyperthermia depending on ambient temperatures.
- Personal Risk

    The data sheet instructs that gloves should be worn when handling medetomidine.
- Low safety

    The data sheet states that medetomidine should not be used in animals 'in poor general health'.
- Muscle relaxation

    Relaxation may cause problems in brachycephalics with redundant oropharyngeal tissue.

Atipamezole. Atipamezole is used to antagonise the effects of medetomidine in companion animals; antagonist dose is the same volume as agonist injected. Its use is desirable because the prolonged effect of medetomidine predisposes recipients to hypothermia and hypostatic lung congestion. However, after painful procedures, antagonism may expose the animal, acutely, to discomfort.

Benzodiazepines

In humans, benzodiazepines like diazepam and midazolam produce anxiolysis, muscle relaxation, sedation, hypnosis and amnesia and have powerful anticonvulsant effects. These effects are not usually seen in animals; paradoxically, intravenous diazepam causes marked stimulation in non-debiliated dogs. Diazepam is water-insoluble and formulated in a way that causes pain on injection and thrombophlebitis. Midazolam is water-soluble and does not cause these problems. It is short-acting; it is approximately twice as potent and is more effective after IM injection.

ADVANTAGES
- Safety

    The drugs have high therapeutic indices and minimal cardiopulmonary effects.
- Drug-sparing effect

    They prolong and enhance effects of other anaesthetics. Anaesthetic doses are lowered and predicted excitement (e.g. recovery after methohexitone increments) is prevented. Effects are better after oral rather than IM administration.
- Muscle relaxation

    Diazepam is used with ketamine to eliminate excitation/convulsions and associated muscle hypertonicity. It is said to control post-operative restlessness.

DISADVANTAGES
- Unpredictable

    In animals, benzodiazepines often stimulate rather than depress but become increasingly effective as the animal's health status deteriorates. In normal, fit dogs, high intravenous doses of diazepam cause marked ataxia, no sedation and violent struggling. Eating is usually stimulated in cats.
- Formulation

    Diazepam causes pain on injection and thrombophlebitis. It should not be drawn up into plastic (polyvinyl chloride) syringes unless used immediately, because the drug 'binds' to PVC.

Flumazenil (Ro 15-1788). A benzodiazepine antagonist used to treat overdosage in people and accelerate recovery in outpatient anaesthesia, this drug is of little benefit in animals as the need to antagonise scarcely arises.

Anti-muscarinic (anti-cholinergic) Drugs

The *routine* use of antimuscarinic drugs like atropine (600 μg/ml solution) and glycopyrrolate (containing 200 mg/ml) for anaesthetic premedication is controversial. In previous times, the widespread use of morphine premedication and diethyl ether anaesthesia in humans justified this practice; morphine causes some vagal slowing of the heart, while diethylether promotes oropharyngeal secretion, bronchosecretion and bronchoconstriction. Modern volatile anaesthetics do not produce excessive secretions and most cause bronchodilation.

ADVANTAGES OF ATROPINE
- Bronchodilates, reduces total airway resistance.
- Rapidly controls intraoperative vagus-mediated bradycardia and bradyarrythmias.
- Protects against adverse vagal effects of anti-cholinesterases during antagonism of neuro-muscular block.

DISADVANTAGES
- Increases metabolic rate.
- Increases heart rate, increases myocardial oxygen consumption.
- Is arrythmogenic, causing bradyarrythmias and, or tachyarrythmias.
- Viscidifies bronchial secretions, promoting peripheral airway collapse.
- Causes gastrointestinal ileus.

Glycopyrrolate (glycopyrronium). This has a slower onset time (and so is of less use in emergencies), a longer duration of action and a greater antisialogogue effect than atropine. Tachyarryhthmias are said to be less likely and cardiovascular stability is better preserved.

It may be wiser to withhold anti-muscarinic drugs from pre-anaesthetic medication, to monitor closely and to use them only when vagal activity (e.g. bradycardia, bradyarrythmias and hypotension) becomes worrying.

Sedation and Environment

Sedative pre-anaesthetic medications work best in quiet environments. After administration, animals should be returned to a calm, quiet kennel. Further stimulation, such as examination of injuries, must be postponed until the animal is unconscious.

Types of Anaesthesia

Regional Analgesia

Intravenous Regional Anaesthesia (IVRA)

Intravenous regional anaesthesia is used for surgical procedures on limb extremities (e.g. digit removal). The limb is first exsanguinated using an Esmarch's bandage, which is then left in place as a tourniquet. Local anaesthetic (e.g. 3–7 ml lignocaine without adrenaline) is then injected into any vein distal to the tourniquet. Surgery may begin after 5 minutes. Anaesthesia persists until the tourniquet is removed.

Conduction block

This involves drug injection in proximity to identifiable nerves, as opposed to nerve endings. The technique requires knowledge of topographical anatomy. Injection is made using sterile needles and syringes. For example, the intercostal nerve (behind each rib) is often blocked with 0.5 ml bupivacaine after thoracotomy. This relieves post-operative chest-wall pain, allowing adequate ventilation.

Neuraxial anaesthesia

Neuraxial anaesthesia refers to anaesthetic injection within the bony confines of the spinal canal. There are two types of neuraxial anaesthesia: extradural and spinal.

Extradural (or epidural) anaesthesia. In this, drug is injected into the space between the dura mater (the thick fibrous outermost covering of the spinal cord) and the periosteum lining the spinal canal. Here, the drug blocks the nerves as they leave the cord. A large spinal needle is used and injection made into the L7–S1 interspace. The technique is useful for pain relief and muscle relaxation during pelvic–limb ortho-paedic procedures in dogs, and less commonly in cats. In current practice, the technique is usually performed on heavily sedated or lightly anaesthetised animals. Lignocaine with adrenaline and bupivacaine are commonly used. Opioid analgesics are increasingly being used in the extradural space. The main advantage of extradural opioids is prolonged analgesia, but not anaesthesia.

Spinal (subarachnoid or intrathecal) injection. This technique has never gained popularity in veterinary anaesthesia. It involves a midline injection at the L5–L6 interspace or, at a higher level, into the CSF-filled space below the arachnoid mater, lying below the dura. Lower doses produce the same effects of extradural injection but there is a slightly greater risk of overdosage.

Local Anaesthetics

Local anaesthetics produce reversible block of nerve impulse conduction.

Mechanisms

Nerve fibres carrying different sensations (e.g. touch, cold and pain) vary in response to local anaesthetics. Because pain fibres are among the most sensitive, and it is possible for local anaesthetics to eliminate pain but allow touch and other sensations to persist. When this occurs, the drug behaves as a local analgesic. If all sensation is lost, the drug is an anaesthetic. Motor fibres are most resistant to local anaesthetics but are usually blocked, resulting in muscle relaxation.

Toxicity

Toxic central nervous signs—convulsions or coma—are seen if high levels of local anaesthetic are absorbed, The former is controlled with diazepam or pentobarbitone. Over dosing is avoided by using low concentrations (the minimum volume required to produce effect) by using regional rather than local techniques (where appropriate) and by adding vasoconstrictors to the injected solution.

Pharmacokinetics

The commonest vasoconstrictor is adrenaline, added to local anaesthetic solutions at 1:100,000 concentration (0.01 mg/ml). This retards drug absorption from the injection site and prolongs block. Solutions containing adrenaline must not be over used in areas with poor or superficial blood flow; vasoconstriction may cause subsequent tissue ischaemia and gangrene.

Onset time of local anaesthetics is related to their molecular structures. These are changed and onset time shortened by adding carbon dioxide to drug solutions.

Uses

- Superficial surgery
  Some minor procedures may be done in the conscious animal using local anaesthetics alone (e.g. skin infiltration for wart removal). More invasive procedures may require moderate sedation, (e.g. intravenous regional anaesthesia for toe amputation).
- Adjunct to surgical anaesthesia
  Local techniques may be superimposed on light general anaesthesia for major surgery. The local technique usually does not affect cardiopulmonary function and so less general anaesthetic is required. This preserves cardiopulmonary performance, making the combined technique useful in high-risk cases. Animals also recover consciousness rapidly and importantly, the surgical site remains analgesic.
- Facilite procedures
  Topical anaesthetics facilitate catheterisation, endotracheal intubation and ophthalmic examination.
- Diagnosis
  Local anaesthetics are used to assist lameness diagnosis in horses.
- Antiarrythmics
  Lignocaine is used to treat certain types of cardiac arrythmia.

Topical

Producing local anaesthesia by localised tissue freezing with ice, aerosol sprays or volatile liquids like ethyl chloride has lost popularity because the effects are very superficial and transient. Local anaesthetics may be applied directly to structures for anaesthesia but absorption is poor if this is skin, and at least 30 minutes application time is required.

Effects on mucous membranes occur more rapidly and are more satisfactory.

Typical applications are shown in Fig. 27.9.

Infiltration

A primary injection of local anaesthetic is made at the surgical site, using as small a needle as possible (22–24 swg). The next injection is made through this site and the process repeated until the surgical area is 'infiltrated' with local anaesthetic. Liberal infiltration must be avoided as overdosage is possible, especially in small animals and birds. Irritant drugs like lignocaine and those containing vasoconstrictors may interfere with wound healing. This is avoided using a field block: nerves innervating the surgical site are blocked along their course by a line of infiltrated anaesthetic.

Haematoma

This technique involves injecting 2–5 ml 2% lignocaine solution into the haematoma adjacent to bone fractures. Scrupulous asepsis must be observed. The technique is suitable as a first-aid measure.

Intrasynovial

Local anaesthetics injected into painful joints and synovial sheaths relieve pain but the effects are not long-acting.

Local anaesthetic drugs

Lignocaine

This is the most commonly used local anaesthetic in veterinary practice. It is available as a gel, topical cream, a spray and in injectable forms. Injections are usually 1% or 2% solutions with or without adrenaline (1:100,000). The drug has a rapid (<5 min) onset of action. It spreads rapidly through tissue and produces almost complete block. The normal duration of action is 50—90 min. Adding adrenaline retards absorption (and toxicity) and prolongs the duration of block. Lignocaine causes tissue irritation after injection.

Bupivacine

This is about 4 times more potent than lignocaine and so is available in lower concentrations (0.25, 0.5 or 0.75%). All contain adrenaline as this accelerates onset and duration of block. It has a slower onset of action (up to 20 min) but may last from 3 to 7 hours. It does not irritate tissue but may cause cardiac arrest if inadvertent intravascular injection is made.

TOPICAL LOCAL ANAESTHESIA		
Site	**Drug**	**Description**
Cornea	Proxymetacaine	'Ophthaine' lasts 15 minutes
Urethra	Lignocaine Gel	Lubrication for catheterisation
Larynx	Lignocaine 10mg	Metered spray

Fig. 27.9. Topical local anaesthesia.

Mepivacaine

This drug is favoured for conduction blocks in the equine limb as it is less irritant than lignocaine.

Injectable Anaesthesia

Injectable anaesthetics may be given in various sites, although irritant drugs must be given by the intravenous route. Intravenous anaesthetics produce unconsciousness in one limb–brain circulation time. Some produce unconsciousness when injected by other routes: pentobarbitone may be given by intraperitoneal injection, while ketamine and 'Saffan' are effective after IM injection.

Pharmacology

The brain has a rich blood supply and receives a high concentration of drug shortly after IV injection. When a critical brain concentration is exceeded, unconsciousness occurs. In time, organs less well-perfused than the brain (such as skeletal muscle) begin to take up drug. Plasma levels fall and this creates a diffusion gradient which promotes movement of drug from brain to plasma. Consciousness returns when brain drug levels fall below the critical level. The duration of action of most modern injectable anaesthetics depends on 'redistribution' of drug from brain to less well-perfused tissues; this depends on factors like cardiac output and the mass of poorly perfused tissue available.

Most anaesthetics are metabolised in the liver by conversion from lipid to water-soluble molecules. These forms are more easily excreted in bile (appearing later in faeces) or urine. Only very small amounts are excreted unchanged in bile and urine as lipid-soluble drug.

The duration of action of drugs which are rapidly metabolised by the liver (e.g. 'Saffan' and methohexitone) depend on a combination of redistribution and metabolism.

Uses

- As sole agents
  For short procedures (e.g. pharyngeal foreign body removal), a single injection of a short-acting drug is used.
  For prolonged procedures, long-acting drugs or combinations may be used although top-up (or incremental) doses of short-acting drugs are preferable. Alternatively, short-acting drugs may be infused. Drugs given by infusion or incremental doses must not accumulate or recovery will be prolonged.
- As induction agents
  Injectable drugs used to induce anaesthesia before maintenance with volatile agents need only eliminate laryngeal reflexes and jaw tone for the purpose of intubation.

- As an adjunct to a mask induction

Barbiturates

Barbiturates like thiopentone, methohexitone and pentobarbitone are hypnotics; they cause unconsciousness but have poor analgesic properties. Muscle relaxation is usually adequate during anaesthesia.

Thiopentone

This thiobarbiturate is available as a sulphurous-yellow powder and requires reconstitution with water. Solutions of various strengths (concentrations) may be made:

A 1% solution contains 1 (g) or 1000 mg in 100 ml. A 1% solution, therefore, contains 10 mg/ml and a 2.5% solution of thiopentone contains 25 mg drug/ml. It is reconstituted by adding 100 ml water to 2.5 g of powder.

Thiopentone is a useful anaesthetic agent for short-duration procedures or for induction prior to maintenance with inhalation agents. Incremental doses should be avoided as they prolong recovery and contribute to 'hang-over'.

The drug is safe in high-risk cases provided the factors which increase patient sensitivity are known. (Many of these apply to drugs other than thiopentone.) Doses are reduced in: hypoalbuminaemia, acidaemia, hypovolaemia, congestive heart failure, azotaemia, toxaemia and obesity. Doses are also reduced when diazepam, (0.5 mg/kg) is injected immediately afterwards.

Note that a 2.5% solution has a pH of 10.4 (strongly alkali) and causes tissue damage when injected outside of the vein. In large animals (but not in companion animal practice), 5% and 10% solution are used.

Special precautions. Thiopentone causes prolonged recoveries in sight-hounds (e.g. whippet, greyhound, saluki) after otherwise uneventful anaesthesia.

The drug should not be used if there is difficulty in achieving venipuncture.

Methohexitone

This oxybarbiturate is available as a dry powder and is reconstituted to produce a 1% solution. Being twice as potent as thiopentone, its dose is halved in all clinical circumstances. Onset time is similar but its duration of action is shorter; extensive and rapid hepatic metabolism occurs in addition to redistribution.

Recoveries are not always smooth, especially when pre-anaesthetic medication is withheld. Excitable recoveries respond to intravenous acepromazine. The drug has been favoured in sight-hounds because it produces rapid recoveries.

Pentobarbitone

This once useful drug has been superseded by newer agents except, perhaps, in laboratory animal anaesthesia. Following injection, its onset of action is relatively slow (related to delay in crossing the blood–brain barrier) and recoveries are prolonged. In companion animal practice it is used as an anti-convulsant and for humane destruction.

Steroid Anaesthetics

'Saffan'

'Saffan' is a mixture of alphaxolone (9 mg/kg) and alphadolone (3 mg/kg). Doses are always expressed in mg of total steroid. The drug has been favoured for some time in cats. The two steroids are water insoluble and the formulation contains cremophor EL (polyethoxylated castor oil). This agent causes histamine release in dogs and cannot be used safely in this species. In cats, it causes mild anaphylactoid reactions and swelling of the pinnae and paws. These are normally of little consequence but very infrequently there is fatal pulmonary oedema. Because the formulation contains no bacteriostat, open ampoules must be discarded.

The intravenous route is preferred because effects are less predictable after intramuscular injection. Predictability is improved when the quadriceps muscle group is used instead of semimembranosus-semitendinosus. The solution is viscous but non-irritant. Frequently, large volumes must be given. The subcutaneous route is unsuitable; the rate of drug metabolism over absorption is high and so anaesthetic levels are not achieved. Apnoea occurs if thiopentone is given after Saffan.

Cyclohexanones

Ketamine

Ketamine is described as a dissociative anaesthetic, producing a unique state of anaesthesia. Protective airway reflexes are maintained, the eyes remain open and the pupil is dilated. Cranial nerve reflexes are less depressed than with other agents although it cannot be assumed that these will remain entirely protective.

Heart rate is increased and blood pressure, is normally maintained. Breathing is modestly reduced, although in overdose an apneustic pattern is seen in which the breath is held after inspiration. Spontaneous muscle movement unrelated to surgery is a disconcerting feature of ketamine anaesthesia but suppressed by other drugs. Ketamine is considered to provide profound somatic analgesia, but controversy exists over its role as a visceral analgesic.

Intramuscular injection is painful although injection volumes are low because the drug is available as a 100 mg/ml solution.

Phenols

Propofol

This water-insoluble phenol derivative (2,6 di-isopropylphenol) is a characteristic milky-white solution solubilised in an egg–phosphatidyl–soyabean oil emulsion. The solution must not be refrigerated, even though cooling is said to reduce the low incidence of pain on intravenous injection. The solution contains no bacteriostat and so opened ampoules must be discarded.

The drug produces dose-dependent levels of unconciousness after intravenous injection. Cats require higher doses than dogs for anaesthesia. The drug is also longer-acting in this species, with induction doses lasting up to 30 minutes.

Propofol has some advantages over thiopentone:

- Recovery is rapid and free from hang-over if a single dose is given. This makes it useful in sight-hounds. This advantage becomes less apparent if inhalation anaesthesia follows.
- Provided oxygen is given, anaesthesia can be maintained with top-up injections with less risk of prolonged recoveries. However, long recoveries occur after infusion.

Occasionally, twitching and spontaneous muscle activity occurs with propofol anaesthesia and excited recoveries have been described.

Combinations and Neuroleptanalgesics

Minor surgical procedures may be performed using neuroleptanalgesic, benzodiazepine/ketamine and α_2-agonist/ketamine mixtures.

Ketamine mixtures

Several drugs are used with ketamine to reduce muscle hypertonicity. These include acepromazine, diazepam, midazolam, xylazine and medetomidine. Some of these also have anti-convulsant effects and render the combinations safe for use in dogs. However, some combinations have adverse physiological effects like hypoventilation and arrythmias.

Opioid mixtures

Opioids are commonly combined with neurolepts such as acepromazine or droperidol to provide conditions for minor surgery. Fentanyl and alfentanil are used to lower the dose of propofol required for anaesthesia. Hypoventilation and bradycardia are serious disadvantages of such mixtures, although analgesia is profound.

Benzodiazepine and opioid mixtures (e.g. midazolam and sufentanil) are favoured in some centres for high-risk cases. The advantages of such combinations over well-administered halothane anaesthesia is often not apparent in companion animals.

Small animal immobilon

This combination injected IV, IM or SC produces profound and prolonged analgesia. Marked hypo-ventilation produces cyanosis, while severe hypotension caused by bradycardia may cause pale mucous membranes. Convulsions and renal failure have followed administration and the drug may recycle; the animal becomes depressed later after apparent restoration of consciousness with the antagonist diprenorphine. The major problem with this formulation is self-administration.

Inhalation Anaesthesia

Volatile and gaseous anaesthetics are used to maintain anaesthesia and, less commonly, for induction. In the past, the 'open method' was popular, consisting of the application of liquid anaesthetic to a gauze swab applied to the patient's nose. The 'semi-open' is similar but the gauze is within a mask through which all inspired gas passes. Ether, chloroform, trichloroethylene and methoxy-flurane were used in these systems. Neither system is acceptable because of pollution and because the inspired gas concentration is difficult to control. The latter is particularly hazardous with anaesthetics like halothane which have high saturated vapour pressures and produce high concentrations at room temperature. Modern techniques require an anaesthetic machine and an anaesthetic breathing system or 'circuit'.

Anaesthetic Machines

Anaesthetic machines produce and deliver safe concentrations of anaesthetic vapour and provide a means of giving oxygen and imposing positive pressure ventilation (PPV) during apnoea or cardiopulmonary arrest.

Understanding the function of anaesthetic machines is needed for the safe administration of volatile anaesthetics and oxygen and for machine maintenance; this prolongs the life of equipment, limits pollution and reduces the risk of equipment failure.

Components

The anaesthetic machine (Fig. 27.10) begins at a carrier gas source (A), passes through a pressure gauge (B), a pressure regulator (C), and flowmeter assembly (D), and ends at the common gas outlet (F), where the anaesthetic breathing system attaches. Vaporisers (E) are usually positioned downstream from the flowmeter assembly. Other features include emergency oxygen valves (a), low oxygen alarms (b), nitrous oxide cut-out devices (c), over-pressure valves (d), and emergency air-intake valves (e).

Gas supply. Cylinders, 'bottles' or 'tanks' are metal containers designed to withstand the pressure of compressed gases. Their size determines the volume of gas contained (in litres) and this is described by letters from AA (very small) to J (large). The volume of oxygen in filled cylinders at room temperature is shown in Fig. 27.11.

- Cylinders are colour-coded:
- oxygen cylinders are black with white shoulders:
- nitrous oxide bottles are blue:
- carbon-dioxide cylinders are grey;
- old machines may have a facility for cyclopropane which is delivered in orange cylinders.

Cylinders are opened by anticlockwise rotation of the spindle. Before attachment to the cylinder yoke, the protective cellophane sleeve is removed from the cylinder valve and the spindle briefly opened to flush away dust that lies in the outlet port. Once connected in the hanger yokes, spindles should be fully opened until resistance is felt and then closed 180° to prevent excessive valve wear.

Cylinder banks. Vertically standing banks of three to five 'J' or 'G' size cylinders are used in busy practices. Two banks for each gas (oxygen and

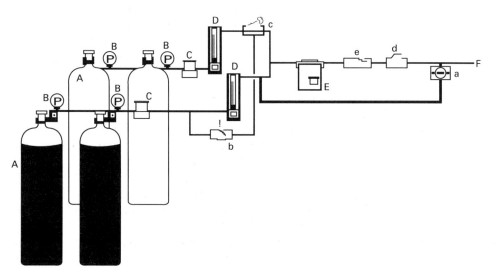

Fig. 27.10. The anaesthetic machine.

CYLINDER SIZES, CONTENTS AND COLOURS				
Cylinder size:	E	F	G	J
Content (L):	680	1340	3400	6800

Cylinders are colour coded:
Oxygen cylinders are black with white shoulders;
Nitrous oxide bottles are blue;
Carbon-dioxide cylinders are grey;
Old machines may have a facility for cyclopropane which was delivered in orange cylinders.

Fig. 27.11. Cylinder sizes, contents and colours.

nitrous oxide) are preferable, with one being 'in use' and the other 'in reserve'. Gas flows to the operating room through pipes in the wall. These end in wall-mounted Schraeder-type sockets which receive probes from the anaesthetic machine. Pipes are colour coded and the probes size-coded so that lines cannot be accidentally crossed.

Low volume cylinders. Low-volume 'E' or 'F' cylinders attached to hanger yokes on the machine suit most practices. Machines usually hold two cylinders of O_2 and two of N_2O. The cylinder valve face has holes which correspond with pins sited within the hanger yoke. The pin and hole pattern constitutes the pin-indexing system and ensures N_2O or CO_2 cylinders cannot be connected to the O_2 yoke.

Pressure/contents gauge. The pressure gauge is indispensable for oxygen, because it indicates the gas volume in the cylinder. This is calculated using Boyles law ($PV = k$).

An 'E' cylinder contains 680 L when filled to 13300 kPa (1935 psi) at 20°C. At the same temperature, a pressure gauge registering 4500 kPa (655 psi) indicates 230 l remain:

$$\frac{4500 \times 680}{13300} = 230 \, l$$

If the calculated oxygen flow rate for the next operation is 4 l/min, then this cylinder will provide gas for 57 minutes:

$$\frac{230}{4} = 57 \, min$$

The N_2O pressure gauge is less useful; the full N_2O cylinder contains liquid and gas and the gauge measures the pressure of gaseous N_2O in equilibrium with liquid. This remains constant until all liquid evaporates, after which pressure falls rapidly. Gas volume in N_2O cylinders is found by weighing the bottle and applying the following formula:

Litres N_2O present

$$= \frac{(net - tare^1) \; weight \, [\varepsilon \, grams] \times 22.4}{44}$$

(^{1}Cylinder tare weight is stamped on the cylinder neck)

Pressure reducing valves or regulators. These produce constant 'downstream' pressure (therefore flow) as cylinder pressure falls with use. Without them, the cylinder valve would need incremental opening to maintain constant flow. They are sited immediately downstream from the hanger yoke and in modern machines, they may be incorporated in the yoke itself and be impossible to find.

Flowmeters. Flowmeters control and measure the rate of gas passing through them. The units are litres per minute (l/min). A freely moving 'float'—either a ball or bobbin—is supported in a transparent, tapered tube by an ascending flow of gas. The flow rate is etched on the tube and read from the top of bobbins and the equator of spheres. The greater the flow, the higher the indicator rises in the glass tube. Flowmeters become inaccurate if dirt or non-vertical positioning makes the float rub against the tube. This is limited by slots machined in the rim of bobbins to encourage rotation. Flowmeters are calibrated for one gas only and so oxygen flowmeters do not accurately indicate the flow of nitrous oxide. Because of this, flow meter control knobs are often colour-coded. Flowmeters control knobs must not be over-tightened.

Vaporisers. Vaporisers dilute the saturated vapour of volatile anaesthetics to yield a range of useful concentrations.

• Uncalibrated vaporisers
The Boyle bottle is simple, inexpensive and easily maintained. However, output concentrations are not guaranteed and they 'drift' despite constant control settings. As liquid anaesthetic cools and the flows increase, the output concentration falls. Concentrations rise when low flows are used, when the vaporiser is agitated or when temperatures rise.

• Calibrated vaporisers
Anaesthetic concentration from 'Tec and other calibrated vaporisers is similar to that 'dialled' on the spindle, provided that the gas flow through the vaporiser and the temperature of liquid anaesthetic are within ranges specific for the model. In Mark III 'Tecs, output is constant between 18–35°C. Dialled and delivered concentrations are similar at flows between 0.2 to 15 l/min.

Vaporisers are agent-specific. Filling with the wrong anaesthetic is prevented by keyed filling ports.

These accept a key-ended tube which only attaches to the corresponding anaesthetic bottle. Used properly, the system also assists pollution control because vaporiser filling occurs without spillage.

• Back bar

Flowmeters and vaporisers may be joined by tapered connectors and attached to a back bar, producing a series of semi-permanent fixtures. The 'Selectatec SM' manifold allows rapid attachment or removal of 'Tec 3 and 'Tec 4 vaporisers and is desirable, facilitating vaporiser removal for refilling out of theatre, servicing and rewarming. In accommodating up to three vaporisers a range of volatile agents may be available.

Common gas outlet (F). This connects the anaesthetic machine to breathing system connectors, ventilators or O_2 supply devices.

O_2 flush. Also known as the bypass or purge valve, this receives O_2 from the cylinder and bypasses the vaporiser. Activation produces high flows of pure oxygen to the common gas outlet. The device is used to provide oxygen in emergency situations and may have a 'lock-in' facility: rotating the valve 90° fixes it in the open position. It is used to flush anaesthetic from breathing systems before patient disconnection, thus lowering pollution.

Nitrous oxide cut-out devices. These devices curtail N_2O flow and sound an alarm when oxygen runs out. The machine's system is checked by means of the following steps:

(1) Switch on both O_2 and N_2O sources
(2) Open the flowmeters to give nominal flows of 2 and 4 l/min O_2 /N_2O respectively.
(3) Close the O_2 cylinder valve.

The N_2O and O_2 bobbins should fall simultaneously while a whistle sounds.

Over-pressure valve. High pressures downstream from the common gas outlet open this valve and sound an alarm. The device is useful for leak-testing breathing systems; the valve's presence is confirmed by occluding the common gas outlet while pressing the oxygen bypass valve.

Emergency air intake valve. When gas flow from the machine accidentally ceases, the patient's inspiratory effort opens an emergency valve which allows room air to enter the breathing system. The valve's opening action is accompanied by a 'whistling' sound. This valve is tested by attaching a pipe to the common gas outlet and applying suction; when sufficient vacuum is present, the valve opens and a whistle is heard.

Checking the machine before use

The anaesthetic machine should receive a major check at the beginning of each working day and a minor check between cases. To ensure that no parts of the test are omitted, a list should be attached to the machine setting out the following steps:

• Ensure that flow control valves (at flowmeter) are 'off'.
• Ensure that cylinders are closed and fit securely on the hanger yoke.
• Press the oxygen flush valve until no gas flow is apparent from the common gas outlet.
• Check that flowmeters and pressure gauges read '0'.
• Open the oxygen cylinder valve slowly, (anti-clockwise) and observe the registered pressure. Open and then close the oxygen flowmeter control valve to ensure smooth function. Press the oxygen flush valve. On machines which carry a second O_2 cylinder, the tested cylinder is closed and the test repeated on the second.
• Label the cylinders 'in use' or 'full' depending on registered pressure.
• Replace bottles that have little remaining gas.
• Open the 'in use' oxygen cylinder and set the O_2 flowmeter control knob at 2 l/min. Examine the status of N_2O cylinders as in step 5. Label N_2O cylinders.
• Check M low-oxygen warning device.
• Ensure that the vaporiser is full, with the filling port tightly closed, and that spindle operation is smooth.
• Check overpressure and emergency air-intake valves.

The testing of machines that receive a service supply from banked cylinders is more complicated.

'Shutting down' the anaesthetic machine

When all surgery is finished, the content status of all cylinders is checked and empty cylinders are removed. (If present, Schraeder probes are removed from the wall sockets and the pipes neatly coiled.) The oxygen flowmeter control knob is then opened to produce flow of 2 l/min. The nitrous oxide cylinder valves are then closed. The nitrous oxide flowmeters are opened and closed once the flow indicator has fallen to '0'. The oxygen bottles are then closed and the O_2 flush valve is activated until no pressure registers on the pressure gauge. Machine surfaces are then wiped with alcohol.

Anaesthetic Breathing Systems

These systems jeopardise animals' lives when used improperly. Each system has both advantages (and disadvantages) in different circumstances, a range should be available to cover most clinical situations.

Circuit classification varies throughout the world and is confusing. In the UK, 'semi-closed' and 'closed' systems are described. The basis of classification lies on whether expired breath is 'rebreathed' or flushed completely from the system by high gas flow.

Rebreathing systems

Expired breath, in comparison with inspired gas, is low in O_2 and anaesthetic but contains more CO_2 and water vapour and is warm. In rebreathing systems (circle and to-and-fro) expired gas passes through soda-lime (absorbent) which removes CO_2. Warm, moist gas is then re-inspired and so rebreathing systems conserve heat and moisture. Fresh gas flow requirements are based on the O_2 and anaesthetic consumption of the patient. Because these values are low (Fig. 27.12) rebreathing systems are efficient.

Absorbent. This absorbs CO_2 and consists of granules of:

- 80% Sodium hydroxide [NaOH] or 'soda'
- 18% Calcium hydroxide [$Ca(OH)_2$] or 'lime'
- Silicates
- pH indicators

Carbon dioxide reacts chemically with the hydroxides to produce carbonates. The reactions require water (derived from expired breath) and produce heat in the process:

$$CO_2 + 2NaOH = Na_2CO_3 + H_2O$$

$$Na_2CO_3 + Ca(OH)_2 = 2NaOH + CaCO_2$$

Silicates used to be included in medical absorbents to increase the hardness and reduce the formation of irritant dust.

pH indicators. These change colour as soda-lime becomes exhausted. Changes depend on the dyes used. Common absorbents turn from pink or lilac to white (although, confusingly, one type turns from white to lilac). The container label describes the colour change its contents undergo and *should be consulted.*

When soda-lime granules are 'spent', they lose their soapy, soft texture and fail to become warm when exposed to CO_2. Opened absorbent containers must be tightly sealed otherwise atmospheric CO_2 enters and causes premature exhaustion.

Soda-lime is irritant (alkali) and gloves should be worn when refilling canisters. The dust must not be inhaled or allowed to contact the eyes.

Soda-lime is contained in canisters, the design of which depends on the circuit involved. The canister contents are approximately 50% granules and 50% air space. Efficient absorption requires an air-space volume in excess of tidal volume (V_t) and so the minimum 'working' soda-lime required is at least 2 V_t. Considerably greater volumes than this are needed because absorbent is inactivated during anaesthesia. Gas flow between the granules is turbulent and when large canisters are filled to capacity resistance to breathing is increased. However, large canisters require less frequent changing.

Soda-lime reacts with trichlorethylene (a once popular volatile agent) to produce phosgene and other toxic gases; trichloroethylene should therefore *not* be used in rebreathing systems.

ADVANTAGES OF REBREATHING SYSTEMS

- Low gas flow requirements.
- Low volatile agent consumption rate.
- 'Closed' or 'low-flow' options.
- Expired moisture and heat conserved.
- Ventilation can be altered (spontaneous to controlled) without changing system performance or efficiency.
- Low explosion risk (when explosive gases are used).
- Less pollution.

DISADVANTAGES

- High resistance to breathing.
- Nitrous oxide cannot be safely used in rebreathing systems.
- Expensive to purchase.
- Regular soda-lime replacement required.
- Inspired gas content undetermined.
- De-nitrogenation required.
- Slow to change level of anaesthesia.
- Cumbersome.

RESPIRATORY VARIABLES IN COMPANION ANIMALS				
Species	Respiratory rate[1] (breaths/min)	Tidal volume[1] (mL/kg)	Minute volume[1] (mL/kg/min)	Oxygen consumption[2] (mL/kg/min)
Dogs >30kg	15–20	12–15	150–250	5.8
<30kg	20–30	16–20	200–300	6.2
Cats	20–30	7–9	180–380	7.3

1 During surgery, factors like pain, pyrexia, light versus deep anaesthesia will affect these.
2 Oxygen consumption depends on factors related to metabolic rate: age, temperature, thyroid status, drugs, muscle tone, response to surgery.

Fig. 27.12. Respiratory variables in companion animals.

'Closed' and 'low-flow'. Rebreathing systems are used in one of two ways. In 'closed' systems, gas inflow precisely replaces anaesthetic and O_2 uptaken by the patient. Approximately 5–10 ml/kg/min is required. Under these conditions the pressure relief valve is shut. When the system is run in a 'low flow' fashion, oxygen delivery is in excess of basal requirements (>10 ml/kg/min) with surplus gas leaking through the partly opened pressure relief valve. This is the easiest system to operate and therefore the most common.

Nitrous oxide. This gas cannot be used safely in rebreathing systems unless inspired oxygen content or arterial-blood gas analysis can be performed.

Denitrogenation. When connected to breathing systems at the onset of anaesthesia, patients expire considerable volumes of nitrogen (which is present in normal air but not in anaesthetic gas mixtures). This may lower circuit O_2 to hypoxic levels unless purged through the pressure-relief valve (denitrogenation). This is achieved by using high flows for the first 10–15 minutes of anaesthesia.

Otherwise, regular 'dumping' of the reservoir bag is required (every 3 minutes in the first 15 minutes, and every 30 minutes thereafter).

Circle system. Circle systems (Fig. 27.13) have valves causing unidirectional gas movement through seven circuit components. These are: fresh gas inflow (1), inspiratory and expiratory unidirectional valves (2 and 4), patient 'Y' connector (3), pressure relief valve (5), reservoir bag (6), and absorbent canister (7).

• Fresh gas inflow (1)
This pipe connects the circuit with the common-gas outlet on the anaesthetic machine.

• Unidirectional valves (2,4)
These are light transparent discs resting on knife-edge valve seats, enclosed within a transparent dome. Units should be easy to dis-assemble for drying and cleaning.

• 'Y' connector (3)
This connects inspiratory and expiratory limbs with endotracheal tube connectors or masks. In paediatric

systems it has a septum dividing inspiratory and expiratory flows, reducing dead space.

• Pressure-relief valve (5)
This is opened to let surplus gas from 'low-flow' systems, during denitrogenation, and closed when lung inflation is imposed. In old systems it was sited at the 'Y' connector which made valve operation difficult. Relief valves should be shrouded for attachment to scavenge hoses.

• Reservoir (rebreathing) bag (6)
This allows PPV; its volume should be 3–6 times the animal's tidal volume. Large bags increase circuit volume, make respiratory movement less obvious and are harder to squeeze. Inadequately sized bags collapse during large breaths and overdistend during expiration. Clearly, a range is required for small animal use.

• Absorbent canister (7)
Canisters for circle systems may have two compartments. When absorbent in one becomes exhausted, it is discarded; after refilling, the canister is replaced in the reverse direction. This allows optimal use of absorbent. Circle system canisters may have a by-pass switch which excludes or incorporates absorbent from the circuit, allowing CO_2 to rise while maintaining ventilation.

• Hoses
These are corrugated to prevent kinking.

Circle systems for small dogs and cats are less popular in the UK than elsewhere because the resistance caused by the absorbent the valves, and the dead space in the 'Y' connector are alleged to be excessive. It is said that circle systems designed for human use should not be used in dogs weighing less than 15 kg although they are useful, efficient systems in larger dogs.

ADVANTAGES OF CIRCLE SYSTEMS INCLUDE
• High gas efficiency.
• Mechanical dead space remains unchanged with use (unlike to-and-fro systems).
• Bronchiolitis unlikely (unlike to-and-fro systems).
• Less circuit inertia than to-and-fro systems.
• Ventilation readily controlled.

DISADVANTAGES
• Expensive.
• Complex, cumbersome and difficult to sterilise.
• Resistance to breathing for animals less than 15 kg.

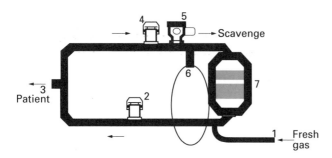

Fig. 27.13. Circle anaesthetic breathing system.

To-and-fro (water's) system. In this system (Fig. 27.14) gas oscillates over absorbent in the Water's canister. Canisters are designed for either vertical or

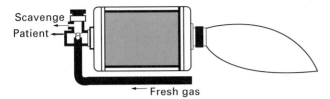

Fig. 27.14. Horizontal to-and-fro system.

horizontal use; only the latter are used with companion animals. Features of to-and-fro systems include:

• Fresh gas inflow
This is situated adjacent to the endotracheal tube connector allowing dialled concentrations of anaesthetic to be preferentially inspired and, therefore, greater control over anaesthesia.

• Filter
A metal gauze screen should be sited at the patient end of the canister to limit inhalation of alkali dust.

• Scavenging shroud
Scavenging waste gas from a to-and-fro system relies on a suitable shroud on the pressure relief valve.

• Canister
Transparent canisters are desirable as they allow soda-lime colour and filling adequacy to be checked. (Canisters in horizontal to-and-fro systems must be filled to capacity, otherwise the expirate will 'channel', i.e. take the low resistance path over the absorbent, retaining CO_2.)

ADVANTAGES OF TO-AND-FRO SYSTEMS

• High gas efficiency.
• Bi-directional gas flow improves CO_2 scrubbing efficiency.
• Greater heat conservation (hyperthermia is possible in high ambient temperatures).
• Lower resistance to breathing than with circle systems (no valves and lower overall circuit length).
• Low circuit volume:
  Denitrogenation achieved rapidly.
  Rapid changes in gas concentration
• Simple, robust construction.
• Portable; easily moved from room to room.
• Readily sterilised.
• Inexpensive.

DISADVANTAGES

• Valve position is inconvenient for positive-pressure ventilation.
• Mechanical dead space increases during surgery as absorbent is exhausted.
• 'Channelling'.
• Bronchiolitis; aspiration of alkali dust from canister may cause chemical injury.
• Considerable drag. The system has much inertia and is inconvenient during head surgery.

Non-rebreathing systems

Non-rebreathing or semi-closed systems rely on high fresh gas flow rates, based on multiples of minute volume, to flush expired CO_2 from the circuit so that it cannot be rebreathed at the next breath.

ADVANTAGES OF SEMI-CLOSED SYSTEMS

• Low resistance; ideal for small animals and birds.
• Simple construction.
• Inexpensive to purchase.
• Soda-lime not required.
• Inspired gas content similar to that 'dialled' at anaesthetic machine.
• De-nitrogenation not required.
• Circuit concentration of anaesthetic can be changed rapidly, allowing more concise control over patient's level of unconsciousness.
• Can be used with trichlorethylene.

DISADVANTAGES

• High carrier gas flow requirements.
• High volatile agent consumption rate.
• Expired moisture and heat usually lost.
• Ventilatory modes affect system performance.
• Different types of non-rebreathing circuits behave differently, and have different flow requirements.

The Magill system. The Magill system consists of a reservoir bag and a corrugated hose which ends at an expiratory (Heidbrink) valve (Fig. 27.15).

Rebreathing is prevented when gas flow equals or exceeds patient minute volume. When N_2O is used, its flow rate is included within this value. For example, a 15 kg dog with a V_m of 3l receives an inspired concentration of 66% N_2O with flows of 1 l/min O_2 and 2 l/min N_2O. Similarly, 1.5 l/min O_2 and 1.5 l/min N_2O provide a 50% mixture.

ADVANTAGES

The Magill is an efficient general-purpose circuit for most companion animal cases. The circuit is readily maintained and sterilised.

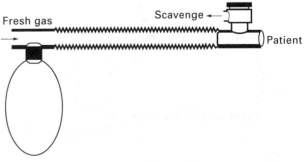

Fig. 27.15. The Magill breathing system.

DISADVANTAGES

Mechanical dead space, inertia and considerable expiratory resistance preclude its usefulness in cats, and in dogs weighing less than 5 kg. Heidbrink valve location is inconvenient for scavenging and operation, especially during surgery on the head. The behaviour of the system changes fundamentally when the reservoir bag is actively squeezed, with expired gas being reintroduced into the lungs rather than expelled through the valve. Consequently, the system must not be used for prolonged positive-pressure ventilation because 'enforced rebreathing' causes hypercapnia.

The Lack system. Inconvenient valve location in Magill circuits is overcome in the co-axial version—the Lack System (Fig. 27.16). In this, a reservoir bag connects to an outer inspiratory limb; this surrounds an inner expiratory tube which ends at the expiratory valve.

The Lack system is slightly more efficient than the Magill. Expiratory resistance is also lower and so the system may be used in smaller animals.

ADVANTAGES

The circuit is lightweight and exerts less drag than Magill systems. Valve position facilitates surgery on the head and scavenging. The system is 1.5 m long, allowing anaesthetic machine positioning away from surgery. Lack systems can be used in lieu of the Magill circuit.

DISADVANTAGES

Older versions had high expiratory (inner limb) resistance and inner hose disconnection, causing considerable rebreathing. The system is stiffer and inconvenient to use in very small animals. Because the Lack system behaves like the Magill, it should not be used for prolonged periods of controlled ventilation.

The Parallel Lack System (Fig. 27.17). Problems of co-axial geometry (disconnection, fracture or kinking of the inner limb) are avoided when the inspiratory and expiratory limbs are juxtapositioned (put side by side) in a parallel configuration. The system is said to behave like a Magill attachment although it has increased drag, thus conferring little advantage in very small animal anaesthesia.

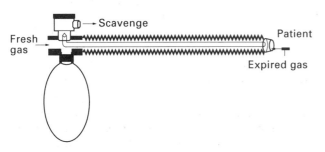

Fig. 27.16. The Lack breathing system.

Ayres' T-piece (Fig. 27.18). Gas flows for T-piece systems must exceed double the minute volume otherwise expired gas is rebreathed ($2 \times V_m$). Rapid respiratory rates may require even higher ($3 \times V_m$) flows. Nitrous oxide is included at 50 or 66% of these levels.

ADVANTAGES

Minimal apparatus dead-space and resistance makes the T-piece ideal for cats, small dogs (below 5 kg) neonates and birds. It is simple, inexpensive and easy to sterilise. Modest drag occurs because two hoses are present. The system is scavenged with appropriate connectors.

DISADVANTAGES

Ventilation is controlled by occluding the distal end of the expiratory limb but gas flow must be increased, otherwise the duration of inspiration is prolonged and limits adequate ventilation.

Ayre's T-Piece With Jackson-Rees' Modification. This circuit is an Ayre's T-piece with an open-ended reservoir bag on the expiratory limb (Fig. 27.18).
Flows of $2.5–3 \times V_m$ are needed.

ADVANTAGES

The bag facilitates PPV and bag movement acts as a useful respiratory monitor. Ventilation is controlled by occluding the bag's end, allowing distension, then squeezing the contents into the patient. The end is then released. The system has the advantages of a T-piece so is used in similar circumstances. Flows need not be increased when PPV is imposed.

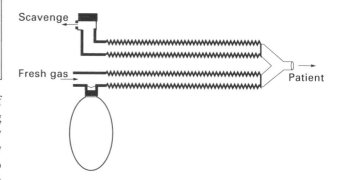

Fig. 27.17. The parallel Lack breathing system.

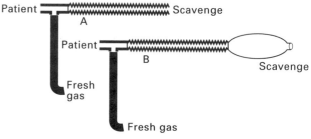

Fig. 27.18. (a) Ayre's T-piece; (b) Jackson–Rees modified Ayre's T-piece.

DISADVANTAGES

Scavenging the system may be complicated; connectors tend to twist and cause rapid over-distension of the bag.

The Bain system. The Bain system is a 'co-axial' (tube within a tube) T-piece with an inner inspiratory limb surrounded by an outer expiratory hose (Fig. 27.19). The expiratory limb ends either in an open-ended tube (Mapleson E), a reservoir bag and expiratory valve (Mapleson D) or an open-ended bag (Mapleson F).

• Gas flow
The circuit probably requires marginally higher flows than corresponding T-piece systems although reports on its performance vary: $2-3 \times V_m$ should be used.

ADVANTAGES

Bain systems without valves (Mapleson E or F) are recommended for cats and very small dogs because of lower expiratory resistance. Ventilation is controlled by occluding the expiratory limb in 'E' systems. In 'D' systems, the expiratory valve is closed and then the bag squeezed. In Mapleson 'F' versions, the reservoir bag is used like a Jackson-Rees modification. The circuit is useful for PPV in small dogs and cats, especially when patient access is limited. The length of the system (1.8 m) allows the anaesthetic machine to be positioned well away from surgery, improving access. Spontaneous ventilation is satisfactory in dogs over 10 kg. The system has low drag and mechanical dead-space; it is easily maintained and sterilised. It is claimed that warm expirate raises the temperature of gas flowing in the inner limb, conserving patient temperature.

DISADVANTAGES

Expiratory resistance with high flows reduces the system's usefulness in spontaneously breathing cats and small dogs. Rebreathing problems caused by inner limb disconnection prompted development of a parallel Bain system. However, inspiratory limb integrity is easily tested by occluding its end with a 5 ml syringe plunger; when gas is flowing the flowmeter indicator falls and,or the machine's over-pressure valve is heard.

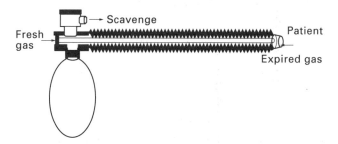

Fig. 27.19. The Bain anaesthetic breathing system.

Other Anaesthetic Equipment

Trouble-free anaesthesia depends on equipment being available and serviceable. Inadequate equipment care causes expensive deterioration and more importantly, may compromise the patient.

Endotracheal tubes

These connect the patient to the anaesthetic breathing system. Most patterns have cuffs at the distal (patient) end which, when filled with air, produce a gas-tight seal. Construction materials confer different properties on the tube. Red rubber tubes have poor resistance to kinking and conform poorly to airway contours. Tubes made of polyvinyl chloride (PVC) are the softest and least irritating to the tracheal mucosa; they have little tendency to kink and they mould to the curve of the airway at body temperature.

Care, maintenance and storage depend on the material of construction. Red rubber tubes are deteriorated by oil and petroleum-based lubricants. After cleaning and sterilisation, tubes should be dried thoroughly and stored in a cool, dry environment. They should not be exposed to direct sunlight.

Before use, check the tubes for patency and establish the cuffs' ability to hold pressure. The endotracheal tube connector should be tight and fit snugly with the chosen breathing system. The tube should be an appropriate length and a range of tube diameters should be made available.

After use, ensure the tubes are rinsed in running water and leave them to soak in detergent solution. Later they should be scrubbed inside and out to remove residual mucus. Rinsing must be thorough to remove detergent.

Sterilising procedures depend on material. Red rubber tubes are deteriorated by heat sterilisation. Polysiloxane tubes can be autoclaved. While most PVC tubes are designed for single use only, they may be safely re-used after cleaning and sterilising. Ethylene oxide must be used cautiously and adequate aeration allowed afterwards (at least 48 hours). Gamma-irradiated single-use items and PVC tubes should not be sterilised with ethylene oxide.

Masks

These are used for administering oxygen, and for volatile anaesthetics when an endotracheal tube is not present. Patterns made of malleable rubber can be shaped to fit the animal's face and minimise apparatus dead-space. Others are made of rigid plastic with a perforated rubber diaphragm; they have high dead-space and so require greater gas flows. However, for birds and laboratory animal species they can be constructed from syringe cases and bits of latex glove. Customised equipment should have minimum dead-space, should be affixable to the animal, should not confer resistance to respiration and should allow the animal to be seen.

Care, maintenance and storage considerations for masks are the same as those for endotracheal tubes.

Masks can be sterilised by soaking in a 0.2% chlorhexidine solution or similar.

Laryngoscopes

Laryngoscopes consist of a handle and a blade and are available in several patterns and sizes. They serve to depress the base of the tongue during intubation; in so doing, they evert the epiglottis. A bulb at the tip of the blade illuminates the oropharynx. Ideally, the bulb should only illuminate when the blade is 'fixed' in the working position.

Before use, it is important to ensure that the bulb is firmly positioned and that the batteries are charged. After use, blades should be wiped clean with a swab soaked in alcohol. Laryngoscopes must not be immersed in water.

Gags

These keep the jaw open and allow safe retraction of the tongue after induction and prior to endotracheal intubation. They are also useful during oral surgery.

Syringes and needles

Disposable plastic syringes have replaced glass except for the use of diazepam. Filled syringes must be labelled. After use the needle should be removed, the syringe discarded and the needle disposed of into a rigid container. If fine (e.g. smaller than 23 swg) needles are used to withdraw drugs from multi-dose vials, they should be replaced before use because they may have become blunted.

Monitors

Stethoscopes. Heart and lung sounds may be heard by applying the stethoscope bell to the animal's chest wall. Because this may be difficult during surgery, an oesophageal stethoscope may be used. This is a hollow, flexible plastic tube which is passed down the oesophagus to the approximate position of the heart base and connected to conventional stethoscope ear-pieces. Its position is then adjusted until heart-sound amplitude is maximum. The device also picks up lung sounds and extraneous vibrations from the breathing system. Small amplifiers may be connected to the device, avoiding the need for ear-pieces. Before use, the tube must be clear of secretion or water, otherwise sounds are damped.

The electrocardiogram (ECG). Through three or more leads connected to the patient, an ECG monitors the electrical activity of the heart. The electrocardiograph is usually displayed on an oscilloscope screen and a microprocessor interprets the signal, generating a numerically displayed heart rate.

Leads from the device connect to the patient by adhesive electrodes or crocodile clips. For a successful signal to be received, patient contacts must be secure and crocodile clips must be clean. Conduction may be assisted with alcohol solutions or electrolyte-conducting gels. In long-coated breeds it may be necessary to clip electrode attachment sites.

Other monitors. In general, electrical monitors should be switched on before use and allowed to warm up. They should be calibrated before attachment to the unconscious patient.

Gases, Vapours and Inhaled Anaesthetics

Inhaled anaesthetics used in animals include nitrous oxide (N_2O) halothane, methoxyflurane, enflurane, isoflurane and diethyl ether. Oxygen and carbon dioxide (CO_2) are used to optimise physiological conditions while O_2 and N_2O, are known as carrier gases because they 'carry' volatile anaesthetics.

Oxygen (O_2)

Oxygen is an odourless, reactive gas that allows combustion and, in the presence of organic material and activation energy (i.e. sparks or naked flames), explosions.

Uses

The gas is given whenever the normal delivery of atmospheric oxygen to active tissue is threatened. This includes anaesthesia (even that produced with injectable agents).

Pure oxygen (100%) is usually given to animals which are anaemic, have pulmonary pathology or are hypoventilating. During inhalation anaesthesia, 100% oxygen may be used as the 'carrier gas' but it is frequently diluted to 50% or 33% concentrations by nitrous oxide.

Oxygen is also supplied during recovery until the animal is capable of maintaining haemoglobin saturation with room air (20% O_2).

Problems

Oxygen does not depress ventilation or cause toxic nervous or pulmonary changes during short periods of exposure. The major hazard is related to the support of combustion.

Carbon Dioxide (CO_2)

Carbon dioxide is supplied in grey cylinders. On British anaesthetic machines, pressure gauges and flowmeters for CO_2 are similarly colour-coded.

Uses

When blood-gas analysis is unavailable and breathing is controlled, it is difficult to know the ventilation level required to produce normal levels of plasma CO_2 (normocapnia). This is avoided by moderately hyperventilating the animal and including 4% CO_2 in inspired gas.

Disadvantages

Excessive CO_2 causes hypercapnia and respiratory acidosis, which stimulates the cardiovascular system and increases blood pressure but at high levels causes depression and arrythmias. Elevated CO_2 stimulates ventilation but high concentrations cause narcosis and depress ventilation.

Nitrous Oxide (N₂O)

Nitrous oxide is an odourless, relatively inert gas with anaesthetic properties. It is non-flammable, but supports combustion.

Nitrous oxide is often combined with oxygen as a carrier gas. It must not be used at concentrations greater than 80% as this lowers O_2 below normal levels. Usually no more than 66% is delivered.

The percentage of gas mixtures is calculated on a flow ratio basis. For example a 50% O_2/N_2O mixture is produced when O_2 and N_2O flows are the same (e.g. 3l/min O_2 and 3 l/min N_2O). Commonly, 66% or 2:1 N_2O/O_2 mixtures are used. These are produced when N_2O flow is exactly twice that of O_2.

Uses

Anaesthetic 'sparing' effect. Nitrous oxide is less potent in animals than in humans but nevertheless lowers the concentration of volatile agent required to produce a given level of anaesthesia. For example, 66% N_2O reduces halothane requirements by about 25%. Because N_2O has minimal effects on cardiac output and ventilation, its inclusion preserves cardiopulmonary performance.

Second gas effect. During induction with N_2O and a volatile agent, the rapid uptake of N_2O from alveoli causes the alveolar concentration of the volatile agent, or second gas, to rise. This accelerates uptake of the second gas and the rate of induction.

Disadvantages

Hypoxia. Whenever N_2O is used, the O_2 content of inspired gas is lowered; this increases the possibility of hypoxia arising from other causes like hypoventilation. Different rates of uptake of N_2O occurs in rebreathing systems and the gas should not be used in circle or to-and-fro systems except in specific circumstances.

Gas-filled viscus. Because N_2O is relatively insoluble in blood, it sequesters to gas-filled organs within the patient—e.g. the dilated stomach of dogs with gastric-dilation–volvulus complex or the pleural space of animals with closed pneumothorax. Nitrous oxide comprises the animal by enlarging, or increasing the pressure within such spaces.

Diffusion hypoxia. When N_2O delivery is ended, its direction of diffusion reverses—from blood into the alveolar space. The volume evolved in the first few minutes after termination may dilute alveolar O_2. If this is low because the animal is breathing air, not 100% O_2, 'diffusion hypoxia' may occur. Therefore on ending N_2O administration, animals must receive 100% O_2 for at least 3 minutes.

Cardiopulmonary effects. N_2O has a very modest stimulant effect on cardiac output and blood pressure. It has no affect on ventilation; when added to volatile agents, ventilation remains unchanged even though anaesthesia deepens.

Other effects. Nitrous oxide crosses the placenta and neonates delivered from a mother receiving N_2O will need inspired O_2 enrichment, otherwise diffusion hypoxia will occur.

Special precautions

Nitrous oxide should not be used in animals whose arterial oxygen tensions are lowered by disease, or where a gas-filled viscus is present.

Pollution. Nitrous oxide is relatively odourless and high atmospheric levels are difficult to detect. There is some evidence that N_2O causes toxic effects like bone-marrow depression after chronic, low-level exposure. It is not absorbed by activated charcoal and so 'canister' scavenging is useless.

Inhalation Anaesthetics

These are delivered into the patient in a 'carrier gas'. This may be pure (100%) oxygen or a mixture of nitrous oxide and oxygen.

The behaviour of inhalation anaesthetics can be predicted and compared if two important features are known. These are the blood/gas solubility coefficient and the minimum alveolar concentration.

Blood/gas solubility coefficient

This value describes the solubility of agents in blood. Drugs with low solubility have low blood/gas solubility coefficients; they cause rapid induction and recovery rates, while 'swings' in levels of anaesthesia on changing vaporiser settings are more rapid. Values for modern anaesthetics with the fastest on the left are:

N₂O > Isoflurane > Enflurane > Halothane
0.47   1.39   1.8   2.4

> Methoxyflurane
12.0

Minimum alveolar concentration (MAC)

Minimum alveolar concentration (MAC) of anaesthetics is the alveolar concentration (expressed as a percentage) that prevents responses occurring to a specified stimulus such as skin incision. It is a measure of potency. Agents with low values have the greatest potency; low inspired concentrations are required for surgery. Many factors alter MAC. The most important being other drugs given during anaesthesia for instance N_2O, analgesics and pre-anaesthetic medication.

Most potent:

Methoxyflurane > Halothane > Isoflurane
0.23   0.8   1.3

> Enflurane > N₂O
2.2   188–220

Uptake and Distribution of Volatile Anaesthetics

Volatile anaesthetics produce anaesthesia when a critical tension is exceeded in the CNS. This tension is achieved by movement of drug molecules down a series of tension gradients, beginning at the anaesthetic machine and ending at the site of action within the CNS. At equilibrium, the tension of drug in the brain mirrors that in arterial blood, which is the same as that in alveoli. Therefore factors influencing alveolar tensions ultimately determine brain tensions.

Alveolar drug levels depend on alveolar ventilation rate and the inspired gas concentration. When these are high, induction of anaesthesia is rapid. The uptake of anaesthetic from alveoli depends on cardiac output, the lipid solubility of the agent in question and tension of anaesthetic in pulmonary venous blood. Alveolar tensions rise rapidly (and induction is rapid) when cardiac output is low, (e.g. in haemorrhagic shock), when insoluble agents like N_2O are used, and when the pulmonary venous tension of anaesthetic is high.

Halothane

Currently the most common volatile anaesthetic in small and large animal anaesthesia, this halogenated hydrocarbon is a sweet-smelling, clear liquid which decomposes in ultra-violet light and so is stored in amber bottles and contains an antioxidant (0.01% thymol). It readily evaporates producing a maximum concentration of 32%. For this reason it must be used from a calibrated vaporiser.

Pharmacokinetics. Halothane is a fast-acting anaesthetic. Up to 12–25% of absorbed halothane is metabolised to bromide, trifluroacetate and chloride by the liver.

Central nervous system. Halothane is a potent anaesthetic; concentrations of 1.0–3.0% may be needed after induction but adequate surgical conditions are obtained with inspired concentrations of 0.75–2.0%. Muscle relaxation is modest but analgesia is poor; adrenergic responses occur until deep levels of anaesthesia are reached.

Cardiopulmonary system. Halothane lowers blood pressure by reducing cardiac output. As a halogenated hydrocarbon, the drug 'sensitises' the myocardium to adrenaline. This is of limited importance in animals that are adequately anaesthetised and ventilated.

Halothane does not reduce systemic vascular resistance although it causes vasodilation in capillary beds of the brain, uterus and skin.

Halothane depresses ventilation in a dose-dependent manner causing decreased tidal volume, increased rate and hypercapnia. It depresses ventilation to a lesser extent than other volatile anaesthetics with the exception of diethyl ether.

Other effects. In people, halothane-associated hepatitis occurs with repeated halothane anaesthetics. The cause is not fully understood but seems related to pre-operative enzyme induction caused by smoking and alcohol consumption, as well as intra-operative hypoxia. The condition has not been conclusively demonstrated to occur in animals during surgical anaesthesia.

Halothane lowers body temperature by inhibiting themoregulatory mechanisms and producing cutaneous vasodilation.

Special precautions. Halothane triggers malignant hyperthermia in sensitive pigs and this genetically determined condition also occurs in man. It has occurred in dogs, horses and cats but is rare.

Methoxyflurane

This fruity-smelling halogenated ether is the most potent volatile anaesthetic. It is non-reactive but decomposes slowly when exposed to soda-lime and ultraviolet light and so it contains butylated hydroxytoluene. The clear liquid changes to a yellow amber colour in the vaporiser but this does not affect potency. Methoxyflurane evaporates poorly—no more than 3% can be delivered at room temperature.

Pharmacokinetics. It has high blood–gas (12.0) and rubber–gas (630) solubility coefficients making induction and recovery very slow. This precludes its use in large animals. Its low volatility allows its use in open or semi-open systems but the use of a calibrated 'Pentec' vaporiser is preferred. Induction requires 1.5–2.5% and maintenance, 0.2–1.25%.

Central nervous system. A potent anaesthetic (its MAC value is 0.16 in humans, 0.29 in dogs, 0.23 in cats and 0.22 in horses) with good muscle relaxant and analgesic properties. Cranial nerve reflexes are lost early and the eye is said to 'centralise' at relatively light levels of anaesthesia.

Cardiopulmonary system. Cardiac output is reduced in a dose-dependent manner, causing hypotension. Heart rate tends to slow. It causes more respiratory depression than halothane.

Special precautions. In people, prolonged methoxyflurane anaesthesia causes renal tubular destruction, polyuria and dehydration lasting several days after administration. This is partly due to fluoride and oxalate ions generated from hepatic methoxyflurane metabolism. While the dog kidney is resistant to flurotoxicosis, acute renal failure has occurred in this species when flunixin has been given peri-operatively.

Methoxyflurane should not be used in animals receiving NSAIDs or other potentially nephrotoxic drugs. Alternatively, these drugs should be withheld from animals in which methoxyflurane anaesthesia is considered desirable. Methoxyflurane is not a good choice when rapid recoveries are desired.

Enflurane

Enflurane, a halogenated ether with a fruity smell has never gained popularity in any branch of veterinary anaesthesia despite some useful features. Chemically it is very stable and contains no preservative.

Pharmacokinetics. Concentrations of 4–6% are needed for induction, with maintenance requirements of 1–3%. It is relatively expensive. Because it is highly volatile (SVP is 171.8 at 20°C) the maximum concentration achievable is 22% (at that temperature) and so the use of an 'Enfluratec' is advisable.

Central nervous system. In humans, deep enflurane anaesthesia causes seizure-type electroencephalographic (EEG) activity which is exacerbated by hypercapnia. Involuntary muscle twitches are seen during anaesthesia and recovery in animals. The MAC in dogs and cats is 2.2% and 1.2% respectively.

Cardiopulmonary system. Enflurane depresses blood pressure to the same extent as isoflurane, but less than halothane. Heart rate is increased in a dose-dependent manner. Cardiac output is reduced. While it is the most potent respiratory depressant, decreasing rate and depth, spontaneous 'sighing' occurs during enflurane anaesthesia.

Other effects. Enflurane produces excellent muscle relaxation and markedly potentiates neuromuscular blockers.

Isoflurane

Isoflurane is an isomer of enflurane, and a recently developed volatile agent. Although it is a halogenated ether, it has an unpleasant pungent smell. Its saturated vapour pressure is similar to halothane and the same (cleaned) precision vaporiser may be used for its administration. At room temperature, the maximum concentration possible is 31.5%.

Pharmacokinetics. Isoflurane has a low blood/gas solubility coefficient and so recoveries are rapid even after prolonged administration. Inductions are not as rapid as predicted because the agent causes breath-holding in some species. After induction, inspired concentrations of 2.5–4.5% are needed. Because it has a lower MAC value than halothane (MAC in dogs and cats is 1.28 and 1.63% respectively) higher inspired concentrations are needed to maintain anaesthesia (1.5–2.5%).

Central nervous system. A potent anaesthetic providing good muscle relaxation and analgesia. Recoveries are rapid but may be associated with transient excitatory effects, especially after painful surgery.

Cardiovascular system. Isoflurane causes a dose-dependent hypotension despite non-dose-dependent increases in heart rate. At 1.0 MAC cardiac output is maintained. Isoflurane is a potent respiratory depressant, but this is partly offset by surgery.

Special precautions. The insolubility of this drug in blood makes it a useful anaesthetic when rapid recoveries are required. The same feature means that 'swings' in level of anaesthesia are greatest with this agent.

Techniques in Anaesthesia

Intravenous Catheterisation

ADVANTAGES
- Reduces risk of extravascular injection, ensures full doses are given and prevents tissue damage with irritant drugs.
- Provides rapid intravenous access for emergency drugs.
- Allows fluids to be given rapidly.
- Allows rapid 'deepening' of anaesthesia with injectable anaesthetics.

DISADVANTAGES

- Vein damage; poor catheterisation technique may damage the vein and preclude further access. This occurs when haematoma or thrombosis form.
- Sepsis; in immunosuppressed animals (e.g. diabetics) poor surgical preparation and management of catheters lead to phlebitis. More severe conditions like bacteraemia may follow.

Technique

Adequate physical and chemical restraint is a prerequisite. The site must receive full surgical preparation. A small skin incision over the vein facilitates catheter introduction in animals with resilient skin (e.g. male cats, dehydrated animals).

Endotracheal Intubation

When animals are rendered unconscious by injectable or inhalation drugs, protective airway reflexes are lost. Endotracheal intubation is one way to prevent related problems.

ADVANTAGES

- Airway protection from saliva and gastric contents.
  If cuffed tubes are not available an oro-pharyngeal pack—layers of moistened gauze laid in a horse-shoe pattern over the tube and 'packed'—may suffice. This is important during dental or oral surgery.
- Allows positive pressure ventilation.
  A leak-proof cuff allows lung inflation without gas escape; this is important if flammable agents are used.
- Reduces waste-gas pollution.
- Reduces anatomic dead-space.

DISADVANTAGES

- Resistance
  Cuffs limit the size of tube that can be introduced atraumatically. Small internal diameters critically increase resistance to breathing.
- Kinking or occlusion
  Overinflated cuffs may compress the underlying tube. Severe occipito-atlantal flexion (e.g. during cisternal puncture) may cause tubes (especially red-rubber types) to kink. If tubes are inadequately cleaned, dried secretions accumulate within the lumen.
- Traumatic laryngitis
  Poor intubation technique or the use of over sized tubes may physically damage the larynx and, or trachea, causing post-operative respiratory embarrasment.

- Chemical/ischaemic tracheitis
  If tubes are inadequately rinsed or irritant sterilants are used, the tracheal mucosa may be irritated. For this reason, tubes must be adequately aired after ethylene-oxide sterilisation.
  Over inflated cuffs left in situ for prolonged periods may produce an ischaemic tracheitis and cause post-operative coughing.
- Apparatus dead-space
  Correctly sized endotracheal tubes reduce anatomic dead-space. However, overlong tubes extending beyond the incisor table constitute apparatus dead-space which should be minimised.
- Endobronchial intubation
  Attempts to reduce apparatus dead-space by advancing the endotracheal tube down the airway may result in endobronchial intubation. In these circumstances, one lung receives no ventilation and blood deoxygenation may occur.
- False security
  The presence of endotracheal tubes does not guarantee a patent airway; they may become kinked, crushed or filled with exudate.
- Interference
  Conventionally placed (orotracheal) tubes interfere with some types of oral surgery. In such cases pharyngotracheal or tracheostomy placement may be required. In some species nasotracheal intubation is practised.

Tube Selection

Ideally, the tube should extend from the incisor table to a point level with the spine of the scapula. Provided that the cuff lies beyond the glottis, the airway will be secure. Surplus dead-space is minimised by cutting off the projecting tube.

Intubation

The jaws must be relaxed (preferably gagged), and laryngeal reflexes suppressed before intubation is attempted. Laryngeal reflexes persist in cats to relatively 'deep' levels of anaesthesia and laryngospasm is not uncommon following tactile stimulation of the glottis. In this species, laryngeal reflexes may be depressed with:

- deep levels of anaesthesia
- succinylcholine
- topical lignocaine by aerosol.

Laryngoscopy is useful during intubation in cats, in dogs with pigmented oral mucosae or in those with surplus soft tissue in the upper airway.

Mask Inductions

Masks are used to provide oxygen in comatose or recovering animals, or for the delivery of volatile anaesthetics when intubation is not performed.

Induction to anaesthesia using masks is a useful technique in high-risk cases because animals receive oxygen during induction; if crisis develop, switching the vapouriser off may prove life-saving.

ADVANTAGES

- Mask inductions do not damage the airway.
- They produce smooth inductions when patients are depressed or heavily sedated.

DISADVANTAGES

- Mask inductions are resisted and cause inelegant inductions in poorly sedated animals.
- Masks increase mechanical dead-space.
- They do not necessarily add to air-flow resistance but, because the airway is not clear, turbulence or obstruction can occur.
- Ventilation is possible with tightly-applied, gas-tight masks. However, some gas inevitably enters the stomach, which inflates and limits diaphragmatic movement.
- Atmospheric pollution is greater with masks. This is reduced by using close-fitting face-masks or eliminating leaks with plasticine.

Chamber Inductions

This technique is useful in laboratory animals and can be used in cats and small dogs. Sedation or depression should be present, otherwise inductions may be violent. Pollution is a problem when the chamber is opened. High inspired oxygen levels are present when consciousness is lost; indeed, the chamber usefully serves as an oxygen-cage for neonates or small animals.

Monitoring

The function of important organ systems—central nervous and cardiopulmonary system—together with body temperature are monitored every 5 minutes in order that deleterious trends may be identified and corrected. Details are recorded on an anaesthetic record.

Monitoring Central Nervous Function

Monitoring central nervous function during anaesthesia, a major component of assessing 'depth' of anaesthesia, is an important skill. Animals should be anaesthetised to a depth that only just prevents obvious responses to surgery. This allows surgery to be performed with minimum cardiopulmonary depression. The depth required depends on:

- The procedure being performed. Laparotomy requires 'deeper' anaesthesia than cutaneous tumour removal.

- The specific activity during surgery. In orthopaedics, the level of anaesthesia adequate for skin incision may prove inadequate for fracture manipulation.
- Surgical experience. Lighter levels of anaesthesia suffice when minimal traction and force are used.

Consequently, monitoring surgical events is an important aid to monitoring the 'level' of anaesthesia. The 'signs' of anaesthesia are based on

- Cranial nerve reflexes:
  Palpebral reflex. A 'blink' occurs when the medial canthus of the eye is stroked with a finger. If the test is repeated too frequently, the reflex becomes sluggish.
  Corneal reflex. 'Blinking' also occurs when the cornea is gently touched with a moistened cotton bud.
  Jaw tone. Tension in the jaws indicates light levels of anaesthesia.
  Tongue curl. During 'light' anaesthesia, the tongue curls when the jaws are opened.
  Eye position. The globe may be ventromedial or central within the orbit.
  Pupillary diameter. Dilation (mydriasis) or constriction (miosis) reflects various levels of anaesthesia.
  Lacrimation. The eye becomes dry at deep levels of anaesthesia.
  Salivation. Profuse salivation indicates inadequate anaesthesia.
- Rate and pattern of respiration
  The rate, depth and pattern of respiration are altered by the level of anaesthesia and the degree of surgical stimulation.
- Autonomic responses
  Heart rate, blood pressure, pupillary diameter and capillary refill time are influenced by the interaction between anaesthetic depth and surgical stimulation.
- Skeletomuscular tone and response to toe pinch.

Stages in Anaesthesia

For convenience, the 'depth' of anaesthesia has been categorised into four-stages although this is somewhat arbitrary because it is based on observations in humans anaesthetised with ether.

Stage I (Stage of Voluntary Excitement or Analgesia)
This begins with induction and lasts until unconsciousness is present. The animal resists induction, shows signs of apprehension and fear but later becomes disorientated. Signs reflect a generalised sympatho-adrenal response to threat. Pulse and respiratory rates are elevated although breath-holding may occur if irritant or pungent vapours are given. The pupil is dilated. Skeletal muscle activity may be marked and hyper-reflexia present. The animal may vocalise, salivate, defecate and urinate.

Stage II (Stage of Involuntary Excitement)

This lasts from the onset of unconsciousness until rhythmic breathing is present. All cranial nerve reflexes are present and may be hyperactive. Initially the eye is wide open and the pupil dilated. Later, eyes begin to rotate to a ventromedial position. Responses to toe pinch reflexes are brisk. Breathing is irregular and gasping but later becomes regular.

Stages I and II are unpleasant for the patient and hazardous for the anaesthetist. They are likely when mask induction is attempted on non-sedated animals or when inadequate doses of injectable anaesthetic are given. An elegant induction passes through these stages rapidly. This is achieved by adequate pre-anaesthetic sedative medication and, or sufficient anaesthetic for induction.

Stage III (Surgical anaesthesia).

This is subdivided into three planes:

Plane I

Respiration is regular and deep. Minute volume is proportional to surgical stimulation. Spontaneous limb movement is absent but pinch reflexes are brisk. Nystagmus, the lateral oscillation of the eyeball, slows and stops by end of Plane I, however it is not always present. Eyeball position in the orbit is ventromedial; opening the eye reveals mainly sclera. The third eyelid moves part way across the corneal surface. Palpebral reflexes begin to slow but the corneal reflex is brisk. Cardiovascular function is only slightly depressed.

This plane is suitable for abscess lancing and superficial surgery like skin suturing and cutaneous tumour removal.

Plane 2

Eye position is ventromedial and the eyelids may be partially separated. The palpebral reflex is sluggish or absent although corneal reflexes persist. The conjunctival surface is moist and the pupil constricted. Muscle relaxation is more apparent. The pedal reflex becomes sluggish and ultimately is lost. Tidal volume is decreased; rate may be increased or decreased. The heart rate and blood pressure may be modestly reduced.

This plane is adequate for most surgery except laparotomy and thoracotomy.

Plane 3

The eyeball becomes central and the eyelids begin to open. The pupillary diameter increases. Respiratory rate increases; tidal volume is decreased. A pause appears between inspiration and expiration (intercostal lag). The pedal reflex is lost and abdominal muscles are relaxed. Heart rate and blood pressure are lowered.

This plane is adequate for all procedures.

Stage IV (overdosage)

Characterised by progressive respiratory failure, which begins when ventilation is achieved by diphragmatic function alone; this eventually ceases. The pulse may be rapid or very slow and becomes impalpable. The eye becomes central, the eyelids open, the pupils are maximally dilated and the corneal surface is dry. Cyanosis progresses to a grey or ashen colour of the mucous membrane. Capillary refill time becomes prolonged. Accessory respiratory muscle activity, indicated by twitching in the throat, represents agonal gasping. This superficially mimics gasping, or inadequate anaesthesia.

Overdosage

Excessive levels of anaesthesia should be avoided because they contribute to prolonged recovery. They also cause unnecessary cardiopulmonary depression, which in turn limits organ perfusion, causing post-operative organ failure. Ultimately it results in cardiac arrest.

Underdosage

Underdosage is equally undesirable. In response to surgery, heart rate increases and respiration becomes rapid and shallow (tachypnoea). Blood pressure rises and increased oozing at the surgical site may be noticed. Capillary refill time may become prolonged and the mucous membranes lose colour. The pupils dilate and spontaneous cranial nerve reflex activity may be seen; lacrimation and salivation may be profuse.

Maintaining inadequate levels of anaesthesia because of inexperience or to ensure that the animal 'stays alive' must be avoided because:

- The animal may recover consciousness.
- Movement will compromise delicate surgery, or the animal may extubate itself.
- Catecholamine release may cause arrythmias, and even cardiac arrest.
- Tachypnoea may impair gas exchange and uptake of anaesthetics. Alternatively, hyperventilation may cause alkalosis.

Monitoring Cardiovascular Function

Assessing cardiovascular variables at 5 minute intervals provides information on the adequacy of anaesthesia, on the effects of surgery (haemorrhage, inadequate anaesthesia, untoward reflexes) and on cardiovascular function itself.

Monitoring can be performed by techniques which do or do not involve invasion of the body cavity. Non-invasive methods, which include clinical observation, are simpler, less expensive and more easily applied but the received information is more subjective.

Heart rate and rhythm

Palpation of superficial arteries. These include the femoral, the lingual, the nasal (in the cheek), the ulnar (medio-caudal carpus), the palmar metacarpal (palmar surface of the paw) the cranial tibial (on the dorso-lateral hock) and the plantar branch of the saphenous (plantar paw) arteries.

Palpation of apex beat. Useful in very small companion animals and laboratory animals, or when hypotension makes peripheral pulses impalpable.

Stethoscopy. Cardiac auscultation gives information on myocardial contractility and valve action as well as rate and rhythm. While heart sounds may be heard with standard (precordial) stethoscopes, these tend to fall off even when adhesive tape is used. Oesophageal stethoscopes are less prone to displacement.

Electrocardiography. Electrocardiograms (ECGs) show the pattern of electrical activity in the heart and demonstrate arrythmias. Unlike heart sounds or pulse palpation, they provide no evidence of mechanical activity or cardiac output (which is more important in terms of O_2 delivery). Heart rate meters are simplified ECGs which register the larger 'R' waves. From this, a heart-rate output is generated in beats per minute and there maybe an audible signal. These devices are prone to counting artefacts and occasionally count large 'T' waves, in which case the displayed rate is double the true rate.

Pulse rhythm may be regularly irregular with respiration, which is normal. Grossly irregular rhythm with pulse deficits may indicate atrial fibrillation or ventricular ectopic activity.

Pulse quality (blood pressure)

Palpation. Arterial pulses are felt at the sites listed above. Nurses should aim to judge pulse quality using small peripheral arteries (like the nasal artery) because pulsations in these are lost at higher pressures than those in larger vessels like the femoral artery. This gives earlier warning of developing hypotension. For this reason routine use of the femoral pulse or apex beat should be reserved for cats and very small dogs.

Oscillotonometry. This non-invasive technique involves a pneumatic cuff which encircles a limb. Modern devices are automated and easily applied but are expensive and not entirely accurate at extremes of blood pressure.

Ultrasonic Doppler/sphygmomanometry. This technique also involves a cuff, but systolic pressures are detected distal to the cuff using an audible signal returned from a Doppler transmitter/receiver.

Transducers. Accurate blood pressure measurement is provided by invasive intra-arterial techniques. An artery is catheterised and connected to a manometer or a 'strain-gauge' transducer.

Capillary refill time

Blanching the oral mucous membrane and waiting for blood to return reflects the capillary refill time (CRT). Normally, this is less than 2 seconds. Intensive vasonstriction or hypotension delays CRT.

Mucous membrane colour

This should be pink. It becomes bright pink in hypercapnia and blue with cyanosis (desaturation of haemoglobin). When blood pressure falls and blood vessels in the oral mucosa constrict, it turns white.

Haemoglobin saturation

Pulse oximetry is a relatively new and readily applied non-invasive monitoring technique that measures the oxygen saturation of haemoglobin (SaO_2 or SpO_2). Measurement involves applying a clip to the animal's tongue or lip. Some devices illustrate the passage of blood between each side of the clip by a bar plethysmograph, the amplitude of this moving column is proportional to the pulse pressure and demonstrates cardiac mechanical activity.

Perfusion

The passage of blood through capillary beds is assessed in a number of ways

Combination of vital signs. Pulse pressure, capillary refill time and pulse oximetry.

Examination of the surgical site. Bright red blood at the surgical site indicates perfusion. Darkly coloured or slowly oozing blood reflects poor perfusion.

Core-periphery temperature difference. Cold ears and extremities may indicate that the animal is hypothermic or that warm blood is being retained at the 'core' and withheld from non-essential tissue like skin. This phenomenum is quantified by the simultaneous use of two calibrated thermistors placed at appropriate sites—e.g. over the base of the heart via the oesophagus and on the lip.

Urine output. Catheterising the urinary bladder and weighing collected urine (1 ml urine weighs 1 gm) indicates urine output. A value in excess of 1 ml/kg/h is held to represent adequate renal perfusion, and therefore vital organ perfusion.

Monitoring Respiratory Function

Respiration is assessed in terms of rate, depth and pattern. Rate and pattern reflect depth of anaesthesia; the combination of rate and depth indicate alveolar ventilation. As a rule, rapid shallow respirations are inefficient for gas exchange. Preferably, breathing should be slow and deep.

Observation

Rate, rhythm and pattern are assessed visually. This is difficult when heavy draping is used but observing the excursions (range of movement) of the reservoir bag helps. Excursions are seen more easily in smaller bags.

Respiratory monitors

Most of these monitors operate on the temperature difference between inspired (cold) and expired (warm) gas. They only indicate rate and give no indication of ventilatory adequacy. They are useful when surgeons must operate without assistance. Some respiratory monitors rely on expired CO_2. The definitive test for respiratory adequacy depends on arterial blood gas analysis.

Monitoring Temperature

Rectal temperature measured with a clinical (mercury in glass) thermometer is the simplest but not the most convenient technique. Flexible thermistor probes inserted per rectum or per os (to the base of the heart) are preferable.

General Management

Other activities during the maintenance period include the following.

Monitoring surgery

Stimulating events should be anticipated. Haemorrhage must be continuously assessed. Liaison with the surgeons is vital during complicated surgery e.g. a thoracotomy.

Monitoring fluid administration

If fluids are being given, administration rates should be checked periodically. If a catheter is in place but fluids are not given, it should be flushed with heparin-saline at 15-minute intervals.

'Sighing'

'Sighing' means delivering a supramaximal lung inflation at 5-minute intervals. It:

- prevents diffuse pulmonary microatalectasis;

- allows appraisal of compliance
  low—surgical instrument, assistants on thorax, kinking of tube.
  high—disconnection, cuff leak.
- reduces hypercapnia and hypoxia.;
- provides the inexperienced with the opportunity to develop manual ventilation skills.

Monitoring the breathing system

The system must be continuously monitored for behaviour, disconnection, soda-lime, valve action etc. The pilot balloon of the endotracheal tube must be periodically checked to ensure the cuff remains gas-tight.

Monitoring gas flows and vaporiser settings

Flowmeters may 'drift' with time and should be constantly checked. Vaporiser fluid levels, settings and temperature should also be monitored. Cylinder contents must be continuously assessed.

Muscle Relaxants

Several types of drug produce muscle relaxation, including general anaesthetics. When absolute relaxation is required, however, neuromuscular blocker agents ('muscle relaxants') are used because they are the most effective and predictable. These drugs, derived from poisons used with blow-darts by indigenous South Americans, act on nicotinic receptors at the neuromuscular junction. They have no direct effect on smooth or cardiac muscle.

Neuromuscular blocking drugs do not cross the blood brain barrier and so do not alter consciousness. However, they eliminate some of the obvious signs of inadequate anaesthesia—movement, ocular position and cranial nerve reflexes,—so that monitoring the level of anaesthesia becomes more complicated. Because the animal cannot respond normally to inadequate anaesthesia, the anaesthetist must ensure the animal is unconscious.

The respiratory muscles (external intercostals and diaphragm) are blocked by relaxants and so ventilation stops. Therefore a means of supporting ventilation must be available, i.e. a cuffed endotracheal tube and a suitable breathing system.

There are two types of relaxant based on their mechanism of action: depolarising and non-depolarising drugs.

Depolarising drugs

Succinylcholine has a rapid onset time (seconds) and is short-acting (3–5 minutes) in horses, pigs, cats and people. It is used to facilitate endotracheal intubation in humans, pigs and cats, or induction of anaesthesia in horses.

Non-depolarising drugs

Many types of non-depolarising drug have been used in veterinary practice and some have more or less fallen out of use:

- D-tubocurarine is seldom used these days because injection causes histamine release in dogs, with vasodilation, hypotension, tachycardia and bronchial spasm.
- Gallamine became unpopular because of tachycardia and hypertension after injection. Prolonged relaxation occurs with animals in renal failure.
- Alcuronium, a long-acting relaxant, is infrequently used nowadays.
- Pancuronium, once the most popular relaxant, with intermediate onset and long duration of action (>30 mins), causes modest tachycardia after injection but remains a useful agent.
- Vecuronium, a popular drug, derived from pancuronium, has an intermediate duration of action (20–30 mins). It has little cumulative effects after repeated doses and little, if any, cardiovascular effects.
- Atracurium is another popular relaxant because of its intermediate duration of action and rapid onset time. Its duration of action is curtailed when the drug molecule spontaneously degrades and so the agent is favoured in animals with diseased elimination pathways (liver and kidneys).

Indications for Neuromuscular Blockade

- High-risk cases.
  Neuromuscular blockers reduce anaesthetic requirements and so cardiopulmonary function is preserved. Positive-pressure ventilation must be imposed.
- Thoracic Surgery and Diaphragmatic Hernia Repair
  Positive-pressure ventilation can be imposed without neuromuscular blockade. In paralysed animals however, reduced rigidity in the thoracic cage (ribs and diaphragm) means lower inflation pressures can be used.
- Laparotomies
  During laparotomy, neuromuscular blockers reduce the amount of traction required to produce exposure, causing less tissue trauma on the wound margins with less post-operative inflammation and pain.
- Microsurgery
  Intraocular and neurological surgery, (which is frequently performed under microscopes) require guaranteed immobility.
- Orthopaedics
  Neuromuscular blocking drugs may facilitate anaesthetic management during surgery but whether surgery itself is facilitated is debatable.

- Inefficient ventilatory pattern
  Joint surgery and other procedures occasionally cause bizarre breathing patterns which are inefficient in terms of gas exchange. In these, relaxants allow positive-pressure ventilation to be imposed without the animal 'fighting the ventilator'.

Monitoring Blockade

The degree of relaxation is measured using peripheral nerve stimulators. Clinical signs must be used when these are unavailable. Because diaphragmatic and respiratory muscles are relatively resistant to neuromuscular blockers, the first sign of a waning block is diaphragmatic 'twitching'.

Monitoring Consciousness

Neuromuscular blockers paralyse facial skeletal muscle and eliminate normal reflexes; after paralysis, the eyelids are open and the eye is central. There are no corneal or palpebral reflexes. In animals which are paralysed but not unconscious, there may be paradoxical jaw tone and mydriasis, lacrimation, salivation, tachycardia and hypertension. When these signs are present, anaesthesia must be deepened by increasing the vaporiser setting or, preferably, by injecting intravenous anaesthetic.

Antagonism

Non-depolarising neuromuscular blockers can be antagonised using one of two combinations of anticholinesterase and antimuscarinic drugs: either edrophonium and atropine or neostigmine and glycopyrrolate.

Perioperative Emergencies

Accidents are generally avoidable problems, affecting patients or personnel and sometimes involving equipment.

Problems may be of minor consequence individually but collectively they may create emergencies.

Emergencies are crises that require rapid responses, as they quickly lead to cardiopulmonary arrest.

Cardiopulmonary arrest occurs when cardiac output fails to meet the body's requirements.

DEFINITIONS
Apnoea: the arrest of breathing
Hypoventilation: reduced aveolar ventilation
Tachypnoea: excessive frequency of respiration
Bradypnoea: excessive slowness of respiration
Hypoxia: lack of oxygen
Hypercapnia: excess of carbon dioxide in lungs or blood
Tachycardia: excessive heart (and pulse) rate.
Bradycardia: excessive slowness of heart (and pulse) rate.
Arrythmia: irregular heart beat (and pulse)
Hypotension: low arterial blood pressure
Haemorrhage: bleeding
Hypothermia: low body temperature

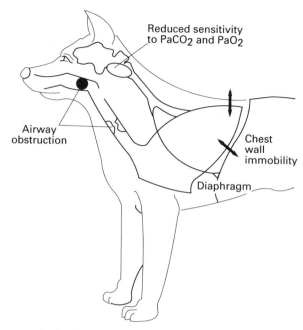

Fig. 27.20. Causes of apnoea and hypoventilation.

Apnoea and Hypoventilation

Apnoea is a dire emergency: severe hypoxia and hypercapnia rapidly cause cardiac arrest. The circumstances in which it occurs are:

- An acute event that prevents breathing (e.g. pneumothorax, upper airway obstruction, intravenous anaesthetic overdose).
- As the end result of progressive hypoventilation.
- As a *sign* of cardiac arrest.

When the heart stops, breathing continues for some seconds until medullary ischaemia causes apnoea.

Signs of apnoea include absence of breathing, or irregular gasping with twitching neck muscles and spasmodic diaphragm contractions.

- In conscious animals the neck is extended, the mouth is wide open, the eyes are staring and the pupil is dilated. Mucous membranes are blue or dirty grey.
- In anaesthetised animals, only ineffectual breathing attempts, discoloured mucous membranes and signs of overdosage may be present.

There are three possible causes of hypoventilation and apnoea (Fig. 27.20) and elements of all three are usually present during surgery:

- Failure of the brain to respond to carbon dioxide or oxygen.
- Airway obstruction (partial or complete).
- Chest-wall fixation.

Failure of the brain to respond to gases

This occurs:

- in severe head trauma;
- when intracranial pressure is raised (for example, by tumours or by inflammatory processes);
- in anaesthetic overdose;
- in severe hypothermia.

The most common cause of hypoventilation is profound anaesthesia, which reduces medullary sensitivity to carbon dioxide and abolishes chemoreceptor stimulation by hypoxia. The deeper the level of anaesthesia, the greater the degree of respiratory depression. Hypoventilation under anaesthesia is exacerbated by hypothermia.

Transient apnoea is common after induction with propofol and thiopentone. While spontaneous respirations resume in the course of time, lung inflations should be imposed if gross signs of overdose or mucous membrane discoloration are observed.

Bradypnoea is caused by:

- deep anaesthesia;
- opioids;
- hypothermia;
- elevated intracranial pressure.

Reduced aveolar ventilation rate results from reduced tidal volume and/or reduced respiratory rate. Conversely, very high respiratory rates with low tidal volumes (tachypnoea) also cause hypoventilation because inspired gas does not reach the alveoli. Tachypnoea results from:

- inadequate anaesthesia;
- pyrexia;
- hypoxia;
- hypercapnia;
- restrictive lung lesions.

Airway obstruction

Airway obstruction in the non-intubated animal contributes to hypoventilation because it causes turbulent gas flow, which increases resistance to breathing. Similarly, undersized endotracheal tubes increase resistance to breathing.

Partial or total obstruction is indicated by inspiratory snoring noises and/or paradoxical thoracic wall movement during inspiration (the abdomen moves outwards and the chest wall inwards). The airway might be obstructed in several ways:

- Soft tissue obstruction
- Blood and gas
- Vomit
- Fluid—pulmonary oedema
- Bronchospasm
- Endotracheal tube problems.

Soft-tissue obstruction. This is likely in brachycephalic breeds whenever sedatives or anaesthetics depress reflex control of oropharyngeal and nasopharyngeal muscles. Sedated brachycephalics must be observed closely and endotracheal intubation performed once consciousness is lost. During recovery, the return of gag reflexes indicates the need for extubation. Thereafter, surveillance must continue because obstruction remains possible.

It must be appreciated that oxygen by mask is ineffective during obstruction. Transtracheal oxygen or tracheotomy is required until the block is relieved.

During recovery, sustained airway protective reflexes may be restored rapidly in cases at risk of obstruction by using drugs with little residual effect, by antagonists, or analeptics.

Blood and gas. Obstruction also results from mycotic or neoplastic lesions, or from blood clots after nasal and dental surgery. After surgery involving the oropharynx, nasopharynx or any part of the upper airway, surgical debris must be cleared before the animal recovers and is extubated.

Vomit. Regurgitation may occur during induction or post-operatively. Rarely, passive regurgitation occurs during surgery.

When there is regurgitation, the animal must be positioned head-down. If it remains conscious, its mouth is gagged and the oropharynx cleared of material. Initially, dry swabs held with towel forceps or haemostats will suffice. Later, moistened swabs may be needed.

If consciousness is lost, cursory pharyngeal lavage must be followed by endotracheal intubation and positive pressure ventilation with oxygen. Endobronchial suction and lavage is then performed. After passive regurgitation in the unconscious animal, oesophageal lavage may be required because debilitating oesophageal strictures may develop later.

Fluid—pulmonary oedema. A froth-filled airway indicates pulmonary oedema which results from end-stage left-heart failure or, rarely, after use of 'Saffan' in cats. Endobronchial suction should be performed, even though the prognosis is poor.

Bronchospasm. Severe bronchospasm (status asthmaticus) is fortunately a rare cause of airway obstruction in companion animals but in theory could occur in response to histamine-releasing drugs—for example high doses of pethidine or morphine given intravenously.

Endotracheal tube problems. The presence of endotracheal tubes does not guarantee an adequate airway. Overinflated cuffs may cause the lumen to collapse, or extreme neck positions may cause kinking. Unless gagged, lightly anaesthetised animals may bite the tube and close the lumen.

Chest-wall fixation

Breathing ceases when the chest wall and diaphragm are immobilised. In pneumothorax, the thorax is expanded to capacity by gas accumulation in the pleural space, resulting in apnoea. Neuromuscular blockers eliminate chest-wall and diaphragmatic activity.

Some breathing systems have expiratory valves. If these are inadvertently left closed, there is a rapid build-up in circuit pressure, preventing expiration and causing rapid death.

In very small animals, breathing may be suppressed when the chest wall is 'stiffened' by heavy drapes, when surgeons rest heavy instruments on the chest, or when the chest wall is covered by adipose tissue. Breathing is also inhibited by restrictive post-operative bandages and by pain after road traffic accidents or thoracotomy.

Treatment of Apnoea or Hypoventilation

If the cause of apnoea or hypoventilation is in doubt, the trachea is intubated and a breathing system is connected. The level of anaesthesia is assessed. Anaesthetic administration is ended if cranial nerve signs indicate overdosage.

The lungs are then inflated at a rate of 8–15 breaths per minute. If this is possible without high pressure being needed, the cause is probably upper airway obstruction or central nervous depression. If the lungs feel 'stiff', there is probably pneumothorax or bronchospasm.

If the animal does not breathe after 5 minutes or so, imposed hyperventilation may have caused hypocapnia. In this case the respiratory rate should be reduced to 2 breaths per minute, and/or the inspired gas should be enriched with 4% CO_2.

Opioid antagonists (naloxone) or analeptics (doxapram) may be considered as a last resort. Doxapram stimulates respiration and elevates consciousness but its use is futile when respiratory embarrassment is caused by chest-wall fixation or airway obstruction. Its effects are short-lived and so the drug is only useful for 'buying time'. It can be infused for a longer effect.

Tachycardia and Bradycardia

The causes and treatment of these two conditions are given in Fig. 27.21.

TREATING TACHYCARDIA AND BRADYCARDIA	
Cause	**Treatment**
Tachycardia	
Inadequate anaesthesia	Increase vaporiser setting or give intravenous anaesthetic.
Hypoxia	End nitrous oxide administration (if used) and ventilate with 100% oxygen.
Hypercapnia	Ventilate with 100% oxygen.
Hypotension	Begin fluid infusion at very rapid rates.
Hyperthermia	Abdominal lavage with ice-cold fluids is indicated.
Drugs	Antimuscarinics and β_1-agonists cause tachycardia.
Bradycardia	
Anaesthetic overdose	Reduce vapouriser setting and ventilate.
Terminal hypoxia	Stop anaesthetics and ventilate with 100% oxygen. Initiate cardiopulmonary resuscitation.
Hyperkalaemia	Ventilate with oxygen and give sodium bicarbonate.
Vagal activity	Check surgeon's activity. If this is related to bradycardia then temporarily suspend surgery and give atropine or glycopyrrolate.
Drugs	α_2-agonists and high doses of opioids produce bradycardia. Anti-muscarinic drugs offset the effects of opioids, but their use with α_2-agonist is controversial. Performing surgery with the animal at light planes of anaesthesia may increase heart rates reduced by drugs.
Hypothermia	End surgery and rewarm as soon as possible.

Fig. 27.21. Tachycardia and bradycardia.

Arrythmias

Irregularities in heart rhythm may reduce cardiac output and cause hypotension. Without treatment some rhythms may deteriorate into more dangerous forms associated with cardiac arrest (e.g. ventricular fibrillation).

Causes

Arrythmias are caused by inadequate anaesthesia *or* overdosage, electrolyte and blood-gas abnormalities, certain surgical procedures and pre-existing heart disease. Certain medical conditions like gastric-dilation–volvulus complex are associated with ventricular arrythmias.

Treatment

This depends primarily on electrocardiography and is based on antiarrythmic drugs. Often, ensuring an adequate level of anaesthesia and ventilation restores normal rhythm.

Haemorrhage

Blood loss during surgery causes hypotension and ultimately haemorrhagic or hypovolaemic shock. In healthy dogs, blood loss results in clinical signs (tachycardia, poor pulse quality, pallor) when 8–18 ml/kg blood has been lost. Blood loss is less well tolerated in cats: 6–12 ml/kg results in clinical signs.

Signs

Obvious signs of shed blood at the surgical site combined with tachycardia, pallor and a weak pulse should raise the suspicion of significant haemorrhage. Loss can be estimated by weighing swabs: 1 ml blood weighs 1.3g. The volume of shed blood can be quantified by deducting the weight of dry swabs from those soaked in blood.

Treatment

Lost blood is replaced with either blood plasma expanders or electrolyte solutions. If blood is used, the volume required equals the volume lost. For blood losses up to 10% circulating volume, electrolyte solutions such as Hartmann's are replaced on a 3:1 basis (3 ml fluids are given for each ml of blood lost). For 10% losses, 7 times the volume lost, are given.

Hypotension

Prolonged hypotension diminishes perfusion in splanchnic and renal vasculature, ultimately causing tissue damage. When hypotension is severe or prolonged, fatal myocardial and cerebral damage occurs.

Low blood pressure results from several factors (Fig. 27.5). Inadequate cardiac output, reduced systemic vascular resistance cause hypotension. Cardiac output falls because of either extremes of heart rate or inadequate stroke volume. The latter results from poor contractility (e.g. anaesthetic overdose) or preload (hypovolaemia). Alternatively, hypotension can occur from loss of systemic vascular resistance when high doses of acepromazine are given.

Treatment

First, fluids should be infused rapidly until improvement is seen. If this does not occur, inotropes (e.g. dobutamine) or α_1-agonists (e.g. methoxamine) may be needed.

Hypothermia

Hypothermia is common under anaesthesia because:

- Hypothalamic thermoregulation is impaired by anaesthetics.
- Skin blood vessels vasodilate.
- Skeletal muscle activity ceases.
- Shivering is inhibited during surgical anaesthesia.
- Visceral surfaces are exposed.
- Inspired gases are cold and dry.

Animals most at risk are those with:

- High ratios of surface area to volume (e.g. neonates, birds and small laboratory animals e.g. mice and hamsters).
- Undeveloped or impaired thermoregulatory reflexes (the very young and old).

There are important adverse effects:

- Reduced alveolar ventilation (V_A).
- Reduced heart rate and cardiac output.
- Haemoglobin binds oxygen more strongly.
- Erythrocytes become stickier; blood viscosity increases.
- During recovery, shivering elevates O_2 consumption and plasma catecholamines.

Consequences

Prolonged recoveries result from reduced elimination of volatile agents, reduced redistribution and retarded metabolism of injectable drugs. This may result in a self-reinforcing cycle.

Cardiac arrest. Ventricular fibrillation is likely when temperatures fall below 28°C.

Prevention

Physical factors

- Increase operating room temperature.
- Do not lay animals on cold, uninsulated surfaces.
- Do not expose to draughts.
- If possible, insulate animals with aluminium foil or bubble wrap.
- Use heated blankets, insulated hotwater-bottles and radiant heat lamps.

Anaesthetic Factors

- Favour the use of short-acting anaesthetics.
- Ensure anaesthetic depth is not excessive.
- Provide adequate but not excessive ventilation.
- Use rebreathing systems where appropriate.

Surgical Factors

- During surgical preparation of high-risk animals, do not unnecessarily wet the animal, clip excessively or use volatile preparations such as alcohol.
- Minimise surgical time.
- Exposed visceral surfaces must be constantly moistened with warm irrigant fluids. Non-surgical areas must not be allowed to get wet. Incision size must be as small as possible. Viscera should be replaced in body cavities as soon as examination or surgery is completed.

Treatment

Post-operatively, the animal should be thoroughly dried using towels and hair driers. Topical heat may then be applied judiciously using 40W light-bulbs, radiant infrared lamps or insulated hotwater-bottles. Small laboratory animals may be placed in plastic bags and their bodies immersed in warm water (they must not be allowed to get wet). If these methods fail, warm-water gastric or rectal lavage may be performed.

Cardiopulmonary Arrest

Cardiopulmonary arrest occurs when cardiac output fails. Failure to initiate effective cardiopulmonary resuscitation (CPR) under these circumstances leads rapidly to death. Sometimes CPR is not appropriate: it is futile when animals with 'terminal' conditions arrest.

Factors predisposing to arrest can develop rapidly (acute arrests) or more slowly (chronic arrests). 'Acute' arrests result from single devastating events occurring in otherwise normal cases (e.g. thiopentone overdose). 'Chronic' arrests result when many derangements develop slowly and remain unnoticed until the cumulative effect is catastrophic. The latter are probably more common in veterinary practice and indicate that close monitoring and rapid treatment of even mildly deteriorating conditions are important. The axiom 'prevention is better than cure' is most important in the context of CPR.

Causes of arrest

- Myocardial hypoxia (e.g. tachycardia, bradycardia, hypotension, myocardial disease).
- Toxins (e.g. toxaemia, azotaemia, anaesthetic overdose).
- pH extremes (e.g. hypoventilation, shock, diabetic ketoacidosis).
- Electrolyte changes (e.g. hyperkalaemia, hypocalcaemia, hypokalaemia).
- Temperature extremes.

Clinical signs of cardiopulmonary arrest

- Blood at surgical site becomes dark and clots easily. Bleeding stops.
- Either 'gasping' ventilation or apnoea is seen (the former resembling 'light' anaesthesia).

- Mucous membranes may become dirty grey, blue or white.
- Capillary refill time becomes prolonged (> 2 s).
- No heart sounds.
- No palpable pulse.
- Central eye position.
- Pupils dilate.
- Dry cornea.
- Cranial nerve reflexes are lost.
- Generalised muscle relaxation.
- Arrythmias. Those normally associated with arrest include ventricular fibrillation and asystole. However, in electro-mechanical dissociation there is a near-normal ECG while mechanical cardiac activity is lost. This is a common cause of arrest in dogs.

Treatment

When these clinical signs are recognised, assistance must be summoned immediately. Simultaneously, preparations are made for CPR, the elements of which are remembered with the mnemonic:

- Airway
- Breathing
- Circulation
- Drugs
- Electric defibrillation
- Follow up.

Before these begin, the animal is laid in right lateral recumbency, positioned against a hard surface and if, possible, in a slight head-down position.

Airway. Effective CPR requires an appropriately positioned, cuffed patient endotracheal tube of suitable size. When assistance is unavailable, tracheal intubation is facilitated by laryngoscopy and is most easily accomplished with the animal in dorsal recumbency. Alternatively, a small-diameter, flexible catheter may be passed to a point proximal to the tracheal bifurcation in preparation for oxygen insufflation.

Breathing. Positive-pressure ventilation (PPV) with oxygen-enriched gas must be imposed. This can be done using any of the following:

- Expired air (containing 16% oxygen).
- An anaesthetic machine and appropriate breathing system flushed with 100% oxygen.
- Self-inflating resuscitation bags (e.g. Ambu resuscitator) which connect to endotracheal tubes and allow manual lung inflation with either air (20% oxygen) or 100% oxygen.

The lungs are inflated using sufficient volume to produce visibly supranormal chest-wall excursions. The lungs are reinflated immediately expiration is ended, but must be allowed to deflate to the normal end-expiratory position.

In single-handed resuscitation attempts, deliver two or three large lung inflations for every 15 chest-wall compressions. Alternatively, insufflate oxygen at high flow rates (5–15 l/min) into the airway.

The femoral pulse, mucous membrane colour and heart sounds should be checked within 30 seconds of beginning ventilation. Thereafter they should be monitored continuously, if assistance is available, or at half-minute intervals. Ventilation alone may restore the pulse but in most cases, circulatory support will be required.

Circulation. When the heart stops, cardiac output must be supported by either compressing the rib-cage (external cardiac compression; closed chest resuscitation) or directly squeezing the surgically-exposed ventricles (internal cardiac compression; open chest resuscitation).

Cardiac output produced by either method depends on adequate venous return. This is enhanced by rapid fluid infusion, posture, abdominal compression and adrenaline.

External cardiac compression. There are two forms of external cardiac compression. The first is most suitable for cats, dogs weighing less than 20 kg, or those with narrow chests (e.g. whippets). The chest wall is compressed in the ventral third of the thorax between the 3rd and 6th rib. This is facilitated if the animal is positioned on a hard surface in right lateral recumbency. For very small dogs, cats and pups, the heart is massaged by compressing the ribs between thumb and forefinger. The compression rate is 80–100 per minute.

The second technique is suited for larger dogs weighing over 20 kg or lighter dogs with 'barrel' chests (e.g. bulldogs). The rib cage is compressed at the widest point—the junction of the dorsal and middle thirds of the 6th to 7th rib—at 60–120 times per minute. If possible, compressions should be made during peak lung inflation.

The efficiency of this second technique is increased by three manoeuvres:

- Abdominal binding
  Applying tight bandages to the hind limbs and then the abdomen directs blood flow (generated by external cardiac compression) towards the head.
- Abdominal counterpulsation (interposed abdominal compression)
  The abdomen is manually compressed during the diastolic or relaxation phase of chest compression to increase coronary perfusion and assists venous return.
- Synchronous lung inflation/chest wall compression
  Cardiac output increases when the chest is compressed on peak lung inflation.

Because ventilation and cardiac compression must never be suspended, abdominal binding and counterpulsation require the presence of a third resuscitator.

The advantages of external cardiac compression are:

- Reasonably effective in certain patients
- Requires little preparation
- Rapidly applied
- Few hazards
- Can be performed by lay staff.

The disadvantage is that it is ineffective in many circumstances.

Signs of effective CPR

Early

- Palpation of pulse during compression.
- Constriction of pupil.
- Ventromedial relocation of the eye.
- Improvement of mucous membrane colour.
- ECG changes.

Late

- Lacrimation
- Return of cranial nerve reflexes like blinking, gagging and coughing.
- Return of spontaneous respiratory activity. Diaphragmatic twitches and irregular breathing appear at first. Then regular deep breathing returns; this is a good prognostic sign.
- Return of special senses: response to sound
- Return of other central nervous function: vocalisation, righting reflexes, purposeful movement.

If early signs are not seen within 2 minutes, two alternative options remain:

- Administer resuscitative (D)rugs and (E)xternally defibrilate (D and E of the mnemonic); or
- Perform emergency thoracotomy and internal cardiac compression.

Nurses can prepare for either eventuality by ensuring that:

- The resuscitation box is fully stocked and that drugs (Fig. 27.22) have not expired. (The VN must know the drugs and equipment required during CPR and be able to reconstitute them).
- Defibrillators are fully charged and paddles are available.

If thoracotomy is planned:

- A rapid clip of the 3rd to 6th intercostal space on the left side may be needed in long-haired dogs. (The appropriate site can be identified by flexing the forelimb so that the olecranon transects the costochondral junction; this point overlies the 5th intercostal space.) However, time must not be wasted in surgical preparation.
- Ensure that a surgical pack containing a scalpel (and blade) and rib-spreaders is available.

EQUIPMENT AND DRUGS REQUIRED FOR CPR	
Drugs	**Equipment**
Adrenaline	Needles and syringes
Atropine	Urinary catheters for intratracheal
Lignocaine	drug administration
Isoprenaline	Emergency surgical pack
Methoxamine	Self-inflating resuscitator bag
Dopamine	Defibrillator
Dobutamine	Internal and external paddles
Propranolol	I/V catheters
Frusemide	Endotracheal tubes
Mannitol	
Methyl prednisolone	
Procainamide	
Calcium gluconate	
Sodium bicarbonate	
Edrophonium or	
neostigmine	
Verapamil	
Doxapram	
Naloxone	
Atipamezole	
A large, clear chart with simple instructions for drug reconstitution should be included.	

Fig. 27.22. Equipment and drugs required for cardio-pulmonary resuscitation.

Accidents

Close monitoring reduces accidents but does not eliminate them. If they do occur, the veterinary nurse must respond appropriately and summon assistance if needed. The time of the accident should be noted and later a report should be entered on the patient's records.

Extravascular Injections

Extravascular injection of irritant drugs like thiopentone result in tissue sloughs. These are painful, take a long time to heal and leave unsightly blemishes. The risk of this is minimised by:

- Effective patient restraint (physical or chemical) before injection.
- Venous catheterisation.
- Using dilute solutions of drug (e.g. 1.25% for thiopentone) in animals with poorly accessible veins.

If extravascular injection does occur, the deposition is enthusiastically diluted with sterile saline or water. There is little advantage in using local anaesthetics or steroids. Large volumes may be safely injected under the skin and massaged. Later a record should be made of the accident.

Drug Overdose

The animal must be intubated and ventilated with oxygen. When inhalation agents are responsible, vaporisers must first be switched off. If pulses are weak or absent, external cardiac compression should be imposed. Intravenous fluids and inotropes (drugs that increase contractility of cardiac muscle) may be considered if circulation fails to redistribute the drug. When available, drug antagonists may be used.

Burns

Burns occur if excess heat is applied to cold animals. This is more likely when skin blood flow is reduced, as in shock, because poorly perfused skin conducts heat less effectively.

Decubital Ulcers

These sores appear when bony prominences remain in prolonged contact with hard surfaces. They are prevented by adequate bedding and frequent turning of the patient.

Hypostatic Congestion

Capillaries in the dependent (lowermost) lung fill with blood and alveoli partially collapse when recoveries are prolonged and cardiac output is low. Both changes result in hypoxia. Prevention is based on frequent (2-hourly) turning.

Equipment-based Accidents

Cylinders

Cylinders contain gas at high pressure (nearly 1935 psi, or 13300 kPa) and will explode if mistreated. They must not be dropped or placed in a position where they may fall or become damaged. They should not be exposed to high temperatures (including direct sunlight). They must be stored in dry conditions away from flammable materials.

When a full O_2 cylinder is exposed to elevated temperatures caused, for example, by naked flames, the pressure within it rises and may exceed the test pressure. Eventually the bottle bursts and releases O_2 that fuels further conflagration.

Explosions and fires

Explosions require a source of fuel (usually carbon-based), oxygen and activation energy (a spark or a naked flame). Once initiated, heat released from the reaction provides further activation energy and the reaction proliferates. Explosions are more likely when fuel–oxygen rather than fuel–air mixtures are present.

For these reasons, 'sticking' valves, or apparatus involved with pressurised oxygen must never be lubricated or sealed with carbon- or petroleum-based lubricants.

In the past cyclopropane and diethyl ether were commonly used for anaesthesia. They lost popularity because of their flammability and explosive properties and their redundancy was accelerated by the introduction of thermocautery and electrical monitoring devices in the operating room. Surgical alcohol remains a possible source of fire and explosion.

Risks of fire and explosion are minimised by keeping the three 'components' separate:

* Inflammable agents must not be used when heat, sparks (from static electricity or electrical apparatus) or naked flames are present.
* If thermocautery is required, cyclopropane and ether must be avoided.
* Naked flames, carbon-based fuels and dust must be minimised.

If fires or explosions occur, the emergency services must be informed that supplies of inflammable material and compressed oxygen are within the vicinity of the accident.

Accidents to personnel

Bites and scratches

These are minimised by suitable physical and chemical restraint techniques, by equipment and by common sense precautions. Fingers should not be placed within the mouth of an ungagged, unconscious animal especially during endotracheal intubation; owners should not normally be allowed to restrain animals in case they are injected accidentally, or bitten.

When an accident occurs, the appropriate report form must be completed. The injured person should report to hospital for examination and tetanus immunisation. If known, details of the animal's condition should be supplied.

Self-administration of drugs

Risks of self-administration are greatest with Immobilon preparations. There is also risk with large-animal sedatives, especially α_2-agonists; toxicity has not yet been reported in humans although the potential is great. Absorption of these drugs across oral mucous membranes is rapid and so placing of needle-caps in mouths is especially hazardous.

Ketamine has been inadvertently self-administered, with ensuing toxic signs.

Whenever drug-based accidents occur, the data sheet or NOAH Compendium should be taken to the emergency room with the injured person. Self-administration can be avoided:

* Ensure that the animal is adequately restrained.
* Do not re-sheath needles but dispose of them immediately after use.

- Do not carry syringes and needles in pockets.
- Do not place syringe caps in the mouth.

When using Immobilon the manufacturer's guidelines must be followed. If drug splashes into the eye or on to skin, the site must be thoroughly irrigated with copious amounts of fresh water. If injection occurs, or if toxic signs follow 'splashing' accidents, the antagonist protocol must be followed. In any event, hospital services must be notified and the data sheet presented to attending clinicians. Many of the guidelines for the prevention of self-administration of Immobilon are appropriate for other potent injectable drugs:

- The needle used for drug withdrawal from vial should be discarded in metal container and a new needle be used for injection.
- Wear gloves.
- Do not pressurise the vial.
- Have eye and skin washes available.
- As assistant capable of giving antagonist should be present.
- The user should brief the assistant on emergency protocol and whether or not diprenorphine (which has a veterinary product licence only) constitutes part of this protocol.
- Naloxone and diprenorphine should always be available.

Exposure to volatile anaesthetics

Atmospheric levels of volatile anaesthetics and nitrous oxide must be kept to a minimum. Exposure has two effects depending on dose and duration of exposure.

- Acute high-level exposure

    Inhaling high levels of expired anaesthetic throughout the working day results in fatigue, nausea, headaches, irritability and, when severe, diminished motor and judgement-making skills.
- Chronic low-level exposure

    Operating-room personnel may be at greater risk of developing certain types of tumour, experiencing reproductive problems and contracting certain diseases. It has not been shown that long-term exposure to low levels of volatile anaesthetics causes these but, until a causative factor is identified, it is prudent to minimise waste gas levels.

Minimising exposure to waste gases

Pregnant women who are concerned about working in areas where anaesthetics are present (including induction and recovery areas where waste levels are frequently higher than in theatre) should consult a gynaecologist about risk.

Improved ventilation. Increasing the air-change rate in theatres has an important lowering effect on pollution levels. Opening the windows has the same effect but may promote undesirable cooling in patients.

Machine performance. The anaesthetic machine, and especially breathing systems, must be leak-tested before use. Leaking bags and hoses should be discarded.

Endotracheal tubes, chambers and masks. Chambers and masks are useful for induction on occasion but should be reserved for deserving cases When used, room ventilation should be increased and the chamber closed as soon as the unconscious animal is retrieved. Whenever possible, anaesthesia should be induced with injectable agents and maintained either with injectable drugs or with inhaled anaesthetics administered via an endotracheal tube.

Vaporisers. Spillage of anaesthetic is reduced if vaporisers have a key-indexed filling system. 'Selectatec' back-bars allow easy disconnection of vaporisers which can then be taken from the working environment and filled elsewhere—outside or in a well-ventilated room.

Procedure. Applying common sense when administering anaesthetics will limit pollution.

- Do not open flowmeters until the breathing system is connected to the endotracheal tube and the cuff inflated.
- Flush breathing system with oxygen for 30–60 seconds before deflating the cuff and disconnecting the patient.

Scavenge. 'Scavenging' is the removal of expired waste-gas (from expiratory valves, pressure-relief valves or expiratory limbs of breathing systems) to a site distant from the working environment. All anaesthetic circuits must have expiratory valves that connect easily to a scavenging hose. Gas scavenging systems are of two types: passsive and acute.

In **passive systems**, expired gases are moved by the combined effects of gas flowing into the breathing system from the anaesthetic machine, expiratory effort and elastic recoil in reservoir or rebreathing bags. Passive systems must not incorporate excessively long scavenging hose or there will be resistance to expiration. Passive systems empty either to the atmosphere through ducts in walls, or into a canister of activated charcoal attached to the anaesthetic machine. Activated charcoal does not adsorb nitrous oxide.

In **active systems**, gas is moved by negative pressures generated by an extractor fan from a shrouded expiratory valve to an air brake receiver (ABR). This has two functions: it prevents the extractor fan exerting excessive negative pressure on the patient circuit and it prevents build-up of excess pressure if the evacuation system fails. It also allows several systems to be scavenged without affecting the performance of the extraction unit. From the ABR, gases are vented to the atmosphere.

Under COSHH regulations there is now an obligation for veterinary practices to protect themselves and their staff 'adequately' against exposure to hazardous substances. The Health and Safety Executive (HSE) inspects premises to see that regulations are being obeyed.

Token sampling for anaesthetic gases should be performed every 6 months.

The Recovery Period

Poor attention to recovering animals contributes to post-operative mortality. Problems are probably more likely at this time because attention relaxes, the perceived high-risk periods of induction and maintenance having passed. Responsibilities during recovery include the following:

- Monitoring vital signs and keeping records.
- Keeping animals calm and dry, and surgical sites and orifices clean.
- Attending to wounds and preventing interference.
- Providing post-operative medication.
- Monitoring fluid and energy balance.
- Reporting recovery problems.

Pain

Several factors determine the magnitude of post-operative pain (see Chapter 2).

Surgical procedures

The degree of post-operative pain depends on surgery and the condition with which the animal presents. Victims of road-traffic accidents may be in severe pain but surgery, in repairing damage, represents an analgesic step. In these cases, post-operative discomfort may require treatment although the animal may, for the first time since injury, feel relatively comfortable.

Some animals experience only low-grade chronic pain on presentation (e.g. osteoarthritis) but are in considerable discomfort after surgery (femoral head arthroplasty). Aggressive treatment may be required in these cases.

Medical conditions (e.g. neoplasia or patent ductus arteriosus) cause little pre-operative discomfort but post-operative pain may be profound. After thoracotomy, special attention must be paid to the adequacy of ventilation.

Patient demeanour can be misleading. Some breeds are more hardy than others but the absence of discomfort does not exclude the presence of pain.

Poor surgical techniques characterised by slowness, indelicate tissue handling, excessive traction and poor attention to wound hydration contribute to post-operative discomfort.

Unnecessarily light anaesthesia allows muscle tonicity; greater surgical traction is then required.

Perioperative analgesics

The efficacy of perioperative analgesics can be affected by the type of drug, the dose used and the timing of administration.

Drugs used. Possibly because opioids produce sedation, the quality of analgesia they confer appears superior to that produced with NSAIDs. Of the opioids, pure agonists (e.g. morphine) seem to produce 'higher quality' analgesia than partial agonist drugs (e.g. buprenorphine). Some drugs are relatively short-acting; if these are not redosed frequently then analgesia will be incomplete.

Dose used. Fear of side-effects promotes a tendency to underdose opioids. As a rule, higher doses can be given with little, if any, risk to cases in which high levels of discomfort are anticipated.

Timing of first dose. Optimally, post-operative analgesics are given before recovery begins because:

- The clinical impression of many is that superior quality analgesia of longer duration is achieved if analgesics are given before the animal appreciates pain, i.e. recovers. This is termed 'pre-emptive analgesia'.
- Some opioids have a slow onset of action; the onset time of morphine and buprenorphine is about 15–30 minutes.

Sequential analgesia. Problems with the side-effects of analgesics are in theory reduced by giving low doses of drugs from groups which act at different levels of the pain pathway.

Assessing post-operative discomfort

Behavioural signs of post-operative pain or inadequate analgesia depend in part on the species. 'Autonomic' signs like tachycardia are common to all species. Common signs of pain are listed in Fig. 27.23.

Dogs in pain have an anxious, 'hangdog', dejected or cringing appearance. The tail is held between the legs. Animals may be aggressive but are usually submissive.

Cats in pain appear depressed; ears are flattened and they adopt a 'cringing' posture. The head and neck are tucked in.

Any suspicion of post-operative pain must be reported immediately, as rapid, rather than delayed intervention is more likely to be successful.

COMMON SIGNS OF PAIN IN ANIMALS
Failure to respond to normal stimuli
Vocalisation (periodic or continuous)
Attention to surgical site
Panting
Abnormal posture (huddling)
Shivering
Disinterest in food and water
Failure to groom
Dilated pupils
Tachycardia
High or low blood pressure
Faecal and urinary incontinence or constipation and urinary retention
High temperature

Fig. 27.23. Common signs of pain in animals.

After prolonged procedures, or when prolonged recovery period is anticipated, the urinary bladder should be catheterised to prevent the bladder from becoming distended and causing discomfort.

Prolonged Recoveries

Causes

After 'analgesic' surgery, animals with painful injuries may rest comfortably for the first time since presentation. These cases are recognised because cranial nerve reflexes are brisk although overt signs indicate depression. Such animals should be monitored but not unduly disturbed.

Pain is likely to stimulate, rather than depress consciousness. However, depression may indicate very severe pain.

Persistent drug activity

The fact that overdose has occurred may only become apparent after review of the anaesthetic record. Acepromazine may cause slow recoveries in certain breeds of dogs (e.g. rough collies, brachycephalics) and in dogs with diminished liver function. Drug retention may result from inadequate perfusion or failure of the liver or kidney. In these cases, haemodynamic support with fluids may be required. Persistent drug activity can be countered if the suspect agent has an antagonist:

Agonist	Antagonist
Opioids	Naloxone, nalbuphine
Benzodiazepines	Flumazenil
α_2-agonists	Atipamezole

However, the use of antagonists cannot always be justified because endogenous pain-systems may also be antagonised.

Hypothermia causes retarded expiration of volatile agents and the redistribution and metabolism of injectable agents. The rectal temperature should be taken and recorded throughout recovery.

The fundamental approach to prolonged recovery is based on nursing (e.g. raising temperature) and creating a diffusion gradient from the drugs site of action to the organ of elimination.

Excitation

Bad recoveries characterised by excitation, hyperaesthesia, vocalisation, exaggerated responsiveness and excessive activity may result from pain, emergence, pharmacological phenomena and epilepsy/convulsion.

Pain

This responds to analgesic administration.

Emergence

Some animals recover after non-painful surgery as if in pain. Disconcerting signs are normally short-lived. The incidence is higher with certain drugs (e.g. Saffan) but may be reduced if sedative premedications are used and recovery occurs in a quiet environment.

Pharmacological phenomena

Cats often 'recover' poorly irrespective of the anaesthetic. In dogs it seems more common after thiopentone 'top-ups' and after propofol.

Convulsions/epilepsy

Post-operative convulsions traditionally followed myelographic investigation with certain contrast media. Epileptic patients may be at increased risk of post-operative seizures.

Hypoxia

Although extubation must be performed when gagging, 'bucking' and other cranial nerve reflexes are restored, it is not safe to assume that O_2 delivery may be safely discontinued. Nor is it safe to give 5 mins O_2 arbitrarily after the anaesthesia ends. Hypothermia, residual anaesthetic drug activity and lung changes may combine to diminish blood oxygenation, while shivering and pain increase O_2 consumption. Oxygen (100%) should be delivered until animals can maintain satisfactory oxygenation on room air. If extubation is necessary before this time, O_2 should be given by:

- Mask
- Intranasal catheter
- Tracheostomy tube
- Transtracheal catheter.

Oxygen must be given for at least 3 minutes after the discontinuation of N_2O in order to avoid diffusion hypoxia. Animals incapable of maintaining sternal recumbency should be repositioned every 2–4 hours to prevent hypostatic congestion of the lungs.

Respiratory depression caused by persistent drug activity is alleviated by antagonising drug effects under certain circumstances, enhancing drug elimination or giving analeptics. Because of the short duration of action, doxapram must be repeated at 10–15 minute intervals or given as an infusion.

Hypothermia

Low body temperature initiates shivering and prolongs recovery rate. Rectal temperature should be monitored at frequent intervals. Failure of temperature to rise should be countered by high ambient temperatures (25°C) supplemented with heater blankets, infra-red lamps or hot water-bottles. Evaporative and convective losses should be minimised; animals must be kept dry and in a draught-free environment. Severe depression of core temperature may necessitate more complex steps such as gastric, peritoneal or rectal lavage.

Topical heat application can have adverse consequences in addition to burns. Cutaneous blood vessel dilation caused by topical heat may lower systemic vascular resistence and cause hypotension. This is more likely in hypovolaemic animals.

Animals which have normal body temperatures may shiver post-operatively; in humans, this is associated with halothane anaesthesia. Oxygen should be supplied.

Discharge

Animals must not be discharged before full recovery from anaesthesia and surgery. Some drugs (e.g. Small Animal Immobilon) may 're-cycle' and owners must be warned of this. The client must also be forewarned of other anaesthetic and surgery-related complications such as haemorrhage.

References

Morton, D. B. and Griffiths, P. H. M. (1985) Guidelines on the recognition of pain, distress and discomfort in experimental animals and an hypothesis for assessment, *Veterinary Record* **116**, 431–436.

28
Radiography

RUTH DENNIS

Radiography is an integral part of veterinary practice and is a procedure in which most nurses become actively involved. The production of diagnostic films requires skill in the use of radiographic equipment, in patient positioning and in the processing of the films. At the same time the procedure must be carried out safely without hazard to the handlers or patient.

This chapter summarises the use of radiography in small animal practice. All parts of the veterinary nursing part II examination syllabus are covered but it is hoped that the chapter will also prove useful for day-to-day reference.

Basic Principles of Radiography

X-rays are produced by X-ray machines when electricity from the mains is transformed to a high voltage current, converting some of the energy in the current to X-ray energy. The intensity and penetrating power of the emergent X-ray beam varies with the size and complexity of the apparatus; portable X-ray machines are capable only of a relatively low output whereas larger machines are far more powerful.

X-rays travel in straight lines and can be focused into an area called the **primary beam**, which is directed at the patient. Within the patient's tissues some of the X-rays are absorbed; the remainder pass through and are detected by photographic X-ray film producing a hidden image. When the film is processed chemically a permanent picture or **radiograph** is produced and the image may be viewed.

The Electromagnetic Spectrum

X-rays are members of the **electromagnetic spectrum**, a group of types of radiation which have some similar properties but which differ from each other in their **wavelength** and **frequency** (Fig. 28.1). Electromagnetic radiations consist of energy in small, discrete packets called **photons** or **quanta**. The energy in a photon of a given type of radiation is **directly** proportional to the frequency of the radiation and **inversely** proportional to its wavelength. X-rays and gamma rays are similar types of electromagnetic radiation which have high frequency, short wavelength and therefore high energy. X-rays are produced by X-ray machines and gamma rays by the decay of radioactive materials.

Members of the electromagnetic spectrum have the following features in common:

- They do not require a medium for transmission and can pass through a vacuum;
- They travel in straight lines;
- They travel at the same speed—3×10^8 m/s in a vacuum;
- They interact with matter by being absorbed or scattered.

X-rays have some additional properties which mean that they can be used to produce images of the internal structures of animals; they are also used in engineering for detecting flaws in pipes and construction materials. Their extra properties are:

- **Penetration**—Because of their high energy they can penetrate substances which are opaque to visible ('white') light. The X-ray photons are absorbed to varying degrees depending on the nature of the substance penetrated and the power of the photons themselves. Some may pass right through the patient, emerging at the other side.
- **Effect on photographic film**—X-rays have the ability to produce a hidden or latent image on photographic film which can be rendered visible by processing (film in cameras is damaged by exposure to X-radiation).
- **Fluorescence**—X-rays cause crystals of certain substances to fluoresce (emit visible light), and this property is utilised in the composition of intensifying screens which are used in the recording of the image.

X-rays also produce biological changes in living tissues by altering the structure of atoms or molecules or by causing chemical reactions. Some of these effects can be used beneficially in the radiotherapy of tumours, but they are harmful to normal tissues and constitute a safety hazard. Aspects of radiation safety are considered later in the chapter.

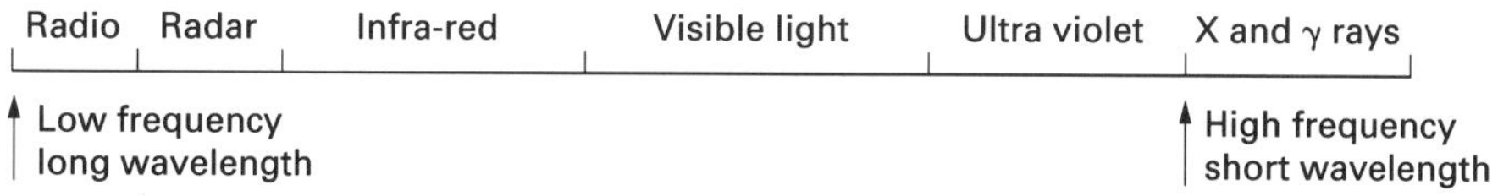

Radio	Radar	Infra-red	Visible light	Ultra violet	X and γ rays

↑ Low frequency
long wavelength

↑ High frequency
short wavelength

Fig. 28.1. The electromagnetic spectrum.

Production of X-rays

X-ray photons are packets of energy which are released whenever rapidly-moving electrons are slowed down or stopped. Electrons are present in the atoms of all elements and in order to grasp the fundamentals of simple radiation physics it is necessary to understand the structure of an atom (Fig. 28.2). Atoms contains the following particles:

- **Protons**: positively-charged particles contained in the centre or nucleus of the atom.
- **Neutrons**: particles of similar size to protons which are also found in the nucleus but which carry no electrical charge.
- **Electrons**: smaller, negatively-charged particles which orbit around the nucleus in different planes or 'shells'.

The number of electrons normally equals the number of protons and so the atom as a whole is electrically neutral. The number of protons (or electrons) is unique to the atoms of each element and is called the **atomic number**. If an atom loses one or more electrons it becomes positively charged, and may be written as X^+ (where X is the symbol for that element). If an atom gains electrons it becomes negatively charged (X^-). Atoms with charges are called **ions** or are said to be ionised. **Compounds** are combinations of two or more elements and usually consist of positive ions of one element in combination with negative ions of another, e.g. silver bromide (in X-ray film emulsion) consists of silver (Ag^+) and bromide (Br^-) ions.

In an X-ray tube head, X-ray photons are produced by collisions between fast-moving electrons and the atoms of a 'target' element. Tungsten is usually used as the target material because it has a high atomic number and its atoms are therefore large and efficient at impeding the incident electrons. Electrons which are completely halted by the tungsten atoms give up all of their energy to form an X-ray photon, whereas those which are merely decelerated give up smaller and variable amounts of energy, producing lower-energy X-ray photons. The X-ray beam produced therefore contains photons of a range of energies and is said to be **polychromatic**. If the number of incident electrons is increased, more X-ray photons are produced, and the **intensity** of the X-ray beam increases. If the incident electrons are faster-moving, then they have more energy to lose and so the X-ray photons produced are more energetic; the X-ray beam's **quality** is therefore increased and it has greater penetrating power.

The intensity and quality of an X-ray beam can be altered by adjusting the settings on the machine, and the practical effect of this will discussed in greater detail later.

The X-ray Tube Head

The X-ray tube head is the part of the machine where the X-rays are generated. A diagram of the simplest type of X-ray tube, a **stationary** or **fixed anode** tube, is shown in Fig. 28.3.

The X-ray tube head contains two electrodes: the negatively-charged **cathode** and the positively-charged **anode**. Electrons are produced at the cathode, which is a coiled wire filament. When a small electrical current is passed through the filament it becomes hot and releases a cloud of electrons by a process called **thermionic emission**. Tungsten is used as the filament material because (a) it has a high atomic number (74) and therefore has many electrons; and (b) it has a very high melting point and so can safely be heated. The current required to heat the filament is small and so the mains current is reduced by a **step-down** or **filament transformer** which is wired into the X-ray machine. (A transformer is a device for increasing or decreasing an electric current.)

Next, the cloud of electrons needs to be made to travel at high speed across the short distance to the target. This is done by applying a high electrical potential difference between the filament and the target so that the filament becomes negative (and therefore repels the electrons) and the target becomes positive (and attracts them). The filament therefore becomes a cathode and the target an anode. The electrons are formed into a narrow beam by the fact that the filament sits in a nickel or molybdenum **focusing cup**, which is also at a negative potential and so repels the electrons. The electron beam constitutes a weak electric current across the tube, which is measured in **milliamperes (mA)**.

The potential difference applied between the filament and the target needs to be very high and many times the voltage of the mains supply, which is 240 volts in the U.K. In fact it is measured in thousands of volts, or **kilovolts (kV)**, and is created from the mains using a **step-up** or **high tension transformer**, which is also part of the electrical circuitry of the X-ray machine.

The stream of electrons impinges at high speed on to the target or anode. Tungsten or rhenium–tungsten alloy is used as the target material because its high

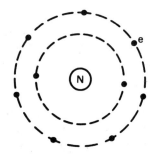

Fig. 28.2. The structure of an atom. N = nucleus (protons and neutrons); e = electron (dotted lines represent electron shells).

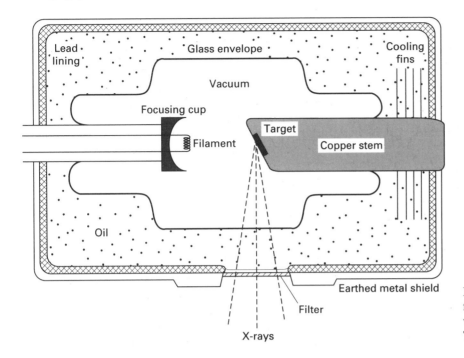

Fig. 28.3. Diagram of a stationary or fixed anode X-ray tube (reproduced with the permission of Baillière Tindall Limited, London).

atomic number renders it a relatively efficient producer of X-rays. Unfortunately the process is still very inefficient and more than 99% of the energy lost by the electrons is converted to heat, so that the anode must be able to withstand very high temperatures without melting or cracking. Tungsten's high melting point is therefore useful in the target as well as in the filament.

In a simple type of X-ray tube as shown in Fig. 28.3 the target is a rectangle of tungsten set in a copper block. Copper is a good conductor of heat and so the heat is removed from the target by conduction along the copper stem to cooling fins radiating into the surrounding oil bath, which can absorb heat.

The target is set at an angle of about 20° to the vertical (Fig. 28.4). This is so that the area of the target upon which the electrons impinge (and therefore the area over which heat is produced) is as large as possible. This area is called the **actual focal spot**. At the same time the angulation of the target means that the X-ray beam appears to originate from

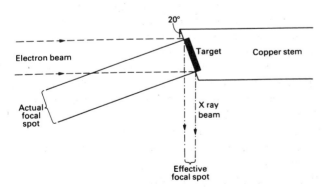

Fig. 28.4. Diagram to show how angulation of target produces a large actual focal spot and a small effective focal spot.

a much smaller area and this is called the **effective focal spot**. The importance of having a small effective focal spot—ideally a point source—is explained below.

Some X-ray machines allow a choice of focal spot size using two filaments of different sizes at the cathode:

- The smaller filament, or **fine focus**, produces a narrower electron beam and hence smaller effective and actual focal spot. The emergent X-ray beam arises from a tiny area and will produce very fine radiographic definition. However, the heat generated is concentrated over a very small area of the target and so the exposure factors that can be used are limited
- The larger filament produces the **coarse** or **broad focus** with larger effective and actual focal spot sizes. Higher exposures can be used but the image definition will be slightly poorer due to the 'penumbra effect', a blurring of margins related to the geometry of the beam (Fig. 28.5). In practice, fine focus is selected for small parts when fine definition is required (e.g. the limbs), and coarse focus when thicker areas are to be radiographed (e.g. the chest and abdomen).

The cathode, the anode and part of the copper stem are enclosed in a **glass envelope**. Within the envelope is a vacuum, which increases the speed of the electrons. The glass envelope is bathed in oil, which acts as both a heat sink and an electrical insulator, and the whole is encased in an earthed, lead-lined **metal casing**. X-rays are produced in all directions by the target but only one narrow beam of X-rays is required, and this emerges through a **window** in the casing, placed beneath the angled target. This is the **primary** or **useful beam.** X-rays

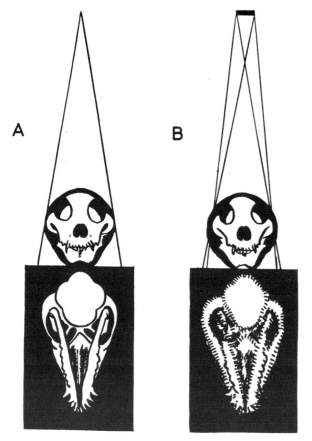

Fig. 28.5. Diagram to show the effect of focal-spot size. In (A) the spot is a pin-point and the projected image is sharp. In (B) the rays from a focal-spot of large dimensions cause a penumbral effect which blurs the projected image. (Reproduced with the permission of Baillière Tindall Limited, London.)

produced in other directions are absorbed by the casing.

Within the X-ray beam are some low-energy or 'soft' X-ray photons which are not powerful enough to pass through the patient but which may be absorbed or scattered by the patient and therefore represent a safety hazard. They are removed from the beam by an **aluminium filter** placed across the tube window; these filters are legally required as a safety precaution and must not be removed. Old X-ray machines must be checked by an engineer to make sure that an aluminium filter is present.

In stationary anode X-ray tubes, the X-ray output is limited by the amount of heat generated at the target. Such tubes are found in low-powered, portable X-ray machines. More powerful machines require a more efficient way of removing the heat and this is accomplished by using a **rotating anode** (Fig. 28.6). In such tubes the target area is the bevelled rim of a metal disc whose rim is set at about 20° to the vertical, as in a stationary anode X-ray tube. The target area is again tungsten or rhenium–tungsten. During the exposure the disc rotates rapidly so that the target area upon which the electrons impinge is constantly changing. The actual focal spot

is therefore many times greater than in a stationary anode X-ray tube and the heat generated is spread over a much bigger area allowing larger exposures to be made, whilst the effective focal spot remains the same. The disc is mounted on a molybdenum rod and is rotated at speeds of up to 10,000 revs/minute by an induction motor at the other end of the rod. Molybdenum is used because it is a poor conductor of heat and therefore prevents the motor from overheating. Heat generated in the anode is lost by radiation through the vacuum and the glass envelope into the oil bath.

The size of the emerging X-ray beam must be controlled for safety reasons otherwise it will spread out over a very large area. This control is achieved using a **collimation device**, preferably a light beam diaphragm. Methods of collimation are described later.

The X-ray Control Panel

X-ray machine control panels vary in their complexity, but some or all of the following controls will be present.

On/Off Switch

As well as switching the machine on at the mains socket, there will be an on/off switch or key on the control panel. Sometimes the line voltage compensator (see below) is incorporated into the on/off switch, which therefore performs both functions. When the machine is switched on a warning light on the control panel will indicate that it is ready to produce X-rays, or, in the case of panels with digital displays, the numbers will be illuminated. In some old machines the filament is heated continually whilst the machine is on, and may burn out. Such machines should always be turned off when the exposure is terminated. X-ray machines must always be switched off when not in use, so that accidental exposure cannot occur when unprotected people are in the room.

Line Voltage Compensator

Fluctuations in the normal mains electricity output may occur resulting in an inconsistent output of X-rays. The images produced may appear under- or over-exposed despite using normal exposure factors. In larger machines these fluctuations are automatically corrected by an **autotransformer** wired into the circuit, but in smaller machines they are controlled manually. A voltmeter dial on the control panel will indicate the incoming voltage which can be adjusted until it is satisfactory. The line voltage should be checked before each session of radiography.

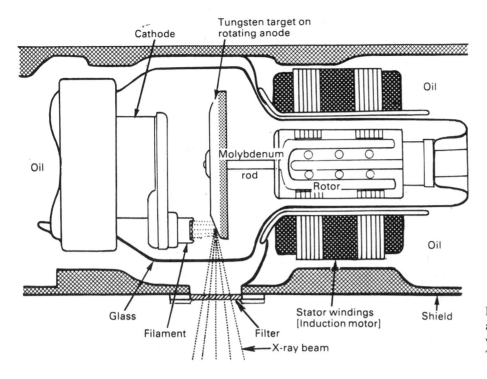

Fig. 28.6. Diagram of a rotating anode X-ray tube. (Reproduced with the permission of Baillière Tindall Limited, London.)

Kilovoltage (kV) Control

The kilovoltage control selects the kV (potential difference) that is applied across the tube during the instant of exposure. It determines the speed and energy with which the electrons bombard the target and hence the quality or penetrating power of the X-ray beam produced. Depending on the power and sophistication of the X-ray machine, the kV is controlled in various ways. Ideally it is controlled quite independently of the mA, often in increments of 1kV, and the kV meter is either a dial or a digital display.

In smaller machines the kV is linked to the mA so that only lower kVs can be used if a higher mA is selected. Often there is a single control knob for both kV and mA and the mA available drops as the kV is increased. This is not ideal since, for larger patients, a high kV and high mAs may be required at the same time, meaning that long exposure times are needed. In very basic machines the kV and mA are fixed, and only the time can be altered.

Milliamperage (mA) Control

The milliamperage is a measure of the quantity of electrons crossing the tube during the exposure (the 'tube current') and is directly related to the quantity of X-rays produced. Moving electrons constitute an electrical current which is measured in amperes, but the tube current is very small and is measured in 1/1000 amperes or milliamperes (mA). Adjusting the mA control alters the degree of heating of the filament and hence the number of electrons released by thermionic emission, the tube current and the intensity of the X-ray beam.

Timer

The quantity of X-rays produced depends not only on the mA but also on the length of the exposure, and so a composite term, the **milliampere-seconds** or **mAs**, is usually used. A given mAs may be obtained using a high mA with a short time or a low mA for a longer time. The two numbers are multiplied together; e.g.

$$30 \text{ mAs} = 300 \text{ mA for } 0.1 \text{ seconds}$$

or $\qquad$ 30 mA for 1.0 seconds.

The effect on the film is the same except that the longer the exposure the more likely it is that movement blur will occur. It is always preferable therefore to use the largest mA allowed by the machine for that kV setting, in order to minimise the exposure time. It will now be appreciated why the type of machine in which kV and mA are inversely linked is less than ideal.

Clockwork timers are found on old, small machines and also incorporate the exposure button. A dial is 'wound up' to an appropriate time setting and runs back to zero whilst the exposure button is depressed. The time must be reset between exposures. These timers are not only inaccurate and noisy but also they do not usually allow the exposure to be aborted if, for instance, a manually-restrained patient moves, pulling the holder into the primary beam. For this reason they are now discouraged and ideally should be replaced.

Electronic timers are found on all larger machines and on modern portables. They are situated on the control panel. They are quiet and accurate and do not need to be reset between exposures.

Exposure Button

The exposure button must be at the end of a cable which can stretch to more than 2 m to enable the radiographer to be distanced from the primary beam during the exposure. Alternatively, the button may be on the control panel itself provided that the panel is at least 2 m from the tube head. Most exposure buttons are two-stage devices: depression of the button to a halfway stage ('prepping') heats the filament and rotates the anode if a rotating anode is present; after a brief pause further depression of the button causes application of the kV to the tube and an instant exposure to be made. Some machines have only a single-stage exposure button; in this case there is slight delay between depression of the button and exposure during which time the patient may move or breath deeply. In old machines with single-stage exposure buttons the filament may be constantly heated while the machine is switched on and in these there is a risk of burning out the filament.

Types of X-ray Machine

X-ray machines can conveniently be divided into three broad types.

Portable Machines (Fig. 28.7)

These are the commonest type of machine found in general practice. As their name suggests they are relatively easy to move from site to site for large animal radiography and many come with a special carrying case. The electrical transformers are located in the tube head and the controls may be either on a separate panel or on the head itself. Portable machines are low-powered, producing only about 20–60 mA and often less. In most the kV and mA are inversely linked. Although portable machines are widely used, their relatively low output means that longer exposure times are needed, and chest and abdomen radiographs of larger patients are often degraded by the effects of movement blur.

Mobile Machines (Fig. 28.8)

These are larger and more powerful than portable machines but can still be moved from room to room on wheels, some having battery-operated motors. The transformers are bulkier and are encased in a large box which is an intergral part of the tube stand. Mobile machines usually have outputs of up to 300 mA and are likely to produce good radiographs of most small animal patients. Although they are more expensive to buy new, they can sometimes be obtained second-hand from hospitals, where they will have had relatively little use yet been well cared for.

Fixed Machines (Fig. 28.9)

The most powerful X-ray machines are built into the X-ray room, screwed to the floor or mounted on rails or overhead gantries. The transformers are situated in cabinets some distance from the machine itself,

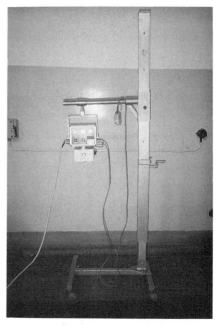

Fig. 28.7. Portable X-ray machine.

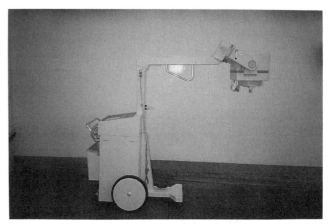

Fig. 28.8. Mobile X-ray machine.

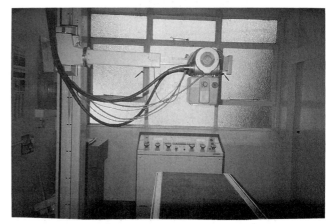

Fig. 28.9. Fixed X-ray machine.

and connected to it by high-tension cables. The largest fixed machines can produce up to 1250 mA and produce excellent radiographs of all patients but (because of the high cost of purchase, installation and maintenance) they are rarely found outside veterinary institutions and large equine practices. However, several companies are now producing smaller, fixed X-ray machines especially for the veterinary market and these are much more affordable.

Formation of the X-ray Image

The X-ray picture is essentially a 'shadowgraph', or a picture in black, white and varying shades of grey, caused by differences in the amount of absorption of the beam by different tissues and hence in differences in the amount of radiation reaching the X-ray film and causing blackening (Fig. 28.10).

The degree of absorption by a given tissue depends on three factors:

(1) **The atomic number (Z)** of the tissue. Bone has a higher effective atomic number than soft tissue and so absorbs more X-ray photons, producing whiter areas on the radiograph. Similarly, soft tissue has a higher effective atomic number than fat. The effective atomic number is the average of the different atomic numbers present in the tissue.

(2) **The specific gravity of the tissue.** This is the density or mass per unit volume. Bone has a high specific gravity, soft tissue a medium specific gravity and gas a very low specific gravity. Hence gas-filled areas absorb few X-rays and appear nearly black on the radiograph.

Combination of effective atomic number and specific gravity produces five characteristic shades to be seen on a radiograph:

Gas—very dark.
Fat—dark grey.
Soft tissue or fluid—mid grey.
Bone—nearly white.
Metal—white, as all X-rays are absorbed.

Note that solid soft tissue and fluid produce the same radiographic appearance; therefore fluid within a soft tissue viscus (e.g. urine in the bladder or blood in the heart) cannot be differentiated from the tissue that surrounds it. Note also that fat is less radio-opaque (darker) than soft tissue and fluid, and so fat in the abdomen is helpful in surrounding and outlining the various organs.

(3) **Thickness of the tissue.** Overlap in the ranges of grey shades on the radiograph occurs because thicker areas of tissue absorb more X-ray photons than thinner areas. Hence a very thick area of soft tissue may actually appear more radio-opaque (whiter) than a thin area of bone.

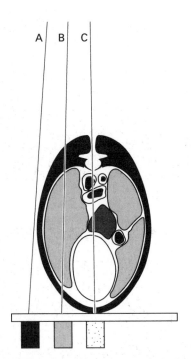

Fig. 28.10. Diagrammatic cross-section of a thorax to show formation of an X-ray shadowgraph. X-ray photons passing along path C are largely absorbed, and result in white areas on the radiograph. X-ray photons passing along path B are partly absorbed and produce intermediate shades of grey on the radiograph. (Reproduced with the permission of Baillière Tindall Limited, London.)

Selection of Exposure Factors

Kilovoltage (kV)

The kV controls the **quality**, or **penetrating power** of the X-ray beam. A higher kV is required for tissues that have a higher atomic number or specific gravity, or that are very thick. Both the nature and depth of the tissue being X-rayed must therefore be taken into consideration when selecting the appropriate kV setting.

Milliamperage (mA)

The mA setting determines the tube current and therefore the quantity of X-rays in the emergent beam, also known as its **intensity**. Altering the mA will **not** affect the penetrating power of the beam but **will** change the degree of blackening of the film under the areas that are penetrated.

Time

The product of milliamperage and length of exposure produces the mAs (milliampere-seconds) factor or total quantity of X-rays used for that particular exposure.

Increasing the kV will cause greater penetration of all tissues and hence a blacker film. Too high a kV will overpenetrate tissues resulting in a dark film with few different shades; this is called a 'flat' film or is said to be 'lacking in contrast'. Too low a kV will underpenetrate tissue (especially bone) which will appear white, on a black background. This type of appearance is sometimes called 'soot and whitewash'; its contrast is too high. Figure 28.11 shows the effect of alterations in the kV.

Increasing the mAs will produce more X-ray photons to blacken the film, though they have no more penetrating ability. The contrast between adjacent tissues (the difference in shades of grey) will not change, but the overall picture will be darker. Figure 28.12 shows the effect of alterations in the mAs.

Although kV and mAs can be seen to govern different parameters of the X-ray beam, in the diagnostic range of exposures they are linked, in that pictures which appear similar can be produced by raising the kV and at the same time lowering the mAs, or vice versa.

A useful and simple rule is that for every 10 kV increase, the mAs can be halved (Fig. 28.13). Conversely if the mAs is doubled, the kV must be reduced by 10. In practice, the time factor is usually paramount and so it is normal to work with as high a kV as possible, allowing the mAs to be kept small.

Focal–Film Distance (FFD)

The FFD is the total distance between the focal spot and the X-ray film. It is important because although the **quality** of the X-ray beam remains constant as it travels from the tube head, the **intensity** falls with increasing distance as the beam spreads out over a larger area. Figure 28.14 shows that if the FFD is doubled, the intensity of the beam over a given area is reduced to one quarter, and the film will appear underexposed unless the mAs is raised. Conversely, if the FFD is reduced, the film will appear

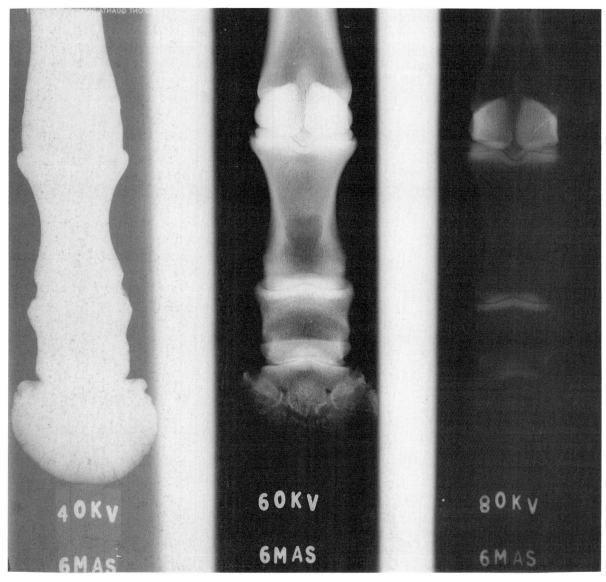

Fig. 28.11. The effect on subject penetration of altering the kV and keeping the mAs constant.

overexposed. The rule governing this effect is called the **Inverse Square Law,** which states that **the intensity of the beam varies inversely as the square of the distance from the source.** Thus a long FFD requires a higher mAs than a short FFD. The exact figure can be calculated mathematically from the equation:

$$\text{new mAs} = \text{old mAs} \times \frac{\text{new distance}^2}{\text{old distance}^2}.$$

It is normal practice to work always at a given, measured FFD; a suitable distance for a portable X-ray machine is 75 cm. However, there may be occasions when the FFD is unavoidably altered, especially in large animal radiography.

Exposure Charts

In order to avoid wastage of film and time in repeating radiographs, it is necessary to build up an exposure chart for each machine. An exposure chart is a list of the kV and mAs required for radiography of various areas of different-sized patients. For the exposure chart to be accurate all other parameters must be kept constant (i.e. line voltage, FFD, film-screen combination, use of a grid and quality of processing). The chart may be compiled for patients of different types (e.g. cats; small, medium, large and giant dogs) or may be made more accurate still by measuring the thickness of the part to be X-rayed using calipers. The exposure chart can be built up over a period by recording in the X-ray day book all the exposures made, with comments.

Exposure charts are not usually interchangeable between types of machine and may not be accurate even for other machines of the same make and model because of the varying factors listed above.

X-ray Tube Rating

The maximum kV and mAs produced by an X-ray tube are determined by the amount of heat

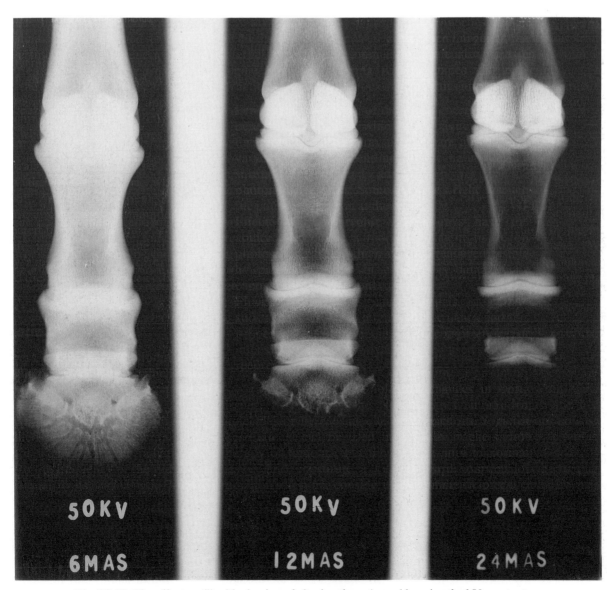

Fig. 28.12. The effect on film blackening of altering the mAs and keeping the kV constant.

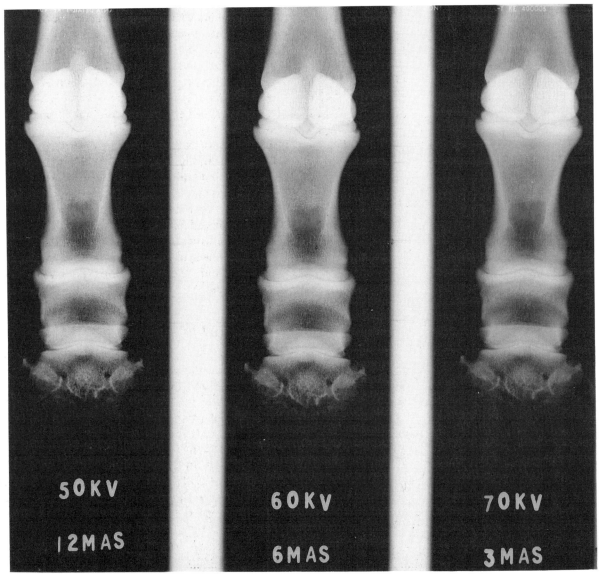

Fig. 28.13. The interplay between kV and mAs; if the kV is increased by 10 and the mAs is halved, the effect on the film is almost identical.

production which it can withstand. If this heat production is exceeded, the tube is said to be 'overloaded' and damage may occur. The majority of X-ray machines, including all modern models, have built-in fail-safe mechanisms which prevent these limits from being exceeded: if too high an exposure combination is selected a warning light will come on and the machine will fail to expose. However, this may not be the case in old machines and so care should be taken to work within the machine's capabilities by consulting the manufacturer's details of maximum safe combinations of kV, mA and time. These details are known as **ratings charts**.

Scattered Radiation

Although most of the X-ray photons entering the patient during the exposure are either completely absorbed or pass straight through, a certain proportion undergo a process known as **scattering**. Scattering occurs when incident photons interact with the tissues, losing some of their energy and 'bouncing' off in random directions as photons of lower energy (Fig. 28.15). At lower kVs and when thin areas of tissue are being radiographed, the production of **scattered** or **secondary radiation** is small and most is reabsorbed within the patient. Scatter is therefore not a problem when cats, small dogs and the skulls and limbs of larger dogs are being radiographed. However, when higher kVs are required in order to penetrate thicker or denser tissues, the amount and energy of the scattered radiation increases and substantial amounts may exit from the patient's body. The problems associated with this scattered radiation are two-fold:

- Scatter is a potential hazard to the radiographers, as it travels in all directions and may also ricochet off the table top or the floor or walls of the room. This remains a problem in the radiographic

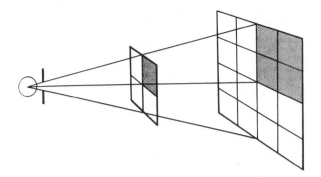

Fig. 28.14. The inverse square law. The intensity of the beam falling on a given area is reduced to one quarter by doubling the distance from the point of source. (Reproduced with the permission of Baillière Tindall Limited, London.)

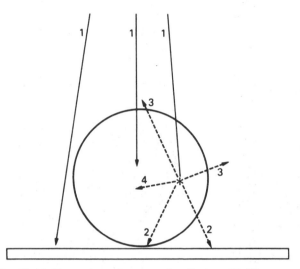

Fig. 28.15. Formation of scattered radiation. (1) Photons of the primary beam. (2) Scatter in a forward direction causing film fogging. (3) Scatter in a backwards direction which is a safety hazard. (4) Some scatter is absorbed by the patient.

examination of equine limbs, although it should be less serious in small animal radiography where patients are usually artificially restrained and radiographers stand further away.

- Scattered radiation will cause a uniform blackening of the X-ray film unrelated to the radiographic image, and will detract from the film's contrast and definition. The blurring which results is called **fogging**.

The amount of scattered radiation produced may be reduced in several ways:

- Collimation of the primary beam (i.e. restriction in the size of the primary beam using a device such as a light beam diaphragm) has a very large effect on the production of scatter. The primary beam should therefore cover only the area of interest, and tight collimation on to very small lesions (such as areas of bone pathology) will greatly improve the quality of the finished radiograph.

- Compression of a large abdomen using a broad radiolucent compression band will reduce the thickness of tissue being radiographed and will also reduce the amount of scattered radiation produced. Compression band devices may be attached to X-ray tables but should be used with caution in animals with abdominal pathology such as uterine or bladder distension.
- Reduction of the kV factor will reduce scattered radiation and the lowest practicable kV should be selected; but this is not always feasible, as in lower-powered X-ray machines the priority is usually to keep exposure time down using a low mAs factor and hence a large kV.
- Reduction of back-scatter from the table top, by placing a sheet of lead or lead-rubber between the cassette and the table top, is now a legal requirement.

The Use of Grids

Even when the above precautions are taken, scattered radiation is still often a significant problem. The amount of scatter reaching the film can be greatly reduced by using a device known as a **grid**, which is a flat plate placed between the patient and the cassette. A grid consists of a series of thin strips of lead alternating with strips of a material which allows X-rays through, such as plastic or aluminium. X-ray photons that have passed undeflected through a patient will pass through the radiolucent plastic or aluminium strips ('interspaces') but obliquely moving scattered radiation will largely be absorbed by the lead strips (Fig. 28.16). Thus there will be a

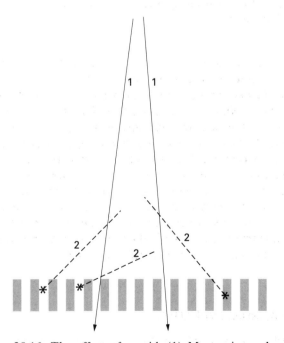

Fig. 28.16. The effect of a grid. (1) Most primary beam X-ray photons pass through the grid. (2) Obliquely-moving scattered radiation is absorbed by the strips of lead.

reduction in the degree of film fogging and an improvement in the image. Significant amounts of scattered radiation are produced from depths of solid tissue greater than 10 cm (or a 15 cm depth of chest, which contains much air), and so the use of a grid is usually recommended for areas thicker than this. Various types of grid are available, and there are two broad groups; **stationary** and **moving grids**.

Stationary Grids

Stationary grids are either separate pieces of equipment or are built into the front of special cassettes. Various sizes are available, but it is advisable to buy a grid large enough to cover the biggest cassette used in the practice. Grids are expensive and fragile and should be treated with care as the strips may be broken if the grid is dropped. There are several types:

- Parallel grids are the simplest and cheapest type of grid. The strips are vertical, and parallel to each other (Fig. 28.17a). This means that, since the X-ray beam is diverging from its very small source, the X-ray photons at the edge of the primary beam may also be absorbed by the lead strips, as well as scatter. There may therefore be some reduction in the quality of the film around the edges; this is called 'grid cut-off'.
- Focused grids should prevent grid cut-off as the central strips are vertical but those on either side slope gradually, to take into account the divergence of the primary beam (Fig. 28.17b). A focused grid must be used at its correct focus-film distance (which is usually written on the front of the grid), and should not be used upside down. The X-ray beam must be centred correctly over the grid and be at right angles to it. Focused grids are considerably more expensive than parallel grids.
- Pseudo-focused grids are intermediate between parallel and focused grids in efficiency and price. The slats are vertical but get progressively shorter towards the edges, so reducing the amount of primary beam absorbed (Fig. 28.17c). Pseudo-focused grids should also be used at the correct focus-film distance.
- Crossed grids contain strips running in both directions and so remove much more scattered radiation (most grids contain strips aligned only in one direction and therefore scattered radiation travelling in line with the strips will not be absorbed). The strips may be either parallel or focused. Crossed grids cost several hundred pounds and are likely to be used only in establishments that routinely X-ray equine spines, chests and pelvises.

Moving Grids

The use of a stationary grid results in the presence of visible parallel lines on the radiograph. These lines may be eliminated by the use of a grid which moves slightly during the exposure. This requires an electronic connection between the X-ray machine and the moving grid or 'Potter-Bucky diaphragm', which is built into the X-ray table. Moving grids are used in larger veterinary institutions and moving grid tables may sometimes be available for purchase second-hand from human hospitals.

Grid Parameters

- Grid factor. The use of a grid means that it will absorb some of the useful primary beam as well as scattered radiation. The mAs must therefore be increased when using a grid (this increases the quantity of radiation) by an amount known as the grid factor. This is usually 2.5 to 3, but will be specified for each grid. In most cases it will require that a longer exposure time is used, as the X-ray machine will probably already be set at its maximum mA output. The increase in time may increase the risk of movement blur on the film, and the radiographer will have to decide whether or not this is outweighed by the advantages of using a grid.
- Lines per cm (lines per inch). The greater the number of lines/cm, the finer are the grid lines on the film and the less the disruption to the image; coarse grid lines may be very distracting. The usual number is about 24 lines/cm for grids used in general practice. Grids with finer lines are more expensive.
- Grid ratio. This is the ratio of the height of the strips to the width of the radiolucent interspace. The larger the grid ratio the more efficient it is at absorbing scatter, but the more expensive the grid and the larger the grid factor. Practice grids usually have a ratio of 5:1 to 10:1. Grids used with more powerful machines may have a ratio of 16:1.

Recording the X-ray Image

Once the X-ray beam has passed through the subject and undergone differential absorption by the tissues, it must be recorded in order to produce a visible and permanent image. This is done using X-ray film which has some properties in common with photographic film, including its sensitivity to white (visible) light. It must therefore be enclosed in a light-proof container (either a metal or plastic cassette or a thick paper envelope) and handled only in conditions of special subdued 'safe lighting' until after processing.

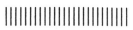
(a) Parallel grid

(b) Focused grid

(c) Pseudo-focused grid   Fig. 28.17. Types of stationary grid.

Structure of X-ray Film

The part of the film which is responsible for producing the image is the **emulsion**, which coats the film base on both sides in a thin, uniform layer. The emulsion gives unexposed film an apple green, fawn or mauve colour when examined in daylight (obviously an unexposed film examined in this way will then be ruined for X-ray purposes!). The emulsion consists of gelatin in which are suspended tiny grains of **silver bromide**. The silver bromide molecules are sensitive to X-ray photons and to visible light, both of which change their chemical structure slightly. During a radiographic exposure, X-ray photons passing through the patient will cause this invisible chemical change in the underlying film emulsion, but the picture is not visible to the naked eye and the film will still be spoilt by blackening ('fogging') if exposed to white light. The picture is therefore a hidden or 'latent' image and must be rendered visible to the eye by chemical processing or development. When the film is developed the chemical change in the emulsion continues until those silver bromide grains which were exposed lose their bromine and become grains of pure silver, appearing black when the film is viewed.

The emulsion layers are attached to the transparent polyester film base by a sticky 'subbing' layer, and the outer surfaces are protected by a supercoat (Fig. 28.18).

Intensifying Screens

Unfortunately, X-ray film used alone requires a very large exposure to produce an image and the use of film in this way is unacceptable in most circumstances. It was discovered many years ago that the exposure time could be greatly reduced for the same degree of blackening if some of the X-ray photons emerging from the patient were converted into visible light photons by using crystals of phosphorescent material coating flat sheets held against the X-ray film. These devices are known as **intensifying screens** (because they **intensify** the effect of the X-rays on the film) and for many years the most common phosphor used in the construction of intensifying screens was **calcium tungstate**, which emits blue light when stimulated by X-rays. More recently a new group of phosphors has been used in intensifying screens; these are the **rare-earth** phosphors, some of which produce blue light and others green light. It is important that the X-ray film being used is sensitive primarily to the right colour (blue or green) and for this reason some film–screen combinations are incompatible. The advantage of rare-earth screens is that they are more sensitive to the primary beam than are calcium tungstate screens and so exposure factors can be markedly reduced, producing less scattered radiation and images with less movement blur.

Screens consist of a stiff plastic base covered with a white reflecting surface and then with a layer of the phosphor. Over the top is a protective supercoat layer. The screens are usually used in pairs and are enclosed in a light-proof metal or plastic box (a **cassette**) with the film sandwiched between. For good detail the film and screens must be in close contact and so the cassette contains a thick felt pad between the back plate and the back screen. Poor screen–film contact causes blurring in that part of the film. The top of the cassette must be radiolucent (i.e. allow X-rays through), and the bottom is often lead-lined to absorb remaining X-rays and prevent back-scatter. The cassette must be fully light-proof with secure fastenings (Fig. 28.19).

Care of Intensifying Screens

Intensifying screens are expensive and fairly delicate and should be treated gently. Scratches or abrasions will damage the phosphor layer permanently, resulting in white (unexposed) marks on all subsequent radiographs produced in that cassette. Screens should not be splashed with chemicals or touched with dirty or greasy fingers. Any dust particles or hairs falling on the screens will prevent light from reaching the film from the screens and will produce fine white specks or lines on the film. Screens should therefore be cleaned frequently.

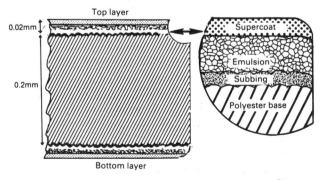

Fig. 28.18. Section of X-ray film, showing emulsion coats bound to the base by subbing layers and protected by supercoats. (Reproduced with the permission of Baillière Tindall Limited, London.)

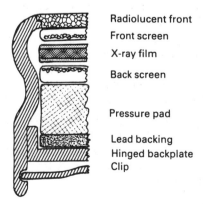

Fig. 28.19. Exploded section through an X-ray cassette. (Reproduced with the permission of Baillière Tindall Limited, London.)

Types of X-ray Film

Non-screen film

This film is designed for use without intensifying screens, i.e. the image is solely due to X-rays. Its use is normally limited to intra-oral views especially for examination of the nasal chambers. The patient will be anaesthetised for this type of study and so the very long exposure time required is not a problem, as the radiographer can retire to a safe distance and movement blur should not occur. Non-screen film produces very fine bone detail and is commonly used in human dentistry. It comes wrapped in a thick paper envelope.

Screen film

This is designed for use in cassettes and is used for all other studies. The detail produced is less than with non-screen film, as the visible light produced by the phosphor crystals spreads out in all directions and will result in blackening of a larger number of silver halide grains than the initial X-ray photon would have done—an effect called 'screen unsharpness' (Fig. 28.20). **Monochromatic** or blue-sensitive film is used with calcium tungstate or blue-light emitting rare-earth screens; it is sensitive only to visible light in the blue part of the spectrum. For use with green-light emitting rare-earth screens, the sensitivity of the film emulsion is extended to include green as well as blue light; this is called **orthochromatic** film. It can therefore be appreciated that, whilst green-sensitive film can be used with blue-light emitting screens as well (since it is sensitive to both colours), blue-sensitive film can only be used with blue-light emitting screens.

Film and Screen Speed

The **speed** of a film, a screen or a screen–film combination is related to the exposure required for a given degree of blackening. A fast film or screen requires much less than a slow system. The speed is due to the size and shape of the phosphor crystals in the screens and the silver bromide grains in the film emulsion, as well as to the thickness of the layers. Fast film–screen combinations require less exposure but produce poorer image definition (the image is more blurred), whereas slow film–screen combinations produce finer detail and are often called **high**

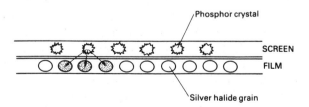

Fig. 28.20. Screen unsharpness. The arrows show how visible light emitted from each phosphor crystal may affect several silver halide grains resulting in some loss of definition of the image.

definition. In practice, a medium speed system is usually the best compromise for keeping exposure times down and still getting reasonable quality images. Rare-earth systems give better definition at the same speed. Different manufacturers describe their various films and screens with different terms, which makes comparison difficult, but most produce three speeds of film and screen: slow (high detail), medium and fast. If a choice of speeds of film–screen combinations is available in the practice, then a slow, high-definition combination may be used where exposure times are not a problem (e.g. for bone detail in limbs and skulls) but a faster combination should be used where it is important to keep exposure times short in order to reduce movement blur (e.g. for the chest and abdomen).

Films, screens and cassettes come in a range of sizes from 13×18 cm ($5 \times 7''$) to 35×43 cm ($14 \times 17''$). It is wise to have several different sizes available so as not to waste film by radiographing small areas on large plates. Hangers of corresponding size must be available if the films are processed manually.

Storage of X-ray Film

As unexposed X-ray film is sensitive to light, it must be stored in a light-proof container. This may be either the original film box or a light-proof hopper. Film boxes and loaded cassettes should be kept away from the X-ray area in case they are fogged by scattered radiation; they may be kept in lead-lined cupboards if stored near a source of radiation.

Films are also sensitive to certain chemical fumes and of course to chemical splashes, and so good darkroom technique is essential. They may be damaged by pressure or folding: they should be stored upright and handled carefully, without being bent or scratched. In hot climates, high temperature or humidity may be a problem and film should be refrigerated.

Finally, film has a finite shelf life which varies with the type of film. It is wise to date the film boxes and use them in sequence, within their expiry dates.

Processing the Film

The invisible or **latent** image on the exposed X-ray film is rendered visible and permanent by a series of chemical reactions known as **processing**. As with photographic film, this must be carried out under conditions of relative darkness because the X-ray film is sensitive to blackening by white light (**fogging**) until processing is complete. There are five stages in the procedure of manual film processing: development, intermediate rinsing, fixing, washing and drying.

Development

The main active ingredient in the developing solution is either **phenidone-hydroquinone** or **metol-hydroquinone**. These chemicals convert the exposed crystals of silver bromide into minute grains of black, metallic silver whilst the bromide ions are released into the solution. This process is known as **reduction** and the developer acts as a **reducing agent**. The length of time for which the film is immersed in the developer (usually 3–5 minutes) is critical, since longer development times will allow some of the unexposed silver bromide crystals to be converted to black, metallic silver as well, causing uniform darkening of the film (**chemical** or **development fog**: see section on film faults). The developer must also be used at a constant and uniform temperature (usually 20°C/68°F) and ways of achieving this are considered later. Precise times and temperatures for developing films are given in the manufacturer's instructions along with some indication of how the development time may be altered to compensate for unavoidable changes in the temperature of the solution.

Other chemicals present in the developing solution include an **accelerator** and a **buffer**, to produce and maintain the alkalinity of the solution necessary for efficient development, and a **restrainer** to reduce the amount of development fog.

X-ray developing solutions are purchased either as concentrated liquids or as powders, to be made up by the addition of the required amount of water. If powders are used, mixing should be performed outside the darkroom to prevent dust from contaminating the working area. Occasionally, skin irritation may be observed after handling processing solutions, usually due to an allergic reaction to metal. If this occurs, clean and intact rubber gloves should be worn when the chemicals are handled. If the problem is marked, a doctor should be consulted and informed of the chemicals involved.

During the development of each film a certain quantity of the developer will be absorbed into the film emulsion and so the level in the developer tank will gradually fall. On no account should the solution be topped up with water, as this will cause dilution and subsequent underdevelopment of films. The original developer solution may also be unsuitable for topping up, as the proportions of the different chemical constituents of the developer change with each film that is developed and the solution becomes imbalanced. Instead, some manufacturers produce special **developer replenisher** solutions which compensate for imbalance. Eventually, however, the developer will become exhausted as the active ingredients are used up and the solution becomes saturated with bromide ions.

Developer will also deteriorate with time by the process of **oxidation**, which will again result in underdevelopment of films. This process can be slowed by keeping the developer tank covered or by keeping the solution in dark, stoppered bottles. Whether or not the developer is actually used, it is unlikely to be fit for use after three months and the general rule is to change the developer completely either every three months or when an equal volume of replenisher has been used, whichever is the sooner.

Rinsing

After the appropriate development time, the film and hanger are removed from the solution and quickly transferred to the rinse water tank. Surplus developer should not be allowed to drain back into the developer tank because it will be saturated with bromide ions and will contribute to developer exhaustion. The film should be rinsed for about 10 seconds to remove excess developer solution and prevent carry-over into the fixer tank. Ideally the rinse tank will be situated between the developer and the fixer to prevent splashes of developer falling into the fixer.

Fixing

Following immersion in the developer, the film is still sensitive to white light and so the image must be rendered permanent by a process known as **fixing**, which removes the unexposed silver halide crystals, leaving the metallic silver image that can be viewed in normal light. The fixer contains **sodium** or **ammonium thiosulphate** which dissolves the unexposed silver halide, causing the emulsion to take on a milky-white appearance until the process is complete. The time taken for the removal of all of the unexposed halide is called the **clearing time** and depends on the thickness of the film emulsion, the temperature and concentration of the solution and the degree of exhaustion of the fixer. The fixer becomes exhausted as the amount of dissolved silver halide builds up within it, and exhaustion of fixer will occur more quickly than exhaustion of developer.

Fixer temperature is not critical but warm fixer will clear a film faster than cold fixer. However, staining may occur above 21°C/70°F and so the fixer should not be overheated. Fixing can also be speeded up by agitating the film slightly in the fixer. After the film has been immersed in the fixer for 30 seconds it is safe to switch on the darkroom light. The film may be viewed once the milky appearance has cleared. The total fixing time should be at least twice the clearing time—a total of about 10 minutes.

A second function of the fixer bath is to harden the film emulsion (a process known as **tanning**) to prevent the film from being scratched when handled. As well as the fixing agent (thiosulphate) and the **hardener**, the fixer solution also contains a **weak acid**, to neutralise any remaining developer, a **buffer** to maintain the acidity and a **preservative**.

Fixing solutions are made up from concentrated liquids or powders by the addition of water according to manufacturer's instructions, as are developing solutions. They should be changed when the clearing time has doubled.

Washing

Following development and fixing the film must be washed thoroughly to remove residual chemicals that would cause fading and yellow-brown staining of the film. Washing is best achieved by immersion of the film and hanger in a tank with a constant circulation of water so that the film is properly rinsed; static water tanks are much less satisfactory. Washing time should be 15–30 minutes.

Drying

Following adequate washing the films should be removed from their hangers for drying. Films left in hangers of the channel type will not dry adequately around the edges. The usual method is to clip the films to a taut line over a sink, taking care that they do not touch each other. The atmosphere should be dust-free with a good air circulation. Drying frames and warm-air drying cabinets are also available and are useful if film throughput is high.

Processing of Non-screen Film

As the emulsion of non-screen film is thicker than that of screen film, it takes longer for the developing and fixing chemicals to penetrate the emulsion and act on the silver halide crystals. Development time should normally be increased by about one minute and clearing time in the fixer will be several minutes longer.

Darkroom Design

Requirements

The darkroom is an important part of the radiography set-up within each practice. The following factors should be considered in its construction:

- Size. Ideally it should be of a reasonable size to allow for satisfactory working conditions, and should not be used for any other purpose.
- Light-proofing. The darkroom must be completely light-proof, and this must be checked by standing inside the darkroom for about 5 minutes until the eyes becomes dark-adapted, as small chinks of light may go unnoticed. The room must be lockable from the inside to prevent the door being opened inadvertently whilst films are being processed. Light-proof maze entrances or revolving cylindrical doors are used in busy hospital departments so that radiographers have free access to the darkroom.
- Services. There should be a supply of electricity and mains water and a drain.
- Ventilation. If the room is used often, some form of light-proofed ventilation is essential.

- Walls, floor and ceiling. The walls and ceiling should be painted white or cream (not black) so as to reflect the subdued lighting, making it easier for those working inside to see what they are doing. The walls and floor should be washable and resistant to chemical splashes; it may be wise to tile any wall areas likely to be splashed.

Safe Lighting

Since X-ray film is sensitive to white light until the fixing stage, illumination must be achieved using light of low intensity and a specific colour from **safe-lights**, which are boxes containing low-wattage bulbs behind brown or dark red filters. The colour of light produced must be safe for the type of film being processed, as green-sensitive films require different filters to blue-sensitive films. If the wrong filter is used, the films will become uniformly fogged whilst being handled in the darkroom. To check the efficiency of the safe-lights, lay a pair of scissors or a bunch of keys on an unexposed film on the work bench for periods of up to 2 minutes and then process the film. If significant fogging is occurring the metal object will be visible on the film. It should be noted that no safe-light is completely safe if the films are exposed for too long or if the safe-light is too close to the handling area. Film manufacturers will advise on the correct filter colour for particular types of film.

Two types of safe-light are available: **direct safe-lights** shine directly over the working area and **indirect safe-lights** produce light upwards which is then reflected from the ceiling. The number of safe-lights required varies with the size of the room but should allow efficient film handling without fumbling.

Dry and Wet Areas

The darkroom should be divided into two working areas: the **dry area** and the **wet area** (Fig. 28.21). If the room is large enough, these areas may be separated by being on opposite sides of the room. Where this is not possible they must be separated by a partition to prevent splashes from the wet area reaching the dry bench and damaging the films or contaminating the intensifying screens.

- Dry area. In this area the films are stored in boxes (preferably in cupboards) or in film hoppers, loaded into and out of cassettes and placed in the film hangers prior to processing. Sometimes films are also labelled at this stage. Dry film hangers should be stored on a rack above the dry bench and there may also be a storage area for cassettes.
- Wet area. The processing chemicals are kept and used here. There should be a viewing box with a drip tray for initial examination of the films, a wall rack for wet hangers and some arrangement for allowing films to dry without dripping over the floor or other working areas.

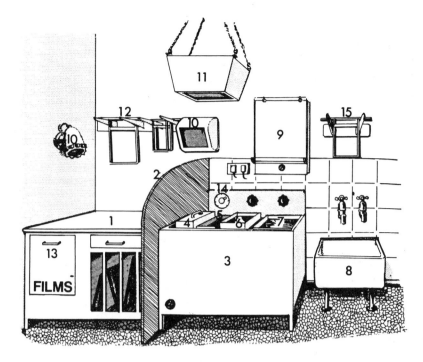

Fig. 28.21. A simple darkroom layout. (1) Dry bench. (2) High partition between dry and wet benches. (3) Wet bench—manual processing unit. (4) Developer tank with lid. (5) Rinse water tank. (6) Fixer tank. (7) Wash tank. (8) Sink. (9) Viewing box. (10) Direct safe-light. (11) Indirect/direct ceiling safe-light. (12) Film hangers on wall rack. (13) Film hopper. (14) Thermostatic control and temperature gauge for processing unit water jacket. (15) Wall rack for wet hangers. (Reproduced with the permission of Baillière Tindall Limited, London.)

Usually, the processing solutions are contained in tanks. Ideally the intermediate rinse water is held in a separate tank situated between the developer and the fixer so as to prevent splashes of developer falling into the fixer. The rinse water should be changed frequently. The final wash tank should contain running water if possible and should be at least four times the size of the developer tank. The developer tank should have a well-fitting lid to slow down the rate of deterioration of the developer due to oxidation by the atmosphere.

In a busy radiography unit, the tanks should be housed together in a larger container filled with water and maintained at a constant temperature (usually 20°C/68°F) (Fig. 28.22). This water bath ensures that the chemicals are always at the correct, uniform temperature for processing and saves time as well as helping to avoid underdevelopment of films. It is not essential to heat the fixer but inclusion in the water bath will prevent fixing from slowing down in very cold weather. Water bath arrangements may be purchased as special units or may be self-constructed, using an immersion heater and a thermostat.

If a water bath is not available the tanks should sit in a shallow sink to prevent wetting the floor. In this case the developer must be heated prior to use, by means of an immersion heater with a thermostat or a thermometer—the latter requires constant checking (Fig. 28.23). The solution must not be allowed to overheat and must be thoroughly mixed before the film is placed in the tank as an uneven temperature in the solution will result in patchy development and a mottled appearance to the film.

If few radiographs are processed, the chemicals may be kept in dark, stoppered bottles and poured into shallow dishes for use (as in photography). Cat litter trays make ideal processing dishes for radiographs. The correct development temperature is achieved either by heating the solution prior to use or by placing the dish on an electric heating pad. The solutions are usually discarded after use, as the developer oxidises rapidly.

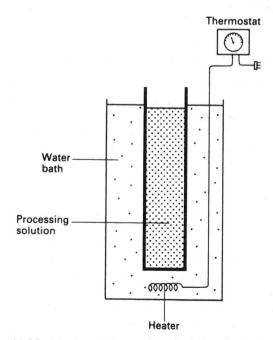

Fig. 28.22. Heating the processing solutions: water bath method.

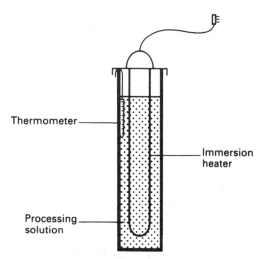

Fig. 28.23. Heating the processing solutions: immersion heater method.

Other Equipment

Film hangers are available in two types: **channel hangers** and **clip hangers**. Each type has its advantages and disadvantages. Channel hangers are easier to load but may result in poor development of the edges of the film. Films must be removed for drying and attached to the drying line using clips. The hangers should be washed after the films are removed, otherwise chemicals may build up in the channels and cause staining of subsequent films. Very large films may not be held securely in channel hangers. Clip hangers avoid these disadvantages but they are more fragile, they are more cumbersome to use and they may tear the films if not used correctly.

A **timer with a bell** should be present in the darkroom so that the period of development can be timed accurately. Ideally the timer should be capable of being pre-set to a given time.

A **hand towel** and a **waste-paper bin** are also useful additions to the darkroom.

General Darkroom Procedure

Most film faults arise during processing and often radiographs which have been carefully taken are spoilt by careless darkroom technique. Competent handling of the films during this stage is therefore vital to the success of radiography within the practice, and it is a duty usually delegated to the veterinary nurse.

General Care of the Darkroom

The darkroom should be kept tidy, clean and uncluttered, with all the equipment in its correct place. Cleanliness is particularly important as undeveloped films handled with fingers which are dirty or contaminated with developer, fixer or water will show permanent finger prints. Splashes of liquid falling on to undeveloped films result in black (developer), grey (water) or white (fixer) patches on the film. Splashing onto open cassettes will contaminate the screens and result in patches on subsequent films due to interference with light emission. Specks of dust or hairs falling into open cassettes during unloading or reloading will become trapped between the screen and the film resulting in small bright white specks or lines on the radiographs. (Even minute particles will prevent the visible light from the intensifying screens from blackening the film in that area although they will not, of course, interfere with the passage of X-rays.) Screens should therefore be cleaned periodically by wiping them gently with cotton wool in a circular motion using mild soap or a proprietary screen-cleaning liquid. The cassettes are then propped open in a vertical position to allow the screens to dry naturally.

Attention must also be paid to the maintenance of the processing solutions, as underdevelopment is the single most common film fault. They should be topped up when their levels fall and they should be changed regularly with a record being kept of the date on which they are changed. Separate mixing rods should be used for developer and fixer and should be cleaned after use. Chemicals splashing on to the walls or the floor should be wiped up, as they produce dust when dry and they may corrode the surfaces. The chemical solutions may also stain clothing and so aprons should be worn while they are being mixed. The temperature of the solutions should be checked regularly and the heater or thermostat adjusted if necessary.

Other important points are to ensure that the cassettes are always reloaded ready for use when the previous film is removed and to ensure that a sufficient number of film hangers are always clean and dry.

X-ray Film Processing Sequence

In order to ensure that no mistakes are made a strict protocol should be adhered to and all those involved in film processing must be familiar with it. The following steps should be carried out.

Preparation

(1) Check that the developer and fixer are at the correct level. Check that the developer is at the required temperature and is adequately stirred.
(2) Ensure that hands are clean and dry.
(3) Select a suitable film hanger and check that new films for reloading the cassette are available.
(4) Lock the door, switch on the safe-light and switch off the main light.

Unloading the Cassette

Open the cassette and take hold of the film gently in one corner between finger and thumb. Shaking the cassette gently first may help to dislodge the film. Remove the film and close the cassette to prevent dirt falling into it.

Identifying the Film

If labelling has not been performed during radiography, label the film using a light marker if available or by writing on the film in pencil.

Loading the Hanger

Load the film into the hanger, handling it as little as possible and touching it only at the edges. With the channel type of hanger, the film is slid gently down the channels from the top, engaged in the bottom channel and then the top hinge is closed (Fig. 28.24). With the clip type of hanger, the film is attached to the bottom clips first with the hanger upside down, and then the hanger is placed upright and the film attached to the top clips so that it is held taut (Fig. 28.25).

Processing the Film (Fig. 28.26)

(1) Remove the developer tank lid, insert the film and hanger and agitate gently to remove air bubbles from the film's surface.
(2) Close the lid and commence timing. The lid is kept on for two reasons: firstly it reduces the amount of oxidation of the developer by the atmosphere and secondly the developing film is still sensitive to fogging by prolonged exposure to the safe-light.
(3) The film may be agitated periodically during development to bring fresh developer into contact with the film surface and prevent streaking.

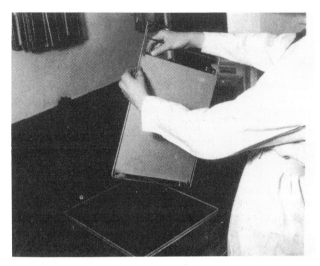

Fig. 28.25. Loading a clip hanger. (Reproduced with the permission of Baillière Tindall Limited, London.)

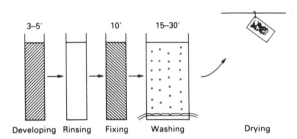

Fig. 28.26. Processing routine.

(4) At the end of the development period, remove the film and transfer quickly to the rinse tank.
(5) Immerse and agitate the film in the rinse water for about 10 seconds.
(6) Transfer the film to the fixing tank. After 30 seconds the light may be switched on or the door opened. The film may be examined briefly once the milky appearance has cleared but it should be fixed for at least 10 minutes to allow hardening to take place.
(7) Wash in running water for half an hour. (If running water is not available in the darkroom the film may be washed elsewhere.)
(8) Dry the film by hanging it on a taut wire in a dust-free atmosphere. Films in channel hangers must be removed first and hung by clips. Films must not touch each other during drying.

Reloading the Cassette

This stage may be performed whilst the film is developing.

(1) Ensure hands are clean and dry.
(2) Open the cassette.
(3) Remove a new film from the film box or hopper. Handle carefully without excessive pressure or bending as unprocessed films are susceptible to damage by pressure.

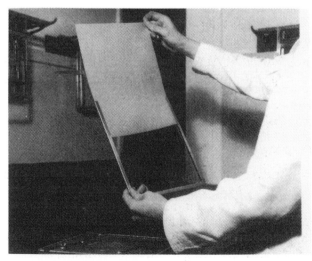

Fig. 28.24. Loading a channel hanger. (Reproduced with the permission of Baillière Tindall Limited, London.)

(4) Lay the film in the cassette and, with a fingertip, ensure that it is seated correctly and will not be trapped when the cassette is closed.

Viewing the Radiograph

Although the radiograph may be examined whilst it is still wet for technical quality, a provisional diagnosis or the need for a contrast study, the image will be somewhat blurred due to swelling of the two layers of wet emulsion. Full examination must be delayed until the film has dried, when the emulsion will have shrunk and the image is clearer. Films should be examined on clean viewing boxes (not held up to a window) in a dim area to allow the eyes to pick out detail on the film without distracting glare from elsewhere. If the film is small, the rest of the viewer may be masked off with black card—a simple procedure that will allow very much more detail to be appreciated. Relatively over-exposed areas should examined with a special bright light.

Automatic Processing

Automatic film processing has several advantages over systems of manual film development as it saves considerable time and effort and produces a dry radiograph that is ready to interpret in a very short space of time (as low as 90 seconds with some machines). In addition, the films are processed to a consistently high standard.

Automatic processors are used in human hospitals and in veterinary institutions. They are becoming more popular in general practice as small table-top processors are now available for about £3,000. A darkroom is still required to unload and reload the cassettes, but only a dry bench is necessary. The processor may be entirely within the darkroom, or the feed tray may pass through the darkroom wall to a processor which is located outside.

Construction of an Automatic Processor

An automatic processor consists of a light-proof container enclosing a series of rollers which pass the film through developer, fixer, wash water and warm air (Fig. 28.27). The intermediate rinse is omitted as excess developer is removed from the films by squeegee rollers. The chemicals are used at a higher temperature (about 28°C/82°F) to speed up the process, and the solutions are pumped in afresh for each film at a predetermined rate; there is therefore no risk of poor processing due to the use of exhausted chemicals. A considerable amount of water needs to flow through the unit for the final rinse and so there must be an adequate water supply and adequate drainage. Finally, the films are dried by a flow of warm air. If the film through-put is high, a silver recovery unit may be attached to the processor to retrieve silver from waste chemicals.

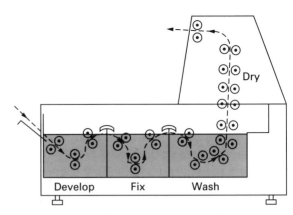

Fig. 28.27. The essential features of an automatic processor. (Reproduced with the permission of Baillière Tindall Limited, London.)

Maintenance of the Automatic Processor

Automatic processors usually require a warm-up period of 10–20 minutes prior to use (longer in cold weather). Films processed before the machine has reached its operating temperature will be under-developed. During the warm-up period an old, clean, processed film may be passed through to check the correct functioning of the processor and to remove any dried-on chemicals from the rollers. At the end of the working day the machine should be switched off and the superficial rollers wiped or rinsed to remove any chemical scum. Once a week the machine may be given a more thorough clean according to the manufacturer's instructions.

The chemicals required are produced specially for automatic processors and are not usually interchangeable with solutions for manual processing as they are formulated for use at higher temperatures. Since the chemicals are pumped in afresh for each film and then discarded, there is no need for developer replenisher solution. The chemicals are made up by mixing concentrated solutions thoroughly with water; in the case of the developer there are two concentrates, one acting as a 'starter' solution.

The automatic processor should be regularly serviced by the manufacturer's engineers as breakdowns can be very inconvenient. Most engineers will also operate an emergency service but nevertheless it may be wise to have the facility to process by hand, should the occasion arise.

Disposal of Waste Chemicals

Waste processing chemicals are currently allowed to drain into the mains, but it is very likely that in the near future legislation will be enforced which will require them to be collected and disposed of separately.

Film Quality with Automatic Processing

Although automatic processing will produce films of a consistently good standard, there is always a slight loss of contrast compared with the best that can be achieved by perfect hand processing. However the latter is not often achieved and so the automatic processor is usually of great benefit to the practice and likely to increase the enthusiasm of the staff for radiography.

Assessing Radiographic Quality

Films must be of high technical quality if a radiographic examination is to produce maximum information about the patient. Errors can arise both during radiography and in the darkroom and the radiographer should be able to assess the film for its quality, recognise any faults and know how to correct them.

Before film faults can be recognised, it is necessary to understand the terms **density**, **contrast** and **definition**.

Density

Radiographic **density** is the degree of blackening of the film and is determined by two factors: the **exposure** used and the **processing technique**:

- Exposure. Film blackening is affected by the quantity of X-rays passing through the patient and reaching the film. It is influenced by both the kV and the mAs. If the patient's image is generally too dark, then the film is **overexposed** and the exposure factors should be reduced; conversely, if it is too light, then it is **underexposed** and they must be increased.
- Processing. Radiographic density can also be affected by processing. **Underdevelopment**, due to the use of diluted, exhausted or cold developer or development for too short a time will cause all areas of the film to be too light, including the background. Development can be tested by performing the 'finger test', i.e. putting a finger between the film and the viewer in an area where the film was not covered by the patient and which should therefore be completely black. If the finger is visible, the film is underdeveloped. Underdevelopment is the commonest film fault in practice, and should be corrected by topping up the developer with replenisher and not water, by changing the solution regularly and by ensuring that it is used at the correct temperature and well mixed. **Overdevelopment** may occur if the developer is too hot or if the film is inadvertently left in the solution for too long. In this case some of the unexposed silver halide crystals will be converted to black metallic silver leading to uniform darkening of the film or **development fog**.

Overexposure and **overdevelopment** may be hard to differentiate as both will cause an increased radiographic density. However, areas covered by metal markers during exposure will remain white if the fault is overexposure but will darken if the film is overdeveloped.

Underexposure and **underdevelopment** can usually be easily differentiated. Underdevelopment will produce a grey background using the finger test; with underexposure the background should still be black but the area covered by the patient will be too pale.

In general, films which are too dark are to be preferred to those which are too light, as they may yield more information when examined under a bright light.

Contrast

Contrast is the difference between various shades or densities seen on the radiograph. A film that shows a white image on a black background with few intermediate grey shades has a very high contrast ('soot and whitewash') and is due to the use of too low a kV with insufficient penetrating power. A film without extremes of density showing mainly grey shades has a very low contrast and is called a 'flat' film. Poor contrast is usually due to underdevelopment, in which case the background will be grey (use the finger test). Overexposure, overdevelopment and various types of fogging will also produce a flat film but in this case the background density will be black and the remainder of the film will also be very dark.

Definition

Definition refers to the sharpness and clarity of the structures visible on a radiograph. Good definition is usually essential if the film is to be diagnostic.

Definition may be affected by a number of factors:

- Movement blur. This is the most common cause of poor definition on chest and abdominal radiographs and is usually due to respiration or struggling by the patient. It may also occur if the tube stand is unstable or if the cassette moves (the latter is applicable only to equine radiography). Patient movement is minimised by the use of sedation or general anaesthesia and by adequate artificial restraint using sandbags etc. The exposure time should be kept as low as possible.
- Scattered radiation. Scattered radiation produced when thick or dense areas of tissue are X-rayed will produce random darkening of the film resulting in loss of definition and contrast. Its effects may be reduced by collimating the beam and by the use of a grid.
- Fog. Fogging is darkening of the film unrelated to the radiographic image and has a number of causes. These include scattered radiation, accidental exposure of the film to radiation or

white light prior to or during processing, the use of an unsuitable safe-light filter, prolonged storage and overdevelopment. The result is a loss of definition and contrast.

- Poor screen–film contact. Poor contact between the intensifying screen and the film within the cassette due to shrinkage of the felt pad will cause blurring of the image in the affected area. It will be present in the same place on all films taken in that cassette.
- Film and screen speed. Fast film–screen combinations require a smaller exposure for a given degree of film blackening than do slower combinations, but the definition of the image is poorer due to the larger size of the phosphor crystals in the intensifying screens and to the characteristics of the film emulsion.
- Focal spot size. Some machines allow a choice of focal spot size. **Fine focus** produces finer radiographic detail but the exposure factors available are limited. **Coarse focus** allows higher exposure factors but, since the effective focal spot is larger, some detail is lost by the penumbra effect (Fig. 28.5). The penumbra effect is reduced by keeping the object–film distance as small as possible and by using a reasonably long focus-film distance (Fig. 28.28).
- Magnification and object–film distance. Since the X-ray beam diverges from the focal spot, the geometry of the X-ray beam results in some degree of magnification of the image. In order to reduce this effect, the part being radiographed should always be positioned as close as possible to the film, with the focus-film distance as long as is practicable for that machine (Fig. 28.28).

The more common film faults and their remedies are summarised in Figure 28.29.

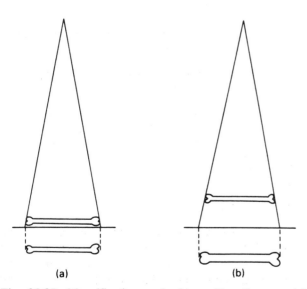

(a)   (b)

Fig. 28.28. Magnification and object—film distance: (a) object close to film so reproduced accurately on radiograph; (b) object not close to film so image is magnified.

Labelling of Films

All radiographs should be permanently labelled with the case identification (name or number), the date, a right or left marker if appropriate and any other relevant details (e.g. time after administration of a contrast medium). Labelling of the paper sleeve or film envelope only is inadequate and liable to cause mix-ups, especially on busy days.

Films can be labelled at one of three stages:

- Labelling of film during exposure. Films can be identified during radiography by placing lead letters on the cassette or by writing details on special lead tape which is then stuck to the cassette. Care should be taken to ensure that the whole of the information appears on the film after processing and is neither lost on the edge of the film or overexposed. Right or left markers should be used at this stage and not substituted for by the use of personal codes such as scissors or keys!
- Labelling in the darkroom. Films may also be identified by labelling in the darkroom prior to processing. The most efficient method is to use a light marker, which is a small device that prints information, written or typed on paper, on to the corner of the film, using white light. A small, rectangular area in the corner of the film must therefore be protected from exposure to X-rays by the incorporation of a piece of lead in the cassette to act as a blocker and leave a space on the film on which these details may be printed. If no light marker is available, case details may be temporarily inscribed on the film in pencil but must be reinforced after processing.
- Labelling of the dry film. Information may be written on the film after processing using a white 'Chinagraph' pencil, white ink or a black felt-tip pen. Such identification may not be acceptable for films used in legal cases.

Identification of Films for the BVA/KC Hip Dysplasia Scoring Scheme

The requirement for submission of films to the Hip Dysplasia Scoring Scheme is that they must be identified with the dog's Kennel Club number during radiography, i.e. using lead letters or tape. Subsequent labelling is not acceptable. The date and a right or left marker must also be present.

Filing of Radiographs

Radiographs may be required for retrospective study or as legal documents and so should be clearly labelled and carefully filed. Many films can accumulate within a short space of time in a busy practice and the filing system must be simple and fool-proof.

COMMON FILM FAULTS AND THEIR REMEDIES		
Fault	**Cause**	**Remedy**
Film too dark	overexposure overdevelopment fogging	reduce exposure factors check developer temperature time development accurately (see below)
Film too pale	underexposure (background black but image too light) underdevelopment (background pale)	increase exposure factors check developer temperature time development accurately change developer
Patch film density	developer not stirred film not agitated in developer	correct development technique
Contrast too high ("soot and whitewash" film)	kV too low	increase kV
Contrast too low ("flat film")	overexposure underdevelopment overdevelopment fogging	reduce exposure factors correct development technique (see below)
Fogging	scattered radiation from patient scattered radiation from elsewhere exposure to white light before fixing stage storage fog (prolonged storage) chemical or development fog	collimate beam; use grid change storage area for films/cassettes check darkroom, film, hoppers, cassettes, safelights use films before expiry date correct development techniques
Image blurring	patient movement tube head movement cassette movement scattered radiation fogging poor screen-film contact	as for causes
Extraneous marks (artefacts): small, bright marks white, grey or black patches scratches	dirt on screens chemical splashes on film or screen careless handling of unprocessed film	clean screens correct darkroom techniques clean screens handle film carefully prior to fixing and hardening
Black or white crescentic crimp marks	bending of unprocessed film	handle film carefully
Fingerprints	handling with dirty fingers	clean hands handle through paper if film individually wrapped
Static marks (branching black lines)	static electricity	handle unprocessed film carefully use anti-static screen cleaner
Chemical staining: yellow-brown patches borders around films dichroic fog (pink-green) Grid lines too coarse	insufficient fixing or washing use of dirty channel hangers insufficient washing; exhausted fixer X-ray beam not perpendicular to grid focussed or pseudo focussed grid upside down or at wrong F.F.D.	correct fixing or washing procedure clean hangers correct washing procedure; change fixer correct use of grid

Fig. 28.29. Common film faults and their remedies.

Films processed manually must be completely dry before filing, otherwise they will be damaged by sticking to paper. Films may be stored in their original paper folders or in special X-ray envelopes, with case details (e.g. owner's name, patient information and date) marked clearly on the outside. These may then be kept in film boxes, files or filing cabinets depending on the number of films involved. Films may be stored either chronologically or in alphabetical order of owner's name, with films from each year being kept separately. Films of special interest or good examples of normals may be mounted in plastic sleeves and kept for reference.

Radiation Protection

The Dangers Associated with Radiography

Exposure of the human or animal body to radiation is not without hazard because of the biological effects which X-rays have on living tissues via cellular chemical reactions. X-rays have four properties which mean that the danger from them may be seriously underestimated:

* They are **invisible.**
* They are **painless.**
* Their effects are **latent**, i.e. they are not evident immediately and may not manifest until some time later.
* Their effects are **cumulative**, so that repeated very low doses may be as hazardous as a single large exposure.

Large doses are unlikely to occur in human or veterinary radiography but may be seen after nuclear accidents. It is the danger arising from repeated exposure to small amounts of radiation that concerns people working with veterinary radiography.

The adverse effects of radiation on the body may be divided into three groups: Somatic, carcinogenic and genetic.

* Somatic effects. These are direct changes in body tissues which usually occur soon after exposure. They include changes such as skin reddening and cracking, blood disorders, baldness, cataract formation and digestive upsets. The latter cause severe dehydration which is the usual cause of death following nuclear accidents and bombs. Different tissues vary in their susceptibility to this type of damage, with the developing foetus being particularly susceptible. The somatic effect is used to advantage in the radiotherapy of tumours.
* Carcinogenic effects. These are the induction of tumours in tissues that have been exposed to radiation. There may be a considerable time lag before these tumours arise, which may be as long as 20 or 30 years in the case of leukaemia.
* Genetic effects. These occur when gonads are irradiated and mutations are induced in the chromosomes of germ cells. The mutations may give rise to inherited abnormalities in the offspring.

Despite these hazards, it is possible to perform radiography in veterinary practice with no significant risk to any of the people involved, providing that adequate precautions are taken.

Sources of Radiation Hazard

During an exposure, there are three potential sources of X-rays that may be hazardous to the radiographers (Fig. 28.30).

* The tube head. Although the tube head is lead-lined (except at the window where the primary beam emerges), older machines may have suffered cracks in the casing, which allow X-rays to escape in other directions. For this reason the tube head should never be held or touched during an exposure. Checks on the efficiency of the casing can be made by engineers but a simple test may be performed by taping envelope-wrapped non-screen film to the tube head, leaving it for a few exposures and then processing it. Any cracks in the casing will cause black lines to appear on the film, where it has been exposed.
* The primary beam. The beam of X-rays produced at the anode is directed out of the tube head through the window. This primary beam constitutes the greatest safety hazard, since it consists of high energy X-rays. It may be visualised using a **light beam diaphragm**, a device attached to the tube head which produces a light over the area covered by the X-ray beam (Fig. 28.31). The light beam diaphragm usually contains crossed wires which produce a shadow in the illuminated area showing the position of the centre of the beam (the **central ray**). Movable metal plates operated by knobs allow the area covered to be adjusted to the size required, a procedure known as **collimation**. Collimation should always be as 'tight' as possible (i.e. to as small an area as possible) and the accuracy of the light beam diaphragm should be checked periodically.

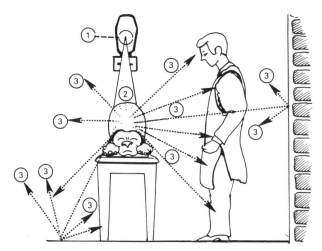

Fig. 28.30. The spread of scattered radiation. (1) The tube head. (2) The primary beam. (3) Scattered radiation. (Reproduced with the permission of Baillière Tindall Limited, London.)

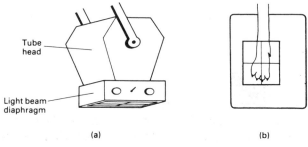

Fig. 28.31. (a) Light beam diaphragm. (b) Centring and collimating a paw.

An alternative method of collimation is to use conical or cylindrical devices or **cones** attached to the tube window to produce a circular primary beam of varying diameter. Cones are much less satisfactory than light beam diaphragms since the area covered by the primary beam is merely estimated. Metal plates with holes of varying sizes can also be placed over the window to restrict the primary beam but these are even less accurate than cones and should be avoided. Whichever method of collimation is used, the area covered by the primary beam should be no larger than the size of the cassette, and so the borders of the beam should be visible on the processed radiograph.

No part of any handler should come within the primary beam, even if protected by lead rubber clothing. In the rare cases where animals have to be held for radiography, a light beam diaphragm **must** be used to ensure that the primary beam is safely collimated. To prevent the primary beam from passing through the table and scattering off the floor or irradiating the feet of any handlers the table-top should be covered with lead or else a lead sheet placed underneath the cassette.

The use of a horizontal X-ray beam is especially hazardous as the primary beam may pass through doors, windows and thin walls. This procedure should only be performed with great care.

- Secondary or scattered radiation. Scattered radiation is produced in all directions when the primary beam strikes a solid object, and so it arises from the patient and the cassette. It is produced by the table or floor if the table-top is not lead lined and it can also bounce off walls and ceilings and travel in unexpected directions. It is, however, of much lower energy than the primary beam and is absorbed by protective clothing. Its intensity falls off rapidly with distance from the source (due to the Inverse Square Law). The best protection against scatter is to stand as far from the X-ray machine and patient as possible.

Ways of reducing the amount of scatter produced (as already discussed in the section on Scattered Radiation) include tight collimation of the primary beam, compression of large areas of soft tissue, reduction in the kV where possible and the use of lead-backed cassettes and a lead-topped table. Protection against scatter is also afforded by protective clothing. The rotation of staff involved in radiography is advisable.

Legislation

In 1985 the law governing the use of radiation and radioactive materials was revised and updated with the publication of **The Ionising Radiations Regulations 1985**. This legal document covers all uses of radiation and radioactive materials, including veterinary radiography. As it is written in legal terms and is somewhat lengthy, a second booklet was published at the same time which attempted to explain the Regulations, and is called the **Approved Code of Practice for the Protection of Persons against Ionising Radiation arising from any Work Activity**. The Code of Practice does contain some specific references to veterinary radiography but is also rather long-winded and so easy-to-read guidance notes explaining the law as it applies to veterinary radiography were published in July 1988 (**Guidance notes for the protection of persons against ionising radiations arising from veterinary use** ISBN 0 85951 300 9 H.M.S.O.). These cover premises, equipment, personnel and procedures and aim to minimise radiation doses received by veterinary staff. A summary of the legislation is given in the following paragraphs.

Principles of Radiographic Protection

Protection follows three basic principles:

(1) Radiography should only be undertaken if there is definite clinical justification for the use of the procedure.
(2) Any exposure of personnel should be kept to a minimum.
(3) No dose limit should be exceeded.

The aim is to avoid exposure at all times, but failing this a high standard of protection will exist if the advice contained in the Guidance Notes is followed.

Notification of the Health and Safety Executive (HSE)

All practices using X-ray machines must notify the HSE that they are doing so, by filling in Form F2522 9/85. They may then be subject to periodic visits by HSE inspectors to ensure that they are complying with the law.

Practices which are failing to do so may be served with compulsory improvement orders or even prosecuted.

Radiation Protection Supervisor (RPS)

An RPS must be appointed within the practice and will usually be the principal or a senior partner. The RPS is responsible for ensuring that radiography is carried out safely and in accordance with the Regulations, and that the Local Rules (see below) are obeyed, but need not be present at every radiographic examination.

Radiation Protection Advisor (RPA)

Most practices also need to appoint an external RPA The qualifications necessary to act as an RPA are laid down in the Approved Code of Practice and include veterinary surgeons who hold the Diploma in Veterinary Radiology and who have a knowledge of radiation physics, and medical physicists with an interest in veterinary radiography. The RPA will give advice on all aspects of radiation protection, the demarcation of the controlled area and the drawing up of Local Rules and Written Systems of Work.

The Controlled Area

A specific room should be identified for small animal radiography and should have sufficiently thick walls that no part of the controlled area extends outside it (single brick is usually adequate; thin walls may be reinforced with lead ply or barium plaster). The room should be large enough to allow people remaining in the room to stand at least 2 m from the primary beam. If this is not possible, a protective lead screen must be provided. Unshielded doors and windows may be acceptable if the work load is low and the room is large enough. Special recommendations are made for flooring in rare cases where there may be an occupied area below the radiography room.

Technically, the **controlled area** is the area around the primary beam within which the average dose rate of exposure exceeds a given limit (laid down in the Regulations). The controlled area for a typical practice is within a 2 m radius from the beam but usually needs to be defined by the RPA. Since the controlled area must be physically demarcated and clearly labelled, it is usually simpler to designate the whole X-ray room as a controlled area and to place warning notices on its doors to exclude people not involved in radiography. When the radiographic examination is completed the X-ray machine must be disconnected from the power supply; the room then ceases to be a controlled area and may be entered freely.

A warning sign should be placed at the entrance to the X-ray room, consisting of the radiation warning symbol and a simple legend (Fig. 28.32). For permanently installed equipment there should also be an automatic signal at the room entrance indicating when the X-ray machine is in a state of readiness to produce X-rays. This signal usually takes the form of a red light or an illuminated sign. Whilst not a legal requirement for portable and mobile X-ray machines (which comprise the majority of practice X-ray machines) many practitioners have installed red lights outside their radiography rooms to warn when radiography is in progress and prevent accidental entry, and this is to be recommended.

In addition, all X-ray machines should have lights visible from the control panel indicating (a) when they are switched on at the mains and (b) when exposure is taking place.

X-ray Equipment

Radiation safety features of the X-ray machine should be regularly checked by a qualified engineer. Leakage radiation from the tube housing must not exceed a certain level and the beam filtration must be equivalent to not less than 2.5 mm aluminium. All machines must be fitted with a collimation device, preferably a light beam diaphragm. The exposure button must allow the radiographer to stand at least 2 m from the primary beam which means either that it must be at the end of a sufficiently long cable or else that it should be on the control panel which is placed well away from the tube head. The timer should be electronic rather than clockwork as exposures cannot usually be aborted with the latter, should the patient move.

Suppliers of X-ray machines have a responsibility to ensure that they are safe and functioning correctly, and they should provide a report to this effect when installing the equipment. Servicing of X-ray machines is a legal requirement and should be carried out at least once a year.

The X-ray table must be lead-lined, or else a sheet of lead 1 mm thick and larger than the maximum size of the beam should be placed on the table and beneath the cassette to absorb the residual primary beam and reduce scatter. Many practices now use purpose-built X-ray tables which are not only lead-lined but also fitted with hooks to aid in patient positioning.

Practices performing equine radiography also require cassette holders with long handles for supporting cassettes during limb radiography and various types of wooden blocks for positioning the lower limbs with the minimum of manual restraint.

Film and Film Processing

The Regulations recommend the use of fast film–screen combinations in order to reduce exposure times. They stress the importance of correct processing techniques in order to minimise the number of non-diagnostic films and avoid the need for repeat exposures.

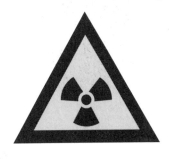

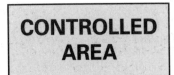

Fig. 28.32. Radiation warning signs.

Protective Clothing

Protective clothing consists of aprons, gloves and sleeves and is usually made of plastic or rubber impregnated with lead. The thickness and efficiency of the garment is described in millimeters of lead equivalent (L.E.), i.e. the thickness of pure lead which would afford the same protection. It is important to remember that **protective clothing is only effective against scatter and does not protect against the primary beam.**

Lead aprons should be worn by any person who needs to be present in the X-ray room during the exposure. They are designed to cover the trunk (especially the gonads) and should reach at least to mid-thigh level. Their thickness should be at least 0.25 mm LE; many are 0.35 or even 0.5mm LE although the latter are rather heavy to wear. Single-sided aprons covering the front of the body but with straps at the back are cheaper but provide less protection than double-sided aprons covering both front and back, and are also less comfortable to wear for long periods. Aprons are expensive items and should be handled carefully; when not in use they should be stored on coat hangers or on rails and they must never be folded as this can lead to undetected cracking of the material (Fig. 28.33).

Lead gloves and hand shields are available for use in those cases where manual restraint of the patient is unavoidable. They are also required for equine radiography when a limb or a cassette holder may need to be held. Lead sleeves are tubes of lead rubber into which the hands and forearms may be inserted as an alternative to gloves. Single sheets of lead rubber draped over the hands are not adequate as they do not protect against back-scatter. Gloves, handshields and sleeves should be of at least 0.35 mm LE and must never appear in the primary beam since they offer inadequate protection against high energy X-rays. It is important to remember that, although a lead glove may appear completely opaque on a radiograph, the film is being protected by two layers of lead rubber but the hand by only one (Fig. 28.34).

All items of protective clothing should be checked frequently for signs of cracking. A small defect may not allow many X-rays through but will always be over the same area of skin. If in doubt, the garment may be X-rayed to check for cracks (Fig. 28.35).

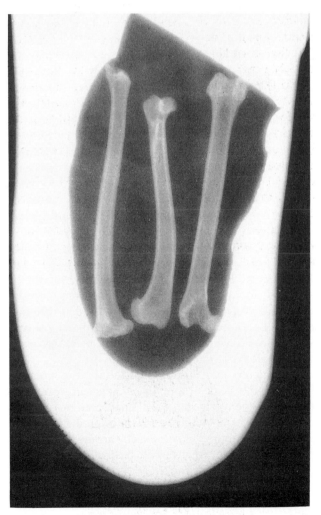

Fig. 28.33. Correct storage of a lead apron. (Reproduced with the permission of Baillière Tindall Limited, London.)

Fig. 28.34. Radiograph of bones covered by a single thickness of lead rubber; compare with the edge where there are two layers of lead rubber.

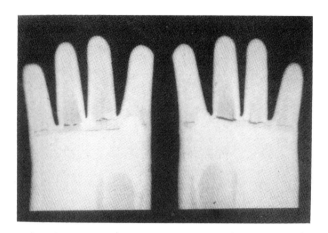

Fig. 28.35. Cracking of the lead rubber at the usual site—the base of the fingers. (Reproduced with the permission of Baillière Tindall Limited, London.)

Mobile lead screens with lead glass windows are also useful as the radiographer can stand behind them during the exposure and still see the patient. Unfortunately they are very expensive.

Dosimetry

All persons who are regularly involved in radiography should wear small monitoring devices or **dosemeters** to record any radiation to which they are exposed. Dosemeters should be worn on the trunk beneath the lead apron, though an extra dosemeter may be worn on the collar or sleeve to monitor the levels of radiation received by unprotected parts of the body. Each dosemeter should be worn only by the person to whom it is issued, and it must neither be left in the X-ray room whilst not being worn nor exposed to heat or sunlight. Two types of dosemeter are available: **film badges** contain small pieces of X-ray film and are usually blue; **thermoluminescent dosemeters** (TLDs) contain radiation-sensitive crystals and are usually yellow. They are obtained from dosimetry services such as the National Radiological Protection Board and they should be sent off for reading every one to three months, depending on the radiographic caseload. If animals are likely to be held for radiography (e.g. equine work), special finger badges may also be worn inside the lead gloves to monitor the dose to the hands.

Dosemeters may also be used to monitor radiation levels in the X-ray room or in adjacent rooms by mounting them on the wall. They can be used to check the adequacy of protection offered by internal walls and doors. The exact arrangements for dosimetry in the practice will be made in consultation with the RPA.

Maximum Permissible Dose (MPD)

Maximum permissible doses are amounts of radiation which are thought not to constitute a greater risk to health than that encountered in other walks of life. Legal limits have been laid down for various categories of person and for different parts of the body. MPDs are laid down for the whole body, for individual organs, for the lens of the eye and for pregnancy. 'Classified' persons are those working with radiation who are likely to receive more than three-tenths of any relevant MPD. However, in veterinary practice these levels should not be reached and so veterinary workers rarely need to be designated as classified persons providing that they are working under a Written System of Work (see below).

MPDs are laid down only as guidelines and should not be considered 100% safe. Ideally no readings should be recorded on dosemeters. If any member of staff receives a reading, the procedure for radiography should be reassessed.

Staff Involved in Radiography

The Local Rules will include a list of names of designated persons authorised to carry out exposures. It should be remembered that nurses and other lay staff aged 16 or 17 have a lower MPD than do adults aged 18 or over and therefore their involvement in radiography should be limited. Young people under 16 years of age should not be present during radiography under any circumstances. Owners should not routinely be present as they are members of the general public and so have a low MPD, although it may be necessary in emergency situations. The Local Rules should ensure that doses to pregnant women are also well within the legal limit, but nevertheless it is wise to avoid the involvement of pregnant women in radiography whenever possible.

The general rule is that the minimum number of people should be present during radiography. When the patient is artificially restrained only the person making the exposure need be present, and this should be the case in the majority of radiographic studies. Often the radiographer will be able to retire behind a wall or even outside the room during the exposure.

Local Rules and Written Systems of Work

The **Local Rules** are a set of instructions drawn up in consultation with the practice's RPA which set down details of equipment, procedures and restriction of access to the controlled area for that practice. They include the method of restraint of patients for radiography and the precautions to be taken should manual restraint be necessary. They contain an assessment of the maximum dose of radiation likely to be received by people in the practice, and this will normally be zero. A copy of the Local Rules should be given to anyone involved in radiography (including the nurses) and should also be displayed in the X-ray room.

The Local Rules include a subsection, the **Written System of Work**, which describes the step-by-step procedure to be followed for radiography.

Radiographic Procedures

Whenever possible, the beam should be directed vertically downwards on to an X-ray table. The minimum number of people should remain in the room and they should either stand behind lead screens or wear protective clothing. All those present must obey the instructions given by the person operating the X-ray machine. The beam must be collimated to the smallest size practicable, and must be entirely within the borders of the film. Grids should only be used when the part being X-rayed is more than 10 cm thick, as their use necessitates an increase in the exposure.

The method of restraint of the patient is of paramount importance. Many practices previously held all their patients for radiography but this should now be discontinued as it is not only dangerous but also illegal. The Approved Code of Practice states that 'only in exceptional circumstances should a patient or animal undergoing a diagnostic examination be supported or manipulated by hand'. These exceptional circumstances may include severely ill or injured animals for whom a diagnosis requires radiography but for whom sedation, anaesthesia or restraint with sandbags is dangerous (e.g. congestive heart failure; ruptured diaphragm or other severe traumatic injuries). In these cases the animal may be held providing that those restraining it are fully protected and providing that no part of their hands (even in gloves) enters the primary beam. A light beam diaphragm is essential for manual restraint. The majority of patients may be positioned and restrained artificially under varying degrees of sedation or general anaesthesia, and sometimes with no chemical restraint at all.

Large Animal Radiography

Special consideration is given to large animal radiography using a horizontal beam. The investigation may need to be undertaken outside the X-ray room, when it should preferably take place in a walled or fenced area with the primary beam directed at a wall of double brick. The extent of the controlled area should be identified using portable warning signs, in order to prevent people not involved from being accidentally irradiated. Everyone taking part in radiography must wear protective clothing and dosemeters. The extra hazards posed by the use of a horizontal beam must be remembered and care must be taken not to irradiate the legs of anyone assisting in the procedure.

Contrast Studies

Although much information about soft tissues can be gained from good quality radiographs, certain structures may be unclear either because they are radiolucent or because they are masked by other structures. In addition, the inner lining (the mucosal surface) of hollow, fluid-filled organs cannot be assessed because it is of the same radiographic density as the fluid contained within the organ. A good example is the urinary bladder, which appears simply as a homogenous pear-shaped structure of soft tissue/fluid density.

Contrast studies aim to render these structures and organs more apparent and to outline the mucosal surface where appropriate, either by changing the radio-opacity of the structure itself or by altering that of the surrounding tissue. Both procedures increase the contrast between the structure of interest and the surrounding tissues, allowing assessment of its **position, size** and **shape**. If serial films are taken over a period, it may also be possible to gain some idea of the **function** of the organ (e.g. rate of stomach emptying).

Many contrast techniques are possible, but only those of most relevance to veterinary radiography will be discussed.

Types of Contrast Media

Two broad groups of contrast media exist: positive and negative.

- Positive contrast agents contain elements of high atomic number which absorb a large proportion of the X-ray beam and are therefore relatively radio-opaque, appearing whiter on radiographs than do normal tissues. They are said to provide **positive contrast** with the soft tissues. The agents most commonly used are compounds of barium (atomic number 56) and iodine (atomic number 53).

  (i) **Barium sulphate preparations**
     Barium sulphate is a white, chalky material which may be mixed with water to produce a fine colloidal suspension. It is available as a liquid, a paste or a powder which is made up to the desired thickness by the addition of water. It is used almost exclusively in the gut and is not suitable for injection into blood vessels. Being inert, it is non-toxic and well-tolerated by the patient and it produces excellent contrast. Its main disadvantages are that if it is aspirated it may cause pneumonia and if it leaks through a perforated area of gut into the thoracic or abdominal cavities it may provoke the formation of granulomas or adhesions.

(ii) Water-soluble iodine preparations

The iodine compounds are water-soluble and may therefore be safely injected into blood vessels. They are then excreted by the kidney and outline the upper urinary tract. They are also safe to use in many other parts of the body. Intravascular injection of these media usually causes nausea and retching and so the patient must be heavily sedated or anaesthetised. Despite being radio-opaque, they appear clear to the eye (unlike barium).

Being water-soluble, the iodine preparations are absorbed by the body and so should be used in the gut in preference to barium if there is a possibility of perforation. However, due to their high osmotic pressure they absorb fluid during their passage through the gut with the result that they become progressively diluted, so that the pictures they produce have much less contrast than those obtained using barium and there is a risk of collapse in a dehydrated patient. They are therefore not routinely used for gut studies.

Many different water-soluble iodine preparations are available but most contain diatrizoate, metrizoate or iothalamate as the active ingredients. For myelography special iodine media with lower osmotic pressures must be used to avoid irritation of the spinal cord and these are iohexol and iopamidol.

- Negative contrast agents are gases which, because of their low density, appear relatively radiolucent or black on radiographs, providing **negative contrast** with soft tissues. Room air is usually satisfactory but oxygen, carbon dioxide and nitrous oxide from pressurised cylinders can also be used.

Studies on hollow organs may utilise both a positive and a negative agent in a **double contrast study**. In these cases a small amount of positive contrast agent is used to coat the inner lining of the organ, which is then distended with gas. This provides excellent mucosal detail and prevents the obliteration of small filling defects, such as calculi, by large volumes of positive contrast. Examples of commonly performed studies are double contrast cystography (bladder) and double contrast gastrography (stomach).

Patient Preparation

Adequate patient preparation is essential before many of the contrast studies. Prior to a barium study of the stomach or small intestine, the animal must be starved for at least 24 hours to empty the gut of residual ingesta. If food remains in the gut it will mix with the barium, mimicking pathology. Patients should also be starved prior to studies on the kidneys, as a full stomach may obscure the renal shadows. However, most patients are anaesthetised for these studies and so will have been starved anyway.

The presence of faeces in the colon will also obscure much abdominal detail and so an enema is often required prior to the contrast study. This is particularly important before investigations of the urinary tract as faeces may obscure or distort the kidneys, ureters, bladder or urethra. The colon must be completely empty of faeces if a barium enema is to be performed as even a small amount of faecal material will produce filling defects, giving the appearance of severe pathology. The patient should therefore be starved for 24 hours and the colon must be thoroughly washed out with tepid saline or water.

Plain films must **always** be taken and examined before the contrast study commences. They are assessed for the following factors:

- Any pathology previously overlooked.
- Correct exposure factors, to avoid the need to repeat films after the contrast study has begun.
- Adequacy of patient preparation.
- Assessment of the amount of contrast medium required.
- Comparison with subsequent films (to show whether any shadows on the radiographs are due to contrast media or were already present).

A brief description of common contrast studies is given below. More detailed information can be found in Chapter 13 of *Principles of Veterinary Radiography*, 4th edition, by Douglas, Herrtage and Williamson.

Gastrointestinal Tract

Oesophagus (Barium Swallow)

Indications: regurgitation, retching, dysphagia (difficulty in swallowing).

Preparation: no patient preparation required; plain films.

Equipment: barium paste is usually preferred since it is sticky and adheres to the oesophageal mucosa for several minutes. Barium liquid may be used if paste is not available (5–50 ml depending on patient size). Oral water-soluble iodine preparations should be used if a perforation is suspected or if the patient is severely dysphagic and aspiration is likely. Liquid barium mixed with tinned meat should be used if a megaoesophagus is suspected on plain films, as paste or liquid alone may fail to demonstrate the full extent of the oesophagus.

Restraint: moderate sedation; heavy sedation or G.A. is contraindicated because of the possibility of regurgitation and aspiration.

Technique: barium paste is deposited on the back of the tongue barium or iodine liquids should be given slowly by syringe, into the buccal pouch, allowing the patient to swallow a small amount at a time to avoid aspiration. Barium/meat mixture is usually eaten voluntarily as animals with megaoesophagus tend to be hungry.

Radiographs are taken immediately after administration of the contrast medium. Lateral views are usually sufficient but VDs may also occasionally be indicated. Two separate radiographs may be needed to cover the cervical and thoracic areas of the oesophagus.

Stomach (Gastrogram)

Two techniques are used: barium only or barium and air (double contrast gastrogram). The latter gives better mucosal detail.

Indications: persistent vomiting, haematemesis, displacement of stomach, assessment of liver size.
Preparation: 24 hours starvation enema if necessary; plain films.
Equipment: barium liquid (20–100 ml depending on patient size). N.B. barium paste and barium/meat mixtures are not suitable and oral water soluble iodine preparations should be used if a perforation is suspected. Syringe or stomach tube plus three-way tap. Glucagon, for double contrast gastrogram.
Restraint: moderate sedation (to allow positioning); acepromazine has least effect on gut.
Technique: (i) barium only: administer the required dose of barium liquid by syringe or stomach tube. Roll the patient to coat the gastric mucosa. Take four radiographs; DV, VD, left and right lateral recumbency. Take further films as indicated e.g. to follow stomach emptying.
(ii) double contrast gastrogram: give the required dose of glucagon intravenously to relax the stomach allowing distension, and to delay stomach emptying. Stomach tube the patient. Give liquid barium, using the syringe and three-way tap, roll the patient (with the stomach tube still in place) and then distend the stomach with room air. Remove the stomach tube and immediately take four views of the stomach as above.

Method (ii) is preferred if a definite gastric lesion is suspected, but follow-up films cannot be made to assess the small intestine due to the action of the glucagon and the presence of the air.

Small Intestine (Barium Series)

Indications: persistent vomiting, haematemesis, abdominal masses, weight loss, malabsorption, intestinal dilation (usually unrewarding in cases of chronic diarrhoea).
Preparation: as stomach.
Equipment: as stomach.
Restraint: as stomach.
Technique: administer liquid barium by syringe or stomach tube. Take serial lateral and VD radiographs to follow the passage of barium through the small intestine (usually at intervals of 15–60 minutes, plus a 24-hour film) depending on pathology seen.

Large Intestine

Three techniques are used: air only (pneumocolon), barium only (barium enema) and barium and air (double contrast enema). A pneumocolon will outline soft tissue masses within the colon and the use of barium alone will demonstrate displacement or compression of the colon; but for most purposes a double contrast enema is indicated as it yields maximum information about the colonic mucosa.

Indications: tenesmus, melaena, colitis, identification of certain abdominal masses.
Preparation: 24 hours starvation; thorough enema, using tepid water or saline until no faecal matter returns; plain films.
Equipment: cuffed rectal catheter or Foley catheter. For pneumocolon: three-way tap and large syringe. For barium and double contrast enemas: gravity feed can and hose or a proprietary barium enema bag; barium sulphate liquid diluted 1:1 with warm water.
Restraint: moderate to deep sedation (to allow positioning) or general anaesthesia.
Technique: (i) pneumocolon: position the rectal catheter and inflate the colon with room air, using the syringe and three-way tap, until air leaks out around the catheter. Take lateral and VD radiographs without removing the catheter.
(ii) barium enema: position the rectal catheter and allow barium to flow into the colon under gravity, until it just begins to leak out around the catheter (usually 10–20 ml/kg is required). Take lateral and VD radiographs without removing the catheter.
(iii) double contrast enema: as (ii) for initial radiographs.

Then allow excess barium to drain out and re-inflate with air. This can be a very messy procedure unless a special barium enema bag is used; when the bag is lowered to the floor the barium drains back down the tube into the bag. If the bag is then compressed, the air within it will inflate the colon (Fig. 28.36). Repeat the lateral and VD radiographs after the introduction of the air

Urogenital Tract

Kidneys and Ureters (Intravenous Urography, Excretion Urography)

Contrast radiography of the upper urinary tract involves the intravenous injection of a water-soluble iodine preparation which is subsequently excreted by, and opacifies, the kidneys and ureters. Two methods are used: rapid injection of a small volume of a very concentrated solution (**bolus intravenous urogram**) and a slow infusion of a large volume of a weaker solution (**infusion intravenous urogram**). The bolus IVU produces excellent opacification of the kidneys. The infusion IVU is preferred for investigation of the ureters, as it produces more ureteric distension by inducing a greater degree of osmotic diuresis.

Indications: identification of kidney size, shape and position, haematuria, urinary incontinence.

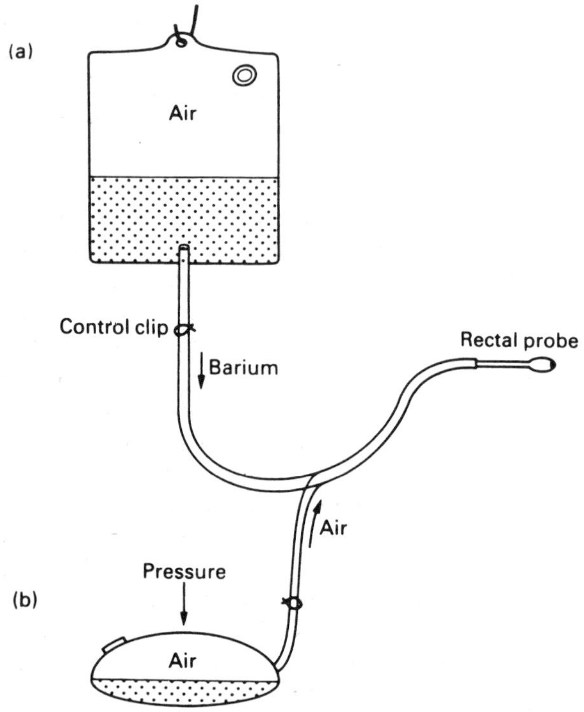

Fig. 28.36. Barium enema bag. In position (a) barium flows under gravity into the colon. In position (b) barium empties from the colon into the bag and then pressure on the bag will distend the colon with air for the double contrast effect.

Preparation: 24 hours starvation; enema; plain films.

Equipment: intravenous cannula (perivascular leakage of contrast medium is irritant).
For bolus IVU: syringe and three-way tap; concentrated contrast medium (300–400 mg iodine/ml) at a dose rate of up to 850 mg iodine/kg body weight, i.e. about 50 ml for a 25 kg dog. For infusion IVU: drip giving set; weaker contrast medium (150–200 mg iodine/ml) at a dose rate of up to 1200 mg of iodine per kg body weight i.e. about 200 ml for a 25 kg dog. Concentrated solutions may be diluted with saline for this study if necessary.

Restraint: general anaesthesia to prevent patient nausea and allow positioning.

Technique: (i) bolus IVU: warm the contrast medium to body temperature to reduce its viscosity and make it easier to inject. Inject the whole amount as quickly as possible. Take lateral and VD films immediately and at 2, 5, 10 minutes and so on as indicated by the initial pictures.
(ii) infusion IVU: if the patient has urinary incontinence and the position of the ureteric endings is being assessed, a pneumocystogram should be performed first to produce a radiolucent background. Infuse the total dose over 10–15 minutes. Take lateral and VD films once most of the contrast medium has run in. Oblique films are also useful for ureteric endings.

Bladder (Cystography)

Direct or retrograde cystography may be performed in three ways: using negative contrast (**pneumocystogram**), positive contrast (**positive contrast cystogram**) or a combination of the two (**double contrast cystogram**). Pneumocystography is quick and easy but gives poor mucosal detail and will fail to demonstrate small bladder tears, as air leaking out will resemble intestinal gas. Positive contrast cystography is ideal for the detection of bladder ruptures but will mask small lesions and calculi. Double contrast cystography is usually the method of choice as it produces excellent mucosal detail and will demonstrate all types of calculi. A positive contrast cystogram will also be seen following an IVU, if the patient cannot be catheterised for any reason. Excreted contrast should be mixed with urine already present in the bladder by rolling the animal. This type of cystogram is not ideal as adequate bladder distension cannot be ensured.

Indications: haematuria, dysuria, urinary incontinence, urinary retention, suspected bladder rupture, identification of bladder if not visible on plain film, assessment of prostatic size.

Preparation: enema, if many faeces are present; plain films.

Equipment: appropriate urinary catheter; syringe and three-way tap; dilute water-soluble iodine contrast medium for positive and double contrast cystogram.

Restraint: sedation or general anaesthesia to allow catheterisation and positioning.

Technique: catheterise bladder and drain completely of urine (obtaining sterile urine sample if required).

(i) pneumocystogram: inflate bladder slowly with room air, using syringe and three-way tap.

The bladder should be inflated until it is felt to be moderately firm by abdominal palpation (usually requires 30–300 ml air depending on patient size)

(ii) positive contrast cystogram; as for (i), but using diluted iodine contrast medium instead of air. However, for detection of bladder rupture, a much smaller quantity is required

(iii) double contrast cystogram: inject 2–15 ml iodine contrast medium at a concentration of about 150 mg iodine/ml into the empty bladder via the catheter. Palpate the abdomen or roll the patient to coat the bladder mucosa. Inflate with air until taut. The bladder wall will be lightly coated with positive contrast, and residual contrast will pool in the centre of the bladder shadow, highlighting calculi and other filling defects. Lateral radiographs are usually more informative, but VD views may be taken if required

Urethra (Retrograde Urethrography—Male Animals: Retrograde Vaginourethrography—Female Animals)

Indications: haematuria, dysuria, urinary incontinence, urinary retention, prostatic disease, vaginal disease.

Preparation: enema, if faeces likely to obscure urethra on either view; plain films.

Equipment: appropriate urinary catheter; syringe; dilute iodine contrast medium (150 mg I/ml) (may be mixed with equal amount of KY Jelly for studies on male dogs, to increase urethral distension); gentle bowel clamp (for bitches).

Restraint: sedation (dogs) or general anaesthesia (bitches).

Technique: (i) retrograde urethrography (males): insert the urinary catheter into the penile urethra. Occlude the urethral opening manually, to prevent leakage of contrast. Inject 5–15 ml contrast or contrast/KY mixture slowly. Release the urethral occlusion and stand back prior to exposure. Lateral views are most useful and should be taken with the hind legs pulled forwards for the ischial arch and backwards for the penile urethra.

(ii) retrograde vaginourethrography (female): snip off the tip of a Foley catheter, distal to the bulb. Insert the catheter just inside the vulval lips, inflate the bulb and clamp the vulval lips together with the bowel clamp to hold the catheter in place. Inject up to 1 ml/kg body weight of iodine contrast medium carefully (vaginal rupture has been reported).

Lateral views are most informative, and demonstrate filling of the vagina and urethra

Spine (Myelography)

A narrow gap surrounds the spinal cord as it runs along the vertebral column; this is called the **subarachnoid space** and it contains **cerebrospinal fluid (CSF)**. It may be opacified by the injection of positive contrast medium and will then demonstrate the spinal cord, showing areas of cord swelling (e.g. tumours) or cord compression (e.g. prolapsed intervertebral discs) not evident on plain films. This technique, which is called **myelography**, requires the use of special water-soluble iodine preparations which have lower osmotic pressures than do the other iodine media and which are therefore less irritant to nervous tissue. The two low osmolar contrast media currently in use in human and veterinary myelography are iohexol and iopamidol.

Two approaches may be made to the subarachnoid space: The one most commonly used in veterinary radiology is the **cisternal puncture**, where the needle is inserted into the cisterna magna—the cranial end of the subarachnoid space just behind the skull. Myelography may also be performed by injection in the lumbar area via a **lumbar puncture**, which is more commonly used in humans. Lumbar myelography involves passing the needle through the cord and injecting into the ventral subarachnoid space. Both techniques involve practice and skill and the patient must be anaesthetised to prevent movement during needle placement or injection.

Indications: spinal pain, spinal neurological signs (ataxia, paralysis), identification of prolapsed intervertebral discs prior to surgery.

Preparation: clip relevant area, i.e. caudal to skull or over lumbar spine.

Equipment: spinal needle of suitable length depending on patient size; contrast medium, warmed to body temperature to reduce viscosity and ease injection (dose rate 0.3 ml/kg of 200–300 mg iodine/ml solution, up to a maximum of 9 ml. Dose administered depends on size of patient and expected site of lesion); syringe; sample bottles for CSF if required for analysis; some means of elevating the head end of the table for cisternal punctures, to aid flow of contrast along the spine.

Restraint: general anaesthesia.

Technique: (i) cisternal puncture: elevate table to about 10° tilt. Cleanse injection site. Flex head to 90° angle with neck. Insert needle carefully into cisterna, between skull and atlas (Fig. 28.37), advancing the needle slowly until CSF drips out of the hub.
Collect several ml of CSF.
Inject warmed contrast medium slowly. Remove needle and extend head again. Take serial lateral radiographs until contrast reaches lesion, when VD films may also be taken.
(ii) lumbar puncture: cleanse injection site. Flex the vertebral column by pulling the hind limbs forwards. Insert the needle carefully (usually at L4–5 or L5–6); as it passes through the cord the animal's hind legs will twitch slightly. Little or no CSF will appear, so inject warmed contrast immediately, slowly. Remove the needle, extend the spine and take radiographs as above.

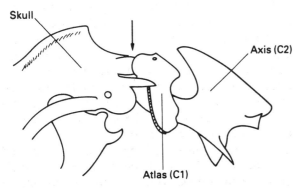

Fig. 28.37. Myelography: site for cisternal puncture.

Other Contrast Techniques

Some other contrast techniques occasionally performed in veterinary practice are described briefly.

Angiocardiography

Angiocardiography is used to demonstrate both congenital and acquired cardiac disease. It involves the opacification of the heart chambers and major vessels by the injection of a bolus of concentrated water-soluble iodine contrast medium. The procedure requires general anaesthesia to prevent patient discomfort or movement. The contrast medium may be injected into the jugular or cephalic vein (**non-selective angiocardiography**) or deposited directly into the heart chambers and major vessels via catheters inserted surgically into the jugular vein and carotid or femoral arteries (**selective angiocardiography**). The latter will also allow blood pressure and blood gas measurements to be made if the appropriate high-technology equipment is available.

Although a single film may provide a diagnosis, it is desirable to obtain a number of radiographs taken over a very short space of time in order to follow the bolus of contrast around the heart and lungs. This is best performed using a special rapid film changing angiography table, but can also be achieved using a home-made cassette tunnel with several cassettes lined up on a piece of wood and pushed through the tunnel at the appropriate speed.

Portal Venography

Portal venography is used to diagnose certain types of liver disease (e.g. congenital porto-systemic shunts, cirrhosis) by demonstration of the vascular system within the liver parenchyma. Under general anaesthesia a laparotomy is performed and a splenic or mesenteric vein cannulated. A small quantity of concentrated iodine contrast medium is injected as a bolus and a single film taken at the end of the injection. The contrast medium enters the liver via the hepatic portal vein and in the normal animal shows branching and tapering portal vessels throughout the liver.

Bronchography

Bronchography is opacification of part of the bronchial tree using specially prepared iodine-containing medium, propyliodine. This medium is rather thicker than the other iodine media, to prevent alveolar flooding. Each study may only demonstrate the left or right bronchial tree; if both sides are to be investigated then two studies must be performed several days apart. The patient is anaesthetised and placed in lateral recumbency with the side to be investigated down. The contrast medium is injected down the endotracheal tube via a dog urinary catheter. The patient is manipulated to ensure that the contrast has entered all of the bronchi on the side of interest and several films are taken over about 10 minutes.

Bronchography may demonstrate bronchial foreign bodies, **Oslerus osleri** nodules, bronchial tumours, lung lobe torsion and bronchiectasis. It has, however, been largely superseded by bronchoscopy.

Arthrography

Arthrography is the demonstration of a joint space using negative contrast (air), positive contrast (iodine) or double contrast techniques injected under sterile conditions. The joints most amenable to arthrography in small animals are the shoulder and stifle. General anaesthesia is required as the procedure is uncomfortable. Arthrography will demonstrate joint capsule distension or rupture and defects in the articular cartilage, which is normally radiolucent.

Fistulography

Fistulography is the opacification of sinus tracts and fistulae using water-soluble or oily iodine contrast media. Fistulography will demonstrate the extent and course of these lesions and may outline radiolucent foreign bodies such as pieces of wood.

Positioning

In order to produce radiographs of maximum diagnostic value it is necessary to position the patient carefully and to centre and collimate the beam accurately. Poor positioning, with rotation or obliquity of the area being radiographed, will result in a film that is hard to interpret or misleading or that fails to demonstrate the lesion.

There are several general rules that should be adhered to when positioning the patient:

- Place the area of interest as close to the film as possible in order to minimise magnification and blurring and to produce an accurate image.
- Centre over the area of interest, especially if it is a joint or a disc space.
- Ensure that the central ray of the primary beam is perpendicular to the film otherwise distortion and non-uniform exposure of the structures will result. If a grid is being used, accurate alignment of the primary beam is essential to prevent grid faults.

- Collimate the beam to as small an area as possible, to reduce the amount of scattered radiation produced.
- Since a radiograph is a two-dimensional image of a three-dimensional structure, it is usually necessary to take two radiographs at right angles to each other in order to visualise the area fully.

Oblique views may then be taken to highlight lesions seen on the initial films.

Restraint

Small animals should be held for radiography **only in exceptional circumstances**, when a radiograph is essential for a diagnosis but their condition renders other means of restraint unsafe. In practice, patients rarely need to be held and most views may be achieved using a combination of chemical restraint and positioning aids.

Simple lateral views of chest, abdomen and limbs may be possible on placid animals without any form of sedation. Other views require varying degrees of sedation or general anaesthesia and the positioning requirements and the temperament of the patient must be taken into consideration when assessing the depth of sedation required. It is also important to handle patients gently, calmly and firmly during radiography and to reassure them with touch and voice.

Positioning Aids

With the skilful use of positioning aids and the correct degree of sedation, almost any radiographic view may be achieved. The following positioning aids should be present in the practice:

- Troughs. Radiolucent plastic or foam-filled troughs are essential for restraining animals on their backs. They are available in a variety of sizes.
- Foam wedges. When lateral views are required, these are placed under the chest, skull or spine to prevent rotation and to ensure that a true lateral view is achieved. They are also useful for accurate limb positioning. They are radiolucent and may therefore be used in the primary beam. It is useful to have several, in different shapes and sizes, and to cover them with plastic for easy cleaning.
- Sandbags. Long, thin sandbags of various sizes may be wrapped around limbs or placed over the neck for restraint. They should only be loosely filled with sand, so that they can be bent and twisted. As they are radio-opaque they should not be used in the primary beam. They should be plastic-covered for easy cleaning.
- Tapes. Cotton tapes are looped around limbs and may then be tied to hooks on the edge of the table or wrapped around sandbags, for positioning of the limbs. Sticky tape may also be useful at times.

- Wooden blocks. Wooden blocks are used to raise the cassette to the area of interest, for certain views (e.g. dorsoventral skull). They are radio-opaque and so should not be placed between the patient and the film.

Nomenclature

Each radiographic projection is named by a composite term describing first the point of entry and then the point of exit of the beam; e.g. a **dorsoventral (DV)** view of the chest involves the X-ray beam entering through the spine (**dorsally**) and emerging through the sternum (**ventrally**). An exception is the lateromedial or mediolateral view, which is commonly just called the **lateral** view. A standardised nomenclature has been devised for veterinary radiology and the naming of the various body regions is shown in Fig. 28.38. Note that the terms 'anterior' and 'posterior' are no longer used in veterinary radiology as they are not appropriate to four-legged creatures. Instead, anteroposterior (AP) and postero-anterior (PA) views of the limbs are called **cranio-caudal (CrCd)** or **caudocranial (CdCr)** above the radiocarpal and tibiotarsal joints, and **dorsopalmar (DPa)/palmarodorsal (PaD)** or **dorsoplantar (DPl)/plantarodorsal (PlD)** below. The newer terminology will be used throughout this section. **Dorsal recumbency** describes an animal lying on its back and **sternal recumbency** describes the crouching position.

Positions for Common Views

The following notes describe in brief the positioning for the more common views performed in veterinary practice. Further details are found in Principles of Veterinary Radiography (see further reading). Anatomy texts and radiological atlases should be consulted for identification of normal anatomical structures.

Thorax

Lateral view. (Fig. 28.39). The right lateral recumbent position is usual as the heart outline is more consistent in shape. When assessing the lungs it is useful to perform the left lateral view too, as the uppermost lung field is better aerated and is therefore more likely to show pathology.

Pad up the sternum with a foam pad to raise it to the same height above table-top as the spine. Draw the forelimbs forwards with tapes or sandbags to prevent them from obscuring the cranial thorax. Restrain the hind limbs with a sandbag and place a further sandbag carefully over the neck. Centre on the middle of the fifth rib and level with the caudal border of the scapula. Collimate to include lung fields and expose on inspiration for maximum aeration.

Identify the trachea, heart, aorta, caudal vena cava, diaphragm, bronchovascular lung markings and skeletal structures. The oesophagus is not normally visible on plain films.

Dorsoventral view (DV) (Fig. 28.40). The dorso-ventral view and not the ventrodorsal must be used for assessment of the heart because in the latter position the heart may tip to one side. Position the patient in sternal recumbency, crouching symmetric-ally. Push the elbows laterally to 'prop' up the dog or cat. Drape a sandbag over the neck to keep the head down shaking the sand into either end to produce a sparsely-filled area in the middle of the sandbag. It may be useful to rest the patient's chin on a foam pad or wooden block. Centre in the midline between the tips of the scapulae. Collimate to include the lung fields and expose on inspiration.

Identify the structures visible on the lateral view.

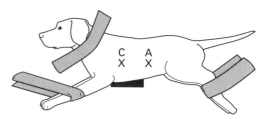

X = centring points (C = chest; A = abdomen)

Fig. 28.39. Positioning for lateral chest/abdomen views. X = centring points; C = chest; A = abdomen.

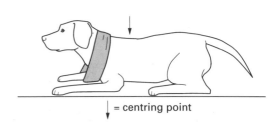

↓ = centring point

Fig. 28.40. Positioning for dorsoventral chest view. ↓ = centring point.

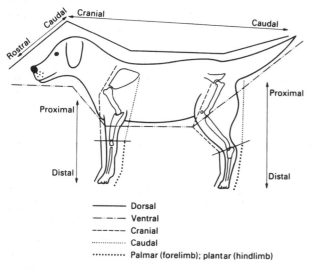

— — — Dorsal
— · — · — Ventral
- - - - Cranial
··········· Caudal
·········· Palmar (forelimb); plantar (hindlimb)

Fig. 28.38. Standardised nomenclature for body regions.

Ventrodorsal view (VD) (Fig. 28.41). Patients must never be placed on their backs if pleural fluid, pneumothorax or a ruptured diaphragm is suspected as this may cause respiratory embarrassment.

Position in dorsal recumbency using a radiolucent trough or sandbags around the hind end. Ensure that the patient is lying straight and not tipped to one side. Draw the forelimbs forwards with tapes or by placing a sandbag gently over them. Secure the hind limbs too if necessary. Centre on the mid-point of the sternum, collimate to the lung field and expose on inspiration.

Identify the same structures as on the lateral and DV views.

Abdomen

Lateral view (Fig. 28.39). Position the patient in lateral recumbency and pad up the sternum if necessary. Restrain the fore and hind limbs with sandbags, ensuring that the hind limbs are pulled well back so that they do not obscure the caudal abdomen. Place a further sandbag over the neck (sometimes one end of the sandbag placed around the forelimbs can be used for this). Centre over the area of interest and collimate as necessary. Expose on expiration to give a more 'spread out' view of the abdominal viscera.

Identify the liver, spleen, kidneys, bladder, stomach, small and large intestine and skeletal structures.

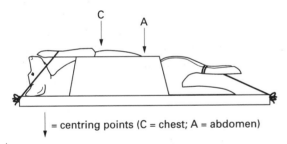

Fig. 28.41. Positioning for ventrodorsal chest/abdomen views. ↓ = centring points; C = chest; A = abdomen.

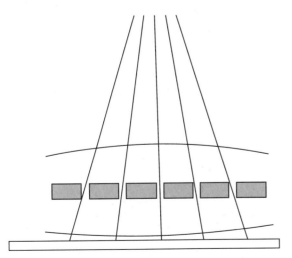

Fig. 28.42. Radiography of disc spaces.

Ventrodorsal view (VD) (Fig. 28.41). Position in dorsal recumbency using a trough, or by placing sandbags on either side of the chest. Sandbag or tape the fore and hind limbs if necessary. Centre and collimate as required and expose on expiration. **Dorsoventral** views of the abdomen are rarely performed as the viscera are usually compressed and distorted but may be all that is possible if the patient is dyspnoeic.

Identify the same structures as on the lateral view.

Skull

Skull views generally require general anaesthesia.

Lateral view. Position the animal in lateral recumbency, using foam wedges under the nose and mandible to ensure that the line between the eyes is vertical and that the midline is horizontal and parallel to the table. The degree of padding depends on the shape of the patient's skull. It may also be necessary to pad the neck and sternum. Centre and collimate as required.

Identify the cranium, frontal sinuses, nasal chambers, teeth, mandibles and tympanic bullae.

Dorsoventral view (DV). Place the animal in a crouching position, with the chin resting on a wooden or foam block, on which is placed the cassette. Secure the head with a sandbag over the neck if necessary. Ensure that the line between the eye is horizontal. Centre and collimate as required. If an endotracheal tube is being used, it may require removal before exposure so as not to obscure any structures in the midline.

Ventrodorsal view (VD). Place the animal in dorsal recumbency in a trough, with the head and neck extended. Put foam pads under the neck and nose. Hold the nose down using a tape placed behind the upper canine teeth, or using sticky tape.

Oblique view for tympanic bullae. Place the animal in lateral recumbency with the side to be radiographed down. Using foam pads, rotate the skull about 20° around its long axis, towards the VD position (this will skyline the tympanic bulla nearest the table). Centre and collimate by palpation of the bulla. It is usually necessary to repeat the procedure for the other bulla, either to give a normal for comparison or to check if it is also affected. Care should be taken to ensure that the positioning is the same for the two sides.

Intra-oral DV (occlusal) view for nasal chambers. This view always requires general anaesthesia. Place the animal in sternal recumbency with the chin resting on a wooden or foam block. Insert an envelope-wrapped, non-screen film into the mouth above the tongue, placing it corner first so as to get it as far back in the mouth as possible. Ensure that the head is level. Centre and collimate over the nasal chambers.

Non-screen film is usually used for this view as it provides the excellent detail required for investigation of nasal disease. Remember that non-screen film requires a much larger mAs factor than screen film. Screen film in cassettes may also be used but gives poorer detail and is harder to place in the mouth.

Many other views of the skull are possible but their description is beyond the scope of this chapter. They include the intra-oral VD for the mandibles, special obliques for temporomandibular joints, obliques for dental arcades and the frontal sinuses, skyline views of the frontal sinuses and cranium and the open-mouth view for tympanic bullae and the odontoid peg.

Vertebral column

Spinal pathology is often undramatic and therefore requires particularly careful positioning, especially if disc spaces are under scrutiny. It is not possible to get an accurate picture of the entire spine on one film, since the X-ray beam is diverging and will not equally penetrate all disc spaces, and so it is usually necessary to take serial radiographs of small areas. In medium and large dogs, up to six films may be required for a spinal survey as follows:

cervical C1–C6
cervico-thoracic C6–T3
thoracic T3–T11
thoraco-lumbar T11–L3
lumbar L1–L7
sacral and coccygeal (caudal) L6–Cd4

Once a lesion is suspected, collimated views taken over the area of interest should be made. For disc disease, only the few disc spaces in the centre of the film are fully assessable (Fig. 28.42). If the animal is in pain and muscle spasm, then general anaesthesia may be required in order to obtain diagnostic films.

Lateral views. Ample use of foam pads is required to prevent the spine sagging or rotating (Fig. 28.43) and to ensure that it forms a straight line parallel to the table top. Centre and collimate to the area of interest by the palpation of bony landmarks (in obese animals the spine may be some distance below the skin surface).

Ventrodorsal views (VD). The patient is positioned in symmetrical dorsal recumbency using a trough or sandbags. The limbs are secured as appropriate. Centre and collimate over the area of interest. For VD views of the cervical spine and cervicothoracic junction, the X-ray beam must be angled 15° to 20° towards the patient's head in order to pass through the disc spaces.

The forelimb

Lateral scapula. Lie the animal on the side to be radiographed. Pull the lower limb backwards and the upper limb forwards, flexing it towards the head and securing it with a tape. Centre and collimate to the lower scapula by palpation.

Caudocranial scapula (CdCr). Lie the animal on its back in a trough, tipping it slightly over to the side not under investigation. Draw the limb forwards and secure in maximum extension with a tape. Centre and collimate by palpation.

Lateral shoulder (Fig. 28.44). Lie the animal on the side to be radiographed. Draw the lower limb forwards and secure it; pull the upper limb well back out of the way. Extend the head and neck. Centre and collimate to the shoulder joint by palpation.

Caudocranial shoulder (CdCr). As for caudocranial scapula but centre on the shoulder joint.

Lateral humerus (Fig. 28.44). As for the lateral shoulder but centre on the humerus.

Caudocranial humerus (CdCr). As for caudocranial scapula but centre on the humerus.

Craniocaudal humerus (CrCd). Lie the animal on its back and pull the affected limb caudally, securing with a tape. The humerus should lie parallel to the

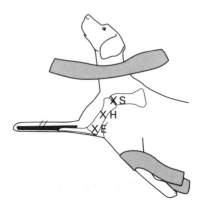

Fig. 28.44. Positioning for lateral forelimb views. X = centring points; S = shoulder; H = humerus; E = elbow.

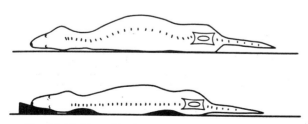

Fig. 28.43. Use of foam pads for spinal radiography.

film. It may not be possible to use a trough for this view.

Lateral elbow. **Extended view**: as for lateral shoulder but centre on the elbow (Fig. 28.44).

Flexed view (more useful for assessing degenerative joint disease): as for lateral shoulder but flex the lower limb at the elbow so that the paw comes up to the patient's chin. Secure with a tape or sandbag (Fig. 28.45a).

Craniocaudal elbow (CrCd). Position the animal in sternal recumbency with both forelimbs extended and pulled forwards. Turn the head and neck to the non affected side and restrain by draping a sandbag over the neck. Take care that the affected elbow does not slide sideways. Centre on the elbow joint, angling the beam about 10° to the patient's tail (Fig. 28.45b).

Caudocranial elbow (CdCr). As for caudocranial shoulder but centre on the elbow joint.

Lateral forearm (radius and ulna), carpus and paw (Fig. 28.44). Lie the animal on the affected side, drawing the lower limb forwards and the upper limb backwards out of the way. Ensure that a lateral position is achieved using foam pads or sticky tape. Centre and collimate to the appropriate area.

For individual toes, it may be useful to separate them by drawing the affected one forwards and the others backwards with tapes.

Craniocaudal forearm (CrCd) and dorsopalmar carpus and paw (DPa). As for craniocaudal elbow, but centre and collimate to the appropriate area and use a vertical beam.

The hindlimbs

Lateral pelvis. Position the patient on its side, using foam pads under the spine and sternum to achieve a true lateral position. Centre on the hip joints.

Ventrodorsal pelvis (VD). **Extended hip position**: This position is described in some detail as it is required for official assessment of hip dysplasia in dogs. It requires general anaesthesia or a reasonable degree of sedation.

Place the patient on its back in a trough, ensuring that it is perfectly upright and not tipped to either side. Extend the forelimbs cranially and secure them with tapes; a sandbag may also be draped over the sternum, taking care not to impair respiration. Extend the hind limbs caudally using tapes looped just above the hocks and tied to hooks on the edge of the table. The femora should be parallel to each other and to the table-top, and the stifles should be rotated inwards by means of a further tape tied firmly around them (Fig. 28.46). Centre on the pubic symphysis. Perfect positioning may be achieved in this way without the need for manual restraint.

For submission to the BVA/Kennel Club Hip Dysplasia Scoring Scheme the film must be permanently identified with the patient's Kennel Club number, the date and a right or left marker. Use lead letters and numbers taped together and placed on the cassette or write on lead tape. Films labelled during or after processing will not be accepted by the scheme.

Identify the various anatomical areas of the hip joint assessed under the scoring scheme.

Flexed or frog-legged view: This view allows some assessment of the hips but is not as satisfactory as the extended view. The hind limbs are flexed and allowed to fall to either side. Sandbags may be used to steady the hind paws.

Lateral femur. Two methods are used, both requiring the patient to lie on the affected side. In the first method the uppermost limb is pulled upwards so that it is roughly vertical, and secured with tapes or

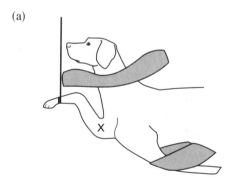

(a)

X = centring point

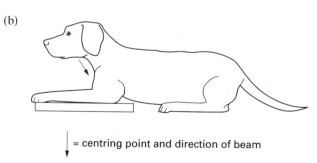

(b)

↓ = centring point and direction of beam

Fig. 28.45. (a) Positioning for flexed lateral elbow. (b) Positioning for craniocaudal elbow view.

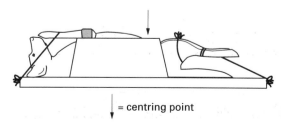

↓ = centring point

Fig. 28.46. Positioning for assessment of hip dysplasia.

sandbags. It may be difficult to prevent super-imposition of part of this limb over the femur under investigation and so an alternative is to pull the lower hind limb forwards and the upper hindlimb back. In this case the lower femur is radiographed through the soft tissues of the abdomen.

Craniocaudal femur (CrCd). As for the extended view of the hips, but centering and collimating to the femur.

Lateral stifle (Fig. 28.47). Position the animal with the affected side down. Move the other hind limb upwards or caudally so that it is not superimposed over the lower stifle. Ensure that a true lateral projection is obtained by placing a small pad under the hock. In obese animals, the mammary tissue or sheath may obscure the stifle joint; this may be prevented by tying a tape around the caudal abdomen to act like a corset. Centre and collimate on the stifle by palpation.

Craniocaudal stifle (CrCd). Similar to ventrodorsal pelvis (extended view) by positioning in dorsal recumbency and extending the affected limb. The other hind limb may be left free. It may be useful to tilt the patient slightly away from the affected side to ensure a true craniocaudal view.

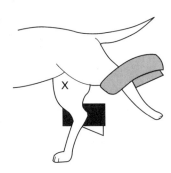

X = centring point

Fig. 28.47. Positioning for lateral stifle view.

Caudocranial stifle (CdCr). Position in sternal recumbency and extend the affected limb caudally.

Lateral tibia, hock and paw. Lie the patient with the affected side down. Draw the upper limb forwards or backwards to prevent superimposition. Use sandbags to achieve a true lateral position if necessary. Centre and collimate to the required area.

Craniocaudal tibia (CrCd) and dorsoplantar hock (DPl). As for craniocaudal stifle, but centre and collimate to the appropriate area. For the hock, the tape is looped around the paw. To reduce the object–film distance for the hock view, it may be necessary to raise the cassette from the table with a wooden block.

Dorsoplantar paw (DPl). Two methods are available. Firstly, the patient may be positioned as for craniocaudal stifle, but with the paw held down to the cassette with strong radiolucent tape. Alternatively, the animal may crouch, with the affected paw pulled slightly outwards and resting on the cassette.

Further Reading

Dennis, R. (1992) The right X-ray machine for you? *In Practice* July, 181–184.

Douglas, S. W., Herrtage, M. E. and Williamson, H. D. *Principles of Veterinary Radiography* 4th Edn; Baillière Tindall.

Guidance Notes for the Protection of Persons against Ionising Radiations arising from Veterinary Use; ISBN 0 85951 300 9, HMSO, 49 High Holborn, London WC1V 6HB.

Manual of Radiography and Radiology in Small Animal Practice; Lee, R. (ed). BSAVA.

Ryan, G. D. *Radiographic Positioning of Small Animals*; Baillière Tindall.

Ticer, J. W. *Radiographic Technique in Small Animal Practice*; W. B. Saunders Co.

Appendix
Guide to Professional Conduct for Veterinary Nurses

Introduction

Under the Veterinary Surgeons Act 1966, the Royal College of Veterinary Surgeons is responsible for all ethical matters relating to veterinary practice within the United Kingdom. That responsibility encompasses the work of both veterinary surgeons and veterinary nurses.

This Code is issued to assist veterinary nurses in maintaining acceptable professional standards. Matters of concern should be raised first with their employer and thereafter if not satisfactorily resolved, with the BVNA.

General Standards

- Veterinary nurses should be mindful that they are only permitted to act under the supervision or direction of a veterinary surgeon.
- They should be familiar with and work within the RCVS 'Guide to Professional Conduct'.
- They are personally responsible for their own professional standards and negligence.

They shall act at all times in the best interests of the animal while taking into consideration the wishes of the owner/keeper and employer and in such a manner as to justify the trust and confidence of the public and to uphold the good standing of the veterinary profession.

Acknowledgement of Limitations

- Veterinary nurses are expected to maintain their professional knowledge and competence.
- They are equally expected to acknowledge any limitations in knowledge or competence, and, where relevant, to make these known to their employer.
- Similarly an employer should not ask a veterinary nurse to undertake any task above and beyond their known level of competence.

Relationship with Veterinary Colleagues

- Veterinary nurses should cooperate fully with veterinary surgeons, assisting them in the provision of veterinary care.

- They should encourage and help colleagues to develop their professional skills.

Conscientious Objections

Veterinary nurses should discuss with any employer and/or prospective employer any conscientious objection which they may have to any treatment of any species of animal. Nevertheless it must be recognised that the welfare of the animal is always paramount and that there will be circumstances when this overrides any conscientious objection.

Confidentiality

Veterinary nurses must keep confidential any information relating to an animal, owner, an employer or fellow employee, acquired in the course of their work.

Such information must not be disclosed to anyone except where:

- They are required to do so in a court of law or
- Where animal welfare or the wider public interest would be endangered by non disclosure.

Health and Safety

Veterinary nurses should be mindful of their responsibility to report to their employer any circumstances where the health and safety of staff or animals is put at risk.

Promotion of Products or Services

Veterinary nurses employed in veterinary practice should not permit their professional qualification to be used as a means of promoting commercial animal related products or services to the public, nor should they allow commercial considerations to override their professional judgement.

Copies of the *Guide to Professional Conduct for Veterinary Nurses* are available from the RCVS; a postage charge may apply.

Index

I